Health Care Management

To Walter J. McNerney, M.H.A.,
our teacher, friend, and colleague,
for his enormous contributions
to health policy and practice

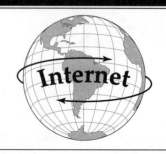

Health Care Management

ORGANIZATION DESIGN AND BEHAVIOR

FOURTH EDITION

Stephen M. Shortell, PhD
Blue Cross of California
Distinguished Professor of Health Policy and
Management and Professor of Organization Behavior,
School of Public Health
University of California, Berkeley, California

Arnold D. Kaluzny, PhD
Professor of Health Policy and Administration and
Director of the Public Health Leadership Program,
School of Public Health, and Senior Research Fellow,
Cecil G. Sheps Center for Health Services Research
University of North Carolina at Chapel Hill
Chapel Hill, North Carolina

and Associates

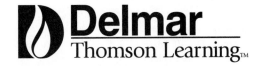

Africa • Australia • Canada • Denmark • Japan • Mexico • New Zealand • Philippines
Puerto Rico • Singapore • Spain • United Kingdom • United States

NOTICE TO THE READER

Publisher does not warrant or guarantee any of the products described herein or perform any independent analysis in connection with any of the product information contained herein. Publisher does not assume, and expressly disclaims, any obligation to obtain and include information other than that provided to it by the manufacturer.

The reader is expressly warned to consider and adopt all safety precautions that might be indicated by the activities herein and to avoid all potential hazards. By following the instructions contained herein, the reader willingly assumes all risks in connection with such instructions.

The Publisher makes no representation or warranties of any kind, including but not limited to, the warranties of fitness for particular purpose or merchantability, nor are any such representations implied with respect to the material set forth herein, and the publisher takes no responsibility with respect to such material. The publisher shall not be liable for any special, consequential, or exemplary damages resulting, in whole or part, from the readers' use of, or reliance upon, this material.

Delmar Staff:
Health Care Publishing Director: William Brottmiller
Acquisitions Editor: Marion Waldman
Executive Marketing Manager: Dawn F. Gerrain
Channel Manager: Nicole L. Benson
Project Editor: Christopher C. Leonard

Production Coordinator: Barbara A. Bullock
Art/Design Coordinator: Jay Purcell

Printed in the United States of America
1 2 3 4 5 6 7 8 9 10 XXX 05 04 03 02 01 00

For more information, contact Delmar, 3 Columbia Circle, PO Box 15015, Albany, NY 12212-0515; or find us on the World Wide Web at http://www.delmar.com

You can request permission to use material from this text through the following phone and fax numbers. Phone: 1-800-730-2214; Fax 1-800-730-2215; or visit our Web site at http://www.thomsonrights.com

Library of Congress Cataloging-in-Publication Data
Health care management : organization, design, and behavior / [edited
   by] Stephen M. Shortell, Arnold D. Kaluzny and associates. --4th
   ed.
      p.   cm. -- (Delmar series in health services administration)
   Includes bibliographical references and index.
   ISBN 0-7668-1072-0
   1. Health services administration.   I. Shortell, Stephen M.
(Stephen Michael), 1944–   . II. Kaluzny, Arnold D.   III. Series.
   [DNLM: 1. Health Services Administration.   W 84.1 H4364 2000]
RA393.H38   2000
362.1'068--dc21
DNLM/DLC
for Library of Congress   99-31968
                                                              CIP

INTRODUCTION TO THE SERIES

This Series in Health Services is now in its second decade of providing top-quality teaching materials to the health administration/public health field. Each year has witnessed further strengthening of the market position of each of the principal books in the Series, also reflecting the continued excellence of the products. Each author, book editor, and contributor to the Series has helped build what is widely recognized as the top textbook and issues collection of books available in this field today.

But we have achieved only a beginning. Everyone involved in the Series is committed to further expansion of the scope, technical excellence, and usability of the Series. Our goal is to do more for you, the reader. We will add new books in important areas, seek out more excellent authors, and increase the physical attributes of the book to make them easier for you to use.

We thank everyone, the authors and users in particular, who have made this Series so successful and so widely used. And we promise that this second decade will be dedicated to further expansion of the Series and to enhancement of the books it contains to provide still greater value to you, our constituency.

Stephen J. Williams
Series Editor

DELMAR SERIES IN HEALTH SERVICES ADMINISTRATION

CONTRIBUTORS

Jeff Alexander, PhD
Richard C. Jelenek Professor of Health Management and Policy
School of Public Health
University of Michigan
Ann Arbor, Michigan

James W. Begun, PhD
Professor
Department of Healthcare Management
Carlson School of Management
University of Minnesota
Minneapolis, Minnesota

Lawton R. Burns, PhD
Professor
Department of Health Care Systems
The Wharton School
University of Pennsylvania
Philadelphia, Pennsylvania

Martin P. Charns, DBA
Director
Management Decision and Research Center
Health Services Research and Development Service
Department of Veterans Affairs, and
Professor and Director
Program in Health Policy and Management
School of Public Health
Boston University
Boston, Massachusetts

Thomas A. D'Aunno, PhD
Associate Professor
School of Social Service Administration and Department of
Health Studies, Pritzker School of Medicine
University of Chicago
Chicago, Illinois

William L. Dowling, PhD
Professor and Chairman
Department of Health Services
School of Public Health and Community Medicine
University of Washington
Seattle, Washington

Ann Barry Flood, PhD
Professor
Center for Evaluative Clinical Sciences
Dartmouth Medical School
Hanover, New Hampshire

Myron D. Fottler, PhD
Professor/Director HSA Programs
Graduate and Undergraduate
Health Administration Office
University of Central Florida
Orlando, Florida

Bruce Fried, PhD
Associate Professor
Department of Health Policy and Administration
School of Public Health
University of North Carolina
Chapel Hill, North Carolina

Jody Hoffer Gittel, PhD
Assistant Professor
Harvard Business School
Boston, Massachusetts

Cynthia Carter Haddock, PhD
Professor
Graduate Program in Hospital and Health Administration
School of Community and Allied Health Professions
University of Alabama
Birmingham, Alabama

Robert S. Hernandez, PhD
Professor
Graduate Program in Hospital and Health Administration
School of Community and Allied Health Professions
University of Alabama
Birmingham, Alabama

Arnold D. Kaluzny, PhD
Professor of Health Policy and Administration and Director of
the Public Health Leadership Program
School of Public Health, and
Senior Research Fellow
Cecil G. Sheps Center for Health Services Research
University of North Carolina at Chapel Hill
Chapel Hill, North Carolina

John R. Kimberly, PhD
Henry Bower Professor of Entrepreneurial Studies
Department of Management
The Wharton School
University of Pennsylvania
Philadelphia, Pennsylvania

Peggy Leatt, PhD
Chief Executive Officer
Health Services Restructuring Commission
Toronto, Ontario, Canada

Beaufort B. Longest, Jr., PhD
Professor and Director
Health Policy Institute
Graduate School of Public Health
University of Pittsburgh
Pittsburgh, Pennsylvania

Roice D. Luke, PhD
Professor
Graduate Program in Health Administration
School of Allied Health Professions
Medical College of Virginia
Richmond, Virginia

Laura L. Morlock, PhD
Professor and Associate Chair for Health Management Program
Department of Health Policy and Management
Johns Hopkins University
Baltimore, Maryland

Margaret A. Neale, PhD
Professor
Graduate School of Business
Stanford University
Stanford, California

Stephen J. O'Connor, PhD
Associate Professor
M.S. Program in Health Care Management
School of Business Administration
University of Wisconsin, Milwaukee
Milwaukee, Wisconsin

Dennis D. Pointer, PhD
John J. Hanlon Professor of Health Services Research and Policy
Graduate School of Public Health
San Diego State University
San Diego, California

Jeffrey T. Polzer, PhD
Associate Professor
Harvard Business School
Harvard University
Boston, Massachusetts

Mary L. Richardson, PhD
Associate Professor and Director
Graduate Program in Health Services Administration
School of Public Health and Community Medicine
University of Washington
Seattle, Washington

Thomas G. Rundall, PhD
Professor
Division of Health Policy and Management
School of Public Health
University of California
Berkeley, California

Julianne P. Sanchez
Principal
Dennis D. Pointer & Associates
San Diego, California

W. Richard Scott, PhD
Professor
Department of Sociology
Stanford University
Stanford, California

Stephen M. Shortell, PhD
Blue Cross of California Distinguished Professor of Health Policy
and Management
Professor of Organization Behavior
Division of Health Policy and Management
School of Public Health
University of California, Berkeley
Berkeley, California

Sharon Topping, PhD
Associate Professor of Management
University of Southern Mississippi
Hattiesburg, Mississippi, and
Former NIMH Postdoctoral Fellow at
Sheps Center for Health Services Research at the University of
North Carolina at Chapel Hill

Stephen L. Walston, PhD
Associate Professor and Director
Graduate Program in Health Administration
School of Public and Environmental Affairs
Indiana University
Indianapolis, Indiana

Gary J. Young, J.D., PhD
Senior Researcher
Management Decision and Research Center
Health Services Research and Development Service
Department of Veterans Affairs
Boston, Massachusetts, and
Associate Professor and Co-Director Program in Health Policy
and Management
Boston University School of Public Health

Edward J. Zajac, PhD
James F. Beré Professor of Organization Behavior
J.L. Kellogg Graduate School of Management
Northwestern University
Evanston, Illinois

Jacqueline Zinn, PhD
Associate Professor
Department of Risk, Insurance and Health Care Management
Fox School of Business and Management
Temple University
Philadelphia, Pennsylvania

Howard S. Zuckerman, PhD
Professor and Director
Center for Health Management Research
Department of Health Services
University of Washington
Seattle, Washington

CONTENTS

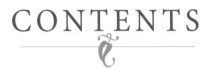

FOREWORD

Today's health care executives may be faced with the most challenging managerial assignments in America. In a high-pressure environment where consumer demands for comprehensive services, payors' insistence on efficiency and cost control, tensions between the health professions, requests for the latest technologies, and a renewed emphasis on quality care all converge, managers must pursue strategic goals and objectives to ensure survival as well as progress. This necessitates a sound balance of performance-based management and imaginative leadership that embraces customer mindedness, product line breadth, market and financial strength, and a focus on productivity. It is to these challenges that this new edition of *Health Care Management* is addressed.

Since the third edition was published in 1994, the field of health care management has acquired added layers of complexity, largely as a result of the explosive growth of the health care industry (of the 10 million individuals employed in this sector, managers and administrators number approximately 450,000). Fueled by virtually insatiable public demands for enhanced services and leading-edge technology, the national health bill has skyrocketed to well over $1 trillion, or 14 percent of the nation's gross domestic product, in contrast to $42 billion in 1965, the watershed year that witnessed the passage of Medicare and Medicaid.

Managed care and related forces have exerted a profound impact on the way that health care organizations are designed, structured, and controlled, as well as the manner in which patient care is financed and delivered. Substantial organizational and sector-wide transformations have occurred, analogous to those that dramatically changed health care in the 1960s, requiring major adaptations by patients, the health professions, and managers. Increased demands for information regarding the quality and outcomes of care and improved information systems technology will undoubtedly lead to enhanced accountability standards. These and other measures will in turn create a further mandate for reinvigorated approaches to health care management and leadership.

Professors Shortell and Kaluzny have brought together a set of chapters by a distinguished panel of authors that promises to inform and stimulate thinking and discussion among students and educators, as well as health executives and professionals. The chapters deal with the art and science of management in health care organizations, and the selections provide the reader with practical assessments, approaches, and insights for understanding these organizations.

Perhaps the main concerns of this book are the key environmental and technological changes that are now taking place, and that will inevitably result in further advances in the years ahead. For example, the manager of the twenty-first century will be faced with having to engage in planning for the care of populations and in the design of planned health care campuses that will offer arrays of sophisticated preventive and diagnostic services as well as rehabilitative, long-term care, and wellness programs. New organizational designs and methods of implementing staff participation and teamwork at all levels will require managers who are expert in human resource management and are highly skilled in negotiation techniques and conflict resolution.

With a principal focus on effective management and leadership, the content of the book admirably reflects a balanced concern for organization theory and behavior as well as the improvement of management practices. The text provides numerous suggestions and examples of creative ideas and ways of managing and problem solving. The editors and authors offer many illustrations of specific tasks and decision-making strategies that will help prepare the reader for future contingencies.

Obviously, no work can be a comprehensive handbook that guarantees managerial excellence. But this volume does provide a thorough examination and analysis of the most important structures, processes, checkpoints, and preferred futures that figure prominently in high-performance organizations. It recognizes that in the real world, suboptimal solutions are often necessary and that there are no royal roads to attainment of quality, only deliberately improved ones.

The editors and authors are to be commended for providing the field with this thoughtfully conceived and carefully revised and updated treatment of health care management for the twenty-first century.

Samuel Levey, Ph.D.
Gerhard Hartman Professor
Division of Health Management and Policy
College of Medicine
The University of Iowa
Iowa City, Iowa

PREFACE

This book is intended for those interested in a systematic understanding of organizational principles, practices, and insights pertinent to the management of health services organizations. While based on state-of-the-art organizational theory and research, the emphasis is on application. While the primary audience is graduate students in health services administration management and policy programs, the book will also be of interest to undergraduate programs, extended degree programs, executive education programs, and practicing health services executives interested in ready access to the latest developments in organizational and managerial thinking. It is also intended for students of medicine, nursing, pharmacy, social work, and other health professions who will assume managerial responsibilities or who want to learn more about the organizations in which they will spend the major portion of their professional lives.

This fourth edition of the text continues a number of popular features from the third edition. These include:

- An explicit list of topics provided at the beginning of each chapter.
- Specific behaviorally oriented learning objectives highlighted at the beginning of each chapter.
- Each chapter includes a list of key terms that readers should be able to define and apply as a result of reading each chapter.
- Each chapter opens with an "In The Real World" column describing a practical situation facing a health services organization. Many chapters contain several "In The Real World" columns to illustrate the major principles and lessons of the chapter.
- Most chapters incorporate a section called "Debate Time," which poses a controversial issue or presents divergent perspectives to stimulate the reader's thinking.
- A set of comprehensive managerial guidelines concludes each chapter.

All chapters have been updated and revised. The book is organized in five sections or parts. Part One provides an overall perspective on the study of health services organizations and the associated managerial role. Part Two deals with fundamental building blocks of managerial activity involving motivation, leadership, conflict management, and negotiation. Part Three deals with largely internal organizational issues including work design, coordination and communication, and managing power and political processes. Part Four focuses on performance issues related to organization design, strategic alliances, innovation and change, and managing for efficiency and effectiveness. The final section focuses on strategic issues and attempts to anticipate future issues that will challenge health services leaders. With the exception of Part One, which should be read first by all readers because it provides the groundwork for chapters that follow, the remaining sections can be read in any order depending on instructor and course objectives.

We believe that the major strength of the text is the diversity of the talented authors involved. They have brought multiple perspectives, experiences, skills, and expertise to bear on each chapter. As a result, each chapter is at the frontiers of knowledge with clear applications that illuminate the practice of health services management. We hope that readers enjoy this richness as much as we and our colleagues continue to have in creating it.

Stephen M. Shortell
Berkeley, California

Arnold D. Kaluzny
Chapel Hill, North Carolina

ACKNOWLEDGMENTS

This fourth edition has benefitted greatly from feedback from students and faculty over the past five years too numerous to mention. Appreciation is expressed to Alice Schaller and John Troidl at the University of California, Berkeley, and Glen Mays, Adriane Terrel, Marleen Sturgill, Ruben Fernandez, and Lynette Wyche at the University of North Carolina at Chapel Hill for their overall assistance in manuscript preparation and organization. We also acknowledge the assistance of Barbara Bullock and Marion Waldman at Delmar and Michael Jennings at Carlisle Publishers Services for their overall guidance and suggestions in the production of this fourth edition.

Stephen M. Shortell
Berkeley, California

Arnold D. Kaluzny
Chapel Hill, North Carolina

ABOUT THE AUTHORS

Stephen M. Shortell, Ph.D., is the Blue Cross of California Distinguished Professor of Health Policy and Management, and Professor of Organization Behavior in the School of Public Health, University of California, Berkeley. He also holds appointments at the Haas School of Business, the Department of Sociology, and is an affiliated member at the Institute for Health Policy Studies at the University of California, San Francisco.

Dr. Shortell received his undergraduate degree from the University of Notre Dame, his masters degree in public health and hospital administration from UCLA, and his Ph.D. in the behavioral sciences from the University of Chicago.

He has been the recipient of the Baxter Allegiance Prize for Health Services Research, the Gold Medal Award from the American College of Healthcare Executives, the Distinguished Investigator Award from the Association of Health Services Research, and the American Hospital Association Honorary Life Member Award.

He is an elected member of the Institute of Medicine of the National Academy of Sciences; has served as President of the Association for Health Services Research; and has served as Chairman of the Accrediting Commission for Graduate Education in Health Services Administration. He serves as a consultant and advisor to a number of private and public organizations.

He is currently conducting research on the strategy, structure, and performance of integrated health systems, and physician group practices, is assessing the implementation and impact of continuous quality improvement/total quality management on U.S. health care organizations, and is involved in evaluations of community health-improvement efforts.

Arnold D. Kaluzny is Professor of Health Policy and Administration, and Director of the Public Health Leadership Program, School of Public Health, as well as a Senior Research Fellow in the Cecil G. Sheps Center for Health Services Research and a member of the Lineberger Comprehensive Cancer Center at the University of North Carolina at Chapel Hill.

He is a consultant to a number of private research organizations and various international, federal, and state agencies, including Project HOPE, the World Health Organization, the National Cancer Institute, the Joint Commission on the Accreditation of Healthcare Organizations, the Department of Veterans Affairs, and the Agency for Health Care Policy and Research. From 1991 through 1995, he was a member of the Board of Scientific Counselors for the Division of Prevention and Control at the National Cancer Institute and served as Chairman from 1993 to 1995.

Dr. Kaluzny was a member of the Advisory Panel for Public Health, Pew Health Professions Commission, and chaired the Commission's Advisory Panel for Health Care Management. He also served as Chairman of the Accrediting Commission for Graduate Education in Health Services Administration.

His research has focused on the organizational factors affecting implementation and change of a variety of health care organizations, with specific emphasis given to cancer treatment and prevention and control, continuous quality improvement initiatives in both organizational and primary care settings, and most recently, the study of alliances within health care. In all these endeavors, a major focus has been to strengthen the science base of policy and practice.

Dr. Kaluzny received his undergraduate degree from the University of Wisconsin at River Falls, his Master's degree in Hospital Administration from the University of Michigan Graduate School of Business, and his Doctorate in Medical Care Organization-Social Psychology from the University of Michigan.

PART

1

Organizations and Managers

THE NATURE OF ORGANIZATIONS: FRAMEWORK FOR THE TEXT

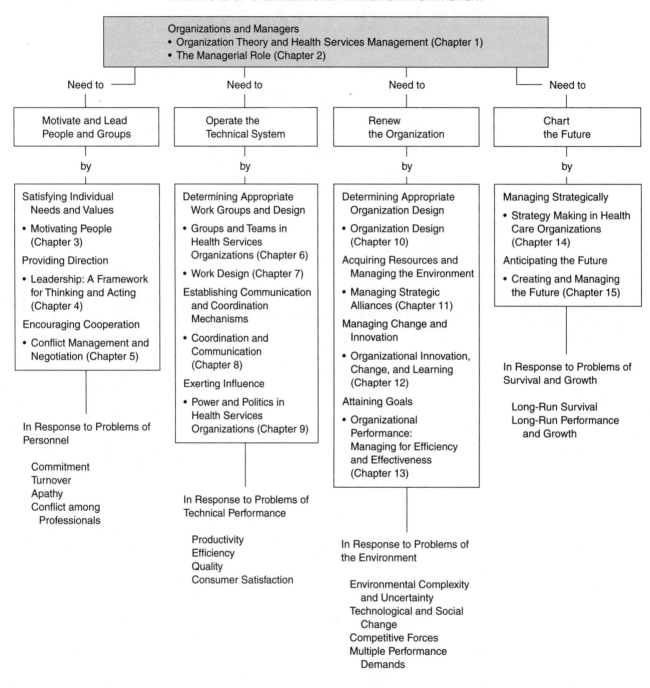

The unrelenting changes in the health care environment are increasing the demand for organizational and managerial expertise. There is an increased need to manage across organizational boundaries in responding to new treatment technologies, payment mechanisms, consumer preferences, and accountability. The two chapters in this first section take up this challenge by laying the groundwork for the remainder of the book.

Chapter 1, "Organization Theory and Health Services Management," addresses the following kinds of questions:

- What are the main forces influencing the organization and delivery of health services?
- What are the major conceptual frameworks and perspectives for thinking about health services organizations?
- What are the major units of analysis that require managerial attention?

The first chapter suggests the importance of viewing health services organizations from different perspectives drawing on a number of different metaphors to stimulate thinking.

Chapter 2, "The Managerial Role," focuses on the following kinds of questions:

- What are the major ways of viewing the manager's role?
- What new roles are called for to meet the challenges of the changing health care environment?
- What new skills and knowledge are needed by health services managers to be successful?

This chapter emphasizes the need for leaders who can build consensus and negotiate compromises in an increasingly turbulent environment.

Upon completing the first two chapters, readers should have a clearer understanding of the complexity of the health services manager's role and the need for comprehensive frameworks and approaches that recognize the complexity of the role.

CHAPTER
1

Organization Theory and Health Services Management

Stephen M. Shortell, Ph.D.
Arnold D. Kaluzny, Ph.D.

Chapter Outline

- The Changing Health Care System
- Ecology of Health Services Organizations
- Key Dimensions of Health Services Organizations
- Health Services Organizations as Systems
- Areas of Managerial Activity
- Major Perspectives on Health Services Organizations
- Metaphors of Health Services Organizations
- Organization Theory and Behavior: A Framework for the Text

Learning Objectives

After completing this chapter, the reader should be able to:

1. Identify the major forces affecting the delivery of health services.
2. Understand how these major forces affect the role of the health services manager.
3. Identify some of the commonalities and differences among major types of health services organizations.
4. Identify and understand the basic processes that must be accomplished by any organization.
5. Identify and understand the different areas of managerial activity.
6. Identify, understand, and apply the major perspectives and theories on organizations to real problems facing health services organizations.
7. Identify, understand, and apply major metaphors of organizations to the challenges facing health services organizations.

Key Terms

Adaptation Function
Biological Organisms
Boundary Spanning Function
Brains
Bureaucratic Theory
Change
Closed System
Contingency Theory
Continuous Improvement
Differentiation
External Environment
Governance Function
Health Networks
Health Systems
Holograms
Human Relations School
Innovation
Interorganizational Relationships
Institutional Theory
Machines
Macro Approach
Maintenance Function
Management Function
Managing Across Boundaries
Micro Approach
Mission/Goals
Open System
Organization Behavior
Playing Fields
Political Systems
Population-Based Management
Population Ecology Theory
Production Function
Psychic Prisons
Resource Dependence Theory
Scientific Management School
Strategic Management Perspective
Tyrants

Chapter Purpose

The health services management challenge of the new millenium is to create value for an increasingly diverse and demanding citizenry. *Value* is created when for a given cost or price to the purchaser additional quality features desired by the purchaser are provided or, conversely, when a given level of quality services can be provided at a lower cost or price relative to others from whom purchasers can obtain the services. Providing greater value is a challenge for all health services organizations and to the professionals—both clinical and managerial—associated with them. As noted in a Pew Commission Report on Education for the Health Professions:

> Health services management will become even more challenging, because it is the point where increasing service demands, cost containment strategies, interprofessional tensions, technological change pressures, guidelines implementation, and quality improvement mandates all converge. The managerial function in health services is unique because of the relative autonomy of providers and the complexity of assessing the quality of the services rendered. (Pew Commission, 1993)

The challenges facing Sutter Health in the accompanying "In the Real World" are representative of those facing any health care organization. This chapter sets the stage for addressing some of these challenges. We discuss the major forces that influence the health care system; describe the great variety of organizations involved; highlight key approaches, dimensions, perspectives, theories, and metaphors; and indicate how each of the succeeding chapters will address the complex issues that are raised.

THE CHANGING HEALTH CARE SYSTEM

Ultimately the goal of health services managers is to help maintain and enhance the health of the public. While individual citizens hold primary responsibility for their health status, there is much that health services managers working in concert with physicians, nurses, other health professionals, and community leaders can do to assist in the process. This goal may seem strange to some and unrealistic to others. After all, isn't it sufficient simply to care for those who come to you for help and make sure that one's organization

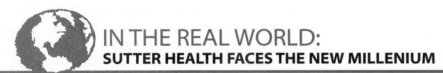

IN THE REAL WORLD:
SUTTER HEALTH FACES THE NEW MILLENIUM

The public's ongoing fascination with the health care sector and especially the larger players in that sector fairly leaps from the headlines: "State agency rules against hospitals' governing policies" (1996), "Sutter Health, PacifiCare sign systemwide alliance" (1997), and "Sutter Health's HMO woes mirror national trend" (1998).

Sutter Health is a major health system in what is considered one of the most advanced managed care markets in the United States. Founded as a for-profit doctors' hospital in 1923, Sutter converted to nonprofit status in the early 1940s and remained a very local, two-hospital enterprise through the 1960s and early 1970s. Significant expansion in the 1980s and 1990s led to a system that in 1999 included 26 acute care hospitals with 5,211 beds, 722 affiliated medical group physicians, 4,198 independent practice associations (IPA) physicians, long-term care, home health, and occupational and hospice services. Sutter Health employed more than 35,000 people.

The impetus for the growth strategy was articulated by the Sutter board in 1980 in the following closing paragraph of the then mission statement:

> *A proactive philosophy of constant controlled growth facilitates any human organization in attracting the best clinical and managerial talent available. It prevents mediocrity in performance and, eventually, organizational senility and decay. In this context, a no-growth policy is inconsistent with the Sutter Community Hospitals' commitment to high-quality, patient-centered health care. Sutter Community Hospitals is committed to a policy of planned, orderly, but constant growth in providing health services and in peripheral areas that promote the general health of the citizens of northern California and the western United States (Sutter Health Annual Report, 1980).*

Notwithstanding its stunning growth, Sutter has formidable competitors in the northern California marketplace in which it operates. One of these, Catholic Healthcare West, is about the same size as Sutter and has similarly developed an integrated system of services over the past twenty years. Kaiser HMO and its affiliated Permanente Medical Group are also, dominant players in the

marketplace, and the UC Davis Medical Center has the strategic advantages (and disadvantages) of being the only academic medical center in the dominant central region.

The Sacramento market is heavily impacted by evolving market economics with nearly 100% of the nongovernmental health insurance offered in a managed care mode. CalPERS (California Public Employees Retirement System) is a powerful purchaser, as is the state of California generally, and both act to constrain price inflation by tough negotiations with the major providers of care.

By the late 1990s, the economy in the region has begun a resurgence, and the population continues to grow due to favorable climate and housing prices. An "aging boom" is taking place in Sacramento as more seniors move to the area after selling their homes in a more expensive part of the state.

Among the major issues facing Sutter in the decade ahead are:

1. Lack of profitability
   According to Moody's Investor's Service, Sutter Health suffered operating losses in 1992, 1993, 1994, and 1996. The Sacramento Business Journal reports that in 1997 there was better financial news with a $7 million operating profit. Unfortunately, that profit was wiped out by one-time charges of $7.1 million related to its merger, acquisition, and liquidation strategies. Fortunately, the stock market was booming that year, as Sutter's investments contributed $60 million in nonoperating income. In 1996 Moody's lowered Sutter's bond rating to reflect the riskiness of its expansion strategy.
2. Problems with payers
   On May 15, 1998, the Sacramento Bee announced that Sutter Health and Blue Cross had come to an impasse in their contract negotiations and that "Tens of thousands of Blue Cross members in Northern California will be unable to attend Sutter Health hospitals starting today following the collapse of contract negotiations between the two health care giants" (Sutter Health to drop Blue Cross patients: Contract talks stall over money, 1998).

This contract represented $60 million worth of business from an insurer that provides coverage for over 4.4 million Californians. By June 6, though, the Bee told of the corporate "reconciliation": ". . . [I]n a significant reversal, Sutter Health hospitals and Blue Cross have smoothed over a contract dispute that threatened to disrupt health care for hundreds of Northern Californians this month" (Sutter, Blue Cross ink new contract: Hospital given higher payments, 1998).

3. Problems with other providers

On Christmas Day 1997, it was announced that Sutter and UC Davis Medical Center had "signed an agreement that expands medical services in the Auburn area" (Sacramento Business: Sutter, UCDMC ink agreement, 1997) which arranged for cross-provider coverage for acute care, OB-GYN medical care, and pediatric care between the two systems. Seven months later in a much less cooperative mood, Sutter announced that it was suing the medical center over "exorbitant and unconscionable" charges for trauma care for Sutter patients at the medical center. Frank Loge, then CEO of the medical center described Sutter as ". . . Very poor public citizens . . . now they are trying to badger UCDMC, which is a good corporate citizen with public responsibility."

4. Problems with subsidiaries

In attempting to model themselves after Kaiser as an integrated health care system, Sutter has been an investor/owner of two HMOs. In 1992 Sutter bought into Omni Healthcare in order to have a "captive" health insurance product. Despite spending $20.8 million to make a go of it in the HMO business, Omni has not grown as Sutter had hoped and is now for sale.

Omni lost $1.1 million on revenues of $30.7 million in 1997 in providing coverage for 170,000 lives. This investment in an HMO is the second time around for Sutter. They sold their interests in Foundation Health Plan in 1994. Omni is not the only subsidiary that has been a money loser for Sutter. In December 1997 the corporation announced that it was selling its long-term care units, citing losses of over $3 million per year as the cause.

5. Challenges in governance

In late July 1998, the Auburn Community Health Care Watch Committee (Auburn, California) issued its report on the health needs of the 80,000+ residents of the Auburn area. This report principally deals with the services provided by Auburn Faith Hospital, which became a Sutter subsidiary in 1989. The first of the list of 10 findings is: "The Memorandum of Understanding (MOU) resulting from the transfer in 1989 of the Auburn Faith Community Hospital to Sutter Health included several promises which have not been fulfilled, including $6 million in capital improvements." The first recommendation of the committee is to

Create a local Auburn Faith Community Hospital board composed of people interested in having local input. This is a requirement of the Memorandum of Understanding signed by Sutter Health at the time of the transfer of Auburn Faith Community Hospital to them in 1989.

It is clear that Sutter faces significant challenges and opportunities as it positions itself for the future. What should it do? What can it do? How and where can it create value? Where will the resources come from? How much time does it have? Welcome to the real world!

retains its financial health in order to provide the requested care? The answer is no. Economic, political, and social forces have moved the health services system beyond the largely reactive acute care paradigm to a more holistic paradigm emphasizing population-based wellness. Some of the major economic, political, and social forces that will influence health care delivery in the next five to ten years are highlighted in Table 1.1. These forces are causing a fundamental shift in the way in which health care is viewed. The major elements of this *paradigm shift* are outlined in Table 1.2.

At the core of this shift is the movement away from episodic treatment of acute illness events to the provision of a coordinated continuum of services that will enhance the health status of defined populations. In the evolving health care system of greater capitated payment, global budgets, and expenditure targets, organizations win by helping health care professionals

Table 1.1. Nine Forces Influencing Health Care Delivery and Their Implications for Management

External Force	Management Implication
1. Capitated payment, expenditure targets, or global budgets for providing care to defined populations	• Need for increased efficiency and productivity • Redesign of patient care delivery • Development of strategic alliances that add value • Increased growth of networks, systems, and physician groups
2. Increased accountability for performance	• Information systems that link financial and clinical data across episodes of illness and "pathways of wellness" • Effective implementation of clinical practice guidelines • Ability to demonstrate continuous improvements of all functions and processes
3. Technological advances in the biological and clinical sciences	• Expansion of the continuum of care, need for new treatment sites to accommodate new treatment modalities • Increased capacity to manage care across organizational boundaries • Need to confront new ethical dilemmas
4. Aging of the population	• Increased demand for primary care, wellness, and health promotion services among the 65 to 75 age group • Increased demand for chronic care management among the 75 plus group • Challenge of managing ethical issues associated with prolongation of life
5. Increased ethnic or cultural diversity of the population	• Greater difficulty in understanding and meeting patient expectations • Challenge of managing an increasingly diverse health services workforce
6. Changes in the supply and education of health professionals	• Need for creative approaches in meeting the population's need for disease prevention, health promotion, and chronic care management services • Need to compensate for shortages in some categories of health professionals (i.e., physical therapy, pharmacy, and some areas of nursing) • Need to develop effective teams of caregivers across multiple treatment sites
7. Social morbidity (AIDS, drugs, violence, "new surprises")	• Ability to deal with unpredictable increases in demand • Need for increased social support systems and chronic care management • Need to work effectively with community agencies
8. Information technology	• Training the health care workforce in new information technologies • Increased ability to coordinate care across sites • Challenge of managing an increased pace of change due to more rapid information transfer • Challenge of dealing with confidentiality issues associated with new information technologies
9. Globalization and expansion of the world economy	• Need to manage cross-national and cross-cultural tertiary and quaternary patient care referrals • Increasing the competitiveness and productivity of the American labor force • Managing global strategic alliances, particularly in the areas of biotechnology and new technology development

Table 1.2. Transformation of Health Care

Old Paradigm	New Paradigm
Emphasis on acute inpatient care	Emphasis on the continuum of care
Emphasis on treating illness	Emphasis on maintaining and promoting wellness
Responsible for individual patients	Accountable for the health of defined populations
Emphasis on tangible physical assets	Emphasis on intangible knowledge/relationship-based assets
All providers are essentially similar	Differentiation based on ability to add value
Success achieved by increasing market share of inpatient admissions	Success achieved by increasing the number of covered lives and keeping people well
Goal is to fill beds	Goal is to provide care at the most appropriate level
Hospitals, physicians, and health plans are separate	Virtual and/or vertically integrated delivery system
Managers run an organization	Managers oversee a market
	Managers operate services across organizational boundaries
Managers coordinate services	Managers actively pursue quality and continuous improvement

provide services at that point in the continuum of care where the greatest value (i.e., cost-benefit) is provided. They do not win by filling hospital beds or continuing to have key professionals working at cross purposes with each other. These kinds of changes require new and different ways of organizing and managing health care services. Among the most important are the following:

- Emphasizing intangible knowledge-building/relationship-building assets.
- Being accountable for the health of defined populations. This might be termed **population-based** or denominator-based **management.**

- **Managing across** organizational **boundaries.**
- Actively managing quality and **continuous improvement.**
- Emphasizing knowledge and relationship-building assets requires a shift in thinking about how to create value in health care delivery. In the past, value was largely created through investment in physical assets involving bricks and mortar (e.g., hospitals, research labs, clinics). But with the information and knowledge explosion brought on by the computer revolution and the increased emphasis on customer satisfaction, value is now primarily created through the development and application of intellectual capital. Thus, health care executives must give greater attention to investments in the human capital represented by the physicians, nurses, and other professionals with whom they work and by all employees. They must also give greater attention to customer service and retention. Further, to meet the new demands for accountability and continuous quality improvement, greater investment must be made in information systems ranging from the computerized patient record to data banks that can store information on large numbers of patients over time.

Population-based or denominator-based management is illustrated by Group Health Cooperative (GHC) of Puget Sound, as discussed in the accompanying "In the Real World." The keys are assessing the health needs of the population to be served; understanding how the community uses health and social services; organizing relationships among providers, health plans, and payers to ensure continuity of care; and developing an outcomes reporting system for purposes of internal continuous improvement and external accountability.

An example of actively managing quality of care and continuous improvement in processes is provided by Intermountain Health Care in Salt Lake City, Utah. Using guidelines developed through computer-assisted decision-support systems, Intermountain increased the percentage of patients who received appropriately timed preoperative antibiotics from 40% to 99% while reducing antibiotic-associated adverse drug events by 30% (Pestonick, Classen, Evans, & Burke, 1996). Other examples of the application of

IN THE REAL WORLD:
GROUP HEALTH COOPERATIVE (GHC) AND POPULATION-BASED HEALTH CARE

Group Health Cooperative (GHC) of Puget Sound is a large HMO with a 55-year history of serving residents of the Pacific Northwest. It has approximately 25% of the insured market. In its Olympia, Washington, service area, GHC administrators have begun to emphasize population-based health care approaches in their formal strategic planning process. The structure of a staff-model HMO has long provided the organization with the ability to monitor trends in health status and service utilization across its population of enrollees. Expanding information systems are now greatly improving GHC's capabilities in this area.

An example of GHC's population-based approach to health care can be found in its strategies for diabetes management. Until recently, management of enrollees with diabetes occurred solely through medically oriented, one-on-one visits with clinicians. Over time, GHC recognized that patient learning could be enhanced by conducting group sessions with a team of clinicians that included a physician, nurse, pharmacist, and dietitian. In this setting, patients could learn from each other as well as from the clinicians, and behavioral change could be reinforced by the perspectives of multiple people participating in the group session. Since starting the group sessions, GHC has realized greater patient compliance with clinical self-monitoring guidelines and reduced incidence of retinopathy and foot necrosis.

As another population-based strategy, GHC carefully monitors its hospital readmission rates, which tend to range between 4% and 5% of total admissions. The or-ganization has begun targeting interventions for certain high-readmission population groups, such as enrollees with congestive heart failure and diabetes. It hopes to reduce readmission in these groups by improving their outpatient medical management through the use of regular telephone follow-up. GHC views the improved management of high-risk population groups as a key component of its strategy to remain competitive in the growing managed care marketplace.

A third population-based strategy underway at GHC involves influenza vaccinations for senior citizens. GHC Olympia has struggled with this performance criterion, since only about 70% of its senior membership receives annual influenza vaccinations, compared with 72% for the corporation as a whole and 80% as its target. To achieve greater success, GHC Olympia recognizes the need for a larger, community-wide campaign to encourage vaccination. As part of this effort, GHC combines with the local health department in sponsoring flu shot clinics held at various community locations during influenza season. Additionally, GHC solicits the participation of other private providers by persuading them to offer reduced-cost vaccinations to community members. The organization has met with some resistance to this effort but continues to work on expanding the number of providers who participate in the program.

Adapted with permission from, Managed Care and Public Health, Halverson, P. K., Kaluzny, A. D., McLaughlin, C. P., Mays, G. P.: pp. 226–227, © 1998 Aspen Publishers, Inc.

continuous improvement are discussed throughout the text, particularly Chapter 13.

Drawing on examples such as these, this book focuses on *the new attitudes, the new ideas, the new skills, the new behaviors, and the new mind-sets required to manage a continually changing health care system.*

The book is divided into three parts. Part 1 lays the foundation with chapters that discuss the manager's role, motivational forces, and leadership issues. Part 2 emphasizes the knowledge, skills, and understanding required to manage interdependent professional work teams in the provision of services across the continuum of care. Areas covered include negotiation and conflict management, work groups, work design, coordination and communication, and power and influence. Parts 3 and 4 deal with the challenges posed by issues of organization design, the development of interorganizational networks and strategic alliances, the demands for change and innovation, the emphasis on performance accountability, and the importance of positioning the organization strategically. The book concludes with a discussion of the future issues that will challenge health services executives.

ECOLOGY OF HEALTH SERVICES ORGANIZATIONS

An organization is formally defined as a group of people who come together to pursue a specific purpose. Most organizations will embody both formal properties reflected in rules, policies, procedures, reporting relationships, and informal properties as expressed by customs, norms, beliefs, values, rituals, and celebrations. Figure 1.1 depicts the great number and variety of organizations engaged in the process by which services are ultimately delivered to patients. Those organizations most directly involved in services to patients, enrolled populations, or the communities at large are shown in the innermost concentric circle. These include not only traditional providers such as physicians and hospitals, but also health networks, health systems,

and specialty "carve-out" organizations, such as cancer centers and heart clinics/hospitals, that focus on single diseases. **Health networks** are defined as strategic alliances or contractual arrangements among hospitals, physicians, and other health services organizations that provide an array of health services to the community. **Health systems** are defined as arrangements among hospitals, physicians, and other provider organizations that involve direct ownership of assets on the part of the parent system (Bazzoli, Shortell, Dubbs, Chan, & Kralovec, 1999). Thus, the key distinction is between the looser financial arrangements present in networks versus the unified ownership of health systems. In reality, many systems will have both owned and nonowned components representing "hybrid" organizations. Integrated or organized delivery systems have been defined as a network of organizations that provides or arranges to provide a coordinated continuum of services to a defined population and is willing to be held clinically and fiscally accountable for the outcomes and health status of the population served (Shortell, Gillies, Anderson, Mitchell, & Morgan, 1993).

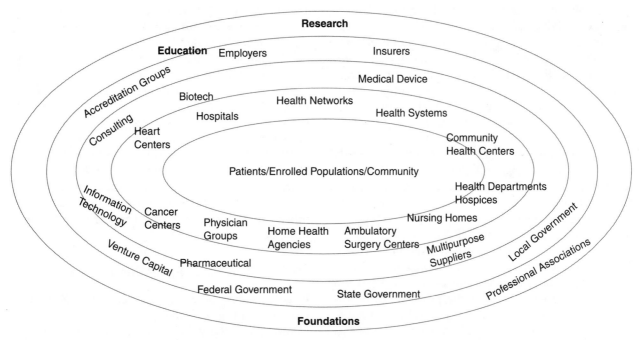

Figure 1.1. The Concentric Ecology of Organizations in the Health Care Sector.

The next concentric circle reflects the major suppliers to those organizations that directly provide services. These include multipurpose suppliers such as Baxter, General Electric, and 3M; biotech companies such as Amgen, Genetech, and Chiron; medical device companies such as Medtronic and information technology companies such as Cerner and SMS; pharmaceutical companies such as Abbott, Lilly, Pfizer, Hoecht-Marion-Roussel, Bristol-Myers Squibb, and Merck; and consulting firms such as Arthur Andersen, Andersen Consulting, Ernst and Young, Deloitte and Touche, Peat Marwick, and numerous health specific consulting firms such as APM and Lewin and Associates.

The third concentric circle reflects the major payers and sources of capital. In addition to private sector employers, business coalitions, and insurers, this group includes federal, state, and local governments and private sector venture capital firms that supply funding to the biotech, medical device, and pharmaceutical companies for research and development. It is also important to note the federal government's important role in funding biomedical, clinical, and health services research as represented in particular by the National Institutes of Health (NIH), the Agency for Health Care Policy and Research (AHCPR), and Centers for Disease Control (CDC). The federal government also plays an important regulatory role as reflected by the Food and Drug Administration (FDA). Also included in this circle are private sector accreditation groups such as the Joint Commission on Accreditation of Healthcare Organizations (JCAHCO) that primarily accredits hospitals, the National Committee for Quality Assurance (NCQA) that primarily accredits health plans, and the Foundation for Accountability (FAACT). Examples of private foundations that provide support for innovations in health care delivery are The Commonwealth Fund, The Hartford Foundation, The Henry J. Kaiser Family Foundation, The Milbank Fund, The Pew Charitable Trusts, The Robert Wood Johnson Foundation, and the W. K. Kellogg Foundation, among others. In recent years, a number of states have used the proceeds from for-profit conversions of not-for-profit Blue Cross plans to establish foundations. Examples include the California Health Care Foundation and the California Wellness Foundation. Note should also be made of the Institute of Medicine (IOM) of the National Academy of Sciences (NAS), which is charged by Congress to offer independent objective analysis of a wide range of biomedical, health policy, and health care delivery issues facing the nation and the world.

What is most significant about Figure 1.1 is the growing *permeability* between the concentric circles. Not only are provider organizations merging and consolidating with each other, but they are also forming linkages with suppliers and payers. Biotech, medical device, and pharmaceutical companies, in turn, are forming alliances with universities. Federal government and private foundation funding is also encouraging the emergence of new partnerships. The clear message for future health care executives is the need for skills, knowledge, and understanding of how to effectively manage such **interorganizational relationships.** Nearly all chapters in this text address this challenge, with Chapters 11 and 14 being particularly relevant.

Figure 1.1 also suggests the immense size, diversity, and complexity of the health care system. On the provider side alone, there are approximately 740,000 physicians, 19,787 medical groups, 1.9 million nurses, 187,000 dentists, 6,200 hospitals, 300 health networks, 300 health systems, 670 health maintenance organizations (HMOs), 17,000 nursing homes, 9,900 home health centers, 4,900 community health centers, 2,000 adult day care centers, and 51 state public health departments. On the education side, there are approximately 125 medical schools, 55 dental schools, 1,500 nursing education programs, and 67 accredited graduate programs in health services management.

While direct health care expenditures comprise about 14% of the gross national product involving more than $1 trillion, the actual impact of health care on the American economy through its linkages with other organizations as shown in Figure 1.1 is even more pervasive.

Are Health Services Organizations Unique?

Health services organizations are often described as unique or at least different from other types of organizations, particularly different from industrial organizations. Further, these differences are believed to be significant in the area of management. Among the most frequently mentioned differences are the following:

- Defining and measuring output are more difficult.
- The work involved is more variable and complex.
- More of the work is of an emergency and nondeferrable nature.
- The work permits little tolerance for ambiguity or error.
- The work activities are highly interdependent, requiring a high degree of coordination among diverse professional groups.
- The work involves an extremely high degree of specialization.
- Organizational participants are highly professionalized, and their primary loyalty belongs to the profession rather than to the organization.
- Little effective organizational or managerial control exists over the group most responsible for generating work and expenditures: physicians.
- Dual lines of authority exist in many health care organizations, particularly hospitals, that create problems of coordination and accountability and confusion of roles.

Upon careful examination, it is possible to refute or at least question each of these allegedly distinctive attributes. For example, universities also have difficulty in defining and measuring their product. Is it the number of students graduated or the number of credit hours produced? Is quality measured by grade point average? If so, how much of that is the contribution of the student or of the faculty? A number of other organizations such as police and fire departments are concerned with highly variable, complex, emergency work. Other organizations also have limited ability to tolerate errors or ambiguities (for example, air traffic controllers). Are work activities any more interdependent in health care than in a symphony orchestra? What about the high degree of specialization of activities in a large legal firm? As for control over professional members, do universities or research institutes have any more control over their faculty or investigators than health services organizations have over physicians? Finally, many business and industrial organizations have dual lines of authority. In fact, as discussed in Chapter 10, many firms have institutionalized dual-authority structures through matrix organization designs. Further, the concept of uniqueness can be harmful if it leads health services managers to believe that their job is so much more difficult or different from others that relatively little can be done to improve performance.

On the other hand, health services organizations may be unusual, if not unique, in that many of them possess all of the characteristics stated above *in combination*. It is one thing to have little control over professionals when they do not need to interact frequently with others in the organization, such as with a number of research and development units in industry. But it is different when physicians, nurses, and other health professionals are highly dependent on each other in providing and coordinating patient care. The independence of professionals from managerial control is also less of a problem in situations where output is readily defined and measured than where clear performance criteria are still under development and yet external bodies hold the organization responsible for the activities of the relatively independent group of professionals. Thus it is the confluence of professional, technological, and task attributes that make the management of health services organizations particularly challenging. Further, health services organizations are highly involved with values on a daily basis. For example, cost containment, which is valued by society at large, may frequently conflict with individual client values, such as the desire to recover one's health at almost any cost. In other cases such as abortion, outcomes valued by different parties may be in conflict.

KEY DIMENSIONS OF HEALTH SERVICES ORGANIZATIONS

Seven key dimensions of health care organizations are its (1) external environment, (2) mission/goals, (3) strategies, (4) level of differentiation, (5) level of integration, (6) level of centralization, and (7) ability to adapt and change. Each of these is discussed in turn.

External Environment

One key to an organization's success is having a good understanding of its **external environment,** defined as all of the political, economic, social, and regulatory forces that exert influence on the organization. Environments differ in their complexity, susceptibility to change, and competitiveness. Depending on these attributes, organizations might choose different strategies, structures, and processes to compete successfully (see Chapters 7, 10, 13, and 14, in particular). For example, in markets characterized by a lower degree of managed care activity, health systems are less likely to own health plans and less likely to have salaried relationships with a large number of physicians. In more heavily penetrated managed care markets, one would expect to see greater ownership of health plans and a greater number of salaried relationships with physicians. The challenge is to appropriately match the organizations' strategies and structures to the demands of the environment. In order to deal with these environmental demands, health services organizations are increasingly forming strategic alliances with each other, resulting in a dense web of interorganizational networks (see Chapter 11).

Mission/Goals

The organization's **mission** and associated **goals** largely dictate the major tasks to be carried out and the kinds of technologies and human resources to be employed. Organizations, of course, differ widely in their mission and goals. Three examples of mission statements and statements of values are shown in Table 1.3. An organization's mission and goals have both an external and internal purpose. Externally they communicate what the organization is about to those who may want to use its services (e.g., patients) or in some other way have contact with the organization (e.g., regulators and third-party payers). They help to provide legitimacy, which, in turn, assists in helping the organization acquire needed resources (see Chapter 13). Internally goals serve as a source of motivation and direction (see Chapters 3 and 4).

Strategies

Strategies are plans for achieving the organization's mission and goals and primarily involve positioning the organization to succeed in its environment relative to its competitors. Chapters 11, 13, and 14 emphasize the importance of the manager's role in the development and implementation of strategy. It is believed that in fast-paced turbulent environments characterized by considerable change, flexible, "emergent" strategies are needed, drawing on the best thinking of those closest to the customers. In more stable environments, a more top-down formal planning process may be effective. In reality, most organizations engage in and require both approaches to strategy development and implementation.

The generic content of strategies that health care organizations may adopt include being (1) low-cost providers or (2) differentiating on high quality. Either of these can be done across-the-board or targeted to specific market niches or customer segments (Porter, 1985). Others have characterized an organization's strategies as being those of a prospector (i.e., almost always first to do anything), analyzer (approaches new developments cautiously with an emphasis on well-thought-out plans), defender (is seldom an innovator; emphasizes cost effectiveness), and reactor (doesn't have a coherent strategy) (Miles & Snow, 1978). Existing research suggests that in the fast-paced health care environment, organizations using prospector and analyzer strategies appear to do better than those using defender and reactor strategies (Shortell, Gillies, Anderson, Morgan-Erickson, & Mitchell, 1996).

Differentiation

The major way in which organizations compete is through the array of products and services that they offer. This is referred to as **differentiation** and involves the development of specialized knowledge, functions, departments, and viewpoints (Lawrence & Lorsch, 1967). Some pharmaceutical/biotech companies, such as Merck, offer a broad array of drugs across a wide spectrum of diseases, while others, such as Amgen, have a more narrow "pipeline," focusing

Table 1.3. Three Examples of Mission and Value Statements

Detroit Medical Center Mission

The Detroit Medical Center (DMC) is committed to improving the health of the population served by providing the highest quality health care services in a caring and efficient manner.

Together with Wayne State University (Detroit, Michigan), the DMC strives to be the region's premiere health care resource through a broad range of clinical services, the discovery and application of new knowledge, and the education of practitioners, teachers, and scientists.

DMC Values
- Community welfare
- Quality
- Respect and involvement
- Teamwork
- Communication
- Innovation and education
- Efficient and effective resource use

Cerner Corporation Mission

Cerner's mission is to connect to the appropriate person, knowledge, and resource at the appropriate time and location to achieve the optimal outcome.

Cerner Values
- Excellence in technology
- Investment in people
- Client service

Chiron Mission

Chiron is a global health care company focused on vaccines, diagnostics, therapeutics, and technology development. Its broad expertise enables an integrated approach to preventing, diagnosing, and treating cancer, as well as infectious and cardiovascular diseases. Chiron's approach is supported by scientific strengths in recombinant proteins, gene therapy, small molecule discovery, and diagnostic instrumentation.

on only a few. Some consulting firms offer tax audit information technology and strategic services to their health care clients, while others focus only on strategic services. Some community care networks focus on a wide range of health problems in the community, while others focus on a single problem such as teenage pregnancy or domestic violence (Bazzoli et al., 1997). In general, the greater the degree of differentiation, the greater the managerial challenges to appropriately integrate and coordinate the organization's various products and services offerings. Effective approaches for accomplishing this are discussed in Chapters 5–8, 10, and 13.

Integration

All organizations require some degree of coordination across specialized functions and processes in order to achieve unity of effort. This is referred to as *integration*. Organizations that are more differentiated also require a greater degree of integration. The overall managerial challenge is to appropriately match the levels of differentiation and integration to the demands of the external environment (Lawrence & Lorsch, 1967). While integration has been most studied within individual organizations, health services organizations are increasingly required to integrate their activities across organizational boundaries. This has been particularly true with the growth of health networks and systems, many of which develop complex relationships involving hospitals, physician groups, long-term care facilities, and health plans. The integration challenge within the organization involves issues of work group design (see Chapters 6 and 7), communication and coordination (see Chapter 8), and the overall design of the organization (see Chapter 10). The integration challenge of effectively linking the organization to other organizations involves issues of forging strategic alliances (see Chapter 11) and change and innovation (see Chapter 12). It is important to note that these forms of interorganizational arrangements can be either of a vertical ownership nature or a virtual contractual nature, depending on the costs and benefits associated with each approach (Conrad & Shortell, 1993; Robinson, 1997).

Centralization

Another important dimension of organizations is the extent to which decision making and selected functions are *centralized* or *decentralized.* In a centralized health system, for example, more decisions are made by the top management team of the system than by individual hospitals or physician groups. Also, functions such as strategic planning and marketing would be primarily done centrally rather than within each of the hospitals or physician groups. In a decentralized health system, more decisions, strategic planning, and marketing functions would be primarily done within individual hospitals and physician groups and then "coordinated" at the system-wide level. The degree of centralization has important implications for how quickly decisions get made, how effectively decisions are implemented, the ability of the organization to adapt to change, and how well the organization meets the accountability demands of external groups. The centralization/decentralization issue is further explored in Chapters 9, 10, 12, and 13.

Change/Innovation

As never before, health services organizations are being called on to develop their capacity for **change** and **innovation.** Three points are particularly relevant. First is to recognize that most health care organizations are extremely complex. Hospitals, for example, typically employ up to 260 different professional/occupational groups, each with their own specialized training, norms, beliefs, and views of the world. Second, most health care organizations, particularly on the provider side, are "loosely coupled" (Weick, 1969) in that hospitals, physicians, and health plans often exist through a loose set of contractual relationships rather than ownership of each other's assets. Thus, new ideas, plans, and strategies require negotiation and persuasion involving a rather extensive decision-making process. Third, as the number of interorganizational relationships has grown, the ripple effects of any single organization's change become magnified. For example, problems can be created when a hospital belonging to a given system decides to enter into an arrangement with an HMO that is not the system's own HMO. The accompanying "In the Real World" highlights relevant change management questions for dealing with these kinds of issues within the context of caring for people with chronic illness. These and related issues of managing change in health care organizations are further discussed in Chapter 12.

HEALTH SERVICES ORGANIZATIONS AS SYSTEMS

Health services organizations are complex social systems. In managing these organizations, there is a constant tension between the need for predictability, order, and efficiency on the one hand and openness, adaptability, and innovation on the other. The need for predictability, order, and efficiency is consistent with a **closed system** view of an organization. The closed system view assumes that at least parts of an organization can be sealed off from the external environment. As such, the management challenge is how to use internal design, productivity improvement tools, and incentives to maximize internal efficiency.

The need for openness, adaptability, and innovation is consistent with an **open system** view (Scott, 1981). This view emphasizes that organizations are parts of the external environment and, as such, must continually change and adapt to meet the challenges posed by the environment. The emphasis is on meet-

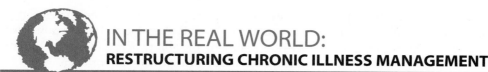

IN THE REAL WORLD:
RESTRUCTURING CHRONIC ILLNESS MANAGEMENT

A number of important questions relevant to assessing an organization's readiness to manage chronic illness must be addressed. Some of these include:

- *Is the effective management of care for chronically ill patients an important part of the organization's overall mission?*
- *Do the goals of functional areas within the organization, and the strategies being used to achieve those goals, support the restructuring of chronic illness treatment processes?*
- *Are purchasers willing to pay for restructured care processes for chronic illness? Is reimbursement for restructured care processes possible under existing payment procedures?*
- *Is the organizational culture supportive of coordinated team approaches to patient care?*
- *Can the existing process of caring for the chronically ill be clearly described? Can its shortcomings be identified? Is the need for restructuring clear in light of these shortcomings?*
- *Can agreement on reasonable performance targets for the restructured care process be reached in light of the perceived shortcomings of the existing process?*

- *Can key individuals within the organization who will be affected by a restructured chronic illness treatment process be recruited to participate in that restructuring?*
- *Is there a "process owner" who will assume leadership responsibility in the restructuring process?*
- *Is there commitment to having patients meaningfully involved in their own treatment?*
- *Will the organization commit the resources to training and education that the restructured care process needs to function effectively?*
- *Do existing compensation systems discourage clinicians from participating in chronic illness treatment teams? Can systems be designed and implemented to reward clinicians and patients for team participation?*

Adapted from Christianson, J. B., Taylor, R. A., Knutson, D. J. Restructuring Chronic Illness Management: Best Practices and Innovations in Team-Based Treatment. *San Francisco: Jossey-Bass, 1998: 163–173.*

ing the needs of external customers and stakeholders with relatively less emphasis given to issues of internal efficiency.

Both approaches are needed to understand and manage health services organizations. While each activity, function, or department of a health services organization can be considered by itself with its unique requirements and expectations, the real payoff lies in recognizing the interdependence of most activities and functions. One set of functions and activities is usually the building blocks for another set, which, in turn, serves as inputs for still others. These sets of functions, activities, and departments serve as internal environments for each other in addition to being influenced by forces in the external environment. The

processes that occur in health services organizations can be described in terms of six primary functions: production, boundary spanning, maintenance, adaptation, management, and governance (Katz & Kahn, 1978).

Production

The **production function** provides the product or service and is at the center of most organizational activity. It is represented by the manufacturing of a new drug in a pharmaceutical company, the diagnosis and treatment of patients in a multispecialty group practice, and the alleviation of pain and suffering in a hospice organization. These core production processes can vary on a number of dimensions including complexity, time, use of labor versus capital, and ease with which results can be measured among others.

Boundary Spanning

The **boundary spanning function** focuses on the interface between the organization and its external environment. It is concerned with new developments in technology, reimbursement, regulation, licensure, changing demographics, customer expectations, competitive threats, and related issues. Depending on the size of the organization and its local market environment, these activities will often vary in their complexity and susceptibility to change. Some organizations will establish certain departments that designate specific individuals or functional areas to carry out boundary spanning activities. In other cases, all employees with managerial responsibilities are required to undertake at least some boundary spanning activities.

Maintenance

The **maintenance function** is concerned with both the physical and human infrastructure of the organization. It includes capital acquisition and maintenance as well as employee growth and development. As the rate of change accelerates and as the external environment becomes more threatening, greater demands are placed on the maintenance functions of health services organizations.

Adaptation

The **adaptation function** focuses on change. Using information obtained from the boundary spanning activities of the organization and with knowledge of the organization's production capability and maintenance support systems, the adaptation function helps the organization to anticipate and adjust to needed changes. This may include the need for new programs and services, deletion or modification of existing programs and services, changes in the organization's structure and design, or major changes in the organization's basic strategy. The adaptation function also emphasizes the health services organization's ability to innovate by actively creating changes in its environment. Given the turbulence of the health services environment, the ability of health services organizations to adapt is of growing importance.

Management

Management is a distinct function that cuts across all the other functions and subsystems. In a sense, it is the "head" that organizes, directs, and oversees all of the other functions. It is represented in most health services organizations by the senior management team and key middle managers.

Governance

Although not usually mentioned in traditional texts, **governance** is added as a sixth distinct function because of the important public trust and social accountability responsibilities of health services organizations. It is the function that holds management and the organization accountable for its actions and that helps provide management with overall strategic direction in guiding the organization's activities. The pressure for greater accountability in regard to patient outcomes, treatment effectiveness, patient satisfaction, cost containment, and ethical use of resources is posing significant challenges to the governance function of health services organizations.

AREAS OF MANAGERIAL ACTIVITY

Figure 1.2 shows the major areas of activity requiring managerial attention. They include the individual, the group/department, the organization as a whole, the network of interorganizational relationships, and the larger environment that interacts with all of the other spheres. The figure also suggests the complexity of the manager's job in attempting to integrate the various levels of activities in positioning the organization to meet its goals and objectives in the face of environmental challenges.

Traditionally, the individual area has been the primary focus of **organizational behavior** or what is sometimes referred to as the **micro approach** to understanding organizations. The emphasis is on exam-

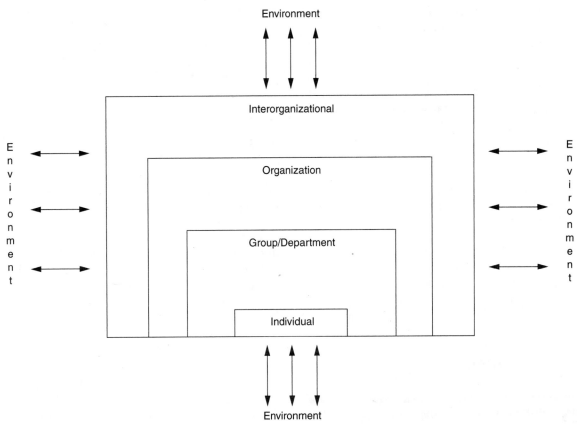

Figure 1.2. Major Areas of Activity.

ining individuals within organizations. Chapters 2–5 deal with clear examples of organizational behavior issues: managers' role relationships, motivation, leadership, and conflict management. The next area shown is the group/department. These activities typically combine both individual issues and organization-wide issues as they influence group behavior. Chapters 6 through 9, dealing with work groups, work design, coordination and communication, and power and politics, address these issues. The organizational and interorganizational areas shown comprise what is often called the **macro approach** to organizational analysis, particularly as they influence and are influenced by the environment. The organizational area issues are the subject of Chapters 9, 10, 12, 13, and 14. Interorganizational issues are explicitly treated in Chapter 11 on managing strategic alliances. It is im-

portant to recognize that these different areas of managerial activity are in reality highly permeable. A large part of the executive's job is to manage the complex, dynamic, interactive relationships among the multiple levels. This is what will be required by the leadership of Sutter Health to deal with the multiple challenges described in the opening scenario of this chapter.

MAJOR PERSPECTIVES ON HEALTH SERVICES ORGANIZATIONS

Everyone has a theory or a perspective on how organizations function. Based on personal experience, we create "mental maps" of what is connected to what and how things happen. In many respects, organization theory consists of the systematic examination of these mental maps of how things work. Over the years, a number of major perspectives of how organizations work have evolved: classical bureaucratic theory, the scientific management school, the human relations school, contingency theory, resource dependence theory, the strategic management perspective, population ecology theory, and institutional theory. These perspectives can be used to gain insight into the structure and functioning of health services organizations.

Bureaucratic Theory

Classical **bureaucratic theory** is consistent with the closed system approach to organizations and is based on five characteristics.

1. The organization is guided by explicit specific procedures for governing activities.
2. Activities are distributed among office holders.
3. Offices are arranged in a hierarchical fashion.
4. Candidates are selected on the basis of their technical competence.
5. Officials carry out their functions in an impersonal fashion (Weber, 1964).

The bureaucratic organizational form can achieve technical superiority over other forms under certain stable conditions. However, a number of investigators have pointed out dysfunctional consequences of bureaucracy, including its lack of individual freedom, rigidity of behavior, and difficulty in dealing with clients (Gouldner, 1954; Merton, 1957; Selznick, 1966). While most health services organizations are organized along bureaucratic lines to some degree, other forms of organization are better at dealing with rapidly changing environments. The manager's challenge is to decide the extent to which some organizational components might best be organized along bureaucratic lines versus other approaches. Chapters 6, 7, and 10 deal explicitly with this issue.

The Scientific Management School

Closely related to the bureaucratic approach is the **scientific management school** (Gulick & Urwick, 1937; Mooney, 1947; Taylor, 1947). This perspective emphasizes span of control, unity of command, appropriate delegation of authority, departmentalization, and the use of work methods to improve efficiency. The scientific management approach consists of

1. programming the job
2. choosing the right person to match the job
3. training the person to do the job

Much of the early work on job design (see Chapter 7) is based on the scientific management school, as are some current work methods' improvement and operations research approaches. Recent interest in "focused factories"—organizations that specialize in the treatment of selected diseases (e.g., cancer, heart disease, and diabetes)—are largely based on the scientific management school (Herzlinger, 1997).

Using quality of care as an example, the bureaucratic and scientific management approaches would suggest that the quality improvement goals be explicitly defined and that the requirements for achieving these goals be spelled out in detail and expressed in terms of specific job positions and necessary skills. People should then be screened and selected on the basis of defined criteria. The quality improvement function would be hierarchically organized with one department reporting to an overall head who in turn would report to an organization-wide coordinating body. Various rules, policies, and practices would exist for what problems to study, how to study them, and what kinds of information should be generated. The bureaucratic and scientific management schools would help to contribute needed structure to an organization's quality improvement efforts.

The Human Relations School

The focus of the **human relations school** is on the individual. Satisfying individual needs is seen as a worthy goal in itself, not merely a means of achieving other organizational goals (Argyris, 1964; Barnard, 1938; Likert, 1967; McGregor, 1960; Roethlisberger & Dickson, 1939). The approach emphasizes the usefulness of participatory decision making that involves the individual in the organization and the role of intrinsic self-actualizing aspects of work. The approach represents the foundation for many applied organization development efforts and for the reemphasis on empowering individuals associated with total quality management and continuous quality improvement efforts. A number of issues associated with the human relations school are discussed in Chapter 3 on motivation and Chapter 4 on leadership.

The human relations school would emphasize the importance of empowering individuals in the organization to take greater responsibility for improving all aspects of their work. Employees would be given greater autonomy to identify and solve problems. They would be provided with the training and tools to function in this role. A major challenge for organizations in implementing this philosophy of management is to get senior and middle managers to let go of the tendency to want to do things themselves to make sure that they get done right. This requires a culture that is consistently supportive of employee empowerment focused on organizational goals (Rundall, Starkweather, & Norrish, 1998).

Contingency Theory

Proponents of the **contingency theory** (Burns & Stalker, 1961; Lawrence & Lorsch, 1967; Perrow, 1967; Rundall, et al., 1998; Thompson, 1967) suggest that a more bureaucratic or "mechanistic" form of organization is more effective when the environment is relatively simple and stable, tasks and technology are relatively routine, and a relatively high percentage of nonprofessional workers are employed. In contrast, a less bureaucratic or more "organic" form of organization is likely to be more effective when the environment is complex and dynamic, tasks and technologies are nonroutine, and a relatively high percentage of professionals are involved. The more organic organizational form involves decentralized decision making, more participative decision making, and a greater reliance on lateral communication and coordination mechanisms to link people and work units. These mechanisms are appropriate when the environment is complex and nonroutine technologies are involved, because the organization has a greater need for information, expertise, and flexibility. Organic forms of design are better able to respond to these needs. In contrast, where no such demands are made, there is less need for flexibility, and the more tradi-

tional bureaucratic approach is likely to be more efficient and effective.

Contingency theorists do not advocate an either/or approach but rather view the process as a continuum from more or less bureaucratic (i.e., mechanistic) to more or less organic. Furthermore, they recognize that different subunits of the organization may be organized differently depending on the specific environments and technologies with which they are involved. Empirical support for contingency theory ideas is mixed depending on whether one is studying the organization as a whole, particular subgroups, or specific individuals (Schoonhoven, 1981). Nonetheless, given the wide variety of health services organizations and different environments in which they operate, the contingency perspective has wide application to health services organizations (Mohr, 1982). The contingency perspective is drawn on throughout this book, including Chapters 7, 8, 10, and 13.

In the case of quality, the contingency perspective would suggest that the quality improvement function might be organized differently depending on the environment faced by each organization, the nature of the clinical problems and other issues being addressed, and the types of employee skills available. For example, in smaller hospitals operating in more stable markets, it may be possible to develop structured approaches to quality improvement and to do so in an orderly fashion by training most employees in quality improvement tools in advance, conducting pilot projects, learning from them, and gradually diffusing them throughout the organization. In more complex hospitals and clinics operating in more dynamic environments, a more flexible approach may be needed. Some of the training may need to occur in a "just in time" fashion, problems may need to be addressed as they arise, and a more flexible structure may need to be used to make rapid changes as required.

Resource Dependence Theory

The **resource dependence theory** emphasizes the importance of the organization's abilities to secure needed resources from its environment in order to survive (Hickson et al., 1971; March & Olsen, 1976; Pfeffer & Salancik, 1978; Strasser, 1983; Williamson,

1981). Those subunits within the organization that have access to key external resources will hold greater power and influence. While organizations desire to maintain their autonomy and remain relatively independent of their environment, they also recognize the need to form certain coalitions or networks to pool resources and reduce transaction costs. The resource dependence perspective, like the strategic management perspective but unlike the population ecology perspective discussed below, assumes that managers can actively influence their environment to reduce unwanted dependencies and enhance survivability. The resource dependence perspective is drawn on in Chapters 2, 9, 11, 13, and 14.

In regard to quality, the resource dependence perspective would emphasize the importance of continuous improvement and total quality management for demonstrating value to purchasers of care. To accomplish this, the organization needs resources from the environment in the form of measurement tools, information systems, and technical expertise to produce valid data on the processes and outcomes of patient care. An organization's ability to exert influence over its environment will depend on how successful it is in demonstrating continuous improvement relative to that of other organizations that patients and purchasers can choose.

Strategic Management Perspective

The **strategic management perspective** emphasizes the importance of positioning the organization relative to its environment and competitors in order to achieve its objectives and ensure its survival (Andrews, 1971; Ansoff, 1965; Ouchi, 1980; Porter, 1980, 1985; Schendel & Hofer, 1979; Shortell & Zajac, 1990). The perspective attempts to link environmental forces, internal organizational design and processes, and the strategy of the firm. It suggests that the firm's strategy needs to be consistent with both the external environmental demands and the organization's internal core capabilities and competencies. It is explicitly concerned with issues of organizational performance, arguing that managers and organizational members have discretion in choosing strategies and structures to match the environment in a way that will enhance

the organization's performance. Major subissues of interest include the different processes by which organizations develop strategies, the extent to which organizations are able to successfully change their strategies, and the extent to which organizations vary in their ability to implement strategies. Chapters 11, 13, and 14 of the text highlight many of these issues.

The strategic management and resource dependence perspectives are illustrated by the "In the Real World" creation of the Somerbridge Community Health Partnership. The likely success of the partnership will depend on its ability to secure needed resources by aligning its strategies and services with the needs of the population, the partnership's own capabilities, and the larger environmental forces affecting the partnership.

Population Ecology Theory

Advocates of the **population ecology theory** (Aldrich, 1979; Delacroix & Carroll, 1983; Hannan & Freeman, 1985, 1989; Kimberly & Zajac, 1985) argue that the environment "selects out" certain organizations for survival. Based on theories of natural selection in biology, the focus is on a given population of organizations rather than on an individual organization. Whether a given organization will succeed depends on where it stands in relation to the population of its competitors and the overall environmental forces influencing that population. As environmental pressures increase, only the stronger, more dominant organizational forms will survive; the weaker forms will cease to exist or will survive only as markedly different forms of organization. In the population ecology approach, unlike the resource dependence and strategic management approaches, there are severe limits on the ability of organizations to adapt. This is expressed in terms of "structural inertia." Thus, in this approach, the ability of managers to successfully influence their environments is subsumed to be relatively minor.

The population ecology approach is based on the principles of variation, selection, and retention. Variation involves the continuous development of new organizational forms that add to the variety and complexity in the environment. In health care, examples include freestanding surgery centers, urgent care cen-

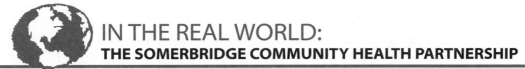

IN THE REAL WORLD:
THE SOMERBRIDGE COMMUNITY HEALTH PARTNERSHIP

MICHAEL E. CAPUANO, Mayor, City of Somerville

ROBERT W. HEALY, City Manager, City of Cambridge

In the aftermath of the failed national health care reform debate, the attention of those committed to health care access has again focused closer to home. For many years, using slightly different methods, health and human service providers and community activists in Somerville and Cambridge have worked on local solutions to the health problems confronted by our communities.

Somerville (Massachusetts) and Cambridge (Massachusetts) have a combined population of 170,000. This population is extremely diverse from a socioeconomic, demographic, and cultural perspective. Both cities have experienced significant growth in immigrant populations, with dozens of languages spoken in the homes of these newly arrived residents. Both communities also have extensive health and human service networks and a high level of community activism.

Both Cambridge Hospital and Somerville Hospital have worked for years in collaboration with their respective communities. Separately, both cities conducted com-

munity needs assessments in partnership with their community hospitals. This work served to strengthen the connection between the hospitals and residents of each city. It also influenced programs and services provided by the hospitals. However, this work was not coordinated between the two cities until the opportunity for closer collaboration was presented through the community care network (CCN) program.

Through the CCN vision, the Somerbridge Community Health Partnership will facilitate this ongoing community health effort across both cities. The three issue initiatives of Somerbridge—substance abuse, geriatric health and immigrant health—were identified as top priorities through the community needs assessment. It is our dream, as chief executives, that this new collaboration will result in greater opportunities for the residents of our cities as cooperation and improvement guide this project. We truly believe that the Somerbridge partnership will serve as a model of collaboration for other communities to replicate.

ters, birthing care centers, hospices, diagnostic imaging centers, and fitness centers.

The selection principle states that some of the new organizational forms will fit the external environment better than others. They will be better able to exploit the environment for resources and will move in the same direction that the environmental trends are moving. In health care, ambulatory surgery centers serve as an example as more surgical procedures are being reimbursed on an outpatient basis, and there appears to be a growing trend for consumers to prefer quicker, more accessible, and convenient services.

Retention involves the preservation and ongoing institutionalization of the new organizational form.

Those that are valued by the environment in the long run will be retained, while others will fall by the wayside. For example, ambulatory surgery centers may experience relatively long survival (at least until it becomes possible to do most surgery in the patient's home), whereas urgent care centers, faced with stiff competition from physician providers, hospital emergency rooms, and growing regulatory requirements, face a less certain future. The winners may be those organizations that manage to carve out specialized market niches viewed as complementary to other organizations and in which they can act as noncompeting sources of patient referrals to other providers.

As health services organizations are faced with increasing cost-containment and competitive pressures, the issues raised by the population ecology perspective become particularly important. In recent years a growing number of general acute care hospitals and HMOs have gone out of business and, as previously noted, a variety of new organizational forms have arisen, including specialty providers in cancer, heart disease, and diabetes and physician management companies. In addition, the hospital industry has been transformed from a largely cottage industry composed of individual hospitals to approximately 600 networks and systems (Bazzoli, Shortell, Dubbs, Chan, & Kralovec, 1999). These entities, both investor-owned and not-for-profit, are working to find specific niches in the marketplace, focusing in particular on the development of regionally and locally integrated networks of care. While the population ecology perspective tends to minimize the manager's role, it adds an important dimension and challenge to the effective management of health services organizations by emphasizing the importance of networking and coalition building and of developing products and services for specific population segments in which the competitive market forces and related pressures are less threatening (Alexander, Kaluzny, & Middleton, 1986; Carroll, 1984). These issues are further discussed in Chapters 2, 9, 12, 13, and 14.

In the case of quality management, the population ecology approach would suggest that efforts at continuous quality improvement are only germane to the extent that they make the organization form more viable in a changing health care environment. It would emphasize the extent to which quality improvement principles are congruent with the current organization's structure and capabilities. It would suggest that the organization has very little flexibility or ability to modify these approaches if they prove to be inconsistent with its culture and capabilities. If the organization experiences difficulty in incorporating the newer continuous quality improvement approaches, the population ecology school would argue that the organization becomes more susceptible to being "selected against" by other organizations with which the new approach is more compatible.

Institutional Theory

Institutional theory emphasizes that organizations face environments characterized by external norms, rules, and requirements that the organizations must conform to in order to receive legitimacy and support (Alexander & Amburgey, 1987; Meyer & Scott, 1983; Scott, 1987). While technical environments reward organizations for effective and efficient performance, institutional environments emphasize rewarding organizations for having structures and processes that are in conformance with the environment. The rules, beliefs, and norms of the external environment are often expressed in the form of "rational myths" (Alexander & D'Aunno, 1990). Such myths are rational in the sense of being reflected in professional standards, laws, and licensure and accreditation requirements but are myths in the sense that they cannot necessarily be verified empirically. They are, nonetheless, widely held to be true. Conformity with these myths helps the organization to gain legitimacy and support. This conformance is often referred to as "isomorphism" and causes organizations faced with a similar set of environmental circumstances to resemble each other (Fennell & Alexander, 1987). Institutional theorists have also addressed issues of organizational change highlighting the role played by institutional processes, social processes, and culture (Fligstein, 1990; Powell & DiMaggio, 1991).

Health services organizations are experiencing a rapid transformation of both their technical and institutional environments. The increased technical pressure for greater efficiency and quality expressed in terms of value is causing health services organizations to change long-established structures. This is reflected in the reorganization of acute care hospitals as they forge new relationships with physician groups and health plans and the development of new norms and beliefs about what constitutes the effective delivery of health care. This transition results in a great deal of internal conflict that must be managed. Chapter 5 addresses the conflict issues. The implications of the institutional theory perspective on health services organization are also discussed in Chapters 9, 11, 13, and 14.

From an institutional theory perspective, efforts at continuous quality improvement might be viewed as a response to newly emerging norms and practices within the health services sector. These are being fostered by the Joint Commission on Accreditation of Healthcare Organizations (JCAHO), which has adopted continuous quality improvement as the basis for new accreditation requirements and by the National Committee for Quality Assurance (NCQA), which has developed quality criteria for health plans. In addition, continuous improvement has been increasingly accepted as a distinguishing feature of an innovative organization with several national awards created to recognize institutions that exert such lead-ership. Thus, it could be argued that an organization's quality effort is not motivated so much by substantive concerns over its quality or efficiency of care in a competitive marketplace but rather by negative perceptions of external groups if it did not pursue continuous quality improvement (DiMaggio & Powell, 1983; Westphal, Gulati, & Shortell, 1997).

Table 1.4 provides a brief summary of how each major theory or perspective would view an organization's quality efforts. It is important to note that none of the perspectives are inherently right or wrong. They are different from each other and incomplete. As such, each represents a *partial* view of organizational dynamics and can provide input for constructive dis-

Table 1.4. How Major Perspectives Would View an Organization's Quality Improvement Efforts

Perspective	Point of Emphasis	Contribution
Bureaucratic and scientific management	Explicit goals; hierarchical organization; detailed specifications	Provide needed structure
Human relations	Employee empowerment	Need for a culture supportive of empowerment
Contingency theory	Structure depends on environment, task, technology, and the contingencies facing each unit	Flexible approach needed; adapt efforts to meet the requirements of the situation
Resource dependence	Ability to secure needed resources	Need to demonstrate value through providing reliable and valid data on patient care processes and outcomes
Strategic management	Achieve fit or alignment between the organization's strategy, external enviornment, and internal structure and capabilities	Need to link quality improvement to core strategies and capabilities of the organization
Population ecology	External environmental pressures are primary determinant of success; little managers can do	Highlights powerful role played by external environment; quality improvement efforts alone may not be sufficient if organization is not well positioned within the environment
Institutional theory	External norms, rules, requirements, and relationships cause organizations to conform in order to receive legitimacy; organizations in a similar institutional environment come to resemble each other (i.e., become isomorphic with the environment)	Quality improvement efforts must take into account regulatory and accreditation pressures and public expectations

DEBATE TIME 1.1: WHAT DO YOU THINK?

In recent years a number of health services organizations including hospitals, medical group practices, and home health care agencies have either merged, consolidated, or gone out of business. How might this be explained? Population ecology theory, of course, would assert that the environmental variables involving reimbursement rates, competitive factors, technological growth, and societal forces are the primary causes of this organizational restructuring. They would further argue that these organizations and their managers could do relatively little to prevent the eventual outcomes. Basically, the organization was no longer "fit" given the changing environmental forces.

In contrast, the resource dependence and strategic management perspectives argue that organizations have considerable control over their destiny. Through actions taken by organization leaders and members, new strategies, policies and procedures, alliances, changes in structure, and hiring of new or different kinds of people can be initiated in order to improve the organization's "fit" with changing environmental forces and to ensure its viability. They point to examples of organizational "turnarounds" that suggest the reasons why some organizations are restructured or closed, while others survive has more to do with the vision and talent of the organization and its members than with externally generated environmental forces. Which view is more correct?

DOES THE LITERATURE HELP?

". . . [T]he corporatization of health care in the United States has been precipitated by a transformation of institutional systems rather than by rational or strategic adaptation by individual organizations to changes in their operating environments." (Morgan, 1986)

"Our view is simply that most relevant environmental forces are, in fact, organizationally created and sustained, and thus are subject to organizational influence." (Alexander & D'Aunno, 1990, p. 79)

"The basic feature of the natural selection perspective is that the environment selects the most fit or optimal organizations. The organization is thus seen as relatively powerless to affect the selection process. But our review of some of the research on health care organizations suggests otherwise. Furthermore, from a managerial perspective it is difficult to accept so much organizational fatalism and inevitability." (Shortell & Zajac, 1990, p. 169)

agreement and debate, an example of which is highlighted in Debate Time 1.1. It is important to understand the basic assumptions and premises of each perspective, as they can be drawn on in various combinations to provide a greater understanding of how health services organizations operate.

METAPHORS OF HEALTH SERVICES ORGANIZATIONS

The above perspectives are enriched by recasting them as metaphors of health services organizations as shown in Table 1.5. The eight metaphors are machines, tyrants, brains, playing fields, psychic prisons, biological organisms, political systems, and holograms.

Machines

Classical bureaucratic theory is reflected in the image of the organization as a **machine.** In fact, workers may speak of the organization as a "well-oiled machine." This metaphor reflects the image of an organization as interlocking parts with clearly defined roles that are appropriately meshed together to accomplish the organization's work. Being a well-oiled machine is important for many of the tasks undertaken by health services organizations including the admission of patients into hospitals, the paperwork associated with billing for patient services, the production of a laboratory test, and the processing of a

Table 1.5. Organizational Perspectives and Metaphors

Organizational Perspectives	Relevant Metaphors
Classical bureaucratic theory ⟶	Machines
	Tyrants
Human relations school ⟶	Brains
	Playing fields
	Psychic prisons
Contingency theory ⟶	Biological organisms
	Brains
Resource dependency theory ⟶	Political systems
	Playing fields
Strategic management ⟶	Biological organisms
perspective	Holograms
Population ecology theory ⟶	Biological organisms
Institutional theory ⟶	Biological organisms

Federal Drug Administration (FDA) application for approval. The downside is that the machines can rapidly become outmoded and inflexible in the face of changing demands and circumstances. An organization whose dominant paradigm is that of a machine sees order and stability where none exists and rapidly becomes technologically and organizationally obsolete.

Tyrants

Organizations can also behave as **tyrants** or as instruments of domination. In pursuit of their missions, they can lose sight of basic human values and exploit their employees and others either unconsciously or by intent. This may be the basis for many physicians' fears of large complex health services organizations such as the growing health services systems and networks. The mental map that many physicians have is that of the organization as tyrant or potential tyrant restricting their freedom and autonomy and making unilateral decisions without soliciting their input. The tyrant metaphor represents the shadow or dark side of organizational functioning that must be carefully guarded against by the organization's leaders.

Brains

The metaphor of organizations as **brains** places emphasis on the importance of learning, intelligence, and information processing. It is based in part on cybernetic theory, which stresses four key principles.

1. Systems have the capacity to sense, monitor, and scan significant aspects of their environment.
2. Systems can relate this information to the norms that guide system behavior.
3. Systems can detect significant deviations from these norms.
4. Systems are able to initiate corrective actions when discrepancies are detected. (Starkweather & Cook, 1988)

When these conditions hold, a continuous process of information exchange is created between an organization and its environment allowing the system to operate in a spontaneous self-correcting manner. This operation is characterized by *double-loop learning,* which involves an ability to take a second look at a situation by questioning the relevance of underlying assumptions (Morgan, 1986, p. 87). The brain metaphor is particularly useful for health services organizations in terms of maximizing the ability of individuals and groups to learn from their environment and make use of the information to create innovative programs and services. It is consistent with the human relations school's emphasis on personal growth and development.

Playing Fields

Organizations can also be viewed as **playing fields** or stages upon which individuals perform their "art." For health services organizations, this frequently involves a complex performance by many different talented individuals. These professionals—physicians, nurses, therapists, technologists, researchers, executives, and many others—have a highly developed sense of professionalism and professional identity. As such, they frequently clash as one culture emphasizes its beliefs and values relative to others in competing for resources. The result is often "tribal warfare," which must be managed (Argyris, 1982). The challenge is to create a larger overall sense of organizational identity and culture that can embrace the individual cultures of the different health professionals. When this is done, the goals articulated by the human relations school are met, and people are able to work effectively in performing interdependent tasks.

Psychic Prisons

Organizations can also be viewed as places where people are trapped by their own perceptions, ideas, and beliefs whether consciously or unconsciously. Often this is reflected in the tendency to avoid conflict, to avoid anxiety-provoking situations, or to strive to maintain one's sense of identity and self-esteem. These issues can be particularly important in health services organizations because, as noted above, individuals identify strongly with their professional disciplines. When these needs are concretized in a way that allows no room for other perspectives or viewpoints, the result is indeed a **psychic prison** stifling organizational learning, innovation, and the ability to adapt. It is the negative side of the human relations school's emphasis on personal growth and development.

Biological Organisms

In recent years it has become popular to think of organizations as **biological organisms;** that is, as different species that must adapt to their environments in the process of birth, growth, decline, and eventual death. It is concerned with the issue of how the organization becomes fit to survive in its environment. As shown in Table 1.5, contingency theory, strategic management perspective, population ecology theory, and institutional theory each contain major aspects of the biological organism metaphor. Contingency theory primarily emphasizes internal organization design and fit, while the strategic management perspective emphasizes the fit of the organization's strategy with its environment. The population ecology approach emphasizes the strength of the external forces that essentially select out various organizational

species for survival. Institutional theory suggests that one way in which organizations can succeed is to mimic or match the values and norms contained in the environment in order to maintain necessary legitimacy and credibility with environmental sources of sanctions and power. The biological organism metaphor highlighting the interplay of the organization with the environment over time can provide many useful insights for health services managers. Organizations of different sizes and at different stages in their existence require different resources and different strategies to ensure success.

Political Systems

Organizations, of course, can also be viewed as **political systems** in which various groups and actors vie for control of important resources. Organizations are ruled by whomever controls these resources and decides how they are used to accomplish the interests of various groups. Given the many different kinds of professionals working in or affiliated with health services organizations, the political system metaphor is particularly salient. Physicians, executives, nurses, researchers, and others often vie for control over important resources to push their own view of what is good for the organization. The political system metaphor is closely aligned with the playing field metaphor in which the organization essentially serves as the playing field or battleground for control. When things get out of control, health services organizations can turn into psychic prisons or tyrants. The resource dependence theory is consistent with the political system metaphor as it focuses on the ways in which organizations acquire and control needed resources.

Holograms

A **hologram** is an object in which each of the parts contains the entire essence of the overall object or image. As a result, the overall object or system can continue to function even when specific parts malfunction or are removed. While this metaphor is often used in conjunction with the brain metaphor and can be considered an important aspect of the brain metaphor, we believe that treating it separately provides some special insights. In a holographic structure the intent is to design the whole into the parts and to create a redundancy of parts so that a range of functions can be performed rather than just a single specialized activity. Designing health services organizations as holograms emphasizes the need for flexibility, creativity, change, and innovation. An organization's culture, its design, and its information-processing capabilities are facilitators of holographic properties. The metaphor is also consistent with the strategic management perspective's emphasis on viewing the organization as a whole in positioning its various elements to deal with outside forces while at the same time recognizing the interplay between those forces and internal organizational components. The idea is to see the organization's strategy as being expressed in the task and function of an individual worker as well as in the accumulation of worker activities across multiple tasks; that is, the "part-whole relationship." Viewing health services organizations as holograms can provide powerful insights contributing to the need for integrating multiple components of health services delivery into a more coherent whole. A micro example is provided by the cross-training of workers such that more functions and activities are contained in a single individual. A macro example is provided by the efforts of some health services organizations to develop regionally based vertically integrated delivery systems to provide more coordinated care across the range of patient needs.

These metaphors are intended to challenge the reader's thinking about health services organizations and to provide a lens for interpreting the chapters that follow. While they are presented in a sequential and categorical fashion, it is important to note that they represent a continuum of perspectives that may overlap each other. Having learned about them, revisit the issues posed in Debate Time 1.1. Have your views of these issues changed?

ORGANIZATION THEORY AND BEHAVIOR: A FRAMEWORK FOR THE TEXT

As discussed in the various perspectives and metaphors above, the essence of management is to motivate people and groups to carry out technical tasks for the attainment of organizational goals and at the same time to renew the organization for long-run survival and growth as it charts the future. These dimensions of the managerial challenge are outlined in Figure 1.3, which provides a basic framework for the book.

The book is divided into five parts. The first is an introductory part that provides an overview of perspectives on the management of health services organizations (Chapter 1) and an analysis of the evolving role of management in these organizations (Chapter 2). This is followed by four parts corresponding to the managerial activities of motivating and leading people and groups, operating the technical system, renewing the organization, and charting the future.

Managers must motivate and lead people to ensure high levels of commitment, stability, and cooperative behavior. This is accomplished by satisfying individual needs and values (Chapter 3), by providing direction (Chapter 4), and by managing conflict and negotiation processes (Chapter 5).

Managers must also operate the technical system in response to challenges of technical performance involving productivity, efficiency, quality, and customer satisfaction. This is accomplished by determining the appropriate work groups and work design (Chapters 6 and 7), establishing communication and coordination mechanisms (Chapter 8), and using appropriate influence processes (Chapter 9).

Organizations operate within a constantly changing environment, and managers must renew the organization by determining effective organizational design (Chapter 10), acquiring resources and managing interorganizational relationships (Chapter 11), managing change, innovation, and learning (Chapter 12), and attaining organizational goals (Chapter 13).

Finally, organizations function through time, and managers must be responsive to the challenges of long-term survival and growth of the organization. This is accomplished by managing strategically (Chapter 14) and anticipating the future (Chapter 15). The framework presented in Figure 1.3 is intended as a departure point, not a point of closure, for the reader's own synthesis of the material that follows.

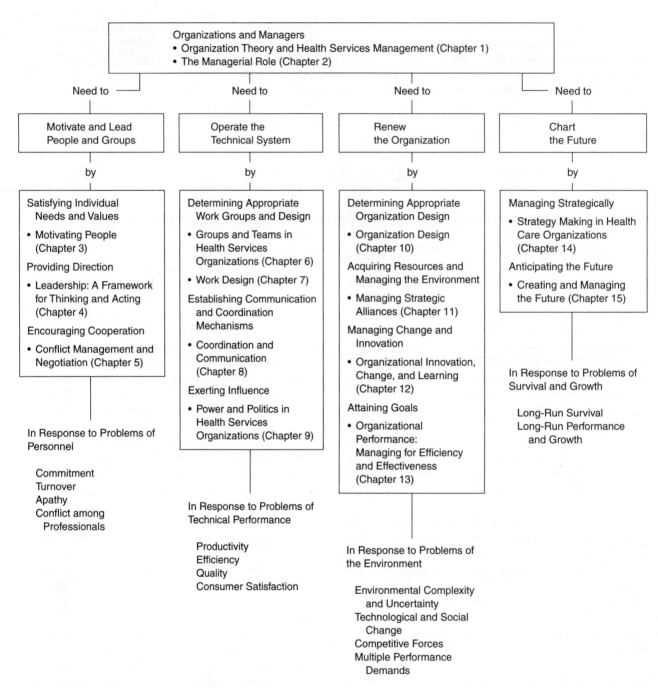

Figure 1.3. The Nature of Organizations: Framework for the Text.

Discussion Questions

1. As you think about the challenges facing Sutter Health in the opening scenario, which of the major perspectives on organizations (bureaucratic, scientific management, human relations, contingency, resource dependence, strategic management, population ecology, and institutional) would offer you the most assistance? Defend your choice.

2. During the past decade, hundreds of hospitals have closed, merged, or entered into various strategic alliances. How would you attempt to explain this reorganization? In addressing this question, refer to Debate Time 1.1 and consider the resource dependence, strategic management, population ecology, and institutional perspectives on organizations.

3. Several community health centers have hired you as a consultant to help them form an umbrella organization that in turn would be merged with the local county health department. Which of the metaphors of organizations (machine, tyrant, brain, playing field, psychic prison, biological organism, political system, hologram) would provide you with the greatest insight as you take on this assignment? Defend your choice.

4. State whether you agree or disagree with the following statement: For the most part, health services organizations are no different from most other organizations. Indicate the specific reasons for your agreement or disagreement and develop at least two reasons in addition to those presented in the chapter.

5. Networks and alliances are marriages of money and convenience. Systems are marriages of commitment and values. Develop arguments and counterarguments for each statement.

References

Aldrich, H. (1979). *Organizations and environments.* Englewood Cliffs, NJ: Princeton Hills.

Alexander, J. A., & Amburgey, T. L. (1987). The dynamics of change in the American hospital industry: Transformation or selection? *Medical Care Review, 44,* 279–321.

Alexander, J. A., & D'Aunno, T. A. (1990). Transformation of institutional environments: Perspectives on the corporatization of U. S. health care. In S. S. Mick and Associates, *Innovations in health care delivery: Insights for organizational theory* (pp. 53–85). Ann Arbor, MI: Health Administration Press.

Alexander, J. A., Kaluzny, A. D., & Middleton, S. C. (1986). Organizational growth, survival and death in the U. S. hospital industry: A population ecology perspective. *Social Science and Medicine, 22,* 303–308.

Andrews, K. R. (1971). *The concept of corporate strategy.* Homewood, IL: Dow Jones-Irwin.

Ansoff, H. I. (1965). *Corporate strategy: An analytic approach to business policy for growth and expansion.* New York: McGraw-Hill.

Argyris, C. (1964). *Integrating the individual and the organization.* New York: John Wiley & Sons.

Argyris, C. (1982). *Reasoning, learning, and action.* San Francisco: Jossey-Bass.

Barnard, C. I. (1938). *The functions of the executive.* Cambridge, MA: Harvard University Press.

Bazzoli, G. J., Shortell, S. M., Dubbs, N., Chan, C., & Kralovec, P. (1999, February). A taxonomy of health networks and systems: Bringing order out of chaos. *Health Services Research, 34.*

Bazzoli, G. J., Stein, R., Alexander, J. A., Conrad, D. A., Sofaer, S., & Shortell, S. M. (1997). Public-private collaboration in health and human service delivery: Evidence from community partnerships. *The Milbank Quarterly, 75*(4), 533–561.

Bogue, R., & Hall, C. H. (Eds.). (1995). *Health network innovation their systems through collaboration.* American Hospital Publishing.

Burns, T., & Stalker, G. M. (1961). *The management of innovation.* London: Tavistock.

Carroll, G. R. (1984). Organizational ecology. *Annual Review of Sociology, 10,* 71–93.

Christianson, J. B., Taylor, R. A., & Knutson, D. J. (1998). Restructing chronic illness management: Best practices and innnovations in team-based treatment. San Francisco, CA: Jossey-Bass.

Conrad, D. A., & Shortell, S. M. (1993, Fall). Integrated health systems: Promise and performance. *Frontiers of Health Services Management,* 13(1), 3–42.

Delacroix, J., & Carroll, G. R. (1983). Organizational foundings: An ecological study of newspaper industries of Argentina and Ireland. *Administrative Sciences Quarterly, 28,* 274–291.

DiMaggio, P. J., & Powell, W. W. (1983). The iron cage revisited: Institutional isomorphism and collective rationality in organizational fields. *American Sociological Review, 48,* 147–160.

Fennell, M., & Alexander, J. A. (1987). Organizational boundary spanning and institutionalized environments. *Academy of Management Journal, 30,* 456–476.

Fligstein, N. (1990). *The transformation of corporate control.* Cambridge, MA: Harvard University Press.

Gouldner, A. (1954). *Patterns of industrial bureaucracy.* New York: Free Press.

Gulick, L., & Urwick, L. (1937). *Papers on science of administration.* New York: Columbia University Press.

Halverson, P. K., Kaluzny, A. D., McLaughlin, C. P., & Mays, G. P. (1998). *Managed care and public health.* Gaithersburg, MD: Aspen Publishers, Inc.

Hannan, M. T., & Freeman, J. H. (1985, April). Structural inertia and organizational change. *American Sociological Review,* 149–164.

Hannan, M. T., & Freeman, J. H. (1989). *Organizational ecology.* Cambridge, MA: Harvard University Press.

Herzlinger, R. (1997). *Market driven health care.* Reading, MA: Addison-Wesley.

Hickson, D. J., Hinings, C. R., Lee, C. A., Schneck, R. E., & Pennings, J. M. (1971). A strategic contingencies theory of intraorganizational power. *Administrative Science Quarterly, 16,* 216–229.

Katz, E., & Kahn, R. (1978). *The social psychology of organizations* (2nd ed.). New York: John Wiley & Sons.

Kimberly, J. R., & Zajac, E. J. (1985). Strategic adaptation in health care oprganizations: Implications for theory and research. *Medical Care Review, 42,* 267–302.

Lawrence, P., & Lorsch, J. (1967). *Organization and environment.* Cambridge, MA: Harvard University Press.

Likert, E. (1967). *The human organization.* New York: McGraw-Hill.

March, J. G., & Olsen, J. P. (1976). *Ambiguity and choice in organizations.* Bergen, Norway: Univeristetsforlaget.

McGregor, D. (1960). *The human side of enterprise.* New York: McGraw-Hill.

Merton, R. K. (1957). Bureaucratic structure and personality. In *Social theory and social structure.* New York: Free Press.

Meyer, J. W., & Scott, W. R. (1983). *Organizational environments: Ritual and rationality.* Beverly Hills, CA: Sage.

Miles, R. E., & Snow, C. C. (1978). *Organizational strategy, structure, and process.* New York: McGraw-Hill.

Mohr, L. B. (1982). *Explaining organizational behavior.* San Francisco: Jossey-Bass.

Mooney, J. E. (1947). *Principles of organization.* New York: Harper & Row.

Morgan, G. (1986). *Images of organization.* Beverly Hills, CA: Sage Library of Social Research.

Ouchi, W. G. (1980). Markets, bureaucracies, and clans. *Administrative Science Quarterly, 24,* 129–141.

Perrow, C. (1967). A framework for the comparative analysis of organizations. *American Sociological Review, 32,* 194–208.

Pestonick, S. L., Classen, D. C., Evans, R. S., & Burke, J. P. (1996). Implementing antibiotic practice guidelines through computer-assisted decision support: Clinical and financial outcomes. *Annals of Internal Medicine, 124,* 884–890.

Pew Commission on Education for the Health Professions, Health Care Administration. (1993). Philadelphia: Pew Charitable Trusts.

Pfeffer, J., & Salancik, G. R. (1978). *The external control of organizations.* New York: Harper & Row.

Porter, M. E. (1980). *Competitive strategy: Techniques for analyzing industries and competitors.* New York: Free Press.

Porter, M. E. (1985). *Competitive advantage: Creating and sustaining superior performance.* New York: Free Press.

Powell, W. W., & DiMaggio, P. J. (Eds.). (1991). *The new institutionalism in organizational analysis.* Chicago: University of Chicago Press.

Robinson, J. (1997, March). Physician-hospital integration and the economic theory of the firm. *Medical Care Research and Review, 54*(1), 3–24.

Roethlisberger, F. J., & Dickson, W. J. (1939). *Management and the worker.* Cambridge, MA: Harvard University Press.

Rundall, T., Starkweather, D., & Norrish, B. (1998). *After restructuring: Empowerment strategies at work in America's hospitals.* San Francisco: Jossey-Bass, Inc.

Sacramento Business: Sutter UCDMC ink management. (1997, December 25). *Sacramento Bee.*

Schendel, D. E., & Hofer, C. W. (1979). *Strategic management: A new view of business policy and planning.* Boston: Little, Brown.

Schoonhoven, C. B. (1981, September). Problems with contingency theory: Testing assumptions hidden within the language of contingency "theory." *Administrative Science Quarterly, 26,* 349–377.

Scott, W. R. (1981). Developments in organization theory, 1960–1980. *American Behavioral Scientist, 24,* 407–422.

Scott, W. R. (1987). The adolescence of institutional theory: Problems and potential for organizational analysis. *Administrative Science Quarterly, 32,* 493–512.

Selznick, P. (1966). *TVA and the grass roots.* New York: Harper & Row.

Shortell, S. M., Gillies, R. R., Anderson, D. A., Mitchell, J. B., & Morgan, K. L. (1993, Winter). Creating organized delivery systems: The barriers and facilitators. *Hospital and Health Services Administration, 38*(4), 447–466.

Shortell, S. M., Gillies, R. R., Anderson, D. A., Morgan-Erickson, K., & Mitchell, J. B. (1996). *Remaking health care in America: Building organized delivery systems.* San Francisco: Jossey-Bass Publishers.

Shortell, S. M., & Zajac, E. J. (1990). Health care organizations and the development of the strategic management perspective. In S. S. Mick and Associates, *Innovations in health care delivery: Insights for organization theory* (pp. 144–180). Ann Arbor, MI: Health Administration Press.

Starkweather, D., & Cook, K. S. (1988). Organization-environment relations. In S. M. Shortell & A. D. Kaluzny (Eds.), *Health care management: A text in organization theory and behavior* (2nd ed.) (p. 352).

State agency rules against hospitals' governing policies. (1996, July 30). *Sacramento Bee.*

Strasser, S. (1983, Winter). The effective application of contingency theory in health settings: Problems and recommended solutions. *Health Care Management Review,* 15–23.

Sutter, Blue Cross ink new contract: Hospital given higher payments (1998, June 6). *Sacramento Bee.*

Sutter Health, *Annual Report.* (1980). Sacramento, CA.

Sutter Health, PacifiCare sign systemwide alliance. (1997, October 17). *Sacramento Bee.*

Sutter Health to drop Blue Cross patients: Contract talks stall over money (1998, May 15). *Sacramento Bee.*

Sutter Health's HMO woes mirror national trend. (1998, May 3). *Sacramento Bee.*

Taylor, F. (1947). *Scientific management.* New York: Harper & Row.

Thompson, J. D. (1967). *Organization in action.* New York: McGraw-Hill.

Weber, M. (1964). *The theory of social and economic organization.* Glencoe, IL: Free Press.

Weick, K. E. (1969). *The social psychology of organizations.* Reading, MA: Addison-Wesley Publishing Co.

Westphal, J. D., Gulati, R., & Shortell, S. M. (1997). Customization or conformity? An institutional and network perspective on the content and consequences of TQM adoption. *Administrative Science Quarterly, 42,* 366–394.

Williamson, O. E. (1981). The economies of organization: The transaction cost approach. *The American Journal of Sociology, 87,* 548–577.

Woodward, J. (1970). *Technology and organizational behavior.* Oxford, England: Oxford University Press.

CHAPTER

2

The Managerial Role

Howard S. Zuckerman, Ph.D.
William L. Dowling, Ph.D.
Mary L. Richardson, Ph.D.

Chapter Outline

- The Role of the Manager
- Implications of New Managerial Roles

Learning Objectives

After completing this chapter, the reader should be able to:

1. Understand the managerial role and how it is derived from alternative perspectives of organizational effectiveness.

2. Recognize the managerial challenges posed by changes in the external environment and within health care organizations.

3. Understand the changing roles of managers in providing vision and leadership, in adapting the organization to its environment, and in designing the organization to enact its mission and to achieve its objectives.

4. Be aware of changing skills and knowledge required by managers in light of environmental and organizational dynamics.

Key Terms

Accountability
Adaptation
Boundary Spanning
Empowerment
External Environment
Innovation
Integration
Internal Environment
Interorganization Relations
Leadership
Learning Organization
Mission and Values
Organization Design
Organization Structure
Organizational Effectiveness
Performance
Power
Shared Vision
Strategy
Transformational Leadership

Chapter Purpose

The reflections from the interviews set the stage for a discussion of the managerial role. They nicely capture the breadth, depth, and complexity of the role, reflecting the manager's responsibilities within the organization and in relating the organization to its environment. The reflections also recognize that the managerial role continues to evolve, as organizations and their environments change. It is acknowledged that the requisite managerial skills and knowledge must also evolve, but there remains a set of core competencies that endure. The purpose of this chapter is to understand the managerial role within health services, identify the contributing factors that influence that role and examine their implications, and specify the skills and knowledge required to meet the challenges of changing environments and organizations.

THE ROLE OF THE MANAGER

The environmental and organizational challenges discussed in Chapter 1 present new opportunities, conflicts, and challenges for managers of health care organizations. The managers of the future, as noted in the following sections, will face a bewildering array of demands and pressures to adapt in a rapidly changing, turbulent, often hostile, external world. At the same time, they will be expected to maintain internally those structures and processes designed to ensure achievement of the organization's purposes and maintain its underlying values.

The basic function of management is to direct the efforts of an organization toward achievement of the organization's goals and maintenance of the organization's viability. What exactly do managers do in carrying out this function? What roles do they play? We will examine alternative conceptions of the management role in relation to the concept of organizational effectiveness. This is the most meaningful starting point, we believe, because most management takes place in organizations, and because the job of managers is ultimately to further the effectiveness and survival of the organizations in which they work. Management, in short, is inextricably linked with organizations.

The goals of organizations vary widely. The ultimate goal of business firms is typically to make a profit. Academic institutions exist to discover and disseminate knowledge. Other organizations exist to further artistic expression. And still others, especially in the health field, exist to meet human needs. To accomplish these goals, organizations must plan and carry out their work, acquire resources, develop and motivate their workers, and adapt to the changing demands of their external environments. Management directs these many and varied activities toward the end of accomplishing the organization's goals.

Over the years, management thinking about the meaning of organizational effectiveness and about how organizations should be managed to enhance effectiveness has evolved. Management scholars and practitioners have offered a variety of definitions of the management role. Some define this role as setting goals for the organization and planning, organizing, directing, and controlling its work. Others see management's job as developing, motivating, and empowering the organization's people to themselves set and achieve goals that contribute to the organization success. Still others have emphasized the "boundary-spanning" role of manage-

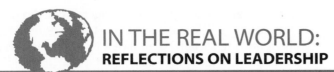

IN THE REAL WORLD:
REFLECTIONS ON LEADERSHIP

**STEPHANIE S. McCUTCHEON, System VP, SSM Health Care
President and CEO, St. Louis Health Care Network**

At SSM Health Care System, we believe that we achieve superior, measurable clinical and business results with the Continuous Quality Improvement (CQI) paradigm. This encourages and allows people to have input in decisions. I have always had tremendous faith and belief in people. There is substantial synergy in individual and collective contributions to well-defined objectives. The role of the leader is to coordinate and synergize action toward a directed outcome.

My leadership style has evolved in a number of ways over the years by becoming more focused on a vision, more committed to communicating it clearly, and working with teams to deliver it day-to-day. We are now more deliberate and purposeful about team alignment, particularly with regard to physician leadership.

I understand, more than ever, the real advantages of a highly motivated group. We are in a tremendous evolution in our field, our reorganization, our system, and our regional organization. People must be motivated and directed, and deliver clear outcomes in turbulent times.

PATRICK G. HAYS, President and CEO, Blue Cross Blue Shield Association, Chicago

They say that age brings seasoning. I am much more trusting of people's good intentions and desire to do a good job now than I was earlier in my career. I know now that most of us show up in the morning wanting to do the best we can. My job in large part is to remove some of the barriers that get in people's way.

During my tenure at Sutter Health, for example, we grew from annual revenues of $69 million to over $1 billion. Clearly I could not have had the same hands-on management style at the end of that 15-year period of growth that I had in 1980. I had to trust my colleagues in management and give them a pretty long leash.

The Blue Cross Blue Shield Association is composed of people of immense talent. In fact, were their lights not hidden under the Blues basket, they would probably be acknowledged as national experts in their own right. Here the challenge has been to bring a management philosophy to the job, as well as a sense of discipline, through objectives that can be measured and for which people are held accountable—and at the same time acknowledge that they know a lot more about their area of expertise than I ever will.

In the earlier part of my career I felt that I had to be the center of all answers. Now it is more a matter of shaping the philosophy and the dialogue, setting the basic strategic directions, and then getting out of the professionals' way.

GAIL L. WARDEN, CEO, Henry Ford Health System, Detroit

Here's what I have learned in 28 years as a health care CEO: 1) The customer is always the boss. 2) Quality and cost go together, and you've got to get it right the first time. 3) The biggest challenge is not in strategy but in execution. 4) Never under-estimate your competition. 5) Most solutions are internal, not external. 6) The hierarchical organization charts of the past are obsolete.

I was appointed to an important job when I was quite young. I was 28 when I was first head of a hospital—Presbyterian-St. Luke's in Chicago—and I was managing people who were in their 50s. Over time, I have become more of a coach and less directive, more flexible about what I expect, more comfortable with ambiguity. On the other hand, though I've always been a consensus kind of manager, today's environment requires more decisiveness.

I've recognized a great need to continue to learn. I have concentrated more on learning for myself in the last 10 years than I did the first 18 years as a CEO, learning about total quality management process improvement, measurement, organizational self-assessment, those kinds of things. The organization has become more complex. You now need skills that you might have been able to manage without in the past.

I have become a better listener. As I become more experienced and comfortable, I become less averse to risk, more open to what I am thinking and feeling. . . . It helps to be willing to admit when you make mistakes. . . . You've got to be a person of your word. If you say that you will do something you either have to do it or you have to have a good reason why you didn't.

THOMAS W. CHAPMAN, Senior Associate VP for Network Development, George Washington University Medical Center, Washington, D.C.

I am more inwardly reflective of challenges than I used to be, and of how they relate to the environment I work in and to the people, both the professionals in the organization and in particular the people that we serve.

I now try harder to integrate the business objectives with the outcome objectives. Often the business objectives are not in tune with the clinical and human objectives. Sometimes they can even be in conflict. For example, providers are now taking some risk and responsibility over the longer term for patient care outcomes and for the benefits people expect. That sure wasn't true when we were in a transactional cash-and-carry mode before we moved into managed care.

[Now] I'm more deliberate, more comprehensive in analysis. The questions and the answers are more multi-dimensional. It's no longer a question of, is this good for the organization, or for the community, or for the customer? The solution has to be good for everybody, on multiple levels. Those kinds of solutions require a lot more thought.

I first became CEO early in my career at Provident Hospital in Baltimore. That was in 1978. The field has obviously changed since then. My style of leadership is now more focused on the relationship of the not-for-profit organization to its community. I understand that neither the leader nor the organization can be everything to everybody. We've got to be more focused, and the leadership has to have a sharper, more concentrated spotlight.

JAMES REINERTSEN, M.D., PRESIDENT and CEO, Caregroup, Boston

After 11 years as a chief executive and of seeing the unexpected results of things that I was really cocksure about

years ago, I realize that things are a lot more complex than I had ever imagined them to be. When I now come to the point of making a decision, I am much less sure of the situation—because I now know a lot more about how complex the world really is.

At first I was under the impression that people looked to me to make decisions. Now I rarely come to a meeting thinking that it's my job to decide anything. It's far more important for me to elicit the best decisions from the group, to see that a decision is made. Now I realize that I don't always know the best course.

Furthermore, the decision is not even necessarily the most important issue. The most important issue is the implementation. For instance, nine years ago I was absolutely certain how to approach improving customer service, and I rolled out a program to do it. Now I must admit that the program had nowhere near the effect that we needed. The reason is that I profoundly underestimated the extent of the change in mind-set, process, and systems that would be required to really achieve this. This flaw was typical of my earlier approach: Underestimating the magnitude of the effort that is involved with any big change or decision.

It's not trivial to make the right decision about what to do—what's important strategically, what's important from a customer perspective, what's important financially for the organization to survive. But I find that I and the organization in general have much less trouble making good decisions and much more trouble implementing them. We need to expend much more energy in understanding how to effect the decision, rather than in worrying about whether it is the most perfect decision.

In my original model, people looked to the leader to do the right thing, to be all-knowing and all-wise. Over my 11 years it has been apparent that this isn't always the case. I have had to learn to admit that I screwed up. A leader must acquire not an air of invincibility, but a very honest vulnerability in front of all the troops. That's hard for a lot of people who are in leadership positions.

Excerpted from Future Focus Forum (Profiles in Leadership) Hospital Research and Educational Trust and J. L. Kellogg Graduate School of Management, Northwestern University, Evanston, IL, May 1997. Reprinted with permission of the Health Research and Educational Trust, copyright May 1997.

ment—keeping up with changes in the external environment, interpreting the implications of these changes for the organization, and adapting the organization to them. How do we reconcile these different views of management? Or are all these roles generic to management?

In answering these questions, we draw on an insightful and useful model or conceptualization of organizations and management—the "competing values framework"—developed by Quinn, Faerman, Thompson, and McGrath (1996). This model brings together and integrates the many perspectives that have influenced management thinking over the years. The model is applicable to different types of organizations and different levels within organizations.

The degree of emphasis on the various dimensions of the managerial role varies, however, as a function of such factors as the stage of an organization's development, its size and resources, and the nature of the environment in which it operates. For purposes of illustration, many of our examples focus on the roles of senior level managers, but are presumed to be generally applicable at other levels as well. We also concur with Mintzberg that the managerial role need not be conceived as being housed within the person of a single individual; rather, the role represents a gestalt involving a number of people whose activities must be integrated in order to result in the full explication of the managerial role (Mintzberg, 1973).

Over the years, academic and practitioner views about how organizations work and how they should be managed have evolved in response to changing economic, social, and political forces; advances in technology; a deepening understanding of human motivation; and shifts in societal values. New perspectives, as they arose, spawned different notions of the roles of management and new principles to guide management practice. Each new perspective, however, only partially replaced earlier perspectives. As a result, we inherit a variety of sometimes contradictory views about management, each of which offers helpful insights, but no one of which is universal in its applicability. The competing values framework provides insight into the nature and relationships among these different views of management.

The starting point of the competing values framework is **organizational effectiveness.** Four different

(i.e., "competing") perspectives of organizational effectiveness are defined in relation to two axes (Figure 2.1).

The vertical axis represents the importance of organizational control (at the bottom) or flexibility (at the top) in achieving effectiveness. Some organizations put great emphasis on (i.e., "value") tight control of everything that goes on in the organization. These organizations exert control by such means as centralized decision making, clear directions, explicit policies and procedures, close supervision, and detailed documentation of work processes and output. Other organizations stress adaptability, change, and innovation; they encourage decentralized decision making and allow for differentiation in work styles and structures in different parts of the organization. The control/flexibility axis suggests an organization's preferences regarding structure. Organizations emphasizing control tend to structure themselves to promote consistency and stability; organizations emphasizing flexibility tend to structure themselves in ways that promote **adaptation** and **innovation.**

The horizontal axis represents the importance of an internal (at the left) or external (at the right) focus of attention in achieving organizational effectiveness. Some organizations tend to look inward, stressing the maintenance or improvement of their own **internal environment** and work processes. Others concentrate on the **external environment** devoting considerable effort to monitoring external forces and to searching for clues about the future. They employ market research to understand consumer needs and demands and pay close attention to the external "stakeholders" on whom the organization depends for clients, resources, or support. Further, they look for ways the organization can adapt to be more responsive to the external signals they identify. Such organizations are often described as "market-driven" or "entrepreneurial," seeking to exploit environmental opportunities through change and innovation.

The major models or schools of thought about organizations and management that have evolved since the turn of the century were briefly described in Chapter 1. Each of these models, reflecting a particular view of organizational effectiveness, fits into one of the quadrants of the competing values framework,

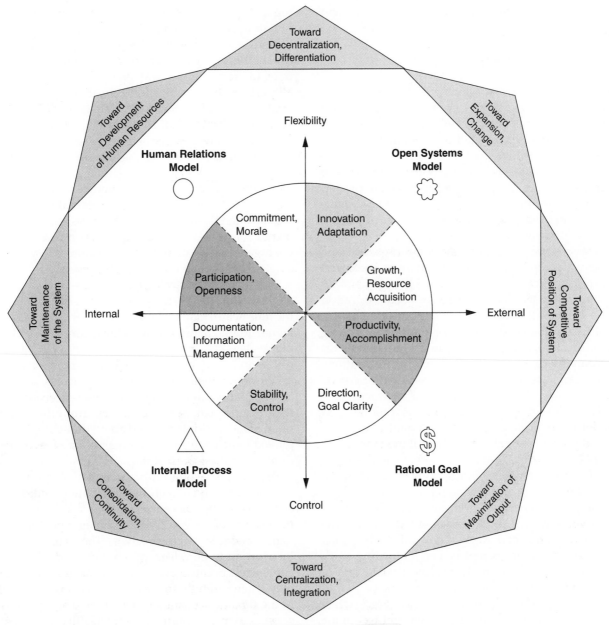

Figure 2.1. Eight General Orientations in the Competing Values Framework. The eight general values that operate in the competing values framework are shown in the triangles on the perimeter. Each value both complements the values next to it and contrasts with the one directly opposite it. Some of these values are shared among roles; these are shown in color.

SOURCE: R. E. Quinn. *Beyond Rational Management.* San Francisco: Jossey-Bass Inc., 1988, p. 48. Used with permission.

with each highlighting a particular view of the management role.

The Rational Goal Model

Scientific management, which emerged in the early 1900s with the work of F. W. Taylor (1911), Henry Gantt (1916), and Frank Gilbreth (1911), fits the control/external focus quadrant. Quinn et al. (1996) label this perspective the "rational goal model," because it advocates the application of rational economic principles in the design and direction of work and in rewarding workers. The goal is to maximize output and productivity to take advantage of external market opportunities.

The rational goal model measures organizational effectiveness by profits and productivity. Profits depend on taking advantage of market opportunities. Management decisions are based on economic rationality: Which alternative will contribute the most to profits? Productivity depends on thorough planning, clear direction, and a work-focused environment. Organizations that evidence the value of the rational goal model are often referred to as "goal-oriented," "all business," "driven," "analyzers," or "focused."

The roles of management in the rational goal model are to set clear goals for the organization, to rationally analyze what actions contribute most to the goals, to plan and organize the work, to define expectations and job responsibilities, to give instructions, to prescribe policies and rules, and to initiate problem solving when necessary. Managers are "in charge," decisive, directive, and task-oriented. They drive themselves and their workers toward the organization's goals. Emphasis is placed on motivating workers to increase productivity and meet goals, and on maintaining a work environment conducive to high productivity. "Management by objectives," which later became a widely used management technique, has its roots in the rational goal model. Quinn et al. (1996) label the management roles associated with this quadrant "director" and "producer" (Figure 2.2).

In health care today, the rational goal model's concept of organizational effectiveness is manifest in the emphasis on "strategic management." Strategic management defines top management's roles as articulating an organization's vision and strategic goals, formulating strategies (consistent with external opportunities and threats and the organization's internal capabilities) that further its vision, deciding on actions to execute these strategies, and seeing to it that all parts of the organization contribute to successful strategy execution. Strategic management, in short, seeks to orchestrate all of the organization's subsystems—its strategies, structures, resources, reward systems, information systems, etc.—in pursuit of the organization's vision. The strategic management view fits the rational goal model (externally focused/control-oriented) because external forces drive organizational strategy, and because top management's role is seen as directing (i.e., controlling) all of the organization's activities and resources toward the single aim of achieving its strategic goals.

Support for the strategic management view of organizational effectiveness is evident in the qualities of the nine health plans selected for the 1995 Sachs HMO Honor Roll (Champions of Satisfaction, 1996). These plans were chosen based on a survey of HMO enrollees in 27 markets nationwide. Respondents were asked about their satisfaction with access, convenience, quality, and the overall value received from their health plan. Senior managers from the highest rated plans were interviewed about the strategies employed to achieve such high marks. The findings indicate that the Honor Roll plans pursue the goal of customer satisfaction with a singularity of purpose. They clearly and forcefully articulate excellence in customer service as central to their vision. They see themselves as driven by this strategic goal and set high standards for themselves. They communicate their vision to enrollees, purchasers, and other constituencies. Because customer satisfaction is the key, they listen carefully to customers and invest heavily in the qualities consumers seek in a health plan. Because plan members equate good health care with satisfaction with their physician, the Honor Roll plans place great emphasis on building positive relationships with physicians, structuring physician compensation to reward customer satisfaction. In short, the winning HMOs demonstrate a singularity of purpose—customer satisfaction—in conducting market research, making quality improvement investments,

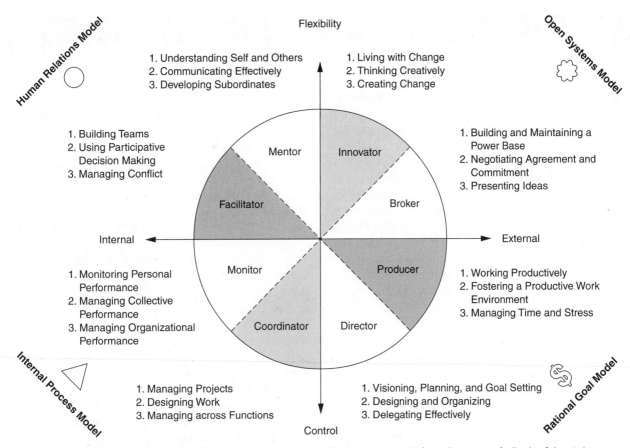

Figure 2.2. The Competencies and the Leadership Roles in the Competing Values Framework. *Each of the eight leadership roles in the competing values framework contains three competencies. They, like the values, both complement the ones next to them and contrast with those opposite to them.*
SOURCE: R. E. Quinn. *Beyond Rational Management.* San Francisco: Jossey-Bass Inc., 1988, p. 48. Used with permission.

designing physician arrangements, and in providing good service. All of the organization's actions are managed with the consumer in mind.

The Internal Process Model

Quinn et al. (1996) call the control/internal focus quadrant the "internal process model." In this model, an effective organization is seen as one that evidences continuity, stability, reliability, and predictability. The focus is internal—on the organization itself—and on control of the processes and resources the organization employs to accomplish its work.

The internal process model reflects the values and principles of "classical bureaucratic theory." Whereas scientific management focused on the jobs of individual workers, bureaucratic theory arose with the growth of larger and more complex factories and business firms. Henri Fayol and Max Weber, the founders of bureaucratic theory, focused on the organization as a whole. Fayol's (1949) principles advocated a clear division of labor, assignment of authority equal to responsibility, unity of command, and subordination of individual interests to the interests of the organization. Fayol saw management functions and skills as generic and learnable, not innate. It was Fayol who

DEBATE TIME 2.1: WHAT DO YOU THINK?

Although we like to think of the top managers of a health care organization as master strategists who envision and lead their organizations to a new and better future, in reality that view of the management role greatly overstates the case. This is because most of what health care organizations do or become is determined not by management but by fundamental external forces and trends. The aging of the population, advances in technology, or changing societal expectations are such fundamental and pervasive forces that health care organizations cannot realistically "envision" or "strategize" direction or roles that are inconsistent with them—at least not if they want to survive. The same can be said of other external forces, like tight-ening reimbursement, the growth of managed care, and the shift to outpatient settings. At most, organizations have a little "wiggle room" in how they adapt to these forces, but adapt they must. Hence, it is more accurate and realistic to take a more limited view of what managers really contribute than what the "experts" and the literature suggest. This more limited view is consistent with some theories that recognize that organizations are open to (i.e., not able to buffer themselves from) external forces and are subject to significant influence from outside, whether they like it or not. This is certainly the case with health care organizations, and so their future is largely determined by the changing environment, not by how they are managed.

first defined management as comprised of the functions of planning, organizing, directing, coordinating, and controlling. Weber (1964) developed a theory of bureaucratic management that addressed the need of complex organizations for efficiency and predictability. He advocated a clearly defined hierarchy governed by formal rules and procedures, clearly defined responsibilities, and clear lines of authority.

In the internal process model, efficiency and predictability are achieved through the application of hierarchical decision making, routinization of work, and the application of formal policies and procedures. Emphasis is placed on measuring, monitoring, and documenting work processes and output. Organizations that exhibit these values are often referred to a "bureaucratic," "top-down," "defenders," or "run by the book."

Quinn et al. (1996) label the management roles associated with the internal process view of organization effectiveness "coordinator" and "monitor." As a technical expert, the manager achieves coordination by defining responsibilities, spelling out the work flow, scheduling, maintaining formal communication and decision-making structures, and tending to logistical support. Managers monitor closely to see that people are following the rules and that performance standards are being met. Attention to detail, documentation, inspections, reviews, and reports are common.

Much of the attention of health care organizations today is directed outward as market demands become ever more intense. Survival depends increasingly on the organization's awareness of external forces and ability to respond. Wise organization leaders spend considerable time outside the organization and invest heavily in building the capacity of their organizations to monitor and interpret external events. But what is it exactly that external stakeholders are demanding? The answer may lie largely in the organization's ability to tightly manage a number of key internal processes. This is illustrated by the 1997 *Hospital and Health Systems* Leadership Survey (Solovy & Sunseri, 1997). This survey, conducted jointly by *Hospitals and Health Systems* and the Medical Group Management Association, queried a national sample of 5,000 senior hospital, managed care, and physician group executives (14% responded) about the issues most critical to the success of their organizations. One part of the survey asked executives to rate the importance of each of 30 issues to their organization's success and then to rate their organization's preparedness to address each issue. The difference between the importance and preparedness ratings represents a "strategic gap."

What are the most troublesome strategic issues? The hospital and managed care executives reported "controlling costs" to be the most challenging issue; physician group executives rated it third out of 30 in importance. "Information technology" had the second largest strategic gap for all three groups. "Measuring quality and outcomes" was the most troublesome issue among physician group executives, and one of the top five for hospitals and health plans. "Improving customer service" was also highly ranked by all three groups. Although the origin of these issues lies outside the organization, effective responses require close management of internal operations and processes. Cost-saving efficiencies, for example, are derived in large part from consistent, stable, reliable functioning of organizational subsystems. Interrelated activities must be closely coordinated and tight control exerted to ensure compliance with "standard operating procedures." Only limited flexibility is allowed, decisions about deviations are centralized, and work is documented and closely monitored.

Even quality improvement, as illusive as this goal has been, is succumbing to appropriateness criteria, treatment guidelines, care paths, and other forms of standardization. Control takes the form of ensuring compliance with protocols. Measurement of outcomes assumes center stage. In short, contemporary pressures on health care organizations to cut costs, improve quality, and increase customer satisfaction have made the coordination and control of operating systems essential to organizational effectiveness. Renewed emphasis is being placed on "running a tight ship"—the focus of the internal process model.

Looking ahead, managing "production functions" will continue to be a major focus for managers of health care organizations. Regardless of the eventual direction of health care reform and changes in the system of financing, managing costs and quality will be fundamental in a competitive environment, in a regulated price structure, or under capitated systems. Managers will further explore means to increase productivity, reduce excess capacity, and improve utilization of physical, financial, and human resources.

Central to the design of organizations will be information systems development and management. Such systems will be crucial for effective management of costs and quality, for analysis of organizational **performance,** and for assessment and monitoring of environmental conditions. It will become increasingly important to integrate clinical and financial information, and shift emphasis to health, consistent with the changing demands of organizational responsibility. Defining information needs and clarifying the role of information technology falls appropriately within the domain of managers (Marting, Dehays, Hoffer, & Perkins, 1991).

The Human Relations Model

The "human relations model" of organization effectiveness fits in the flexibility/internal focus quadrant. Here emphasis is on the organization's people and on the "informal" or "social" side of the organization. The effective organization is characterized by commitment, cohesion, and high morale on the part of its people. Great value is placed on the development of peoples' full potential through training, team building, **empowerment,** participation, and attention to collegial relations. Such organizations are called "people-oriented," "collegial," or "empowering."

Elton Mayo (1933) was one of the first to articulate the concept of the "social man," motivated by social needs, seeking satisfying relationships in the workplace, and influenced more by peer group pressure than by management control. Later, the humanistic psychologists, Chris Argyris (1994), Abraham Maslow (1970), and Douglas McGregor (1960) advanced the notion of "self-actualization" as an important motivating force.

The human relations school of thought gave rise to recognition of the importance of the manager's interpersonal and people-management skills. Understanding group dynamics was seen as the key to building teamwork. People were to be involved in decisions that affected them, with consensus building and conflict-resolution taking center stage. A deeper understanding of the many factors that motivate people led to a new emphasis on meeting the personal and relationship needs of workers. Cohesion, commitment, and morale could be achieved through developing and supporting people and through fostering a collegial work environment.

The manager's roles in the human relations model are "facilitator" and "mentor." Managers foster collective effort, involve employees in decision making, build teamwork, facilitate group problem solving, and manage conflict. Workers are involved and have influence over how things are done. Potentially divisive issues are confronted, and politics takes a back seat to openness. Managers earn the trust of the people with whom they work. In the mentor role, managers develop people through training, job enrichment, and job rotation. They watch over career development and help people reach their full potential. Managers are approachable, caring, empathetic, and supportive, readily conveying appreciation and giving credit. It is through empowered workers, committed to the organization and able to satisfy both their personal needs and the organization's goals through their work, that organizational effectiveness is built.

Health care organizations today are facing intense pressures to change, and change in fundamental ways. The future is unclear, demands are great, resources are insufficient, and critical stakeholders don't see eye to eye on what the organization should do. As a result, the right direction is seldom clear, and every direction poses substantial risks. "Transformational" leaders are needed who can shepherd major change that profoundly affects the organization's values and traditional ways of doing things.

Change is threatening, and people tend to resist. They may fear for their jobs or worry that their present skills will not be up to the new tasks they will be asked to take on. They may resist the breakup of valued relationships as they are moved to new parts of the organization. Repeated downsizings destroy their sense of security, and trust in management erodes. Yet the massive changes that must be made require committed, energized, high-morale people. Involvement and teamwork are essential. Turning resistance into support becomes the key to organizational effectiveness, even survival. And the management roles of facilitator and mentor of the organization's people become paramount.

Health care executives are coming to recognize that changing times demand renewed emphasis on the organization's human resources. This is shown by a national study, "Bridging the Leadership Gap in Healthcare," conducted by The Healthcare Forum Leadership Center (1991). The study found that the management values and competencies health care opinion leaders believed would be essential in the future differed dramatically from the then prevalent management practices. "Managing through the hierarchy" was the most prevalent approach to managing people. But critical to the future would be continuous quality improvement, team learning, a "we" approach, cross-functional structures, and a fostering of commitment to the organization's values, none of which were heavily practiced at the time. The Leadership Center concluded that empowerment would become imperative to organizational success. Critical management competencies call for allowing people to participate in decisions that affect them, encouraging self-direction, helping people find more dignity and meaning in their work, team building, and cross-functional versus hierarchical problem solving.

Commitment to quality is a hallmark of successful organizations. An organization reflects such commitment by taking good care of its customers with superior products and exceptional service, and by constantly innovating. This in turn requires committed people, developed by evidencing trust and respect for the creative potential of each person in the organization (Darling, 1992). Recognizing the centrality of quality not only internally but also in terms of the perceptions and expectations of key external stakeholders is leading health care organizations toward the principles of continuous quality improvement (CQI) and/or total quality management (TQM). These principles represent a paradigm shift from quality inspection and assurance to the continuous and relentless improvement of the processes by which care is provided, not merely the improvement of the performance of individuals (McLaughlin & Kaluzny, 1990). Quality is defined as meeting the needs of customers, which requires broadly based participation throughout the organization. Problems are characterized as typically systemic rather than individual, and changes to operating systems are based on data, use of multidisciplinary teams, and group processes. Health care organizations will come to reconceive the human resource function, seeing it as an investment, not a cost. In so doing, there will be a fuller recognition of the importance of enabling individuals to realize their potential.

The Open Systems Model

The "open systems" perspective of organizational effectiveness emerged in the mid-1960s as the external environment of organizations became more complex, demanding, and uncertain. Rapid change, global competition, exploding information technology, and other forces made it impossible for organizations to remain isolated from external events and be successful. "Systems thinking" was necessary to conceptualize the complex interrelationships among the parts of an organization and between the organization and its environment. Decisions needed to be made quickly, often without complete information, and became riskier. The concept of the manager as a rational decision maker controlling a machinelike organization no longer squared with reality. Adaptability and innovation became the keys to success as organizations sought to respond quickly to the changing demands of the marketplace. They struggled to obtain from external stakeholders the resources and support needed to

survive. Chapter 1 describes this "resource dependence" view of organizations. In the open systems model, organizational success requires being open and responsive to the demands of the marketplace. Competition is intense, yet organizations also collaborate or even merge when competition seems unlikely to lead to success. Internally, organization structures are differentiated to facilitate responsiveness to the many different stakeholders in the organization's environment.

Because of its external focus and emphasis on flexibility, the open systems model fits in the upper right quadrant of Quinn et al.'s (1996) framework. Organizational effectiveness is measured by the organization's ability to adapt and by its ability to acquire support from external stakeholders. These in turn enable the organization to compete and to grow. We call such organizations "adaptable," "entrepreneurial," "growth-oriented," "prospectors," "aggressively competitive" sometimes and "collaborative" at other times.

In the open systems view, the manager is an "innovator" and a "broker." As **boundary spanners,** managers facilitate adaptation and change. They closely monitor changes in the organization's environment, identify opportunities and threats, and envision how

DEBATE TIME 2.2: WHAT DO YOU THINK?

It sounds good to talk about empowering others, sharing power, and teaching people to lead themselves, in part because these ideas appeal to basic values that emphasize the inherent importance of each and every individual. But in the final analysis, the buck has to stop somewhere in organizations, and that's with top management. This is not to say that developing others in the organization and delegating or sharing decisions with them doesn't work. These can be extremely effective management tools in the right circumstances. But in reality, some subordinates just are not comfortable with more responsibility or don't have the skills to solve problems as well as the manager can. In addition, empowering multidisciplinary, cross-organizational teams to grapple with problems, rather than referring them up the management hier-

archy for solution, can be time consuming, creates confusion across departments, and obfuscates who is accountable for results. Perhaps most important, it must be remembered that in the real world, not all the actors in an organization share the organization's goals. Or even if they do, the natural inclination to try to further one's own interests through the organization may be more motivating. As a result, managers could delegate decision-making opportunities only to find the participants "running away with the store." Selective empowerment and carefully proscribed delegation can be effective tools. But organizations work best when top management retains final decision-making authority and everyone knows it, and when the most critical or difficult decisions are not left in the hands of others all over the organization.

the organization should respond. They are creative, intuitive, open to new ideas, visionary, willing to make decisions in the face of uncertainty, and willing to take risks. Above all, the managers of flexible/externally focused organizations need to be able to "manage change."

In the broker role, managers negotiate their organization's position and relationships with consumers, resource suppliers, public agencies, and other parties on whom the organization depends. As the organization's spokespersons, managers need political skills, persuasiveness, and an ability to acquire and use **power.** Strategies for "managing" or influencing the external environment include coalition formation, co-optation, lobbying, and flexibility in responding to external pressures. The manager as broker seeks to sustain the organization's legitimacy, to enhance the organization's image and reputation, and to assure the organization the resources it needs to compete and to grow.

In observing and assessing the environment, managers will expand their field of vision to put health care in a larger context. That is, while health care has many distinctive attributes, it is also true that there are similarities and commonalties with other industries. Other industries, which share structural, strategic, and service characteristics, have undergone transformations not unlike that being experienced by health care. Managers will draw from the lessons, both positive and negative, to be learned from the experience of such other industries. For example, it is instructive to observe the structural and strategic changes in industries such as airlines and banking as they sought to adapt to changing environmental conditions. Structural changes included new entrants, mergers, and consolidations, while strategic shifts involved greater emphasis on cost accounting and cost management, investment in information system development, and use of networking and strategic alliances. In addition, health care managers will employ a variety of techniques, such as game theory and scenario analysis, to assess the environment under differing conditions and seek to understand the organizational implications of alternative strategies.

Health care managers are employing a variety of strategies in response to changing environmental forces. Horizontal integration—linking organizations at the same stage of the production process (e.g., hospital-hospital)—to achieve economies of scale, improve utilization of resources, enhance access to capital, increase political power, and extend the scope of the market will continue. Vertical integration—linking organizations at related stages of the production process through either ownership or contractual arrangements—to ensure sources of supply and/or markets for services and products will expand. Vertical integration enables organizations to move toward providing multiple levels of care and a more comprehensive range of services. Yet a third alternative involves diversified activities that may or may not be related to health care. Diversification, which may focus on new products or services, new production technologies, and/or entry into new markets, seeks to generate new sources of revenue and provide opportunities for growth and expansion (Clement, 1998). Regardless of which strategies or combinations of strategies are selected, adaptation to a changing environment requires a shift away from a product orientation to a market orientation. Strategic managers seek to understand the characteristics, needs, and demands of the various populations that the organization serves. Market research plays a prominent role in answering such questions and provides the bases on which programs, services, and products are developed and marketed.

A key strategic opportunity and challenge for managers lies in the emergence of integrated systems for delivering and financing health care services (Conrad & Shortell, 1996; Shortell, Gillies, & Anderson et al., 1996). As suggested by industry observers, such systems are likely to be local or regional, be organized in relation to natural market areas, and serve a defined population. Emphasis will be placed on health care, and not only medical care. These systems will be integrated vertically as well as horizontally, and clinically as well as administratively. They will be "seamless," designed to enable convenient entry at multiple points. These systems will offer multiple levels of care across a connected continuum of services, enabling the movement of patients up and down the production process to the most appropriate placement both clinically and financially. Financing and delivery increasingly will be linked in order to align incentives for managing care. Governance and management structures, as well as resource allocation decision processes, will reflect the focus on the regional system. Physicians will be key, integral participants in such systems, sharing the risk and the power inherent in such organizations. Information systems will receive substantial attention, designed to reflect the emphasis on health, organized around episodes, and connect or integrate the component units of the organization. Operationally, integrated systems will emphasize continuous quality improvement, development of human resources across the system, and effective management of cost and utilization. There will thus be a unity, symmetry, and synergy in the strategy, structure, and operations of such systems. These integrated organizations will not merely be *structured* as systems, but rather will *function* as systems, thereby building the potential to achieve the benefits of "systemness" (Shortell, 1988). Importantly, such systems should be well-situated for the new and broader accountabilities to be faced by organizations, which will include public **accountability** for the health status of the population served.

The Situational Model and the Search for Balance

In recent years, another view—a "contingency" or "situational" view—of organizational effectiveness and management practice has emerged in response to a growing recognition that none of the historical models apply in all circumstances. The management principles espoused by each model seemed to work sometimes, but not always. There is a need for balance depending on the circumstances. Why, managers ask, does a particular process for employee participation in decision making work well in one situation, but not in another? Why does a highly formal, hierarchical structure work in some circumstances but not in others? The search for answers to questions like this began to show that different processes for participation, different structures, and different **leadership** styles tended to be effective in different situations. An organization's size, resources, and technology; its goals; the variety of products offered; and the complexity, pace of change, and uncertainty of its environment were each found to influence the effectiveness of different management practices.

Management scholars and practitioners began to recognize that there is no "one best way" to manage.

To return to the competing values framework, consistency and stability of work processes generally enhance effectiveness where an organization operates in a simple, stable environment, produces few products, and employs a routine technology. Effectiveness in such situations is most likely to be achieved through control/internally focused management practices. Management's roles are to coordinate and monitor. In contrast, where organizational effectiveness depends on an openness to new ideas, responding quickly to external change, producing multiple products, adapting products and technologies frequently, and competing for resources, flexible/externally oriented management is likely to work best. In this latter case, decision making needs to be more decentralized, the hierarchy flatter, and policies and procedures less formalized. Management's roles are to broker the organization, innovate, and manage change.

The basic logic of the competing values framework is that different management roles are associated with different views of organizational effectiveness. Over the years, new schools of thought have emerged to dominate management thinking, each emphasizing different criteria of effectiveness, different management roles, and different guidelines for management practice. The contingency view argues that the particular roles and practices most likely to be successful in furthering organizational effectiveness depend on the situation. This suggests that managers think in terms of a two-step process, first "sizing-up" the situation and then selecting the approaches most likely to fit that situation.

The Quinn et al. (1996) model offers even greater insight, however. The competing values framework proposes that the different views of effectiveness are not mutually exclusive. That is, they are not conflicting in the sense that one must be chosen over the others. Rather, the management of complex organizations today, more often than not, calls on managers to attend to all four dimensions of effectiveness, often simultaneously. The challenge is one of maintaining appropriate balance among the dimensions. Management needs to "run a tight ship" *and* adapt quickly to changing market demands. Developing an organization's people and gaining their commitment and energy are critical to success in most organizations today. But so are clear goals, explicit directions, and well-developed plans. This might be called a "both-and" versus "either-or" view of management's roles and practices.

> We want our organizations to be adaptable and flexible, but we also want them to be stable and controlled. We want growth, resource acquisition, and external support, but we also want tight information management and formal communication. We want an emphasis on the value of human resources, but we also want an emphasis on planning and goal setting. In any real organization all of these are, to some extent, necessary. (Quinn et al., 1996, p. 14)

The competing values framework proposes that managers, to be fully effective in leading their organizations, must play a range of seemingly conflicting roles. The "master manager" must be able to examine a situation, assess it from contrasting perspectives, and address it employing multiple roles. A particular management role may be the most important in a particular situation, but rarely in the complex situations managers face today will a unilateral view of the organization or a single management role suffice. Every organization, in short, needs to pay attention to goal accomplishment and productivity, people, internal processes, and innovation. What distinguishes organizations is the balance of their values at a particular point in time.

In designing health care organizations for the future, structures must be flexible and adaptive. Organizations face operating environments characterized by increasing turbulence and instability. Consequently, these organizations must develop flexible internal designs that permit them to react to uncertain environmental conditions. Demands from the external environment, coupled with needs of the organization internally, will require that there be a balance of **integration** and differentiation in the design. Health care organizations must strike a balance among facilitating achievement of overall goals, enhancing coordination, and taking advantage of organizational synergies and economies (integration) while encouraging innovation and creativity and enabling rapid response to environmental changes (differentiation). These issues are discussed further in later chapters.

Governance and Physician Involvement in Organizational Leadership

Illustrative of the multiplicities of the managerial role is the changing dynamics of relationships with governance and physicians. Within the organization, new roles, responsibilities, and relationships will emerge among managers, governance, and physicians. Those in governance are finding their roles to be more demanding and challenging (Pointer & Ewell, 1994). In the face of environmental turbulence and organizational complexity, trustees and directors find themselves dealing with conflicting pressures regarding social imperatives, public expectations, community need, cost control, quality improvement, financing, and technological development. As governance evolves, the requisite changes in roles, responsibilities, authorities, and relationships are not always clear. Effective boards will have to manage diverse stakeholders, involve physicians in the governance process, learn to govern emerging organizational forms such as integrated systems of care, and develop greater understanding of strategy formulation and implementation (Shortell, 1989). Boards must actively build assets, be willing to take risk, provide strategic direction for the organization, serve as mentors for management, and be prepared to be held accountable for the activities of the organization (Taylor, Chait, & Holland, 1996). These responsibilities will lead to revisiting such fundamental questions as board membership, structure, operating processes, and expectations (Alexander, Zuckerman, & Pointer, 1995; Pointer, Alexander, & Zuckerman, 1995; Umbdenstock, Hageman, & Amundson, 1990). In many ways, these expanding responsibilities and accountabilities parallel those of managers. Thus, it is anticipated that these two groups will jointly examine such questions as, Do we seek expertise or representation among governance members? How effective are our decision-making processes? Are we sufficiently focused on achieving desired outcomes?

A critical challenge for managers lies in the effective alignment of physician and organizational interests. This will require new models for physician-organization relationships, new thinking about such relationships, and greater involvement of physicians in governance and management of the enterprise (Zuckerman, Hilberman, & Anderson et al., 1998). The imperatives of managing costs, improving quality, enhancing productivity and resource utilization, and of the strategies designed to enable health care organizations to adapt to their environments cannot be achieved without physician involvement. Physicians must play a key role in formulating policy, decision making, allocating resources, and developing and implementing **strategy.** Certainly, the growth of managed care leads organizations and physicians to recognize that they must collaborate, sharing the risks and developing mechanisms to go into the marketplace together. The centrality of physician-organization alignment is being recognized as a factor in the continuing development of integrated systems. A recent national survey of health system executives indicates that 90% believe that physician alignment is critical to a system's success; nevertheless, over half of these executives also see physician alignment as "the most difficult part" of building an integrated system (Japsen, 1997). The destinies of physicians and organizations are inextricably intertwined and while relationships will assume various forms as they evolve, they must be nurtured and cultivated in order to deal with environmental and organizational imperatives.

There is already evidence of physicians playing larger roles in organizational governance and management. In the face of increased competition for patients and market share, physicians see the growing importance of the managerial role and seek to be positioned to influence decision making about the delivery of care (Burns & Thorpe, 1993). This is coupled with a growing disillusion regarding the practice of medicine in the current economic and political environment, and accompanied by changing lifestyle concerns, particularly among newer physicians. The transition into management is not always easy for physicians. Management requires a tolerance for ambiguity, a long-term perspective, and deferred gratification, in contrast to the perspective usually associated with medicine. Further, physician managers often face opposition to their new roles from both physicians and from nonphysician managers. In moving to these new roles, physician managers face the challenge of convincing their physician colleagues that they are still physicians and convincing nonphysician management colleagues that they deserve to be taken seriously as managers (Letourneau & Curry, 1997). Also, new knowledge and skills must be developed to facilitate the transition and to enhance the likelihood that physician managers will be successful in their new roles.

The preceding sections demonstrate how our understanding of organizations, the environments within which they operate, and the roles of managers have changed over time. Our early conceptions of organizations and managers were developed in the context of a relatively stable and placid environment. Thus, the environment as an influence on organizations was given rather little attention in what was essentially a closed-system view of organizational dynamics, with emphasis on internal workings. The role of the manager was, in turn, therefore bounded by the "walls" of the organization. This is clearly exemplified in the traditional conceptions of the managerial role, which focused on planning, organizing, staffing, directing, and controlling or, in the case of the human relations approach, to ensuring that workers were satisfied and happy and that internal processes were free of strain and conflict. Increasingly, today it is recognized that managers and their organizations must interact with their environments. It is clear that a broader view must take into account the responsibilities of managers within the organization—that is, having to do with the workings, operations, processes, and structures of organizations—but must also consider the dynamics of the two-way interplay between organizations and environments. Health care managers of 2000 and beyond will need to manage organizations in new ways, and will need to focus attention on the external environment and its relation to the organization while attending simultaneously to the internal needs as well.

IMPLICATIONS OF NEW MANAGERIAL ROLES

Rosabeth Moss Kanter (1989) argues that new conceptions are required to understand the changing managerial role. As organizations change to adapt to new internal and external pressures, many of the traditional tools of management—hierarchy, motivation, bases of

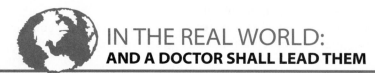

IN THE REAL WORLD:
AND A DOCTOR SHALL LEAD THEM

When physicians talk about their role as leaders it can sound self-serving, but it actually represents a departure from traditional attitudes that assumed the business aspects of health care were beneath the expertise level of those who made the clinical decisions. Dr. Clifford Harris, a founder of one of the early provider groups organized and managed by physicians, says, "If we want to take back medicine, to live up to our compact with the nation, we must [exhibit] leadership." Health system executives are acknowledging and even demanding increased physician leadership in their changing organizations.

As the focus, strategy, and structure of health care organizations have evolved, so have the roles of physician leaders. One health care system that embraced this concept early on was Sutter Health, northern California's largest integrated delivery system. Dr. Thom Atkins, Chief Medical Officer for Sutter Medical Group in Sacramento, says the evolving market is making physician leadership more important than ever. "In a maturing managed care marketplace, our future success depends on our ability to manage care as well as we can," he says. "To do this, we must have capable physician leadership at all levels."

The key here is all levels. Traditionally, physicians were viewed primarily as clinician leaders. They were the keepers of clinical and technical expertise. As such, they tended to be viewed primarily as individual contributors—autonomous and sometimes autocratic experts who focused almost solely on the practice of medicine, leaving the "business" of health care to others. While they held a position in the health care hierarchy, they typically had little control over such tactical issues as hiring and firing, performance review, and budgeting. To the extent they took interest in organizational leadership, physicians often sought board seats, in the belief they could exercise influence, most efficiently, from that vantage point.

Recent market forces such as managed care, mergers, and the integration of services, however, have greatly expanded the roles for which physician leaders are needed. In addition to the more traditional clinician roles, today's organizations need physician managers and executives who can look beyond the more tactical issues of practicing medicine, and help shape both the management of care and the business of delivering that care.

As the roles of physician leaders expand, their focus must change. No longer can they only concern themselves with the quality of care. Now they—like other organization leaders—must add cost effectiveness, patient satisfaction, health policies, and business strategies to the equation. As their focus expands, so too must their scope of influence. To that end, they must quickly break out of the "individual expert" mold, and quickly build relationships with a wide range of decision-makers and leaders in other parts of the organization. In order to make a significant and sustained impact on the system in these new roles, physicians are discovering that their technical skills, while still important, must be complemented by a new set of broader leadership skills.

The transition to such an expanded—and constantly changing—role can be difficult. In customizing its approach, Sutter Health turned to a task force of physician leaders from across its system to help design a competency-based developmental program, which is delivered through what are called "leadership labs." The labs are built around three, Sutter-specific leadership competency models, each focusing on a different leadership arena. These arenas include the hospital medical staff, medical groups and large formal IPAs, and corporate and organizational roles, such as administrative directors or vice presidents of clinical integration. Using expert panels, in-depth behavioral event interviews, and industry research, the physician leadership development task force defined the behaviors of superior performing physician leaders in each of these areas.

The leadership labs provide a developmental environment in which physicians, after building a clear understanding of the competency models, create their own plans to facilitate individual and organizational changes. Using a questionnaire based on the leadership competency model appropriate for their situation, participants are assessed by peers, subordinates, and "influential others." . . . Participants also explore the tenets of leadership, create and refine *their leadership vision and goals, and analyze how their personality preferences influence their leadership behavior. Summaries are provided reflecting their leadership focus and the specific actions to strengthen those areas of behavior most critical to moving their leadership agenda forward.*

Response to the program has been overwhelmingly positive. A number of physicians have described it as a "turning point" in their leadership development, and they consistently report feeling that they have the clearest and most holistic picture of themselves as leaders they have ever experienced. Physician leaders frequently stress

the combined impact of personal insight and practical planning when describing their experiences in the lab program. "It was a turn-around event for me," notes Gary Fields, M.D. "I approached management and leadership situations pretty much the way I dealt with things as a doctor. I was often frustrated that it didn't necessarily get me the outcome I wanted. As a result of my workshop learning, I think I've become a more effective influence."

Excerpts from "And a Doctor Shall Lead Them..." Olson, Scott, Wright-Health Systems Review, 1997.

power, and channels of communication—likewise must change. Indeed, she contends that such tools may no longer be effective. Rather, managers will have to reinvent their profession as they move into "postentrepreneurial organizations" to adapt to these new demands. Her formulation of organizations, and the changing role of managers, calls for the application of flexibility and creativity in order to achieve results. Kanter envisions organizations marked by a greater number and variety of channels for taking action or exerting influence, and in which influence will shift from vertical to horizontal relationships. Such organizations are visualized as flexible clusters of activity rather than as rigid hierarchical and authoritative structures. This view is consistent with that of Peter Drucker (1988), who foresees a shift from control and chain of command models to peer networks and commitment models (Harris, 1993). Likewise, the gap between managers and the managed will shrink as control over information, assignments, and access to external relationships becomes more diffused. External relationships will become a greater source of internal power and influence, recognizing the growing number and importance of linkages between organizations and their environments.

In these postentrepreneurial organizations, there will be shifts of power among and between managers, and alteration of the types of power available. There will be greater reliance on influence without authority, and less on authoritative power based on position in a hierarchy. Managers will recognize the necessity to juggle multiple constituencies, and to negotiate,

broker, bargain, and sell rather than to make unilateral decisions. Success will depend heavily on networking, multiple channels of information, and the ability to span traditional organizational boundaries (Moss Kanter, 1989). Managers will be concerned with their ability to integrate, to facilitate, and to add value to the organization. Managers must ensure that the culture of the organization evolves so as to be consistent with the changing internal and external realities. The importance of external linkages and interorganizational dependencies becomes increasingly apparent but they are, in turn, related to decision-making processes within the organization. Managers must recognize the shift in the role of organizational structure and the need for greater flexibility.

Managers of the future will be called upon to transform their organizations. In so doing, they will need to display, as individuals, a deep personal commitment coupled with the ability to align others with the vision of the organization ("Bridging the Leadership Gap," 1991). Such managers will challenge long-held assumptions, seek new pathways for learning, and craft the organization to promote creativity and participation (Bass, 1990; Matey, 1991; McNeese Smith, 1996). In this context, managerial strength lies "in the ability to maximize the contributions of others by helping them to effectively guide their own destinies, rather than the ability to bend the will of others to the leader's" (Manz & Sims, 1990). Within organizations, Cohen and Tichy (1998) argue that managers will succeed as leaders only to the extent that they are able to articulate their knowledge to others, that is, to teach. As teachers, managers move from a "technician" approach, leading by one's own expertise and ability to show people how to do things, to a "developmental" approach, using opportunities to develop the capabilities of others in the organization ("Leaders of the Pack," 1997). Leading others to lead themselves within organizations will be a particular challenge in health care organizations, where the commitment to one's profession often exceeds commitment to the organization.

> One of the old assumptions used to be that when you teach people to lead, that you teach them to lead other people. The challenge today in healthcare, and for many of our leaders, is just to manage themselves, to manage and lead themselves. And then from there, to truly let go and empower others so that their talents can come to the forefront. ("Bridging the Leadership Gap," 1991)

The concept of **shared vision** is a critical attribute of those who would seek to transform organizations. Vision answers the question, What do we want to become? Shared vision creates a sense of commonality, gives a coherence and connection to diverse activities, and establishes commitment and responsibility because it reflects the individual's personal vision, not merely one handed down from the top. "Visions are powerless unless they are derived from and embraced by those individuals who will collectively achieve them" (Stata, 1988). Thus, **transformational leadership** will foster the nurturing and creation of a shared vision for the organization, and will seek to generate "creative tension" between the current reality and the idealized vision to motivate people to work toward improvement (Senge, 1990). Such creative tension recognizes that "an accurate picture of current reality is just as important as a compelling picture of a desired future." However, managers, in their role as leaders, must continuously strive to maintain the vision of a desired future. It is easy to become discouraged by the seeming difficulty of bringing the vision to reality. The demands of the day can lead people to lose sight of the vision and the connection of those within the organization seeking to achieve the vision. Thus, managers must believe themselves in the vision and in their ability to change

current realities, for vision becomes a living force only when people truly believe they can shape their future" (Senge, 1990).

> Visions are values projected into the future, so if you don't know what you stand for, what you believe in, it's very difficult to develop a compelling vision. A vision should be a very loud pronouncement of what's important to you. Leaders who are involved in helping to set and develop a vision need to have a very clear sense of what their core values are and need to find a way to align those with the values of others. ("Bridging the Leadership Gap," 1991)

In addition to the individual and personal commitment of managers to the notion of shared vision, there is further an organizational dimension that serves to promote the ability of the organization to learn faster than competitors. Learning is seen as being at the heart of an organization's ability to adapt to a rapidly changing environment, the key to being able to identify opportunities that others might not see and to exploit those opportunities rapidly and fully (Prokesch, 1997). Indeed, this may be the only competitive advantage that counts in the future as "over the long run, superior performance depends on superior learning" (Senge, 1990). Such superior learning, however, cannot be simply "adaptive"—that is, focusing only on coping with and responding to an organization's environment. Rather, learning must be "generative," involving seeing the world in terms of interrelated systems and seeking to create and influence the environment. Generative learning emphasizes continual experimentation and feedback as organizations examine themselves and the ways in which they make decisions and solve problems. In building the "social architecture" of an organization, managers must design around the purpose, vision, and core values by which organizational members will live, and ensure that policies, strategies, and structures are consistent to effectively guide the organization. A key element of the architecture is the creation of learning processes, such as scenario analysis and continuous quality improvement, which enable and encourage systems thinking, seeking to examine interrelationships, ongoing processes and patterns, and underlying causes of behavior. In so doing, organizations can become "learning laboratories," characterized by experiential learning, in which management teams learn to learn together (Senge, 1990). "The ability of an organization or manager to learn is not measured by what the organization or manager knows (that is, the product of learning) but rather by how the organization or manager learns—the process of learning" (McGill, Slocum, & Lei, 1992). Thus, building **learning organizations** will require that managers discover how to tap into their organization's commitment and potential and at all levels. Managers must develop individuals who see the organization as a system, who have a personal commitment to a shared vision, and who learn how to experiment and collaboratively reframe problems.

Health care managers also will be called upon to focus on the community and national agenda, playing a key role in developing innovative, long-term solutions for providing affordable health care to the public they serve. In so doing, managers must rethink the ways in which health care is viewed and accomplished. Such rethinking argues that managers be "responsible not only for the productive performance of the organization but also consider the additional dimension of being a citizen of the community" (Miller, 1992). It suggests that organizations will need to refocus attention on the health of the community served, not merely on delivery of medical care. Further, it presumes that health care organizations increasingly will be held accountable for the health status of the populations they serve. Emerging from a series of interviews with current health care

IN THE REAL WORLD:
UNLEASHING THE POWER OF LEARNING: AN INTERVIEW WITH BRITISH PETROLEUM'S JOHN BROWNE

John Browne, head of the giant British Petroleum Company, thinks that all companies battling it out in the global information age face a common challenge: using knowledge more effectively than their competitors do. And he is not talking only about the knowledge that resides in one's own organization. "Any organization that thinks it does everything the best and need not learn from others is incredibly arrogant and foolish," he says.

Prokesch: *Some management thinkers believe we are entering an age of globalization in which building and leveraging knowledge will be the key to success. Do you agree?*

Browne: *Absolutely. Knowledge, ideas, and innovative solutions are being diffused throughout the world today at a speed that would have been unimaginable 10 or 20 years ago. Companies are only now learning how to go beyond seeing that movement as a threat to seeing it as an opportunity.*

Prokesch: *How will the diffusion of knowledge affect the rules of competition?*

Browne: *Learning is at the heart of a company's ability to adapt to a rapidly changing environment. It is the key*

to being able both to identify opportunities that others might not see and to exploit those opportunities rapidly and fully. This means that . . . a company has to learn better than its competitors and apply that knowledge throughout its businesses faster and more widely than they do. The way we see it, anyone in the organization who is not directly accountable for making a profit should be involved in creating and distributing knowledge that the company can use to make a profit.

Prokesch: *What's the most important rule for building an effective learning organization?*

Browne: *A business has to have a clear purpose. If the purpose is not crystal clear, people in the business will not understand what kind of knowledge is critical and what they have to learn in order to improve performance. A clear purpose allows a company to focus its learning efforts in order to increase its competitive advantage. What do we mean by purpose? Our purpose is who we are and what makes us distinctive. It's what we as a company exist to achieve, and what we're willing and not willing to do to achieve it.*

Prokesch: *How did you design an organizational structure to promote learning?*

Browne: *We have built a very flat team-based organization that is designed to motivate and help people to learn. We've divided the company up into lots of business units, and there is nothing between them, and the nine-member executive group to whom they report, which consists of the three managing directors of our business groups and their six deputies. The organization is even flatter . . . because each of the managing directors and his deputies work as a team in dealing with the business units. . . . In addition, we've developed all sorts of networks to encourage the sharing of knowledge throughout the organization. Finally, we've integrated our technology organization with the business units so that it is working with them both to solve the most important business problems and to exploit the most important business opportunities. Previously, the technology organization was a separate fiefdom, focused on invention. In the last five years, we've refocused our technology people on application. Now their mission is to access the best technology wherever it resides inside or outside BP and apply it quickly, cutting costs and time to market.*

Prokesch: *To leverage learning, knowledge must flow among business units. I would think the challenge is to create links among the units to promote that flow without recreating the organizational clutter of the past. How have you tackled that challenge?*

Browne: *Information technology is one solution. In addition, we have made much progress in forming what you might call learning communities. For example, each of the 40 business units that constitute BPX belongs to one of four peer groups. The members of each peer group wrestle with common problems. They have a lot to learn from one another. They share technical staff. And they all are equals.*

Prokesch: *Isn't there a danger that the learning networks you are encouraging will end up creating organizational complexity?*

Browne: *I don't think so. One of the beauties of the networks is that they are not organizational structures per se. In general, we don't think of our business units as permanent structures. We constantly scrutinize them to make sure they serve their business purpose, maximize learning, and help teams perform. If they don't, we change them. We split them up or combine them.*

Prokesch: *What is the role of top management in the learning organization?*

Browne: *The most senior leaders in any company do only a very few things. Ultimately, they have to make decisions on the organizational architecture and the way forward. They set policies, standards, and targets, and create processes to ensure that people achieve or adhere to them. It is while those processes are taking place that learning should take place. What determines whether it does is the questions leaders ask, and the way they approach what is going on. Leadership is all about catalyzing learning as well as better performance. Leaders have to demonstrate that they are active participants in the learning organization.*

leaders is a call for an expanded sense of stewardship and accountability to the community ("Leaders of the Pack," 1997). Organizational leaders are urged to intervene earlier to address health care problems, to develop cooperative relationships among public and private health and community service agencies, and to foster collaboration among health care professionals, public health professionals, managers, and the community.

Maybe what we need is more thought about how as a community we come together to create a better place to live. And I think that is an area where hospitals and healthcare also have a responsibility. I think with the competitive model that has been in place for the last eight years or longer, a lot of the good will toward hospitals and public institutions has evaporated. We are seen as competitive organizations, rather than as organizations whose roots are in nonprofit service. ("Bridging the Leadership Gap," 1991).

This broadening shift in thinking has profound implications for organizations, and may be briefly illustrated in two important areas noted earlier—physician-organization relationships and integrated health care systems. As organizations, their managers, and physicians address the future, fundamental will be the acknowledgment of interdependencies, mutual interests, and shared values. Existing research suggests that effective physician-organization relationships exist in situations where there is a history of cooperation and collaboration, a desire to work together, and recognition of their interdependent destinies (Shortell, 1991). Management stability was found to be important in establishing trust and confidence, as was a genuine respect for and liking of physicians by health care executives. Also identified as successful were those situations in which there was shared decision making, with early physician involvement; an effort to manage change; a commitment to open, honest, and candid communication; and a willingness to admit mistakes and try alternative approaches to problems. Attempts were made to work together as business partners, using an array of structural mechanisms and support of physicians in practice management, information systems, and in enhancing their patient base. Perhaps the most distinguishing characteristic of effective relationships was the strength of physician leadership and commitment to leadership development programs, "helping others to lead themselves." These underlying themes have been reinforced by a recent empirical study examining relationships between physicians and integrating systems and their hospitals. In this effort, key factors leading to successful relationships were trust, physician involvement in governance and management, and physician leadership development (Zuckerman et al., 1998). Managers must recognize that the transition to effective alignment will underscore the interdependence of physicians and organizations and emphasize the sharing of knowledge, capabilities, resources, and risks.

In the development of integrated health care systems, it is presumed that an organization's

ability to continuously improve the effectiveness of managing interdependence is the critical element in

responding to new and pressing competitive forces. Unlike in previous eras, managerial strategies based on optimizing operations within functional departments, product lines, or geographical organizations simply will not be adequate in the future. (Rockart & Short, 1989)

Longest sees organizational integration as leading to greater focus on coordinated continuation of services, accountability for the overall health status of populations served, and involvement in more complex **organizational structures** (Longest, 1998).

Cutting across the managerial roles, these emerging, highly interdependent organizations will lead to greater role complexity as managers must adjust rapidly and more frequently to new situations and cope with ambiguity and fluid structures and decision-making processes. It will often be the case that these systems are not owned or controlled by any one organization; rather, multiple players will be involved and bound together because of commitment to a unifying vision and common values, as well as exigencies of the marketplace. Indeed, managers will need to be skilled in building and maintaining partnerships not only with other health care organizations, but with an array of human service agencies in their communities as well. In such interdependent systems and networks of organizations, there must be managerial commitment to sharing power and sharing risk. Lateral communications, relationships built on trust and respect, extensive sharing of information, joint decision making, and clarity in purpose and expectations will characterize these collaborative efforts (Zuckerman & Kaluzny, 1991). As noted earlier, managers in these organizations will thus balance constituencies rather than control subordinates.

As we have seen, the manager may well seek to transform the organization to meet the new realities of this decade and beyond. Despite the exigencies of external pressures and internal complexity, it will be incumbent on managers to retain a broad view, keep the long-term perspective in mind, and seek to add value to the organization over time. Through all of this, we see that managers play key roles in ensuring that members of the organization know, understand, and accept the core values of the organization. As keepers of the organization's values, managers must

DEBATE TIME 2.3: WHAT DO YOU THINK?

Contrary to what we would like to believe, the manager's personal values and views about what would be best for the organization don't count for much in day-to-day organizational life. This is because management is essentially a political process. The manager's role is to balance (some would say juggle) the many, often contradictory, pressures on the organization from external and internal stakeholders (some of which may be groups or organizations). Each stakeholder has something the organization needs, whether it be dollars, patients, regulatory approvals, a willingness to work for the organization, or whatever. And this enables each stakeholder to make demands on the organization that furthers his or her self-interest. Often, these demands are conflicting. For example, physicians may want a hospital to purchase the latest equipment for them to use in treating their patients, while purchasers want the hospital to cut its costs. Some stakeholders have a lot of power to press for their agendas; others have less. Those that the organization needs the most and those with the most power tend to get more of what they want. The manager has little choice but to respond to these pressures. Skillful managers try to orchestrate the diverse demands so as to accommodate as many as possible while maintaining a reasonable degree of harmony within the organization. This is fundamentally a matter of accommodation and compromise, although sometimes a consensus can be found. The manager's role is essentially political—a broker of power. The manager's job is to balance the competing pressures to maintain harmony in the organization. His or her own goals and values have little to do with it.

live the values of the organization, showing their relevance in decision making and integrating them into the organization's reward system (Rossy, 1987). The extent to which managerial decision making reflects the basic values of the organization is of fundamental importance to its long-term viability. To have meaning, organizational behavior must be consistent with these values; saying so doesn't make it so.

> Phrases such as "the customer comes first," has meaning only if customers are treated with respect and dignity. "We are a people-oriented company" has no meaning if people are treated as expendable. "We are a risk-taking, innovative company" has no meaning if the organization does not reward risk-taking and innovation. (Zuckerman, 1989)

Managers must lead in living the values of the organization, in being responsive to the needs of key stakeholders, and in enacting the mission of the organization. Companies that enjoy enduring success—that is, they are "built to last"—have core values and a core purpose that remain fixed while their business strategies and practices endlessly adapt to a changing world (Collins & Porras, 1996). Indeed, Max DePree

(1994) views organizational leadership as a merger of competence and moral purpose.

In order to transform health care, we must transform our leaders. Believing that health care will be and should be significantly different in the twenty-first century, opinion leaders participating in the Healthcare Forum study ("Bridging the Leadership Gap," 1991) called for a system characterized by greater emphasis on prevention and healing; universal, cost-efficient, community-based managed care; and national health reform with a public/private partnership. Leaders of such a transformation will be called upon to redefine health care, focusing on healing, changing lifestyles, and the holistic interplay of mind, body, and spirit. Such leaders must develop a shared, collective vision of the future, fusing a social mission to the public and the community to organizational goals, objectives, and actions.

> Wouldn't that be marvelous? I mean to keep people healthy, that's what we are supposed to be doing. And wouldn't it be marvelous if we were paid to do that rather than to do procedures, to fix a fender, to replace an engine. I think these are exciting times and I think the next ten years are going to be

dramatic in terms of the direction that healthcare is going. We're talking about healing rather than curing. That's something remarkable isn't it? ("Bridging the Leadership Gap," 1991)

As this chapter has suggested, the role of the health care manager in the 21st century will be complex, multidimensional, and demanding. But it will also be exciting and rewarding, offering opportunities to serve both public and organizational interests while seeking to balance the value orientations of "mission and margin." As suggested by Walter McNerney (1985):

There is more to management than crisp efficiency. In the health field, perhaps more than in any other, management involves moral issues and ethical choices. It involves deep commitment and personal courage. It involves a resolve to be just and right, not only a resolve to win.

List of Suggested Cases

Deal, B., & Tiscornia, J. Hospital Consolidation: Optimal Strategy for a Two-Hospital Town.

Halversen, P., & Kaluzny, A. The Mt. Hope Council: An Emerging Public and Private Community Health Partnership.

Ross, A., & Richardson, M. (1996). *Ambulatory Health Care: Case Studies for Health Services Executive.* Chicago/Englewood, CO: Health Administration Press/Medical Group Management Association.

Zuckerman, H., Torrens, P., Hilberman, D., & Andersen, R. Evaluating Emerging Physician-Organization Integration Arrangements.

 # MANAGERIAL GUIDELINES

1. Conceptualizations (models) of organizations and of the management role help managers make sense of the complex reality in which they work. No one model provides all the answers; rather, different models offer different but useful insights about the context, aims, and functions of management.

2. Managers should look for opportunities to assess their mastery of the competencies and skills associated with the different management roles, and should consciously seek to improve their weaknesses. Managers also should strive to develop a good sense of themselves, and to be introspective about how they react to different types of situations.

3. Managers must consciously "size up" the amount and sources of power of key stakeholders external and internal to the organization, and be aware of the "agendas" each is inclined to press for. The manager then needs to decide how to involve these stakeholders in decision making so that the views of each are balanced with other important perspectives.

4. Translating potential conflicts over desired outcomes into cooperation or collaboration requires that the manager search for common ground among the different interest groups.

5. Organizations need to adapt to the changes in their environment. They must also secure inputs from and sell outputs to external sources. Hence, effective management involves "managing" external interactions, as well as "running a tight ship" internally.

6. The environment of health care organizations is increasingly complex, fast changing, and demanding. Managers must design effective processes and structures for keeping up with external changes affecting the organization, determining their implications, and deciding how the organization should respond.

7. Building consensus, forming coalitions, and negotiating compromises are activities that are becoming more and more important for managers as the number of external and internal parties health care organizations must deal with increases.

8. The difficult issues health care organizations face today require involvement in decision making by representatives of governance, management,

(continued)

MANAGERIAL GUIDELINES

medical staff, and functional or program specialists. Hence, managers should design or find educational opportunities in which all of these parties can learn together as a team.

9. Managers should view the relationships between organizations and their environments as a "two-way street." Each is able to influence the other to some extent. By actively managing external relations, managers should try to make the environment more favorable or moderate external pressures on the organization.

10. Managers must see to it that the organization's information systems encompass external as well as internal information and enable integration of data on demographics, the market, costs, utilization, and quality.

11. Articulation and communication of the mission and values of the organization and a clear sense of direction are critical management responsibilities. Equally important is assessing which parties are "on board" and which do not fully accept the organization's direction.

12. Managers should consciously model and act in concert with the behaviors and values they seek to develop in the organization. Behavior by others consistent with these values should be encouraged and recognized.

13. Managerial training and leadership development should encompass both opportunities to learn about trends and issues in health care and opportunities to strengthen management skills, especially skills that enhance the facilitation of effective interaction with external and internal parties.

14. Managers should establish forums in their organizations where the management team can discuss new concepts of management and the beliefs and values that underlie these conceptualizations.

15. Managers must understand and then act on the knowledge that power or the ability to get things done in the organization of the future will come more from empowering, inspiring, and supporting others and from teamwork, and not so much from the manager's own authority or decisions. It will be through the sharing of power that the manager's effectiveness is enhanced.

16. To inspire and motivate, the organization's mission or vision must be compelling in two respects: It must clearly demonstrate a "fit" between the external demands and organization's direction such that the organization is positioned to be successful, and the mission must be seen as important in the sense of being based on worthy values.

17. Managers must establish a culture, processes, and structures that help the organization become a "learning organization," constantly striving to reexamine old assumptions and old ways of doing things.

Discussion Questions

1. Managers generally respond to the question, "What do you do?" in one of several ways. They may describe their work in terms of generic management functions, the activities or tasks they perform, the ends they seek to achieve, the issues or problems they deal with, or the knowledge and skills they use. Think of several examples pertinent to health services organizations of each way of describing what managers do.

2. Adapting an organization to its environment, articulating and gaining support for a strategic vision and values, and designing the internal structures of the organization are key management roles in health services organizations. Is each role equally important? What determines this? What knowledge and skills do you think are most helpful in carrying out each of these three roles?

3. How important is it for a manager to be proficient in every aspect of management? Can you think of

managers who are particularly competent in some areas but not in others? What do you see as your greatest strengths? Weaknesses? How can managers compensate for areas in which they are not particularly proficient?

4. Assume that you are the chief executive officer of a large urban health system that is struggling for its survival in the face of increasing local competition involving managed care pressures. What role should physicians play in deciding what strategies to pursue? How do you as the leader of the organization facilitate their involvement? What role would other actors play? What are some of the alternative strategies that you might pursue? How are the strategic alternatives facing large urban health systems likely to differ from those encountered by smaller suburban health systems?

References

Alexander, J. A., Zuckerman, H. S., & Pointer, D. (1995, Fall). The challenges of governing integrated health care systems. *Health Care Management Review, 20*(4), 69–81.

Argyris, C. (1994, July-August). Good communication that blocks learning. *Harvard Business Review,* 77–85.

Bass, B. M. (1990, Winter). From transactional to transformational leadership: Learning to share the vision. *Organizational Dynamics,* 19–31.

Bridging the leadership gap in healthcare. (1991). San Francisco: The Healthcare Forum Leadership Center.

Burns, L. R., & Thorpe, D. (1993). Trends and models in physician hospital organizations. *Health Care Management Review, 18*(4), 7–20.

Champions of Satisfaction: Winning Strategies of the Country's Best Health Plans. (1996). Evanston, IL: Sachs Group.

Clement, J. P. (1998, Spring). Vertical integration and diversification of acute care hospitals: Conceptual definitions. *Hospital and Health Services Administration, 33,* 99–110.

Cohen, E., & Tichy, N. (1998, March/April). Teaching: The heart of leadership. *Healthcare Forum Journal,* 20–22, 24, 75.

Collins, J. C., & Porras, J. I. (1996, September/October). Building your company's vision. *Harvard Business Review,* 65–77.

Conrad, D. A., & Shortell, S. M. (1996, Fall). Integrated health systems: Promise and performance. *Frontiers of Health Services Management, 13*(1), 3–40, 57–58.

Darling, J. R. (1992). Total quality management: The key role of leadership strategies. *Leadership and Organizational Development Journal, 13*(4), 3–7.

DePree, M. (1994, Spring). Leadership and moral purpose. *Hospital and Health Services Administration, 39*(1), 133–138.

Drucker, P. (1988, January-February). The coming of the new organization. *Harvard Business Review, 88,* 45–53.

Fayol, H. (1949). *General and industrial administration.* New York: Pitman.

Gantt, H. (1916). *Industrial leadership.* New Haven, CN: Yale University Press.

Gilbreth, F. B. (1911). *Motion study.* New York: Van Nostrand.

Harris, T. G. (1993, May/June). The post-capitalist executive: An interview with Peter Drucker. *Harvard Business Review,* 115–122.

Hospital Research and Educational Trust and J. L. Kellogg Graduate School of Management. (1977, May). *Future focus forum (Profiles in leadership).* Chicago, IL: Health Research and Educational Trust.

Japsen, B. (1997, September 1). The reluctant doctor: Survey finds luring physicians into systems is tough. *Modern Healthcare,* 66, 68.

Letourneau, B., & Curry, W. (1997, Spring). Physicians as executives: Boon or boondoggle? *Frontiers of Health Services Management, 13*(3), 3–25, 43–45.

Longest, B. B., Jr. (1998, March/April). Managerial competence at senior levels of integrated delivery systems. *Journal of Healthcare Management, 43*(2), 115–135.

Manz, C. C., & Sims, H. P., Jr. (1990). *Super leadership.* New York: Berkley Books.

Marting, W. E., Dehays, D. W., Hoffer, J. A., & Perkins, W. C. (1991). *Managing information technology: What managers need to know.* New York: Macmillan Publishing Co.

Maslow, A. (1970). *Motivation and personality* (2nd ed.). New York: Harper & Row.

Matey, D. B. (1991, Winter). Significance of transactional and transformational leadership theory on the hospital manager. *Hospital and Health Services Administration, 36*(1), 600–605.

Mayo, E. (1933). *The human problems of an industrial civilization.* New York: The Macmillan Company.

McGill, M. E., Slocum, J. W., & Lei, D. (1992, Summer). Management practices in learning organizations. *Organizational Dynamics, 21,* 4–17.

McGregor, D. A. (1960). *The human side of enterprise.* New York: McGraw-Hill.

McLaughlin, C. P., & Kaluzny, A. D. (1990, Summer). Total quality management in health: Making it work. *Health Care Management Review, 15*(3), 7–14.

McNeese Smith, D. (1996, Summer). Increased employee productivity, job satisfaction, and organizational commitment: Effective leadership behavior for hospital managers. *Hospital and Health Services Administration, 41*(2), 160–175.

McNerney, W. J. (1985, Summer). Managing ethical dilemmas. *Journal of Health Administration Education, 3,* 331–340.

Miller, I. (1992, Winter). Executive leadership, community action, and the habits of health care politics. *Health Care Management Review, 17*(1), 81–84.

Mintzberg, H. (1973). *The nature of managerial work.* Englewood Cliffs, NJ: Prentice-Hall.

Moss Kanter, R. (1989, November-December). The new managerial work. *Harvard Business Review, 85*–92.

Olson, S. (1997). And a doctor shall lead them. *Wright-Health Systems Review.*

Pointer, D., Alexander, J. A., & Zuckerman, H. S. (1995, Spring). Loosening the gordian knot of governance in integrated health care delivery systems. *Frontiers of Health Services Management, 11*(3), 3–37.

Pointer, D., & Ewell, C. (1994). *Really governing: How health systems and hospital boards can make more of a difference.* Albany, NY: Delmar Publishers.

Prokesch, S. (1997, September-October). Unleasing the power of learning: An interview with British Petroleum's John Browne. *Harvard Business Review,* 146–168.

Quinn, R.E. (1988). *Beyond rational management.* San Francisco, CA: Jossey-Bass Inc.

Quinn, R. E., Faerman, S. R., Thompson, M. P., & McGrath, M. R. (1996). *Becoming a master manager* (2nd ed.). New York: Wiley.

Rockart, J. F., & Short, J. E. (1989, Winter). IT in the 1990s: Managing organizational interdependence. *Sloan Management Review,* 7–17.

Rossy, G. L. (1987, September-October). The executive's role in ethics: The view from business and industry. *Healthcare Executive, 2,* 17–21.

Senge, P. M. (1990). *The fifth discipline.* New York: Doubleday.

Shortell, S. M. (1988, Fall). The evolution of hospitals systems: Unfulfilled promises and self-fulfilling prophesies. *Medical Care Review, 45,* No. 2, 177–213.

Shortell, S. M. (1989, Spring). New directions in hospital governance. *Hospital and Health Services Administration, 34,* No. 1, 7–23.

Shortell, S. M. (1991). *Effective hospital-physician relationships,* Ann Arbor, MI: Health Administration Press.

Shortell, S. M., Gillies, R. R., Anderson, D. A., Erickson, K. M., Mitchell, J. (1996). *Remaking health care in America.* San Francisco: Jossey-Bass.

Solovy, A. T., & Sunseri, R. (1997, August 5 & 20). Leading the way. *Hospitals and Health Systems, 15 & 16,* 30–43.

Stata, R. (1988, May-June). The role of the chief executive officer in articulating the vision. *Interfaces, 18*(3), 3–9.

Taylor, B. E., Chait, R. P., & Holland, T. P. (1996, September-October). The new work of the nonprofit board. *Harvard Business Review,* 4–11.

Taylor, F. W. (1911). *The principles of scientific management.* New York: Harper & Brothers.

Umbdenstock, R., Hageman, W., & Amundson, B., M.D. (1990, Winter). The five critical areas for effective governance of not-for-profit hospitals. *Hospital and Health Services Administration, 35*(4), 481–492.

Weber, M. (1964). *The theory of social and economic organizations.* New York: Free Press of Glencoe.

Zuckerman, H. S. (1989, Spring). Redefining the role of the CEO: Challenges and conflicts. *Hospital and Health Services Administration, 34*(1), 25–38.

Zuckerman, H. S., Hilberman, D. W., Andersen, R. M., Burns, L. R., Alexander, J. A., & Torrens, P. (1998, Spring). Physicians and organizations: Strange bedfellows or a marriage made in heaven? *Frontiers of Health Services Management, 14*(3), 3–34.

Zuckerman, H. S., & Kaluzny, A. D. (1991, Spring). Strategic alliances in health care: The challenges of cooperation. *Frontiers of Health Services Management,* 3–24.

PART

2

Motivating, Leading, and Negotiating

THE NATURE OF ORGANIZATIONS: FRAMEWORK FOR THE TEXT

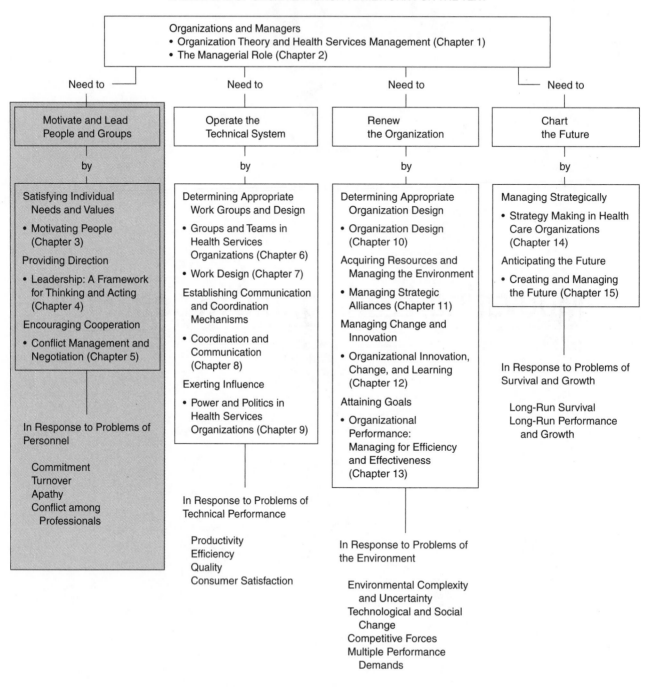

Chapters 3–5 deal with fundamental issues related to motivation, leadership, and negotiation. These processes are fundamental building blocks for working effectively with individuals and groups. Understanding multiple sources of motivation, different approaches to leadership, and various ways of managing conflict and negotiations are key determinants of successful managerial performance.

Chapter 3, "Motivating People," focuses on a variety of issues related to motivation. The chapter addresses the following questions:

- What are some of the common myths associated with motivating people?
- What are the major content and process approaches to understanding motivation?
- What are some of the more effective ways of dealing with motivational problems?

The chapter emphasizes multiple approaches for dealing with motivational issues.

Chapter 4, "Leadership: A Framework for Thinking and Acting," addresses the multiple ways in which leadership has been defined and various approaches to understanding leadership effectiveness. Specific questions examined include:

- What is known about the different perspectives regarding effective leadership?
- What are the special leadership challenges facing health services organizations?

- What skills are needed to be successful health care leaders?

The chapter sets forth an integrative model of leadership for the reader's consideration.

Chapter 5, "Conflict Management and Negotiation," highlights the major forms of conflict that occur in health services organizations and various approaches for dealing with them. Special attention is devoted to structuring and managing negotiation processes. Among the key questions addressed are:

- What are the major causes of conflict in health services organizations?
- What are the pros and cons of different approaches for managing conflict?
- What are the primary concepts and approaches associated with effective negotiation?

The chapter emphasizes multiple approaches to managing conflict and the importance of preparation for effective negotiation.

Upon completing these three chapters, readers should have a fuller understanding of the relationships among motivation, leadership, and conflict management and negotiation. Readers should have a firm grasp of the various approaches to dealing with these issues and understand which approaches are most likely to be effective under different circumstances.

CHAPTER

3

Motivating People

Thomas A. D'Aunno, Ph.D.
Myron D. Fottler, Ph.D.
Stephen J. O'Connor, Ph.D.

Chapter Outline

- Motivation and Management
- Content Perspectives
- Process Perspectives
- Motivating Health Care Professionals
- Motivational Problems

Learning Objectives

After completing this chapter, the reader should be able to:

1. Define *motivation* and distinguish it from other factors that influence individuals' performance.
2. Recognize popular but misleading myths about motivation.
3. Understand that motivation depends heavily on the situations in which individuals work.
4. Understand managers' roles in motivating people.
5. Identify key characteristics of the content of peoples' work that motivates them.
6. Identify important processes involved in motivating people.
7. Assess and deal with motivational problems.

Key Terms

Autonomous Work Groups
Behavior Modification
Empowerment
Equity
Expectancy
Gainsharing
Hierarchy of Needs
Hygiene Factors
Instrumentality
Job Redesign
Motivation
Motivators
Quality Circles
Reinforcement
Self-actualization
Valence

Chapter Purpose

The decision to fire or salvage is a dilemma many health care managers face, and it is not limited to decisions involving lower-level employees. The objective of this chapter is to understand how to motivate individuals to perform effectively in health services organizations. The chapter consists of five major sections. The first section defines *motivation* and distinguishes it from other factors that can affect performance. This section also describes common but misleading myths about motivation. As antidotes to these myths, we emphasize that motivation is situational. That is, there are several characteristics of individuals and the settings in which they work that managers should take into account in trying to motivate people. The section concludes by examining the role that managers can play to maintain or increase motivation. The next two sections identify the most important factors that managers can influence to improve or maintain the motivation of employees and coworkers. The focus is on those approaches that seem most promising, and we refer readers to more extensive reviews (Jurkiewicz, Massey, & Brown, 1998; Kanfer, 1990; Steers & Porter, 1987). Finally, the last section examines common motivational problems and discusses how to assess them. Several alternatives for dealing with motivational problems are explored.

MOTIVATION AND MANAGEMENT

Motivation is a central topic for health services managers, but it can also be an especially difficult one. The types of workers health managers might be expected to motivate can range from highly educated and professional ones such as physicians and nurses, to minimum wage workers such as nurse's aids in long-term care settings (Vance, 1997).

The environment of health care continues to swiftly change and reformulate, requiring regular improvements in productivity while simultaneously requiring cost containment. Health care mergers, layoffs, lower profit margins, increased regulatory demands, cost-cutting pressure, savy purchasers and consumers, and intense competition have all combined to squeeze the expense out of this system, making the workforce health care's most expensive resource (Thomas, 1998). The theories and techniques of motivation that will be described in this chapter are excellent tools for making health care's most expensive resource its most valuable asset. Empirical evidence indicates that human resource practices, such as those that improve motivation, can positively influence an organization's financial performance (Huselid, 1995). Consequently, a highly motivated workforce can serve as a difficult-to-replicate competitive advantage (Zigarelli, 1996).

A primary task of management is to motivate people to perform at high levels toward meeting organizational objectives (Steers & Porter, 1987), but many managers are unclear as to how this should be accomplished (Kovach, 1995; Medcof & Hausdorf, 1995).

In addition to motivating individuals to improve productivity and efficiency, health care managers may wish to motivate workers to reduce absenteeism and tardiness (Mercer, 1988), to improve problem-solving ability, to promote creativity and innovativeness (Colvin, 1998), to work interdependently and cooperatively as team members, to develop consumer-oriented attitudes and behaviors (O'Connor & Shewchuk, 1995), to reenergize those who no longer feel challenged (Kennedy, 1997), to remotivate following a reduction in force (McConnell, 1996), to get people to

IN THE REAL WORLD:
THE DEMOTIVATED ATTENDANTS

St. Mary's Hospital is a Roman Catholic hospital in the Southeast run by the Daughters of Charity system. Until recently, the hospital ran a School of Nursing which had produced about 40 new diploma nurses each year. As a result of the high costs of operating the school, a decision was made to close the school two years ago.

Prior to the closing of the School of Nursing, two attendants (a nurse's aide and a porter) had been in charge of maintenance for 12 years. They received virtually no supervision and the facility was always spotless. During that time period, they were commended verbally and in writing for the high quality of their work. The vice president of Human Resources attributed their high motivation and good work to the pride and ownership they felt in what they viewed as "their" area.

When the School of Nursing was closed, the two attendants were transferred to the hospital. In the hospital they were viewed as new employees, moved around on a regular basis, and no longer had autonomy and ownership of a specific area. The quality of their work suffered. They were written up by supervisors on several occasions for attitudinal problems, lack of motivation, and inade-

quate work performance. Instead of the praise, recognition, and positive reinforcement they had previously received from the director of the now defunct School of Nursing, the two attendants were now receiving criticism from several supervisors.

The vice president for Human Resources faces a dilemma. The easy solution is simply to fire them, as several supervisors have suggested. On the other hand, these have been good and loyal employees of the hospital for many years. Through no fault of their own, their job structure and environment was changed. She would therefore like to salvage them and make them motivated and productive employees once again. Although she's not quite sure how to do it, she realizes the problem is not that the two employees are simply unmotivated by nature since they had demonstrated extremely high motivation for a long period of time prior to their transfer to the hospital.

Adapted from Lutz, S. Employee suggestions net $20 million in savings. Modern Healthcare 1990; 20(9):21–22. Reprinted with permission from Modern Healthcare.

take on added responsibilities (Nordhaus-Bike, 1997), to recruit hard-to-find workers such as information technology professionals (Appleby, 1998), and to motivate moral and ethical behavior (Vidaver-Cohen, 1998).

Defining and Distinguishing Motivation

The beginning of wisdom in motivating people is to recognize what motivation is and is not (Mohr, 1982). We define **motivation** as a state of feeling or thinking in which one is energized or aroused to perform a task or engage in a particular behavior (Steers & Porter, 1987). This definition focuses on motivation as an emotional or cognitive state that is independent of action. This focus clearly distinguishes motivation from the performance of a task and its consequences. No-

tice, too, that motivation can be a state of either feeling or thinking, or a combination of the two. For some individuals, motivation is more a matter of feeling than thinking, while, for others, the reverse is true.

Myths about Motivation—and Some Antidotes

There are several popular but misleading myths about motivating people. Our view is that these myths are more harmful than helpful and, as a result, need to be confronted early in this chapter. Four particular myths are addressed below.

Myth 1: Motivated workers are more productive. To illustrate this myth, consider this conversation (Muchinsky, 1987).

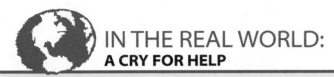

IN THE REAL WORLD:
A CRY FOR HELP

Working and keeping motivated on a busy 24-bed general intensive care unit, a charge nurse tells her story:

ICU nursing is becoming frustrating. It is frustrating to always be there, to work so closely with patients, to do so much to keep them going, and then have someone else get all the credit. The nurses do the work, they act as the eyes and ears monitoring and responding to the patients' condition, but it is always the physician who saves them and gets the accolades.

The ICU is also becoming a more dangerous and scary place to work. In addition to tuberculosis, HIV, and hepatitis, there are more blood borne and communicable diseases than ever before. Patients who come here are often under the influence of drugs or alcohol. They often react badly to pharmaceuticals we administer to them. Because the atmosphere is unfamiliar, they frequently get violent. Even old people can get violent.

Consumerism is rampant in health care. Everyone is an expert. The families continually remind me to wash my hands. Administration has recently been demanding more consumer-friendly behavior from the ICU nurses. They recently instituted wide open, 24-hour visiting hours. They told us, 'You will tolerate someone being here 24 hours a day as long as there is no bonafide reason that they shouldn't be there.' For the most part this is fine with us. We are part of a very family- and community-oriented health system, and families can really help out. They can reassure their kids or make certain their elderly parents or grandparents don't fall out of bed and are comfortable. In some cases, if a family member is not available, we have to hire sitters for $12 an hour to keep an eye on the patient. Generally, the sitters are unskilled people who can't participate in the patient care process. Usually they knit, eat chips, read, listen to the radio, or sleep.

Although the presence of family members can assist us, more often than not, they impede our ability to do our work. We have one 'frequent flyer' who is in here all the time. His wife will not leave. She insists on doing his care. The husband has severe diabetes, and she insists on doing the glucose monitoring and dressing changes. We can't get rid of her. She makes the nurses very uncomfortable. Sometimes you have to take care of the entire family, not just the member in the bed. Many families are already dysfunctional to begin with; they don't usually function any better in the ICU setting.

People who go into ICU nursing go into it because they are more comfortable working with technology than with people. They do best, and I hate to say this, when the patient is paralyzed, sedated, and ventilated. Those really caring nurses go into oncology or the touchy-feelies, not ICU.

Our system has been restructuring lately, and administration has been trying to focus less on financial rewards and more on nontangible rewards. The ICU nurses do receive a higher pay differential, because the work is more demanding and specialized. However, administration wants to get away from differentials because, as they say, 'Everything is getting to be a specialty.' But believe me, money still talks!

A year ago, administration cut back ICU staffing in an effort to save money. Shortly after that time, we went into a 10-month period of very high census and very high acuity. The highest anyone could ever remember, and we were understaffed! Work became horrible. I didn't want to go. Every time it would be hellish. The 24 ICU beds were always full of seriously ill people.

As the demands and stresses became greater, the necessary ICU 'community behaviors' were just put aside. The nurses weren't motivated to work as a team anymore; they began focusing on 'their' patients only. But we all have to keep watch on the telemetry banks and the arrhythmia alarms. Phones ring that have to be answered. The pneumatic tubes [which transport lab results, blood samples, and pharmaceuticals] need to be attended to. These activities are not assigned, but need to be done as a team.

Often, nurses that were scheduled to work eight hours would have to stay for 12. For a while, we had to work every weekend and holiday. To help ease the staffing void, the hospital began to rely on external agency, pool nurses at a higher wage. When the pool nurses come here, they are not 100%. They might be totally unfamiliar with our environment, and we don't necessarily know their skill level. Naturally, these nurses take a lot of orientation and maintenance time. Furthermore, because pool nurses are not given computer passwords, we have to do their computerized charting, which creates more work for us. The pool nurses are hired guns who are paid about $12 more per hour than we are. They also work whenever they want to.

Although we are a nonprofit, we have a gain-sharing plan. Administration thinks money is not an issue with us. They played with the equations. We worked very hard—all out—for 10 months in a very difficult and understaffed environment. We did receive our gain-share checks, but it was practically nothing. Because of the high patient census and acuity, coupled with staff cutbacks, the external agency pool was used heavily. They are paid a premium. Apparently, that is where most of our gain-share went. We didn't feel that the gain-share checks rewarded us at all. In the end, it had nothing to do with all the extra effort. That was our reward for being full-time, committed, extremely hard working, and concerned for quality.

I can go down to the agency tomorrow and make $12 an hour more than I do now.

Supervisor: George just isn't motivated any more!
Foreman: How can you tell?
Supervisor: His productivity has fallen off by more than 50%.

Motivation should not be confused with performance. People can be highly motivated but still perform poorly. Performance depends not just on motivation but also on ability and a host of situational factors such as the availability of resources needed to perform a job well. In other words, motivation is just one of several factors that managers need to consider in trying to improve or sustain individuals' performance. Nonetheless, it is often a critical factor.

Myth 2: Some people are just motivated and others aren't. This myth is based on the view that motivation is a personality trait or characteristic that remains relatively stable from time to time and place to place. If this view were taken to its extreme, it would suggest that managers should carefully select only those employees who have the trait of motivation, for managers could otherwise do little to influence motivation and behavior.

In contrast, we take the view that motivation is more specific to situations (i.e., influenced by factors in an individual's environment) than it is a stable personality trait or characteristic (Kanfer, 1990). There is strong empirical support for the view that situations significantly shape individual behavior (Davis-Blake & Pfeffer, 1989). For example, as illustrated in the case at St. Mary's Hospital, individuals who are motivated at certain times and in particular situations can lose their motivation if their work conditions change.

We argue that, even if motivation were a somewhat stable personality trait, it would still be important for managers to ensure that employees have work conditions that will reinforce their tendency to be motivated or change their tendency to be unmotivated. In short, motivation and behavior are produced by a complex interaction of situational and individual factors.

Myth 3: Motivation can be mass produced. A major myth about motivation is that it can be mass produced (for example, in speeches by charismatic leaders to large groups of people or by placing motivational posters throughout the workplace). Though these approaches sometimes work, most often they do not (Laurinaitis, 1997). Typically, in order to motivate people effectively, managers need to treat them as individuals. Contrary to the myth of mass production, we assert that individuals vary widely from each other in many ways. As a result, it is a central and recurring theme of this chapter that managers must motivate employees and coworkers on an individual basis, taking each person's situation into account. At least three important types of individual and situational differences should be considered:

1. job position or occupation
2. career stage
3. personal factors

Job position or occupation. One of the most distinctive features of health care organizations is the number of different occupational groups and job categories involved. These groups range from nurse's aides and porters to nurses, physical therapists, and physicians. Health care occupations vary along dimensions such as the amount and type of training they require, their power and status, and what types of individuals are attracted to them. Managers should understand how their ability to motivate individuals may vary according to their occupation or job category. For example, union contracts often prohibit certain types of changes in job design and responsibilities; managers need to know what occupational groups are covered by such contracts and how they affect certain approaches to motivation.

Career stage. A second important way in which individuals vary is their career stage. To illustrate, consider a recent graduate of a health services management program. He may be highly motivated by assignments that provide opportunities for learning about the different divisions of a health care organization. In contrast, his colleague who has more experience may wish to work on a single project from start to completion. Managers need to be sensitive to such career stage needs, motives, and values.

Personal factors. Perhaps more than we recognize, people at work are influenced by a variety of factors from their personal lives. For example, personal factors sometimes parallel career stages. A recent graduate may have few family ties that would limit her interest in work that involved travel, whereas a manager with young children may be less motivated by opportunity for travel on the job. Other important personal influences that can affect motivation include family illness, divorce, substance abuse, health problems, child care, and financial stress. These are clearly delicate areas for managers to tread. Yet, managers need to be aware that such personal factors can affect work motivation. On the one hand, it may be harmful to pry into the personal lives of employees and coworkers. On the other hand, it may be very helpful to be sensitive to needs at work that stem from their personal lives.

Myth 4: Money makes the world go 'round. We do not deny that many, if not most, individuals care about and are motivated by money. But too often managers think only of money when trying to motivate people. Unfortunately, money is likely to be in short supply for health care managers, at least in the next several years. Fortunately, money is not always the most important motivator; indeed, it seldom is. In the next sections, the importance of several other factors in motivating people that do not require cash will be discussed.

Manager's Role

The situational perspective described above implies that managers should take an active role in systematically assessing the motivation of their employees and coworkers. Individuals' motivation can vary over time and with the kind of work they are performing. Thus managers need to periodically assess motivation and performance, taking into account the occupational, career stage, and personal factors discussed above. Such assessments should include informal interviews with employees and coworkers in which open-ended questions are asked about individuals' needs, motives, perceptions, and values (Zima, 1983). These assessments need not be lengthy. What matters more is that they are timely; employees feel comfortable in openly expressing their concerns, and managers use the opportunity to do problem solving and goal setting. In short, managers can play a critical role

by not only assessing their employees' motivation but by taking the lead to alter conditions that can increase motivation.

What factors make people energized or aroused to work? Further, what factors influence how individuals' energy is directed and to what tasks, how intense their arousal is, and how long they persist in these states? These are the key questions that managers need to address to motivate people. Research attempts to explain work motivation through two basic types of theories: content and process. *Content theories* are concerned with *what* energizes behavior, while *process theories* focus on *how* behavior is energized.

CONTENT PERSPECTIVES

Content perspectives on motivation focus in large part on needs and need deficiencies. According to content perspectives, motivation can be considered a goal-directed, internal drive, which is always aimed at satisfying needs. A need can be a physical or psychological deficiency that makes specific outcomes or goals attractive. The need, in turn, stimulates individuals' internal drives, which directs them toward those goals that have the capacity to satisfy the need (O'Connor, 1998). Researchers agree that people have a multitude of needs with varying degrees of intensity. Such needs create a state of disequilibrium within the person, which, in turn, creates a desire to meet the need or needs he is experiencing. Consequently, individuals search the environment for potentially satisfying goals. Once attained, these goals will lead to a reduction in the disequilibrium or the fulfillment of their needs. Motivation can be increased to the degree that peoples' needs can be satisfied on the job.

Thus, content perspectives try to answer the question, What factor or factors motivate people? Some assert that motivation is a function of pay, working hours, and working conditions. Others suggest that autonomy and responsibility are the causes of motivation (Kovach, 1987). Still others believe either or both sets of factors could be important in a given situation.

The motivation framework in Figure 3.1 is a good starting point for understanding how needs can motivate people. The motivation process often begins

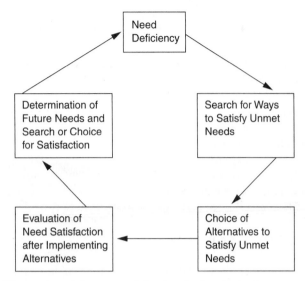

Figure 3.1. A Framework for Employee Motivation.

with needs that reflect some deficiency within the individual. For example, the employee might feel underpaid or lacking recognition *vis-a-vis* other employees. In response to these unsatisfied needs, the employee searches for ways to satisfy them. She may ask for a raise or promotion, work harder to try to earn either, or seek another position outside the organization. Next, she chooses one or more options. After implementing the chosen option or options, she then evaluates her success. If her hard work resulted in a pay raise or a promotion, she will probably continue to work hard. If neither has occurred, she will probably try another option.

The Need Hierarchy

Theory Overview

Many theorists advanced the concept of a need hierarchy, but Abraham Maslow (1943) developed the most popular version in the management field in the 1940s. He proposed that people want to satisfy various needs and that these needs can be arranged in a hierarchy of importance as shown in Figure 3.2.

Maslow's **hierarchy of needs** assumes there are five need levels that must be satisfied sequentially.

The *physiological* needs include such things as air, water, food, warmth, shelter, and sex. They represent basic issues of survival and biological function. In organization settings, such needs are generally satisfied by adequate wages and a satisfactory work environment that provides adequate lighting, temperature, and ventilation.

The *security* needs include a secure physical and emotional environment. Examples include the need to be free from worry about money and job security. In the workplace, security needs are satisfied by job continuity (no layoffs), a grievance system (to protect against arbitrary action), and an adequate health insurance and retirement package (for security against illness and eventual retirement). The latter is especially important, because as the health care environment continues to profoundly change, many employees may fear the loss of their jobs due to mergers, downsizing, or closings.

Because health care organizations have the potential to be fairly hazardous places to work, security needs are frequently important in these settings. The ICU nurses described earlier, for example, feared being subject to violence or of contracting conditions such as tuberculosis, hepatitis, or HIV. AIDs has created a great deal of fear among health care workers (Montgomery & Lewis, 1995).

Belongingness needs involve social processes. They include the need for love and affection and the need to be accepted by one's peers. For most people, they are satisfied by a combination of family and community relationships outside the job and friendships on the job. A manager can promote the satisfaction of these needs by encouraging social interaction and by making employees feel part of a team or work group. Sensitivity to an employee's family problems can also help employees meet this need.

Esteem needs are actually composed of two different sets of needs: the need for a positive self-image or self-respect and the need for recognition and respect from others. For example, the ICU nurses felt they did not receive adequate recognition for what they did on the job. They believed that physicians were getting all the credit. Managers can help address esteem needs by providing signs of accomplishment such as job titles, public recognition, and praise (i.e., extrinsic re-

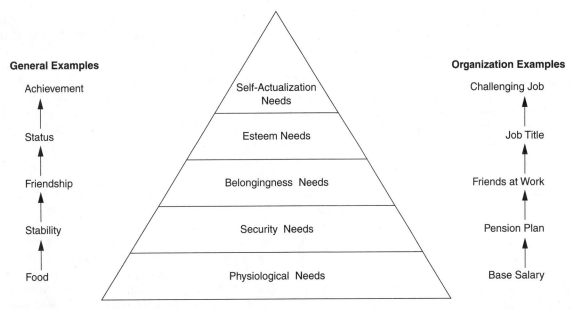

General Examples

Achievement

Status

Friendship

Stability

Food

Organization Examples

Challenging Job

Job Title

Friends at Work

Pension Plan

Base Salary

Self-Actualization Needs

Esteem Needs

Belongingness Needs

Security Needs

Physiological Needs

Figure 3.2. Maslow's Hierarchy of Needs.
SOURCE: Adapted from Maslow, A. H. A Theory of Human Motivation. *Psychological Review.* 1943; 50:370–396.

wards). They may also provide more challenging job assignments and other opportunities for employees to feel a sense of accomplishment.

Self-actualization needs, at the top of the hierarchy, involve realizing one's potential for continued growth and individual development. These are most difficult for a manager to identify and meet due to individual differences in goals. However, allowing employees to participate in decision making and the opportunity to learn new things about their work may promote self-actualization.

Maslow suggests that the five need categories constitute a hierarchy. People are motivated first to satisfy the lower level needs beginning with physiological needs. As long as these remain unsatisfied, the individual is motivated only to fulfill them. When these needs are satisfied, they cease to motivate people and they move up the hierarchy and become sequentially concerned with each higher level in turn. This process is termed *satisfaction-progression*—as an individual satisfies one set of needs, the next higher-level set of needs will dominate. This process will continue until the level of self-actualization is reached.

Research Support and Evaluation

The need hierarchy has a certain intuitive logic, but research indicates various shortcomings in the theory. While the progression principle suggests a systematic approach to satisfying needs from lowest to highest levels, research provides little evidence that a stepwise hierarchy actually exists. For example, some research shows that the five levels of need are not always present and the order of the levels is not always the same as Maslow proposed (Pinder, 1984; Steers & Porter, 1987).

Nor has research confirmed the deficit principle, in which unmet needs systematically motivate behavior (Schwartz, 1983). Needs do not fall into a neat five-step hierarchy (Mitchell & Mowdgill, 1976; Wahba & Budwell, 1976). There are some rather obvious exceptions to the theory to necessitate caution. For example, outstanding artists have continued their creative work while sacrificing health and security. Soldiers risk death for an ideal. Some employees strive for excellence despite their low-wage, dead-end jobs. Others employed in higher-wage jobs offering numerous opportunities for growth and development fail to take advantage of such opportunities. While their lower-level needs are being met, they do not strive to meet higher-level needs identified by Maslow's need hierarchy.

A major reason why the literature shows little support for Maslow's theory is because the needs are ambiguous and overlap, rather than being distinct and independent (Lee, 1980). In some studies, the lower-level needs formed a cluster, and the higher-level needs formed a cluster.

The major problem with Maslow's need hierarchy is that it cannot be turned into a practical guide for managers who are trying to enhance work motivation. The research evidence is just not there to support such rules of thumb as "If you satisfy employees' physiological and safety needs through job security and a competitive compensation system, then employees will be motivated mainly by needs for affiliation or self-actualization." It would be helpful if the advice were accurate, but it is not.

Application

Though managers cannot apply Maslow's needs hierarchy mechanistically, it is not unreasonable to conclude that unmet needs do motivate *most* employees *most* of the time. Maslow did identify some of the major categories of human needs that *may* motivate different employees at different times. In practical terms, organizations should provide employees with wages sufficient for food and shelter; reasonable protection of jobs, health, and safety; a satisfactory physical and social environment at work; and rewards or recognition that reinforce individual esteem. Managers should also recognize and support growth needs by providing opportunities for career advancement, encouraging personal self-development, and creating environments in which individuals can explore their individual talents and dreams.

The major implication of Maslow's theory for management is that organization policies and practices must pay attention to all of these needs if the organization hopes to have employees working up to their full potential. For example, allowing understaffing so that registered nurses work such long hours that they do not get enough sleep probably reduces their de-

sires for providing high-quality patient care (achievement) and creativity. During periods of retrenchment, being arbitrary and capricious about employees' job security interferes with cooperation, initiative, and other desirable behaviors. On the other hand, paying exclusive attention to the more basic physiological and security needs while ignoring the needs for achievement and self-esteem would defeat organizational purposes. Maslow's theory keeps managers aware of employees' higher level needs when considering motivation strategies.

It should also be noted that people's needs change over time. The needs, wants, and desires of individuals in their sixties differ from those of individuals in their twenties. Moreover, all employees have a variety of needs motivating them, and these differ by individual. One study found that the individual's position in the organizational hierarchy affects need satisfaction significantly with lower-level personnel less satisfied with their level of need achievement than higher-level personnel (Hurka, 1980). The manager's task is to develop situations that permit as many employees as possible to satisfy as many wants as possible. The astute manager will recognize what specific needs are important to motivate each individual. When possible, the manager will alter his or her supervisory style, economic and noneconomic rewards, job assignments, and related factors to maximize need fulfillment of as many people as possible.

ERG Theory

Theory Overview

As a result of the above criticisms of Maslow's approach to employee motivation, Clayton Alderfer proposed an alternative hierarchy called the ERG theory of motivation (Alderfer, 1972). The letters *E, R,* and *G* stand for existence, relatedness, and growth. The ERG theory collapses Maslow's need hierarchy into three levels. *Existence* needs correspond to the physiological and security needs of Maslow's hierarchy. *Relatedness* needs focus on how people relate to others and encompass Maslow's need to belong and need to earn the esteem of others. *Growth* needs include both the need for self-esteem and self-actualization.

While the ERG theory assumes a hierarchy of needs as suggested by Maslow, there are three important differences. First, the ERG theory suggests that more than one level of need can motivate behavior at the same time. Unlike Maslow, the emergence of relatedness and growth needs does not require satisfaction of the existence needs. For example, people can be motivated by a desire for money (existence), friendship (relatedness), and the opportunity to learn new skills all at once.

Second, while Maslow's hierarchy functions according to the satisfaction-progression principle, whereby essentially satisfied needs progress to a higher level of needs, the ERG theory has a *frustration-regression* element. Maslow maintained that each lower-level need must be satisfied before an individual can progress to a higher need level. In contrast, the ERG theory suggests that if needs remain unsatisfied at higher levels (i.e., growth), the individual will become frustrated, regress to a lower level, and begin to pursue those things again. For example, an employee receiving "adequate" pay (as defined by the employee) may attempt to seek opportunities for personal growth on the job. If these needs are frustrated, the employee may regress to being motivated to earn more money.

Third, the ERG theory suggests that needs are not fixed. The opportunities available in the organization may affect employee needs. Relatedness and growth needs may become more intense in an organization where there is ample opportunity to meet them (Mitchell, 1984).

Research Support and Evaluation

Research suggests that the ERG theory may be a more valid account of employee motivation in organizations than Maslow's needs hierarchy (Alderfer, 1968; Pinder, 1984), but it, too, has received contradictory reviews when empirically examined (Schneider & Alderfer, 1973). The key insights from both Maslow and Alderfer are that some needs are more important than others and that people may change their behavior after any particular set of needs have been satisfied.

Application

The major managerial implication of the ERG theory is that health care managers should assume that *all*

employees have the potential for continued growth and development. This suggests the desirability of offering ongoing opportunities for training and development, transfer, promotion, and career planning to all employees.

Two-Factor Theory

Theory Overview

Another well-known content perspective on employee motivation is the two-factor theory developed by Frederich Herzberg on the basis of 200 interviews with accountants and engineers in Pittsburgh (Herzberg, 1987; Herzberg, Mausner, & Snyderman, 1959). He asked them to describe occasions when they felt especially satisfied and highly motivated and other occasions when they had been dissatisfied and unmotivated. Surprisingly, he found that entirely different sets of factors were associated with satisfaction and high motivation and with dissatisfaction and low motivation. He found that the key factors in satisfaction and motivation were achievement, recognition, the work itself, responsibility, and advancement. He labeled these factors **motivators** since their presence increases job satisfaction and motivation but their absence does not lead to dissatisfaction. Herzberg also found that if a second group of factors, **hygiene factors,** were negative or absent, dissatisfaction results. These hygiene factors included company policy and administration, supervision, salary, interpersonal relations, and working conditions. The presence of positive hygiene factors, by themselves, prevents dissatisfaction but does not lead to satisfaction and motivation.

Note that the factors influencing the satisfaction dimension—motivation factors—are specifically related to the work content (i.e., intrinsic factors). The factors presumed to cause dissatisfaction—hygiene factors—are related to the work environment. According to Herzberg, changing the environment alone will not enhance employee motivation.

Research Support and Evaluation

Herzberg's two-factor theory has several limitations and weaknesses. His sample was not representative of the general population. His findings may also have been affected by the fact that people often attribute good outcomes (satisfaction) to themselves, and poor outcomes (dissatisfaction) to others. The findings in his initial interviews are subject to different interpretations, some of which differ from the one he offered. Subsequent research often failed to uphold the theory in that some factors, such as salary, appear to be associated with both satisfaction and dissatisfaction (House & Wigdor, 1967; Pinder, 1984; Vroom, 1964). Research also shows that both categories of factors serve to motivate. In one study of managerial and professional workers, the hygiene factors were as frequently associated with self-reports of high performance as were the motivators (Schwarb, Devitt, & Cummings, 1971).

Other researchers question whether the individual factors are mutually exclusive. For example, salary is defined as a hygiene factor, but for many highly paid executives and professionals, salary may be viewed as a form of recognition. Logic suggests that, in reality, these factors do not operate separately from one another in a given person. The desires for advancement and for recognition—both motivators—are connected to feelings and attitudes about salary—a hygiene factor.

Still other researchers criticize the theory for being too simple. Lee (1980) flatly states that "the evidence to date clearly eliminates Herzberg's theory as a general or universal theory of work motivation." Steers and Porter (1987), on the other hand, take a more positive view: "It appears that a fruitful approach to this controversial theory would be to learn from it that which can help us to develop more improved models rather than to accept or reject the model totally."

A recent study examined how 13 variables affected 522 health care managers in motivating them to remain (retention) in their current position, or to be recruited (recruitment) into a new one (Fottler, Shewchuk, & O'Connor, 1998). Of these variables, four were consistently observed to be the most important in making a retention or recruitment decision (see Figures 3.3 and 3.4). These four variables were (1) freedom in decision making, (2) opportunities for personal growth, (3) caliber of the management team, and (4) opportunities for advancement. In keeping with Herzberg's theory, the variable least likely to influence

health care managers in their decision to stay with, or leave, an organization was appearance of the physical work environment. These observed results and others (Alpander, 1985; Longest, 1974) offer some limited corroboration to the greater importance of motivators and the lesser importance of hygienes in terms of what motivates workers in health care settings.

Application

Despite the above criticisms, the two-factor theory has had a major impact by increasing managers' awareness of motivation and its importance. Herzberg argued there are two stages in motivating employees. First, the manager must make sure the hygiene factors are not deficient. Pay and security must be appropriate, working conditions must be safe, and supervision must be acceptable. By providing hygiene factors at an appropriate level, the manager does not stimulate motivation but does avoid dissatisfaction.

The manager should then proceed to stage two— giving employees the opportunity to experience motivation factors such as achievement and recognition. The result is predicted to be a high level of satisfaction and motivation. Herzberg goes a step further than most theorists and describes exactly how to use the two-factor theory in the workplace. Specifically, he recommends that jobs be redesigned and enriched to provide higher levels of the motivation factors. For example, the jobs of some clinical laboratory workers can become extremely monotonous and boring because the work is often highly standardized, which results in exacting routines. As the standardized task is repeated over and over, the work becomes more tedious and less likely to offer potential motivation. Redesigning a job to be horizontally enlarged so that a worker carries out a greater variety of tasks can help in this regard. By further enriching this job, the worker would now have greater control over a wider variety of tasks.

Herzberg's theory has great value for health care managers because it identifies a wide range of factors involved in employee motivation. Consideration of all of these factors is useful in any attempt to enhance motivation and to diminish demotivating factors in an organization. The theory has also had a major influence on job design in many health services organiza-

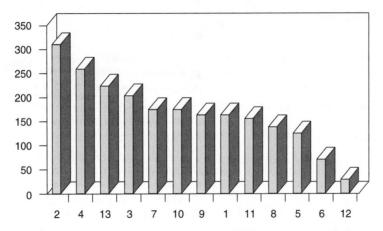

1. Salary (163)
2. Freedom in Decision-Making (311)
3. Opportunities for Advancement (203)
4. Opportunities for Personal Growth (260)
5. Chance to Serve Humankind (124)
6. High Job Profile/Visibility (72)
7. Organization's Reputation (180)
8. Organization's Financial Condition (137)
9. Geographic Location (164)
10. Institutional Mission/Values (177)
11. Corporate Culture (157)
12. Appearance of Physical Work Environment (34)
13. Caliber of the Management Team (223)

Figure 3.3. Relative Perceived Importance of Retention Variables.
SOURCE: Fottler, M. D., Shewchuk, R. M., O'Connor, S. J. What matters to health care executives? Assessing the job attributes associated with their staying or leaving. *International Journal of Organization Theory and Behavior.* 1998: 1(2):223–247, p. 238.

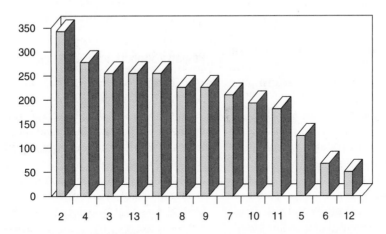

1. Salary (253)
2. Freedom in Decision-Making (344)
3. Opportunities for Advancement (256)
4. Opportunities for Personal Growth (277)
5. Chance to Serve Humankind (127)
6. High Job Profile/Visibility (73)
7. Organization's Reputation (213)
8. Organization's Financial Condition (226)
9. Geographic Location (225)
10. Institutional Mission/Values (194)
11. Corporate Culture (180)
12. Appearance of Physical Work Environment (48)
13. Caliber of the Management Team (255)

Figure 3.4. Relative Perceived Importance of Recruitment Variables.
SOURCE: Fottler, M. D., Shewchuk, R. M., O'Connor, S. J. What matters to health care executives? Assessing the job attributes associated with their staying or leaving. *International Journal of Organization Theory and Behavior.* 1998; 1(2):223–247, p. 238.

tions because it has made managers more aware of the importance of job challenge and responsibility in motivation (also see Chapter 7). The recent trend toward the employment of multiskilled health practitioners is one manifestation of this awareness (Blayney, 1992; Vaughan, Fottler, Bamberg, & Blayney, 1991).

Learned Need Theory

Theory Overview

The theories of Maslow, Alderfer, and Herzberg identify a number of individual needs and then attempt to arrange them in some kind of order of importance. Other content views of employee motivation focus more on the important needs themselves without concern for ordering them. The three needs most often discussed are the needs for *achievement, power,* and *affiliation.* Far more importantly, it has been argued that these needs and the behaviors associated with the efforts to satisfy them can be learned (McClelland, 1961, 1975).

John W. Atkinson (1961) proposed that everyone enjoys an "energy reserve" that can be released depending upon individual incentives to achieve desired goals. He also proposed the above three basic human drives. David C. McClelland (1961) gave form to these three drives and related them to performance in organizations.

The first basic drive is the need for achievement and refers to the individual's need to accomplish complex tasks, compete, and resolve problems. It reflects the desire to achieve a goal more effectively than in the past. People with a high need for achievement are assumed to have a desire for personal responsibility, a tendency to set moderately difficult goals, a need for specific goals and immediate feedback, and a preoccupation with their task.

The second basic drive, a need for power, refers to the individual's desire to influence or control others' behavior. It also represents the desire to control one's environment. Individuals high in power needs are thought to be more suited to management than achievers. In this view, "power" implies being responsible for control of others and for influencing behavior in complex situations (McClelland & Burnham, 1976).

The third drive, the need for affiliation, reflects an individual's desire to associate with others in friendly circumstances. It is similar to Maslow's belongingness need. Those high in affiliation prefer friendly, participative work environments where the quality of group interaction with coworkers is more highly valued than achievements or influence. People with a strong need for affiliation are likely to prefer (and perform better in) a job that entails a lot of social interaction. Few of these individuals manage effectively in most organizations because they tend to emphasize friendship at the expense of organizational productivity and effectiveness. As McClelland and Burnham (1976) state, "[t]he top manager's need for power ought to be greater than his or her need for being liked." However, as teamwork becomes increasingly necessary to carry out administrative functions, somewhat stronger needs for affiliation may be a welcome adjunct for health care managers. By being somewhat more accommodating and cooperative, those managers maintaining slightly greater needs for affiliation may benefit a team-based work setting by reducing dysfunctional conflict and bringing together diverse groups of workers.

Research Support and Evaluation

McClelland concluded that, although the need for achievement is the main motivation for those who wish to start and develop their own small businesses, the need for power is a crucial motivator of top executives in larger, more complex organizations. Most successful managers exercise their power in a controlled and disciplined way on behalf of others and create a strong sense of team spirit among their subordinates. Studies have found that managers as a group tend to have a stronger power motive than the general population and that successful managers tend to have stronger power motives than less successful managers (Holland, Black, & Miner, 1987; McClelland & Burnham, 1976). Other research has shown that people with a strong need for power are likely to be superior performers, have good attendance records, and occupy supervisory positions (Cornelius & Lane, 1984). Chusmir (1986) evaluated 70 health-related job categories relative to the extent they satisfied needs for power, achievement, and affiliation. In his study, the health care jobs best able to satisfy needs for power, and least able to fulfill affiliation needs, are predominantly management roles such as nursing school dean or hospital administrator (Table 3.1).

Persons with high achievement needs tend to flourish in very competitive situations, enjoy challenges, and thrive in complex and stimulating environments such as those found in most health care organizations. McClelland argued that these achievers would be best suited to situations where independent responsibility and autonomy prevail. The implication is that, while many achievers are found in professional positions such as physicians, they are not always among the best managers in highly bureaucratic organizations. Since such organizations are based on diffused authority and group activities, achievers are often uncomfortable in situations of group responsibility and control. The health care occupations in Chusmir's (1986) study that appear best able to fulfill the achievement need are those of technician (dialysis, electrocardiographic, surgical, hematology/serology) and technologist (i.e., medical, radiologic, nuclear medicine).

An important aspect of McClelland's theory is that all three needs are acquired. Individuals develop these needs to varying degrees through life experiences. They are learned drives evolving from one's background and environment. Indeed, since a high need for achievement is important for professional and managerial success in nonbureaucratic organizations, McClelland devised a training program for increasing one's need for achievement. Studies found that employees who complete this achievement training tend to make more money and receive promotions faster than other employees (Kiechel, 1989; Nicholls, 1984). Moreover, achievement training may also affect organizational outcomes. In one case, three different groups of small business employees were given 70 hours of achievement training and assistance. Median profits for these businesses increased from $280 per month to $670 per month (Miron & McClelland, 1979).

Application

Other managerial implications of McClelland's work are far reaching. For individuals already set in their ways, matching work environments with their needs is crucial to their motivation and career success. Employees established in health care organizations undergoing rapid change may need counseling or education to help them adapt to the new environment. For example, an affiliation-oriented manager may not fare well in an entrepreneurial environment that emphasizes achievement.

Further, organizations might focus on identifying and selecting individuals with high levels of achievement motivation or other desired values and behavior. Irvine (CA) Medical Center, for example, uses both psychological testing and structured interviewing in employment selection and promotion decisions (Eubanks, 1991). These approaches determine the prospective candidate's service orientation, performance, motivations, and ability to work as a team member. The result has been a collaborative, achievement-oriented culture with shared values among the employees.

An Assessment of Content Theories

It is well accepted that motivation has important origins in human needs. Need theories of motivation assume that people attempt to satisfy such needs and wants. A simplistic view is that all a manager or supervisor has to do to release his or her employees' motivation potential is to identify their needs and then take steps to satisfy them. Unfortunately, there is no simple set of needs and need satisfiers that would be universally applicable. First, as noted above, people differ on the basis of age, sex, race, and other demographic and background characteristics. No one set of motivators is likely to be appropriate for all employees since their needs will be different. Second, the organizational context and culture differ both across organizations and within organizations. The learned needs of a given individual may vary depending on the incentives present in his or her organization. Third, for a given individual, needs change over time. This has already been implied by the needs hierarchy theorists. The relative importance of various needs are continuously changing, thus forcing managers to aim at a moving target. Fourth, employees in different positions in an organizational

Table 3.1. Health Care Motivation Profiles of over 70 Health-Related Occupations in Terms of the Degree to Which They Satisfy Needs for Achievement, Power, and Affiliation

Job Title	DOT Code	Need Profile	Ach	Aff	Pwr
Hospital administration and operations					
Hospital administrator, superintendent, coordinator rehabilitation services					
Emergency medical services coordinator, sanitarian	117	Pwr	2	1	4
Coordinator auxiliary personnel	127	Pwr	2	1	5
Supervisor, volunteer services, food service, ward service, tray line, floor					
Housekeeper, manager	137	Ach and Pwr	3	2	3
Executive chef	161	Ach	4	1	2
Central supply supervisor	164	Balanced	2	2	2
Medical services administrator, hospital record administrator, communications					
Coordinator, assistant hospital administrator, executive housekeeper,					
Librarian, director food services, director volunteer services, building					
superintendent, laundry superintendent	167	Pwr	3	2	4
Hospital insurance representative	267	Pwr	3	2	4
Hospital collection clerk	357	Ach	4	2	2
Cook	361	Ach	4	2	2
Hospital admitting clerk, cashier, insurance clerk, receiving clerk, ward clerk	362	Ach	4	2	2
Medical record technician, x-ray file clerk, medical service technician	367	Balanced	3	3	3
Ambulance attendant, emergency medical technician	374	Aff	1	4	1
Ward supervisor, ward attendant, psychiatric aide	377	Aff	1	4	1
Linen room attendant, clerk, checker, exchange attendant	387	Aff	2	3	2
Television rental clerk	467	Aff	2	3	2
Food tray assembler	484	Aff	0	3	0
Formula maker, formula room worker	487	Aff	1	3	1
Diet clerk aide	587	Aff	1	2	0
Hospital attendant	674	Aff	0	3	0
Hospital entrance attendant, messenger, admitting office guide, food service worker,					
Tray line worker	677	Aff	1	3	0
Ambulance driver	683	Pwr	1	1	2
Central supply worker, cleaner, clothes room workers	687	Aff	4	0	2
Medical and dental technology					
Medical technologist, teaching supervisor	121	Ach	4	0	2
Medical technologist, chief	161	Ach	5	1	2
Radiologic technologist, chief	162	Ach	5	1	2

(continues)

hierarchy will undoubtedly differ in terms of their configuration of needs and potential motivators. Fifth, resource constraints or lack of such constraints may also impact the relative importance of various needs.

Despite these caveats, content theories of motivation help health care managers focus on individual needs in the motivation process. All provide useful insights into factors that may promote motivation in a given situation. Moreover, they are not separate and discrete views of motivation but share much in com-

mon with one another. Figure 3.5 compares the needs identified by the four content theories described in this section. It should be noted that, while they do not necessarily agree on whether there is a hierarchy of needs or whether individuals attempt to satisfy multiple needs simultaneously, some of their basic concepts are similar and overlap with one another.

Employees in health services organizations have a variety of needs motivating them. For example, one study of registered nurses found achievement, interpersonal relations, and the work itself to be major mo-

Table 3.1. (*continued*)

Job Title	DOT Code	Need Profile	Ach	Aff	Pwr
Medical and dental technology (*continued*)					
Chemistry, microbiology, technologists, orthotist, prosthetist	261	Ach	5	1	2
Cytotechnologist	281	Ach	3	1	1
Medical, nuclear medicine, hematology serology, tissue technologists, orthotist, Prosthetist assistant	361	Ach	4	2	2
Dialysis, electrocardiographic technicians, electroencephalographic, radiology, x-ray technologists	362	Ach	4	2	2
Ultrasound technologist	364	Ach	4	2	2
Surgical technician	374	Aff	1	4	1
Medical and dental technology					
Medical lab assistant or technician, hematology or serology technician	381	Aff	3	2	1
Cephalometric analyst	384	Aff	1	3	1
X-ray developing machine operator	685	Aff	0	1	0
Laboratory assistant	687	Aff	1	2	0
Nursing					
Dean, school of nursing, educational consultant, state board nursing; directors: Community health nursing, educational community health, nursing service, Occupational health nursing, school of nursing, executive director nurses association	117	Pwr	2	1	4
Nurse instructor	121	Pwr	4	0	2
School nurse, community health staff nurse	124	Pwr	1	1	3
Head nurse, nurse supervisor, nurse consultant	127	Pwr	2	1	4
Nurse practitioner, nurse midwife	264	Balanced	2	2	2
Nurse anesthetist	371	Ach and Aff	3	3	1
General duty nurse, office nurse, private duty nurse, staff nurse, licensed practical nurse	374	Aff	1	4	1
Therapists					
Coordinator, rehabilitation services	117	Pwr	2	1	4
Occupational, physical, manual arts, recreational therapists	124	Pwr	1	1	3
Art, music therapists	127	Pwr	2	1	4
Hypnotherapists	157	Ach	4	1	1
Industrial therapists	167	Pwr	3	2	4
Physical therapist assistant	224	Pwr	1	1	3
Corrective or respiratory	361	Ach	4	2	2
Assistant therapy aide	377	Aff	2	4	2

SOURCE: Chusmir L.H. (1986). How fulfilling are health care jobs? *Health Care Management Review*, 11(1), p. 30.

tivators (Longest, 1974), another identified autonomy or personal control, promotion opportunities, and work scheduling (Ford & Fottler, 1992), and yet another found interpersonal relations, work itself, and recognition to be most important (Rantz, Scott, & Porter, 1996). While the specifics differed in all studies, most of the key factors were motivators identified by Herzberg. The task of health care managers is to identify the specific needs of their employees and then develop opportunities that permit these employees to satisfy their needs.

Employees' needs can be identified by attitude surveys and continuous two-way oral communication with various subgroups of employees (Farnham, 1989; Reibstein, 1986). When possible, the manager should also attempt to recognize what needs are important in the motivation of each individual employee and to match those needs to the requirements

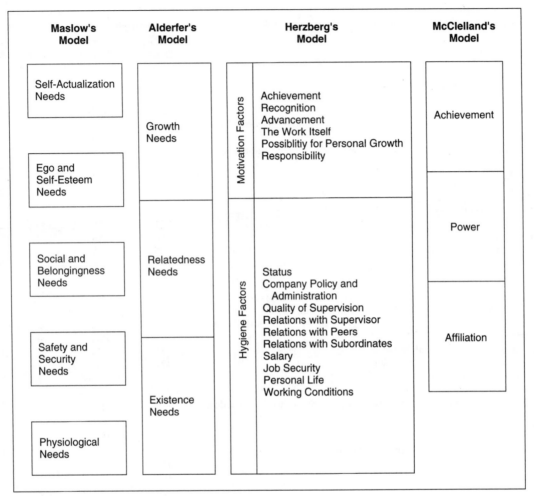

Figure 3.5. A Comparison of Needs Theories of Motivation.

of positions to which those individuals are assigned (Chusmir, 1986). Studies of job redesign typically find significant increases in motivation and performance over time (Hackman & Oldham, 1980; Griffin, 1991). Needs themselves may also be modified by special motivation training courses (Durand, 1983).

Based on identified needs, astute managers will alter their leadership and communication style, economic rewards, noneconomic rewards, job assignments, training and development emphases, and feedback to maximize the need fulfillment of as many subordinates as possible. For example, some will need to be left alone to work independently. Others will need more structure, goals, and feedback. Since employees have different needs, they must be managed in different ways. The following managerial guidelines provide a convenient summary of the managerial implications of content theories.

Though content theories provide useful insights into motivational factors, they do not constitute a complete theoretical or managerial approach to employee motivation. They do not shed much light on the

MANAGERIAL GUIDELINES

1. Employees often have unmet needs that they attempt to satisfy through work. These include physiological, security, social esteem, self-control, power, and achievement needs. Such unmet needs will vary from individual to individual based on a wide variety of factors. No two persons will have the same proportion of each of these needs.

2. At any given point in time, people attempt to satisfy a wide variety of needs. They exchange their labor for rewards that they value because these rewards respond to their needs. Such rewards may be intrinsic or extrinsic to the job. Intrinsic motivation is particularly important for health care professionals.

3. Health care managers can motivate people by determining what needs and rewards they view as most important. This can be accomplished through formal and informal means of communication.

4. Rewards may be both economic and noneconomic. They should be relevant to the priority needs of particular employees or employee groups. What is a hygiene factor for one person may be a motivator for another. However, satisfied needs are not motivators for anyone.

5. Employees should be selected on the basis of how well their needs, motivations, and qualifications match the requirements of each position. Written examinations and oral interviews may be used to assess the degree of job-applicant match.

6. Redesigning jobs is another alternative for increasing this match. Redesigning offers much potential for increased motivation to the extent that it involves building in responsibility, decision making, control, autonomy, challenge, and opportunities for achievement.

7. Training programs that emphasize enhancement of the achievement motive can enhance motivation.

8. Managers should be concerned with both hygiene factors and motivators as defined by the employees themselves.

---

process of motivation. For example, they do not explain why employees might be motivated by one factor rather than by another at a given level or how their different needs might be satisfied. These questions involve behaviors or actions, goals, and feelings of satisfaction that are addressed by various process theories of motivation. It is to these theories that we now turn.

PROCESS PERSPECTIVES

In this section, we examine five approaches to motivation that, although they differ from each other, share a focus on the processes involved in motivation. In contrast to the approaches examined in the previous section that concern the content of work and its influence on motivation, these approaches attend to the context in which work is done as well as individuals' reactions—especially thoughts and feelings—to work.

Equity Theory

Theory Overview

Adams proposed a theory of work motivation that assumes that individuals value and seek fairness, or **equity,** in their relationships with employers (Adams, 1963, 1965). Relationships are fair when people perceive that their outcomes (e.g., pay) are proportionate to their perceived contributions or inputs (e.g., task performance). Further, people evaluate fairness by comparing themselves to others. In other words, people contrast their perceived inputs and outcomes with their perceptions of others' inputs and outcomes. To the extent that this ratio is seen as unequal, individuals experience tension.

Adams proposed two kinds of inequity. Underpayment refers to the case when someone perceives that she is receiving fewer rewards from a job than another person making a comparable contribution. In contrast, overpayment occurs when someone perceives that she is receiving more rewards than another person making a comparable contribution.

Adams also proposed that people are motivated to reduce tensions that result from perceived inequity. The greater the perceived inequity and resulting tension, the greater the motivation to reduce it. In other words, from the perspective of equity theory, work motivation stems from the need to reduce tensions caused by inequity.

Depending on the magnitude of the perceived injustice and individual as well as situational circumstances, people may use one of several approaches to reduce inequity and restore balance in their relationships with employers. These approaches include altering their perceptions of their own or others' inputs or outcomes, changing their inputs or outcomes, getting others to change their inputs or outcomes, and leaving the inequitable situation altogether (Campbell & Pritchard, 1976).

Research Support and Evaluation

There are a relatively large number of studies testing various aspects of Adams's equity theory. Most of these have concentrated on the effects of perceived inequity in pay on quality and quantity of work performance when people are paid either hourly or on a piece-rate. Results from most studies support equity theory's hypotheses about the effects of underpayment (Greenberg, 1982). The results from studies examining hourly payment are also stronger than results from studies examining piece-rate payment (Muchinsky, 1987). One study found experimental support for the "double demotivation" hypothesis—that pay discrepancies decrease work motivation in both lower- as well as higher-paid groups. "Compared with equitably paid workers, employees who felt they were being under- or overpaid reported lower job satisfaction and greater readiness to change jobs" (Carr, McLoughlin, Hodgson, & MacLachlan, 1996).

Despite the empirical support for equity theory, it has several limitations that managers should consider. The theory does not help to identify which of several approaches to restoring equity an individual will take. In actual work situations, there are typically several ways that perceived inequities can be addressed. One can simply convince oneself that an inequity is not worth worrying about or will be reduced at the next annual review.

Further, the theory does not specify who people are likely to compare themselves with to assess their equity with employers. Do people compare themselves more often with immediate coworkers, or are comparisons with colleagues in other organizations equally or more important? For example, do primary care physicians compare their income to that of specialists such as orthopedic surgeons, or do they only consider the pay levels of other primary care physicians?

Another problem is that studies have not examined how perceptions of equity vary over time and how such variation affects motivation (Kanfer, 1990). Most studies take a short-term view of equity issues, and the theory provides little guidance about how to deal with variation over time in work situations. Finally, it is not clear how this theory can be used to motivate people who perceive no important inequities in their work. That is, the theory proposes that people are motivated to reduce tensions created by perceived inequities in inputs and outcomes. It provides no guidance for managers once they have addressed perceived inequities other than to try to be as fair as possible.

Application

Despite the limitations just noted, we believe that equity theory provides some useful guidelines for health care managers. First, it is important to note that people compare themselves to others in many situations and in many ways. Such comparisons affect not only their motivation but other aspects of their behavior as well. When people experience uncertainty, they are especially likely to turn to others, consciously or unconsciously, to provide them with cues about what to do. Equity theory would be useful even if its only contribution were to remind us of the importance of social comparison. The case of the ICU nurses presented earlier is a good example of this. The ICU nurses compared themselves to the external pool nurses who worked alongside them. From this comparison, they felt that they earned $12 per hour less and contributed substantially more.

Second, managers need to directly address perceptions of inequities so that individuals are not motivated to reduce their contributions or inputs or to leave their jobs. It may be that perceptions of inequity can be changed simply by explaining differences between jobs or other conditions that make it necessary to reward or treat people differently. In other cases, managers may need to consider pay raises or increases in other ways to reward people. In still other cases, there may be nothing that a manager can do to restore perceptions of equity. But, if such concerns are not addressed, it is clear that they can be a source of motivational problems.

Finally, we have argued that it is important to motivate people on an individual basis. Equity theory reminds us that even this approach has limits. To the extent that people are treated as individuals, perceptions of inequity are likely to increase because people will be comparing themselves to others who are being treated differently; such differences can trigger perceptions of inequity.

Expectancy Theory

Theory Overview

Expectancy theory has several variations that all trace their roots to cognitive psychology in the early 1950s. Georgopoulos, Mahoney, and Jones and Vroom were the first to apply expectancy theory to work motivation (Georgopoulos, Mahoney, & Jones, 1957; Vroom, 1964). Vroom's expectancy model was particularly influential. Since this early research, expectancy theory has become perhaps the most prominent theory of work motivation. The theory assumes that people are rational decision makers who will expend effort on work that will lead to desired rewards. Further, the theory assumes that people know what rewards they want from work and understand that their performance will determine the extent to which they attain the rewards they value.

Though there are several variations of expectancy theory, they all share four central components (Mitchell, 1982). First, there are *job outcomes*. These include both rewards (e.g., pay raises, promotions, recognition) and negative experiences (e.g., job loss, demotion).

Second, there are *valences*. These are individuals' feelings about job outcomes. Like job outcomes, they can range from positive to neutral to negative, and they vary in strength as well as direction.

The third component is *instrumentality*, which refers to the perceived link between performance and outcomes. In other words, instrumentality is the extent to which individuals believe that attaining a job outcome depends on, or is conditional on, their performance. For example, if a nurse thought that an outcome (pay raise) depended highly on his performance rather than some other factor (hospital patient volume), the instrumentality for the outcome would be high.

Finally, *expectancy* is the perceived link between effort and performance. That is, to what extent do individuals believe that there is a relationship between how hard they try and how well they do.

Using the expectancy theory model, we can illustrate the degree to which the primary care physician described in "In the Real World" will be motivated to vigorously adhere to the HMO's disease-management guidelines. Expectancy is the perceived link between effort and performance. This physician is confident that by following the guidelines, he will be able to do a reasonably good job of controlling the disease among his patients. In other words, the physician has a high expectancy probability for performing effective diabetes disease management. However, the physician knows that due to the higher short-term costs of effectively managing his patients, there is also a high probability that he will not share in any financial bonuses paid out at year's end. Because this is a job outcome he does not favor, it receives a negative valence. Instrumentality, or the probability that performance will lead to outcomes, is fairly high, but the outcome has a forceful negative valence. Because the outcome (no end-of-year bonus) is not related to performance, the physician's motivation to carry out

IN THE REAL WORLD:
MOTIVATING A PRIMARY CARE PHYSICIAN IN AN HMO

Dennis Ralston, M.D., a primary care physician, is employed by a large, staff model health maintenance organization (HMO). Because such a large proportion of his patients are diabetic, he has been intimately involved in the development of a new, long-term diabetic disease management program for his HMO. The HMO wants the disease to be managed in such a way that it is kept under control so that patients can maintain a higher quality of life and longer-term costs do not rise as a result of the need for more extensive medical interventions. Dr. Ralston is very confident that between his own ability and the detailed guidelines for managing the disease developed by the HMO, he will be able to do a good job of keeping his diabetic patients' disease under control. The disease-management guidelines require him to get patients to test their blood sugar levels four times per day using testing strips that cost over $100 per month, and to frequently order relatively expensive laboratory tests, glaucoma screenings, and podiatric referrals throughout the course of a year.

The HMO uses financial incentives to motivate primary care physician behavior, primarily through the use of a "holdback," a bonus pool of dollars from which the physicians can share at the end of the year. The more dollars the physicians save the HMO over the course of the year, the bigger the pool—and the bigger the incentive check at year's end. Although the disease-management guidelines recently went into effect, the HMO's financial incentive system for its primary care physicians has not changed in any way. Dr. Ralston realizes that since a large percentage of his patients are diabetic, if he is to vigorously adhere to the guidelines, he may not receive any incentive dollars at year's end.

Adapted from S. J. O'Connor (1998). Motivating effective performance. In: Ginter P, Swayne L, Duncan WJ, eds. Handbook of Health Care Management. Cambridge, MA: Blackwell Business Publishing, 431–470.

---

high-quality diabetes disease management has been substantially reduced.

Motivation is the end product of valence, instrumentality, and expectancy. People are motivated when a combination of factors occurs: They value an outcome (i.e., valence is high and positive), they believe that good performance will be rewarded with desired outcomes (i.e., instrumentality is high), and they believe that their efforts will produce good performance (i.e., expectancy is high). In contrast, motivation is likely to be low if the components of expectancy theory have low values. If people do not care about their job outcomes, then they have less reason to work for them. Or, if organizations do not link outcomes to performance (e.g., pay raises are linked to seniority rather than performance), then people have less reason to care about their performance. Similarly, if effort and performance seem unrelated, then there is less reason to try hard. Each of these factors can decrease motivation, and if all are present, it is improbable that moti-

vation will be high. The HMO administrator from the "In the Real World" may improve the linkage between outcomes and performance by placing greater emphasis on quality indicators as a condition of participating in the bonus incentive pool.

Research Support and Evaluation

Empirical support from many studies of expectancy theory is quite good (Hom, 1980; Kennedy, Fossum, & White, 1983; Muchinsky, 1987; Stacy, Widaman, & Marlatt, 1990; Tsui, Ashford, St. Clair, & Xin, 1995; Wanous, Keon, & Latack, 1983). Nonetheless, the theory seems to receive more support in studies that examine the levels of effort an individual will expend on different tasks than in studies that examine the strength of motivation across different people (Kennedy, Fossum, & White, 1983).

Expectancy theory rests clearly on the assumption that people are highly rational and consciously engage in decisions to work harder on tasks that they believe will maximize their gains while minimizing their losses. Though this assumption works quite well for many people in many situations, it is not universally valid. People have unconscious motives. Moreover, their calculations about the links between effort and performance and performance and reward are not always accurate. In this regard, the HMO physician may be highly motivated to control diabetes disease among his patients, while fully aware that such outcomes will not be financially rewarded. Most likely this is because he can acquire other valued outcomes such as a sense of personal satisfaction and achievement that derives from being able to effectively help people. People have unconscious motives. Moreover, their calculations about the links between effort and performance and performance and reward are not always accurate.

Further, some studies indicate that the strength of the theory may vary depending on personality factors (Weiner, 1986). For example, the theory may hold more strongly for people who have a high internal, rather than external, locus of control. Such people tend to believe that their lives are under their own control more than the control or influence of external events. As a result, people with a high internal locus of control believe that there are strong links between their efforts and performance and their performance and outcomes. These beliefs, as noted above, are central to the theory's predictions about motivation.

Application

Despite these limitations, expectancy theory (Figure 3.6) provides very useful guidelines for managerial action (Pritchard, De Leo, & Von Bergen, 1976). These include:

1. Incentives or job outcomes should be chosen so that they are attractive to employees. Perhaps the best way to do this is to ask employees directly about their preferences using surveys or interviews.
2. The rules for attaining incentives must be clear to all involved. For example, expected levels of performance should be spelled out in as much detail as possible. Such rules should be stated in job descriptions and employee orientations. These rules should also be reviewed periodically, both informally and formally. We add here a note from equity theory: The rules should be perceived as fair.
3. People must perceive that their efforts will lead to the desired level of performance.

There are many practical limitations involved here simply because several factors can intervene to weaken the link between effort and performance. For example, people may be trying hard but lack the resources (e.g.,

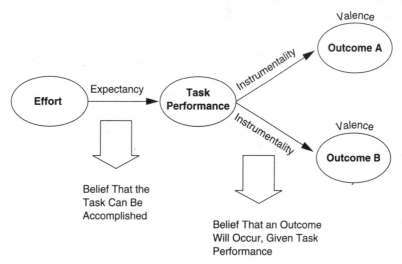

Figure 3.6. Expectancy Theory Process.

equipment) to do well, or as is often the case in health care, there is a great deal of interdependence between people so that performance depends on all their efforts. Work done in groups or teams often has this feature. When this is the case and coworkers' efforts are lacking, an individual's perceptions of the link between their efforts and group or unit performance can be easily diminished. In any case, managers need to make it clear that, insofar as they are able, they will not hold people accountable for performance problems that stem from factors not in their control.

Reinforcement Theory

Theory Overview

Reinforcement theory, also known as operant conditioning or behavior modification, is based on the work of B. F. Skinner. The theory has three components: stimulus, response, and consequence. A stimulus is any condition or variable that elicits a response, such as a request from a supervisor for some information. A response is a behavior performed contingent on a stimulus. A consequence is anything that follows a response that changes the likelihood that the response will occur again following a stimulus.

In turn, there are three types of consequences: rewards (termed *positive reinforcement*), which increase the likelihood of a response; punishments, which decrease the likelihood of a response; and negative reinforcement, which is the removal of a reward or punishment to increase the likelihood of a response.

Further, research shows that four types of connections between responses and consequences can increase the frequency of a response. These include:

1. *Fixed interval.* People are rewarded at a fixed time interval. For example, people paid on an hourly basis are on a fixed-interval reward schedule.
2. *Fixed ratio.* People are rewarded on the basis of a fixed number of responses. For example, physicians who are paid on a fee-for-service basis are rewarded on this schedule.
3. *Variable interval.* Responses are rewarded at some time interval that varies. For example, government safety inspections of hospital oncology units

for the proper storage, handling, and documentation of therapeutic radioactive materials such as iridium and cesium generally occur at any time and are unannounced (i.e., at variable intervals) (O'Connor, 1998).
4. *Variable ratio.* Reward is based on behavior, but the ratio of reward to responses varies. Gambling games such as lotteries and blackjack can be extremely addictive, because they reinforce the player on a variable schedule.

In short, from the perspective of reinforcement theory, motivation results when people are rewarded contingent on performance, based on the above schedules. In general, research indicates that responses are maintained best on ratio schedules.

Research Support and Evaluation

Research from a variety of settings indicates that reinforcement schedules work. As noted, the results may vary depending on the type of reinforcement schedule that is used, but performance is better when rewards are given contingently. This result is, of course, consistent with the views of expectancy theory.

Reinforcement theory has drawn sharp criticism since Skinner (1969) published his first work in this area. One critique is that it encourages managers and others to manipulate employees through the design of reinforcement schedules over which employees have no control. Similarly, if employees have no input into selecting rewards, reinforcement may be ineffective. The antidote for these criticisms seems clear: Employees need to have input into the design of reinforcement systems. Again, this guideline is consistent with an expectancy theory perspective.

A second common critique is that reinforcement theory presents a flat, one-dimensional view of human nature and motivation. That is, the theory says little about human emotion or cognition. People are often portrayed as somewhat mindless robots in pursuit of rewards. This critique is similar to a critique of expectancy theory; that is, it views people as very rational in pursuit of valued outcomes. The difference here is that critics of reinforcement theory argue that it does not even give people credit for thinking.

Application

The primary lesson from reinforcement theory is that performance, if not motivation, is better when rewards are given contingently. The effectiveness of reinforcement schedules will vary; thus it is best to take a pragmatic approach and see what works best in a given situation.

Goal Setting

Theory Overview

Locke (1968) proposed a motivation theory that focuses on the role of goals and *goal setting.* He and his colleagues define a *goal* as something that an individual is consciously attempting to attain (Locke & Latham, 1984, 1990a). Goals are powerful because they direct people's attention, focus effort on tasks related to goal attainment, and encourage people to persist in such tasks. Further, Locke proposed that the more difficult and specific the goal, the greater the motivation will be to attain it. In short, a goal provides guidelines for how much effort to put into work.

Several conditions must be met for goals to have a positive influence on performance. First, people must be aware of goals and know what must be done to attain them. Second, goals must be accepted as something that people are willing to work for. People must be committed to goals. In other words, goals can fail to motivate people if they are seen as too difficult (Sherman, 1995; Tully, 1994) or too easy or if an individual does not know what tasks are required for goal attainment (Muchinsky, 1987).

Research Support and Evaluation

The empirical support for key parts of goal-setting theory is impressive. Nearly 400 studies—mostly experimental—show that specific, difficult goals lead to better performance than specific, easy, vague goals, such as "do your best" or no goals at all (Locke & Latham, 1990a).

There is also support for the view that commitment to goals is critical to effective performance (Erez & Zidon, 1984). In turn, commitment to goals is generally higher when people think they can attain the goals and when they value them (Locke, Latham, & Erez, 1988). Further,

monetary rewards increase goal commitment if people value money and the amount is sufficiently large.

One surprising finding is that assigning goals to individuals generally leads to the same level of commitment and performance as when individuals participate in setting goals or when they set goals for themselves. Perhaps assigned goals work well because they come from authority figures or because assigned goals, if difficult, are more challenging (Locke & Latham, 1990b). We are concerned about applying these results to health care professionals, however, given that many of them are trained and socialized to set their own goals. In this case, managers just need to be sure that goals are specific and difficult regardless of who sets them.

Research also shows that goal setting is more effective, and usually only effective, when feedback is given to individuals so that they can monitor their performance in relation to goals. Indeed, goal setting without feedback seems to have little long-term effect on performance (Becker, 1978). On the other hand, feedback without goal setting is also ineffective. People need both goals and feedback on progress toward goals to be motivated. Furthermore, self-created feedback appears to exert a greater effect on motivation than feedback from external sources (Ivancevich & McMahon, 1982). Finally, for goal setting to be effective, people must have the ability to reach or approach the goals (Locke, 1982). Once again, this result is consistent with the expectancy theory.

The strength of this perspective is its simplicity and ease of application. It seems to be generalizable; its principles can be applied in any circumstance. Moreover, as noted above, it has a very strong base of empirical support.

There are, of course, some important unanswered questions. How do people become committed to goals, and why do they select certain goals and not others (Hollenbeck & Klein, 1987)?

Application

The implications for managers are relatively straightforward:

1. Set or encourage people to set goals that are difficult and specific; revise and update goals as necessary.

Prompts such as daily, weekly, or monthly "to do" lists are examples of useful techniques.

2. Provide timely and specific feedback to people on their progress toward goals.
3. Build commitment to goals by helping people believe they can attain goals and by selecting goals that are congruent with their values.
4. Consistent with the reinforcement theory, rewards should be given contingent on goal attainment.
5. Make sure that individuals have the ability to achieve goals they or you set.

MOTIVATING HEALTH CARE PROFESSIONALS

One key aspect of health care organizations is that they have large numbers of autonomous professionals working within them. These professionals can include a variety of clinical occupations as well as senior managers, information technology specialists, accountants, and so on. Because so much of the day-to-day work in health care is carried out by clinical professionals, from a management perspective, it is instructive to examine how motivation theories may apply to them.

A profession can be characterized in terms of (1) who its members are (selection, licensure, and cohesion), (2) what it is that they know (knowledge base and standards), (3) why they act as they do (service orientation and code of ethics), and (4) how they direct their activities (occupational autonomy and impact on social policy) (O'Connor & Lanning, 1992). Among the various components, autonomy appears to be a key defining characteristic (Haug, 1988).

Professional Economic Incentives: Money Is As Money Does

According to Herzberg's motivation-hygiene theory, money acts as a hygiene. If it is inadequately present, it should serve to dissatisfy and demotivate; however, its ample presence should result in the neutralization of any dissatisfaction, not in satisfaction and motivation. Professionals who view their financial rewards as inadequate compared to their contributions will very likely become dissatisfied. However, an important caution is required: Money has the capability to serve as a motivator, because it can also function as a recognition.

An old saying states that "money is as money does." Well-educated health care professionals who earn fittingly good salaries do not always seek greater financial remuneration solely for what it can purchase for them. Instead, because these individuals often hold very high achievement needs, money can serve as a tangible symbolic recognition of their ability and achievements. Interestingly, research suggests that recognition is one of the most crucial motivational elements for American health care professionals (Alpander, 1985). Far from being a dissatisfier/hygiene, money can become an important vehicle for bestowing recognition. In this sense, money can act as a satisfier/motivator.

Physicians

Health care organizations face continuous pressure to become more productive, innovative, and concerned with quality. Physicians are vitally important to health care organizations because much of the work is carried out at their direction. Managers must be able to motivate physicians to practice high-quality, cost-effective medicine by abandoning detrimental behaviors, such as excessive use of resources (e.g., unnecessary diagnostic testing) and low rates of quality outcomes to resources consumed (O'Connor, 1998).

The task of motivating physicians can be a difficult one indeed. As stated previously, autonomy is a key element of what it means to be a professional, and medicine represents the quintessential profession. Physicians are educated and socialized to think and act with a great deal of individual discretion and autonomy in their day-to-day work. Generally, they resent managerial or organizational forays into their activities (O'Connor, 1996). However, their remarkable traditional autonomy has been receding (O'Connor & Lanning, 1992). For example, the determination of physician salaries, fees, and processes of care delivery have been gradually shifting from the physicians themselves, to a system of hospitals, payers, and managed care organizations (Zimberg & Clement, 1997).

The traditional fee-for-service payment system is a direct reward system: The more work the physician does, the more he bills and collects, and thus, the more he is rewarded. As the fee-for-service physician payment method goes the way of the dinosaur, and more intricate compensation methods become the norm, we must be cautious not to exclusively fixate on new financial schemes to modify physician behavior. "[W]hile compensation is as powerful an extrinsic motivator for physicians as it is for anyone, this incentive operates in the context of other powerful motivational resources, routinely underestimated and ignored by management" (Plume, 1995).

For example, merely inverting the fee-for-service economic reward structure such that physicians who utilize fewer resources receive more economic rewards is probably not a good idea. According to Kongstvedt (1996), such a system—exclusively rewarding reduced resource consumption—ignores other critical activities such as participating in quality management programs, complying with organizational policies, and exhibiting concern for patient satisfaction. Perhaps most disturbing is that such an economic reward mechanism can be unacceptably gamed, resulting in inappropriate underutilization.

Because of their professional socialization and strong achievement needs, physicians want to deliver high-quality excellent medicine to their patients. However, in order for them to know how well they are doing in this regard, they need to be able to assess how well they are doing with respect to their peers, their own past performance, and to benchmark goals. One way of accomplishing this is to develop high-quality information systems that provide feedback on a frequent basis. Such a system can allow medical professionals to know not only how well they are doing, but to also enhance their confidence that they are doing things right (Kongstvedt, 1996).

Feedback can be a powerful tool to assist managers in motivating physician behavior; however, there are several factors that should be considered in order to maximize the feedback effectiveness. First, in order for feedback to have value, physicians must truly see that their behavior needs to change. Second, feedback needs to be frequent, timely, and given at precise time intervals in order to sustain new behaviors. Third, feedback must be useable, consistent, correct, and of sufficient diversity. It should contain various impor-

tant utilization, financial, and quality-related data that are valid representations of what is being measured. Otherwise, behavior problems can intensify as rewards flow to improvements based on flawed feedback data (Charns & Smith Tewksbury, 1993). Last, managers should not portray the feedback as "good" or "bad." Professionals, such as physicians, know when they have missed the goal.

An Assessment of Process Theories

Each process theory has limitations that make it incomplete for understanding and motivating behavior. On the other hand, taken together the theories offer a powerful set of guidelines for health care managers (see Managerial Guidelines). Process theories share the view that the content of work is often not enough to motivate people; they need reinforcement, expectations, fairness, and goals to be energized to perform their best.

Indeed, taken together, process theories suggest a cycle of managerial action as follows:

1. Goals should be set at the time of hiring or at periodic performance evaluations.
2. Expectations about goal attainment and consequences should also be set at this time.
3. Perceptions of fairness should be checked periodically.
4. Reinforcement should be given contingent on performance.

This cycle used in concert with the guidelines suggested from content perspectives can go a long way toward increasing motivation in health care organizations.

MOTIVATIONAL PROBLEMS

Nature and Causes

A major challenge for all health care organizations is to avoid employee motivation problems and to remedy such problems if they do occur. Despite their best efforts, most organizations do experience some problems of employee motivation. The symptoms may

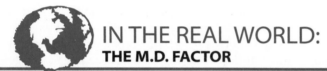

IN THE REAL WORLD:
THE M.D. FACTOR

Manuel Loewenhaupt, M.D., knows doctors. Thousands of them. For nearly a decade, he's been consulting with them, learning from them, and helping them to navigate the troubled waters of change. Now, he's a partner at Deloitte & Touche Consulting Group, Boston. This is his take on changing physician behavior.

Q: *How important to population-based health is a change in the ways physicians practice?*

A: *It's the heart of the whole movement because the bottom line is the way that patient care is delivered. Population-based health is powered by doctors. Without the driver, you have nothing.*

Q: *In what ways does the relationship between health care organizations and doctors complicate change?*

A: *Health systems don't have true authority over doctors. If they don't own them, they can't fire them. In some ways, doctors are like high-level programmers in the computer software industry. If they don't like where they are working, they pick up and find a better place. In health care, the incentives for change don't come through a relationship of control and authority.*

Q: *How does the physician mentality fit in?*

A: *We're trained not to think of teams or collaboration as an ideal way of working. We're trained to rely on our own independent judgment. I recently read a survey in which doctors were asked to list their fictional heroes. The most popular responses were Superman, the Lone Ranger and Maverick, the combat pilot in the movie Top Gun. I can't think of a tougher group of people to try to manage.*

Q: *How well do doctors respond to business management concepts?*

A: *Physicians don't work well with an authority model. In fact, most view themselves as artists, not managers or executives. There attitude often is, "Please don't bother me, please don't irritate me, and please don't try to manage me. Just leave me alone and let me do my thing."*

Q: *What mistakes do health care organizations make trying to motivate doctors to change?*

A: *Too often, administrators couch the message in the wrong terms. Telling a doctor that a new way of working will help the health system thrive may have little motivating effect. Few doctors are lying awake at night worrying about the financial well-being of a hospital or health system. In fact, many doctors may actually fear improved performance of a hospital, because in a reimbursement state of mind, a strong hospital may get that way by reducing its payment to doctors.*

Q: *Are you saying that the best strategy is motivate doctors financially?*

A: *Not necessarily. Most people's first guess is that doctors are motivated by money, and they wouldn't be completely wrong. When doctors rank their priorities, money is in the top five, but not always number one. There are other key motivators, too. Among them are the increased ability to provide excellent care, more time in which to do it, efficiency, and peer recognition. If you want to influence doctors, you need to look at these elements, too.*

Q: *What misconceptions do physicians have about the business of running a health system?*

A: *Most doctors have very little understanding of the way that care is delivered through a system. They view administrators as little more than bean counters. And they don't understand the complicated financial models that drive and influence health care delivery.*

Q: *Specifically, which behaviors need to change?*

A: *First, we have to move away from the solo model of practice to a more collaborative model. Second, we need to work toward eliminating inappropriate variations in care. Most variations are driven not by clinical science, but by a "this-is-the-way-I-was-trained" mentality. And third, we need to get away from reflexive medicine—the kind of medicine that's driven by tradition rather than* *by scientific evidence. We can no longer rely on the "way it's always been done here."*

Q: *Are physicians beginning to "get it"?*

A: *Many are. But there's still a great deal of resistance out there. In some of my meetings with physicians, I do an exercise in which I ask them to describe the ideal practice environment of the future. When I read their responses, I see a lot of descriptions that sound exactly the way things were 10 years ago. People want to turn back the clock. Then I find myself explaining repeatedly that there's probably not going to be a rewind like that.*

Q: *Whose job is it to change the way that health care is delivered?*

A: *It's going to take a real collaboration between health system leaders and physician leaders. Many smaller organizations haven't figured out how to build that collaborative piece, and that's where they're struggling. One of the big problems that they are facing is history. There is still a lot of leftover bad feelings from earlier moves. But everyone is going to have to get beyond all that.*

Q: *What's the first step in moving physicians toward new ways of practicing?*

A: *Awareness. Often, that comes not from a health system, but from the market. In Detroit, for example, when the Ford Motor Company declared that it is going to reduce its health care expenditures by 30%, it was a wake-up call. Ford got aggressive in its contracting, and everyone realized that business as usual was over. There was this instant awareness that it would be crazy to try to achieve different results by doing the same old thing.*

Q: *What's your advice to health care organizations that are trying to influence physician behavior?*

A: *It's a complicated process, and it's not necessarily linear. It's going to happen at a tempo that many business managers will see as too slow. At the same time, doctors are probably going to see it as too fast. But if you work toward a partnership with physicians, and you can achieve a sense of shared investment, shared returns, and shared mission, you can convert physicians from barriers to champions of the cause.*

The M.D. factor, Crossroads: **New directions in health management,** *a supplement to Hospitals & Health Networks, November, 1997, Copyright, 1997, American Hospital Publishing, Inc.*

 MANAGERIAL GUIDELINES

1. Check employees' perceptions of the fairness of their work and rewards. Address perceived inequities as best as possible, given resource constraints. Unfortunately, perceptions of inequity are especially likely when managers try to take individuals' different needs into account.
2. Select rewards that are attractive to employees.
3. Make sure that the rules for attaining rewards are clear to everyone.
4. Make sure that people understand that their efforts will lead to the desired level of performance.
5. Reward people contingent on performance; try various reinforcement schedules to see what works best in your setting.
6. Set or encourage people to set goals that are difficult and specific; revise and update goals as necessary.
7. Provide timely and specific feedback to people on their progress toward goals.
8. Build commitment to goals by helping people believe that they can attain them and by selecting goals that are consistent with their values.

involve apathy, low-quality work, and complaints from supervisors and patients.

The causes of motivational problems often fall into three categories. First, there may be inadequate performance definition. This means the employees do not fully understand what is expected of them. There is no clear definition of what is expected of employees nor any continuous orientation of employees toward effective job performance. Symptoms of this problem include a lack of goals, inadequate job descriptions, inadequate performance standards, and inadequate performance assessment.

Second, there may be impediments to employee performance. Among the most important of these may be bureaucratic or environmental obstacles, inadequate support or resources, and a mismatch between the employee's skills and job requirements. An example is a hospital experiencing significant understaffing in nursing. Since the nursing staff is probably overworked, stressed-out, and burned-out, efforts to provide a motivating environment will fail unless and until adequate staffing is provided. Research has shown that inadequate nurse staffing and consequent high workloads are the major problems motivating nurse turnover (Fottler, Crawford, Quintana, & White, 1995). Obviously, it is difficult to motivate overworked and overstressed nurses to high levels of productivity and service quality.

Third, there may be inadequate performance-reward linkages. Rewards may be economic or noneconomic. Symptoms of this problem are inappropriate rewards that are not valued by employees, inadequate rewards for performance, delay in receipt of rewards, a low probability of receiving rewards, and inequity in the distribution of rewards.

Determining the specific causes of a particular employee motivation problem is difficult. The most effective approach is for health care executives to develop communication skills, interpersonal skills, and interview skills so that two-way communication with employees is continued. The emphasis is on listening and encouraging employees to speak frankly. As a result, the problems and frustrations of particular employees—both individuals and groups—are well-understood by both their immediate supervisors and higher-level managers. Many organizations have found that an upward communication system utilizing interviews has paid off in terms of reduced absenteeism and turnover, increased productivity, and higher profits (Imberman, 1976).

Employee attitude surveys can also be useful in collecting information about employee beliefs and attitudes as long as they are anonymous and there is assurance the results will be acted upon (Fottler et al., 1995; Taglinferri, 1988; York, 1985). First, such surveys are valuable for identifying the problems and impediments to performance that need to be reviewed and modified. Second, they are useful for learning the value that employees attach to a number of different outcomes such as money, recognition, autonomy, and affiliation. Discrepancies between employee and management views provide a basis for exploring ways to modify employee beliefs or job conditions to create a better match of employee values and job attributes. Third, attitude surveys are useful for learning the nature of employee beliefs about contingencies. In particular, surveys should reveal the extent to which employee beliefs about expectancies and instrumentalities (i.e., probability of receiving reward and adequacy in meeting needs) match those that managers believe exist for these employees. Unfortunately, this diagnosis of employee attitudes and needs is deficient in most health services organizations. One survey found only 43% of health care employees felt their organization seeks their opinions and suggestions. Worse yet, only 26% felt their organizations act on their input (Lutz, 1990).

Potential Solutions

Table 3.2 outlines the three motivational problems discussed in the beginning of this section together with potential solutions. It is important to recognize that most motivational problems have more than one cause and more than one solution. In fact, the latest theory and research suggest that successful employee motivation programs should include several integrated and mutually reinforcing motivational approaches (Locke & Latham, 1990b). At a minimum, these approaches should include positive reinforcement with behavior modification if necessary, high challenge or difficult goals, valued rewards contingent upon performance expectancy of success, em-

Table 3.2. Common Employee Motivation Problems and Potential Solutions

Motivational Problems	Potential Solutions
1. Inadequate performance definition (i.e., lack of goals, inadequate job descriptions, inadequate performance standards, inadequate performance assessment) 2. Impediments to performance (i.e., bureaucratic or environmental obstacles, inadequate support or resources, poor employee-job matching, inadequate information) 3. Inadequate performance-reward linkages (i.e., inappropriate rewards, inadequate rewards, poor timing of rewards, low probability of receiving rewards, inequity in distribution of rewards)	• Well-defined job descriptions • Well-defined performance standards • Goal setting • Feedback on performance • Improved employee selection • Job redesign or enrichment • Enhanced hygiene factors (i.e., safe and clean environment, salary and fringe benefits, job security, staffing, time-off-job, equipment) • Behavior modification or positive reinforcement (individual or group) • Pay for performance • Enhanced achievement or growth factors (i.e., employee involvement-participation, job redesign or enrichment, career planning, professional development opportunities) • Enhanced esteem or power factors (i.e., autonomy or personal control, autonomous work teams, self-management, modified work schedule, recognition, praise or awards, opportunity to display skills or talents, opportunity to mentor or train others, promotions in rank or position, information concerning organization or department, preferred work activities or projects, letters of recommendation, preferred work space) • Enhanced affiliation or relatedness factors (i.e., work teams, task groups, business meetings, social activities, professional and community group participation, personal communication or leadership style)

ployee feedback, employee involvement or participation, job redesign, and low situational constraints. The long-run goal should be to develop and retain a "culture of performance."

In situations where motivational problems exist, the cause is often an inadequate linkage between performance and rewards valued by the employee (see Problem 3 of Table 3.2). Empirical research on attitudes of registered nurses indicates a trend toward more negative attitudes toward communication, pay, and promotional opportunities over time (Heckert, Fottler, Swartz, & Mercer, 1993). Apparently, as competition has increased, health care executives have reduced labor costs by restraining the growth of pay and

the opportunity for advancement. While this policy contains costs and makes the organization more cost-competitive in the short run, it also adversely affects employee morale and motivation. One solution is **behavior modification,** a technique for applying the concepts of reinforcement theory in organizational settings (Luthans & Kreitney, 1985). First, the manager specifies behaviors that are to be increased or decreased. Then these target behaviors are measured to establish a baseline against which the effectiveness of behavioral modification will be assessed. The manager then analyzes the situation to ascertain what rewards employees value most and how best to tie these rewards to the target behaviors. Next, rewards are

The leadership of Samaritan Health System, Arizona's largest health care provider, wanted to aggressively position their organization for the future, and in so doing developed a strategic plan to move the system in new and unexpected directions. Howard Rohan, Vice President of Human Resources, looked at the plan "and said, 'my God, our systems were built for the '50s, '60s, and '70s. We can't get to where we want to go with these obsolete systems.'" "For Rohan . . . the prospect was sobering. The organization he saw around him was a reactive, hierarchical, pyramid-shaped confederacy of independent sick-care institutions. The strategic plan . . . demanded a proactive, flattened, team-based wellness organization in which employees could take initiative on behalf of customers."

Next, Samaritans compensation framework was examined. "They trashed the existing pay system because it was a 'built-in' hierarchical pyramid perpetruator." "Rewards flowed from resources a manager controlled, not according to results achieved." "To determine proper compensation, a way to measure performance was needed."

A compensation plan was developed that ties pay inevitably to performance. Annual performance evaluations determine raises. Evaluations are broken down into two parts: functional competencies and core competencies.

Functional competencies refer to the technical skills workers need to fulfill their assigned tasks. To reinforce that employees are responsible for their own development, functional competencies now include initiative, problem solving, supervision required, teamwork, and customer service. These abilities, it was thought, were necessary to help realize the system's larger goals: to let employees make more decisions at the point of service, to improve customer satisfaction, to reduce costs, and to improve clinical outcomes.

Samaritan's new manual says core competencies are the behavior portion of performance management. It's how people do their jobs. Are they polite to coworkers? Respectful to patients? Do they come to work on time? Dress appropriately? Take too many sick days? Do they accept feedback constructively? Finally, in their daily actions, do they contribute to the success of Samaritan Health System?

On the performance evaluation, written by their supervisor, there is a corresponding zone for pay for each level of competence: developing, competent, or master. The biggest raises this year—6%—go to master performers who have been paid in the developing zone. The lowest raises are 3%. Some could get zero. In the future, employees whose performance doesn't measure up to their pay level will see their pay go down. "If they're not performing at an exceptional level, why should we pay them at the top of the range?" Campbell [house compensation expert] asked. "Why shouldn't they be paid at market?"

The new evaluation and compensation process lays out the employees' financial future in front of them and suggests how to do something about it. "It emphasizes the attitudes and behaviors with which the employee must approach the job," Berry [System Director of Pharmacy Services] said. "Customer service and teamwork are now part of the developing functional competency. . . . I've had employees that have cleaned up their act within a month after the assessment."

Sharon Larson, a food service supervisor at Maryvale Samaritan Medical Center, has had the same experience. "It turned on a lot of lights for people. They know they just can't show up for work anymore," she said. Larson has seen the effects of the first evaluation on people's work—their behavior. They realize, "I can't go on being nasty to people. It's going to affect my pay," she said. "As far as attendance, conduct and dress, [in the old days] that would be in the performance appraisal but it didn't affect their wages. Now, we can put a hold on it. All of a sudden, attendance is important."

To keep managers from going too easy on their people, no employee can be judged a master performer without a second signature, by the department director, on the form. That's Samaritan's only leverage to keep managers from gaming the system.

"I was surprised," Berry remarked. "The bell-shaped curve is there.'"

Adopted from Moore, J. D. (1996). Samaritan's revolution: New pay model aims to overhaul how workers think. Modern Healthcare, 26(31), pp. 27, 30, 32–34.

given so that desired behaviors have pleasant consequences and undesirable behaviors have unpleasant consequences. Finally, the target behaviors are measured again to determine the value of the program.

One popular extension of behavior modification is *pay for performance*. This links the desired behavior or outcomes to one specific positive employee outcome—higher pay. In most cases, it applies primarily or exclusively to management personnel.

One way to classify such plans is according to the level of performance targeted—individual, group, or total organization. Within these broad categories, literally hundreds of different approaches for relating pay to performance exist. Failure often occurs because the rewards are too small, the links between performance and rewards are weak, and supervisors resent performance appraisal ("Labor letter," 1980; Lawler, 1989; Rollins, 1987). Successful programs establish high standards of performance, develop accurate performance appraisal systems, train supervisors in the mechanics of performance appraisal and the art of giving feedback, and use a wide range of pay increases.

Well-conceived and well-designed pay-for-performance plans tend to work because they clearly articulate standards of performance and provide a strong motivation for employees to focus on meeting these standards. Health care administrators who have launched pay-for-performance plans have generally found them to have high employee acceptance and to be effective management tools for increasing cost efficiency, productivity, and quality of care (Berger & Moyer, 1991). The goals and performance standards that are rewarded have more intrinsic meaningfulness to employees if they are tied to the strategic goals of the organization (Fottler, Blair, Philips, & Duran, 1990). Samaritan Health System's pay-for-performance plan is an example of this.

Problems with pay-for-performance may result if the organization uses a forced distribution or forced ranking system. Here the organization places limits on how many employees can be placed into each rating group. Typically rating groups are proportionally distributed according to a normal bell-shaped curve. If every worker cannot attain the highest ranking simultaneously, then a "forced" ranking rating system is in place.

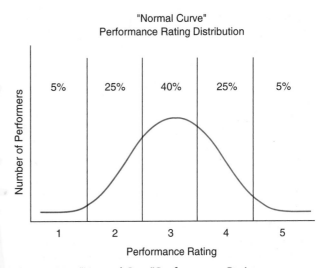

Figure 3.7. "Normal Cure" Performance Rating Distribution
SOURCE: Daniels, A. C. (1994). *Bringing Out the Best in People: How to Apply the Astonishing Power of Positive Reinforcement.* New York, NY: McGraw-Hill, Inc. (p. 153, Figure 18-1).

A forced distribution of any kind creates unhealthy competition among employees. One employee's high rating "forces" someone else to get a lower rating since there can only a limited number in the top group. Employees who continue to try to get to the top rating and end up in the next-to-the-highest group eventually quit trying (extinction).

Proponents of this system say if you measure people on almost any variable, you will get a normal distribution (Figure 3.7). In other words, performance is probably normally distributed, so forced rankings should be fair. The problem with that logic is that organizations don't hire on the basis of a normal distribution (Daniels, 1994).

Unlike many Wall Street brokers who are motivated primarily by money, many health care workers choose their profession for reasons other than salary. Consequently, health care organizations need to identify and respond to a wide variety of noneconomic needs that may motivate their employees (see Table 3.2). There are a wide variety of employee involvement-participation programs that are based on the belief that employees at all levels in the organization can and will contribute useful insights to the effective functioning of the organization given an opportunity. The most common programs are gain-sharing suggestion systems, quality circles, union-management committees, total quality management programs, and autonomous work groups (Cotton, Volrath, Frogett, Lengnick-Hall, & Jennings, 1988; Lawler, 1989). Employee participation in making critical job and organizational decisions is the one common element in all of these programs.

One method of employee participation is to seek employee input into management policies, strategies, tactics, etc., through written employee attitude surveys. These usually cover such topics as supervision, pay, benefits, communication, and policies. However, merely conducting attitude surveys is not sufficient by itself. The results need to be used in organizational decision making, which responds to problem areas identified by employees (Fottler et al., 1995). Otherwise, employees may become angry and cynical if management fails to act on their comments, complaints, and suggestions. Attitude surveys appear to be more effective than exit interviews in identifying employee concerns and problems that may impede employee motivation.

One approach that encompasses many of the participation strategies discussed above is employee **empowerment.** The empowerment process is one of "directed autonomy" whereby employees are given an overall direction yet considerable leeway concerning how they go about following that direction. It also necessitates sharing information and knowledge with employees, which enables them to understand and contribute to organizational performance, and giving them the autonomy to make decisions that influence organizational outcomes (Ford & Fottler, 1995). It is the issue of power that differentiates empowerment from earlier approaches to employee participation (i.e., delegation, decentralization, and participatory management) that tended to emphasize employee input but made no real change in the assignment of power and authority.

Obviously, empowerment is a matter of degree rather than an absolute (Ford & Fottler, 1995). Health care executives could choose to provide higher degrees of empowerment for some individuals and teams doing certain tasks than for others. He or she could empower subordinates in terms of any or all of the following: problem identification, alternative development, alternative evaluation, alternative choice, and implementation. Since employee empowerment has only recently been implemented in most organizations, empirical evidence concerning its benefits to an organization are sparse. However, some researchers have reported extremely positive outcomes for both organizations and employees (Blackburn & Rosen, 1993). Employee involvement-participation appears to be highly desired in health care organizations.

Employees also desire participation linked to incentives. **Gainsharing** encourages employees to find ways to increase productivity and to cut costs in exchange for receiving a share of the savings realized. Gainsharing programs are viewed as innovative approaches to bringing about productivity improvements in developed, labor-intensive industries such as hospitals (Barbusca & Cleek, 1994). To be successful, gainsharing programs require top management to start disseminating relevant information and giving employees the time and tools to get involved.

Quality circles offer another employee involvement-participation option. A quality circle consists of a small number of volunteers, typically 8 to 10 nonmanagement employees from the same department, who meet a few hours each week to examine productivity and quality problems. Members identify a problem, study it, and present their recommendations for change to management. These problems often involve subtle difficulties that may be noticed only by those who actually perform the work.

The research results concerning the effectiveness of quality circles are mixed. In one recent review of the research, about half of the studies of quality circles reported uniformly positive results in all criteria (i.e., productivity, quality, absenteeism, and job attitudes) (Barrick & Alexander, 1987). One-quarter of the studies found some beneficial effects, and the other quarter reported no beneficial changes. Similar mixed results have been found for quality circles in health care organizations (Phillips, Duran, Blair, Peterson, Savage, & Whitehead, 1990). Specific recommendations for increasing the probability of quality circle success include management support for genuine participation, a pilot program, a long-term view, modest expectations, willingness to adapt some proposals, training of participants, voluntary participation, defined scope and limit, and evaluation (Phillips et al., 1990).

Employee recognition programs offer another method of linking employee participation and rewards. Simple recognition practices may include: random and informal public praise for good work, organizing a departmental gathering to honor achievements of one or more employees, and publishing employee accomplishments and complimentary or thank you letters from patients or visitors in the organization's newsletter (Huseman & Hatfield, 1989; McConnell, 1997). Surveys of nonhealth employees show most believe simple positive feedback from management and recognition for a job well done serve as valued rewards capable of motivating employees (Koch, 1990; Rawlinson, 1988). Such feedback and recognition may also take more tangible forms as noneconomic award programs. Examples include trophies, wall plaques, certificates, letters or handwritten personal notes of thanks, visits or telephone calls by top executives, and luncheon invitations (Huseman & Hatfield, 1989). For such awards to be effective motivators, they must recognize only high-performing employees (Blanchard & Bowles, 1998).

Job redesign is yet another strategy that can lead to increased intrinsic motivation (also see Chapter 7). It is based on the premise that altering certain aspects of the job to satisfy employees' psychological needs will motivate them to exert more effort. According to Hackman and Lawler, satisfaction of higher-order needs (which is the essence of intrinsic motivation) occurs when the employee experiences these psychological states (Hackman & Oldham, 1980). First, the job allows the employee to feel personally responsible for a significant segment of his or her work outcomes. Autonomy or personal control is the key job dimension contributing to feelings of personal responsibility for job outcomes. Second, the job involves doing something that is perceived as meaningful by the individual. The three core dimensions that can make jobs more meaningful are task identity (i.e., completion of a whole task), skill variety (i.e., utilization of different skills), and task significance (i.e., substantial impact). Third, the job provides the employee with knowledge of results. Feedback from the job itself or

from another individual is the core job dimension which provides knowledge of results.

Job redesign aims to enrich a job so that the employee is more motivated to do the work. It is most appropriate when there is a demonstrated need to redesign jobs—for example, due to employee downtime, and it is feasible to redesign jobs given the present structure of jobs, legal constraints, technological constraints, and the characteristics and values of employees. Job redesign in health care is feasible but may be subject to more legal and professional constraints than most other industries (Blayney, 1992).

One popular approach to job redesign in health services is the multiskilled health practitioner (MSHP). MSHPs are persons who are cross-trained to provide more than one function, often in more than one discipline. These combined functions can be formed in a broad spectrum of health-related jobs ranging in complexity from the nonprofessional to the professional level, including both clinical and management functions. The additional functions or skills added to the original job may be of a higher, lower, or parallel level. This means the concept includes both job enlargement (i.e., addition of parallel or lower-level functions) and job enrichment (i.e., addition of higher-level functions). Research has shown positive results such as higher patient and employee satisfaction, cost savings, reduced lengths of stay, reduced waiting time, improved patient compliance, improved quality of care, and improved employee retention (Fottler, 1996).

Job redesign may apply to either individual positions or to groups of employees. For employees with high growth needs, job redesign can pay off. Research in both nonhealth care organizations and health care organizations has generally supported the validity of the job characteristics model in enhancing employee motivation for employees who strongly value personal feelings of accomplishment and growth (Alpander, 1990; Guzzo, Jette, & Katzell, 1985). However, the actual success of any job redesign effort is likely to depend on other reinforcing or nonreinforcing factors such as the reward system and top management support (Fried & Ferris, 1987).

One study examined how the level of organizational commitment of nurses and nurse's aides employed in long-term care settings influenced family satisfaction with the quality of services received. The study also examined how the job redesign variables (i.e., autonomy, task identity, skill variety, task significance, and feedback) influenced organizational commitment. Findings indicate that family members' satisfaction with the quality of services received is significantly and positively influenced by organizational commitment, which in turn is significantly and positively correlated with autonomy, task identity, and skill variety. Although feedback and task significance were dropped from the model due to measurement difficulties, this study suggests that redesigning nursing and nurse's aides jobs in long-term care settings can serve to motivate these employees to be more committed to the organization as well as to provide higher levels of perceived service quality (Steffen, Nystrom, & O'Connor, 1996).

In terms of efficiency and practicality, some jobs can be done only by a group. An example is a surgical team in a hospital operating room. Anesthesiologists, surgeons, nurses, and technicians must work interdependently. This is true of most health care occupations. In fact, more organizations in general have implemented work redesign projects for **autonomous work groups** (AWGs) than for individuals (Wall, Kemp, Jackson, & Clegg, 1986). Autonomous work groups are also known as self-managed teams, or high-performance work teams. These groups take on traditional management tasks (Rogers, Metlay, Kaplan, & Shapiro, 1995), and decide how members will work together. Generally when an AWG is created, the group members themselves control the planning and decision-making process within the group, select its own leader, and set its own quality and quantity output levels. AWGs provide opportunities for employees to exercise more control over their daily work life.

While research is sparse, there is some evidence of positive benefits such as job satisfaction and productivity in such groups (Wall et al., 1986). The best known American success story is the Saturn General Motors Plant in Spring Hill, Tennessee, where AWGs emphasize teamwork, efficient use of resources, and a tireless effort to improve quality (Gwynne, 1990).

In contrast to employee involvement-participation approaches, AWGs involve participation together with changes in job design and organization design.

This tends to affect more employees and create a longer-lasting impact on the organizational culture. The specific benefits of AWGs found in certain U. S. corporations include more integration of individual skills, better performance in terms of quantity and quality, reduced absenteeism and turnover, and a growing sense of confidence and accomplishment among team members (Bassin, 1988).

While a large number of experiments are now occurring in health care organizations, most are so recent that empirical evidence of the effectiveness of AWGs is not yet available. There is, however, some evidence to suggest that AWGs will increase employee involvement, commitment, and intrinsic motivation (Alpander, 1990).

Overall Assessment

As we have seen, there are many approaches to dealing with motivational problems among employees. None are foolproof. Whether a particular approach succeeds in a particular setting depends first on whether it was properly matched with the primary causes of low motivation. Second, it depends on how and whether the program was introduced and implemented so that resistance was minimized and commitment maximized. For example, favorable reaction is likely to be greatest if the affected employees have some voice in choosing and implementing a particular motivation program. Third, it depends on whether the program is compatible with other aspects of the organization's culture (Hames, 1991; Mohrmann & Lawler, 1984). The simultaneous introduction of several mutually supportive and mutually reinforcing motivation programs is probably most effective in overcoming motivation problems, assuming they are all relevant to the causes of the problem. An example is the program at AMI Palmetto Hospital in "In the Real World."

Two reviews of the literature have compared the relative effectiveness of several motivation programs. One concluded that financial incentives were most effective, while goal setting was also quite effective (Locke, 1982). Participative decision making and job redesign were relatively less certain to produce significant improvements. The other study suggested that

IN THE REAL WORLD:
A VISION OF EXCELLENCE AT
AMI PALMETTO GENERAL HOSPITAL

AMI Palmetto General Hospital in Hialeah, Florida, recently implemented the Visions of Excellence program to integrate employee relations, customer service, and commitment to patient care quality. Monthly themes and activities are designated by a Visions of Excellence committee to deliver messages to all employees regarding organization goals, communication, customers (i.e., physicians, patients, patient families), challenges, and excellence. Some successful themes and activities have been Physician Appreciation Month, Commitment Pledge Month, Employee Exchange Day, Patient Satisfaction Means Success, and the Employee Honor Roll.

The Visions committee originated as a voluntary task force with the mission of "redefining the organization's culture." This required management to commit to certain beliefs such as recognizing and rewarding employee contributions in a participative environment where individuals are treated with respect and allowed to participate in problem solving. The committee believes that employee commitment to the organization is more likely when all employees are rewarded for attaining specific goals in a participative environment.

Each level of management participates in a series of skills workshops on such topics as identifying supports and barriers to effective teamwork, sharing information, developing action plans based on strategic plans, productivity measures, and the service culture. The purpose of each workshop is to help managers develop mutual goals and plans to achieve success. Each level of management, in turn, is encouraged to train its own team in similar workshops so that everyone is part of the process.

Employees are asked what they want the organization to be and what they are willing to do to get it there. Em-

ployee responses are then integrated into the program document. Volume and quality indicators of performance that are clear and understandable to employees at all levels are preferable to complicated indicators. Each month several employees are selected from employee nominations for recognition as employee achievement award winners. The winner is given a plaque, cash, and a selected parking place for a month.

An employee relations program, a customer service program, and a commitment to excellence have a greater chance of long-term survival if they are interrelated. One of the three without the others will be lame. To expect employees to provide excellent customer service, top management must believe that how employees are treated will affect how they treat customers. Everyone on the organization serves an external customer or an internal customer. A commitment to excellence must be accompanied by an answer to the question, What's in it for me? The employee relations program and the reward system must answer that question. Likewise, good customer service is just window dressing without an excellent technical product to go along with it.

The Visions of Excellence program has demonstrated several benefits. Efficiency, productivity, service quality, employee morale, teamwork, and favorable letters from patients have increased. Costs, physician complaints, and turnover have decreased. The workforce has become focused on what needs to be done for success.

Adapted from Pujol, J. L., Tudanger, E. A vision of excellence. HRM Magazine, 35(6), 112–116.

---

employee training and goal setting were most likely to improve motivation or productivity, followed closely by changes such as AWGs and carefully designed financial incentives (Guzzo, Jette, & Katzell, 1985). Job redesign is less powerful but still has a significant impact on productivity. This review also suggests that combined interventions are more effective than single-method approaches. Yet almost any of these approaches can be effective if they are matched to the motivational problem, are carefully implemented, involve all parties, and are implemented in a culture that emphasizes employee motivation and performance.

MANAGERIAL GUIDELINES

1. The major reasons for low employee motivation are lack of understanding concerning expectations, organizational impediments to performance, and lack of valued rewards for performance.
2. A variety of upward communication methods are available to assist health care managers in determining the nature and causes of employee motivation problems including direct supervisor communication, interviews, and employee attitude surveys.
3. Expectations can be clarified through well-defined job descriptions, performance standards, goal setting, and feedback on performance.
4. Attitude surveys are effective means of identifying and removing motivational impediments as long as management follow-up to concerns occurs.
5. Motivational impediments can be removed by addressing relevant hygiene factors in the environment as well as better matching of employee and job through improved selection and job redesign.
6. Inadequate performance-reward linkages can be addressed through behavior modification, pay for performance, and provision of desired motivators related to achievement or growth or esteem or power needs of employees.

Discussion Questions

1. How can content and process motivation theories best be combined in practice?
2. How can managers distinguish a motivational problem from other factors that affect an individual's performance?
3. How can motivational theories be used to select the best potential solution for a given individual's needs?

References

Adams, J. S. (1963, November). Toward an understanding of inequity. *Journal of Abnormal and Social Psychology, 67,* 422–436.

Adams, J. S. (1965). Inequity in social exchange. In L. Berkowitz (Ed.), *Advances in Experimental Social Psychology, II.* New York: Academic Press.

Alderfer, C. P. (1968). An empirical test of a new theory of human needs. *Organization Behavior and Human Performance, 16*(2), 42–175.

Alderfer, C. P. (1972). *Existence, relatedness, and growth.* New York: Free Press.

Alpander, G. G. (1985). Factors influencing hospital employee motivation: A diagnostic instrument.
Hospital and Health Services Administration, 30(2), 67–83.

Alpander, G. G. (1990). Relationship between commitment to hospital goals and job satisfaction: A case study of a nursing department. *Health Care Management Review, 15*(4), 51–62.

Appleby, C. (1998). Brain drain. *Hospitals and Health Networks, 72*(8), 41–42.

Atkinson, J. W. (1961). *An introduction to motivation.* New York: Van Nostrand.

Barbusca, A., & Cleek, M. (1994). Measuring gain-sharing dividends in acute care hospitals. *Health Care Management Review, 19*(1), 28–33.

Barrick, M. R., & Alexander, R. A. (1987). A review of quality circle efficacy and the existence of a positive finding bias. *Personnel Psychology, 40*(4), 579–592.

Bassin, M. (1988). Teamwork at General Foods: New and improved. *Personnel Administrator, 33*(5), 62–70.

Becker, I. J. (1978). Joint effect of feedback and goal setting on performance: A field study of residential energy conservation. *Journal of Applied Psychology, 63,* 428–433.

Berger, S., & Moyer, J. (1991). Launching a performance-based pay plan. *Modern Healthcare, 21*(33), 64.

Blackburn, R. B., & Rosen, B. (1993). Total quality and human resources management: Lessons learned from Baldridge Award–winning companies. *Academy of Management Executive, 7*(3), 49–60.

Blanchard, K. H., & Bowles, S. M. (1998). Get gung ho. *Success, 45*(5), 30–31.

Blayney, K. D. (Ed.). (1992). *Healing hands: Customizing your health team for institutional survival.* Battle Creek, MI: W. K. Kellogg Foundation.

Campbell, J. P., & Pritchard, R. D. (1976). Motivation theory in industrial and organizational psychology. In M. D. Dunnette (Ed.), *Handbook of industrial and organizational psychology* (pp. 63–130). Skokie, IL: Rand McNally.

Carr, S. C., McLoughlin, D., Hodgson, M., & MacLachlan, M. (1996). Effects of unreasonable pay discrepancies for under- and overpayment on double demotivation. *Genetic, Social, and General Psychology Monograph, 122*(4), 475–494.

Charns, M. P., & Smith Tewksbury, L. J. (1993). *Collaborative management in health care: Implementing the integrative organization.* San Francisco: Jossey-Bass Publishers.

Chusmir, L. H. (1986). How fulfilling are health care jobs? *Health Care Management Review, 11*(1), 27–32.

Colvin, G. (1998). What money makes you do. *Fortune, 138*(4), 213–214.

Cornelius, E., & Lane, F. (1984). The power motive and managerial success in a professionally oriented service company. *Journal of Applied Psychology, 69,* 32–40.

Cotton, J. L., Volrath, D. A., Frogett, K. L., Lengnick-Hall, M. D., & Jennings, K. R. (1988). Employee participation: Diverse forms and different outcomes. *Academy of Management Review, 13*(1), 8–22.

Daniels, A. C. (1994). *Bringing out the best in people: How to apply the astonishing power of positive reinforcement.* New York: McGraw-Hill, Inc.

Davis-Blake, A., & Pfeffer, J. (1989). Just a mirage: The search for disposition effects in organizational research. *Academy of Management Review, 14*(3), 385–400.

Durand, D. E. (1983). Modified achievement motivation training: A longitudinal study of the effects of a condensed training design for entrepreneurs. *Psychological Reports, 52,* 901–911.

Erez, M., & Zidon, I. (1984). Effect of goal acceptance on the relationship of goal difficulty to performance. *Journal of Applied Psychology, 69,* 69–78.

Farnham, A. (1989, December). The trust gap. *Fortune,* 56–78.

Ford, R. C., & Fottler, M. D. (1992). Studies of nurses' attitudes during the 1980's: What have we learned? In D. F. Ray (Ed.), *Proceedings of the annual meeting of the Southern Management Association* (pp. 130–132). Mississippi State, MS: Southern Management Association.

Ford, R. C., & Fottler, M. D. (1995). Empowerment: A matter of degree. *Academy of Management Executive, 9*(3), 21–29.

Fottler, M. D. (1996). The role and impact of multiskilled health practitioners in the health services industry. *Hospital and Health Services Administration, 41*(1), 55–75.

Fottler, M. D., Blair, J. D., Phillips, R. L., & Duran, C. A. (1990). Achieving competitive advantage through strategic human resources management. *Hospital and Health Services Administration, 35*(3), 341–363.

Fottler, M. D., Crawford, M. A., Quintana, J. B., & White, J. B. (1995). Evaluating nurse turnover: Comparing attitude surveys and exit interviews. *Hospital and Health Services Administration, 40*(2), 278–295.

Fottler, M. D., Shewchuk, R. M., & O'Connor, S. J. (1998). What matters to health care executives? Assessing the job attributes associated with their staying or leaving. *International Journal of Organization Theory and Behavior, 1*(2), 223–247.

Fried, Y., & Ferris, G. R. (1987). The validity of the job characteristics model: A review and meta analysis. *Personnel Psychology, 40*(3), 287–322.

Georgopoulos, B. S., Mahoney, B. S., & Jones, N. W. (1957). A path-goal approach to productivity. *Journal of Applied Psychology, 41,* 345–353.

Greenberg, J. (1982). Approaching equity and avoiding inequity in groups and organizations. In J. Greenberg, & R. L. Cohen (Eds.), *Equity and justice in social behavior.* New York: Academic Press.

Griffin, R. W. (1991). Effects of work redesign on employee perceptions, attitudes, and behavior: A long-term investigation. *Academy of Management Journal, 34*(2), 425–435.

Guzzo, R. A., Jette, R. D., & Katzell, R. A. (1985). The effects of psychologically based intervention programs on worker productivity: A meta analysis. *Personnel Psychology, 38*(3), 275–291.

Gwynne, S. C. (1990, October 29). The right stuff. *Time,* 74–84.

Hackman, J. R., & Oldham, G. (1980). *Work redesign.* Reading, MA: Addison-Wesley.

Hames, D. S. (1991). Productivity-enhancing work innovations: Remedies for what ails hospitals? *Hospital and Health Services Administration, 38*(4), 545–557.

Haug, M. E. (1988). A re-examination of the hypothesis of physician deprofessionalization. *The Milbank Quarterly, 66*(Supplement 2), 48–56.

Heckert, D. A., Fottler, M. D., Swartz, B. W., & Mercer, A. A. (1993). The impact of the changing healthcare environment on the attitudes of nursing staff. *Health Services Management Research, 6*(3), 191–202.

Herzberg, F. (1987). One more time: How do you motivate employees? *Harvard Business Review, 65,* 109–120.

Herzberg, F., Mausner, B., & Snyderman, B. (1959). *The motivation to work.* New York: John Wiley.

Holland, M. G., Black, C. H., & Miner, J. B. (1987). Using managerial role motivation theory to predict career success. *Health Care Management Review, 12*(4), 57–64.

Hollenbeck, J. R., & Klein, H. J. (1987). Goal commitment and the goal-setting process: Problems, prospects, and proposals for future research. *Journal of Applied Psychology, 82,* 212–220.

Hom, P. W. (1980). Expectancy prediction of reenlistment in the National Guard. *Journal of Vocational Behavior, 16*(2), 235–248.

House, R. J., & Wigdor, L. A. (1967). Herzberg's two-factor theory of job satisfaction and motivation: A review of the evidence and a criticism. *Personnel Psychology, 20*(3), 369–389.

Hurka, S. J. (1980). Need satisfaction among health care managers. *Hospital and Health Services Administration, 25*(3), 43–54.

Huselid, M. A. (1995). The impact of human resource management practices on turnover, productivity, and corporate financial performance. *Academy of Management Journal, 38*(3), 635–672.

Huseman, R. C., & Hatfield, J. D. (1989). *Managing the equity factor.* Boston: Houghton-Mifflin.

Imberman, W. (1976). Letting the employee speak his mind. *Personnel, 53*(6), 12–22.

Ivancevich, J. M., & McMahon, J. T. (1982). The effects of goal-setting, external feedback, and self-generated feedback on outcome variables: A field experiment. *Academy of Management Journal, 25*(2), 359–372.

Jurkiewicz, C. L., Massey, T. K., & Brown, R. J. (1998). Motivation in public and private organizations: A comparative study. *Public Productivity & Management Review, 21*(3), 230–250.

Kanfer, R. (1990). Motivation theory and industrial and organizational psychology. In M. D. Dunnette, & L. M., Houghlin (Eds.), *Handbook of industrial and organizational psychology* (pp. 75–170). Palo Alto, CA: Consulting Psychologists Press, Inc.

Kennedy, C. W., Fossum, J. A., & White, B. J. (1983). An empirical comparison of within-subjects and between-subjects expectancy theory models. *Organizational Behavior and Human Performance, 32,* 124–143.

Kennedy, M. M. (1997). How to put new life into an old job. *Healthcare Executive, 12*(5), 44–45.

Kiechel, W. (1989, April 10). The workaholic generation. *Fortune,* 50–62.

Koch, J. (1990). Perpetual thanks: Its assets. *Personnel Journal, 69*(1), 72–73.

Kongstvedt, P. R. (1996). *The managed care health care handbook* (3rd ed.). Gaithersburg, MD: Aspen Publishers, Inc.

Kovach, K. A. (1987). What motivates employees: Workers and supervisors give different answers. *Business Horizons, 30,* 58–65.

Kovach, K. A. (1995). Employee motivation: Addressing a crucial factor in your organization's performance. *Employment Relations Today, 22*(2), 93–105.

"Labor letter." (1980, February 20). *The Wall Street Journal,* p. A1.

Laurinaitis, J. (1997). Actions speak louder than posters. *Psychology Today, 30*(3), 16.

Lawler, E. E. (1988). Choosing an involvement strategy. *Academy Of Management Executive, 2*(3), 197–204.

Lawler, E. E. (1989). Pay for performance: A strategic analysis. In L. R. Gomez-Mejia (Ed.), *Compensation and benefits* (pp. 136–181). Washington, DC: Bureau of National Affairs.

Lee, J. A. (1980). *The gold and garbage of management theory and prescriptions.* Athens, OH: Ohio University Press.

Locke, E. A. (1968). Effects of knowledge of results, feedback in relation to standards, and goals on reaction-time performance. *American Journal of Applied Psychology, 81,* 566–574.

Locke, E. A. (1982). Relation of goal level to performance with a short work period and multiple goal levels. *Journal of Applied Psychology, 67,* 512–514.

Locke, E. A., & Latham, G. P. (1984). *Goal setting: A motivational technique that works.* Englewood Cliffs, NJ: Prentice Hall.

Locke, E. A., & Latham, G. P. (1990a). *A theory of goal setting and task performance.* Englewood Cliffs, NJ: Prentice-Hall.

Locke, E. A., & Latham, G. P. (1990b). Work motivation and satisfaction: Light at the end of the tunnel. *Psychological Science, 1*(4), 240–246.

Locke, E. A., Latham, G. P., & Erez, M. (1988). The determinants of goal commitment. *Academy of Management Review, 13,* 23–39.

Longest, B. (1974). Job satisfaction of registered nurses in a hospital setting. *Journal of Nursing Administration, 4*(3), 46–52.

Luthans, F., & Kreitney, R. (1985). *Organization behavior modification and beyond: An operant conditioning approach.* Glenview, IL: Scott, Foresman.

Lutz, S. (1990). Hospitals stretch their creativity to motivate workers. *Modern Healthcare, 20*(9), 20–33.

Lutz, S. (1990). Employee suggestions net $20 million in savings. *Modern Healthcare, 20*(9), 21–22.

Maslow, A. H. (1943). A theory of human motivation. *Psychological Review, 50,* 370–396.

McClelland, D. C. (1961). *The achieving society.* Princeton, NJ: Van Nostrand.

McClelland, D. C. (1975). *Power: The inner experience.* New York: Irvington.

McClelland, D. C., & Burnham, D. H. (1976). Power is the great motivator. *Harvard Business Review, 54*(2), 100–110.

McConnell, C. R. (1996). After reduction in force: Reinvigorating the survivors. *The Health Care Supervisor, 14*(4), 1–2.

McConnell, C. R. (1997). Employee recognition: A little oil on the troubled waters of change. *The Health Care Supervisor, 15*(4), 83–90.

The M.D. factor. (1997). *Crossroads: New directions in health management,* a supplement to Hospitals & Health Networks.

Medcof, J. W., & Hausdorf, P. A. (1995). Instruments to measure opportunities to satisfy needs, and degree of satisfaction of needs, in the workplace. *Journal of Occupational and Organizational Psychology, 68*(3), 193–199.

Mercer, A. A. (1988). Commitment and motivation of professionals. In M. D. Fottler, S. R. Hernandez, and C. L. Joiner (Eds.), *Strategic management of human resources in health services organizations* (pp. 181–205). New York: John Wiley and Sons.

Miron, D., & McClelland, D. C. (1979). The impact of achievement motivation in small business. *California Management Review, 22,* 34–46.

Mitchell, T. R. (1982). Motivation: New directions for theory, research, and practice. *Academy of Management Review, 7,* 80–88.

Mitchell, T. R. (1984). *Motivation and performance.* Chicago: Science Research Associates.

Mitchell, V., & Mowdgill, P. (1976). Measurement of Maslow's need hierarchy. *Organization Behavior and Human Performance, 16*(2), 334–349.

Mohr, L. B. (1982). *Explaining organizational behavior.* San Francisco: Jossey-Bass.

Mohrmann, S. A., & Lawler, E. E. (1984). Quality of worklife. *Research in Personnel and Human Resources Management, 2,* 219–260.

Montgomery, K., Lewis, C. E. (1995). Fear of HIV contagion as workplace stress: Behavioral consequences and buffers. *Hospital and Health Services Administration, 40*(1), 439–456.

Moore, J. D. (1996). Samaritan's revolution: New pay model aims to overhaul how workers think. *Modern Healthcare, 26*(31), pp. 27, 30, 32–34.

Muchinsky, P. M. (1987). *Psychology applied to work: An introduction to industrial and organizational psychology.* Belmont, CA: Wadsworth, Inc., 341–378.

Nicholls, J. G. (1984). Achievement motivation: Conceptions of authority, subjective experience, task chores, and performance. *Psychological Review, 91,* 328–346.

Nordhaus-Bike, A. M. (1997). Cutting with kindness. *Hospital and Health Networks, 71*(2), 62–63.

O'Connor, S. J. (1996). Who will manage the managers? In A. Lazarus (Ed.), *Controversies in managed mental health care* (pp. 383–401). Washington, DC: American Psychiatric Press.

O'Connor, S. J. (1998). Motivating effective performance. In P. Ginter, L. Swayne, and D. J. Duncan (Eds.), *Handbook of health care management* (pp. 431–470). Cambridge, MA: Blackwell Business Publishing.

O'Connor, S. J., & Lanning, J. A. (1992). The end of autonomy? Reflections on the post-professional physician. *Health Care Management Review, 17*(1), 63–72.

O'Connor, S. J., & Shewchuk, R. M. (1995). Service quality revisited: Striving for a new orientation. *Hospital and Health Services Administration, 40*(1), 535–552.

Phillips, R. L., Duran, C. A., Blair, J. D., Peterson, M. F., Savage, G. T., & Whitehead, C. J. (1990). Quality circles in health-care organizations: Pitfalls and promises. In H. Metzger (Ed.), *Handbook of healthcare human resources management* (pp. 137–146). Rockville, MD: Aspen Systems.

Pinder, C. (1984). *Work motivation.* Glenview, IL: Scott, Foresman.

Plume, S. (1995). Redesigning physician compensation mechanisms: A fool's errand. *Motivation & Emotion, 19*(3), 205–210.

Pritchard, R. D., De Leo, P. J., & Von Bergen, C. W. (1976). A field experimental test of expectancy-valence incentive motivation techniques. *Organizational Behavior and Human Performance, 15,* 355–406.

Pujol, J. L., & Tudanger, E. (1992). A vision of excellence. *HRM Magazine, 35*(6), 112–116.

Rantz, M. J., Scott, J., & Porter, R. (1996). Employee motivation: New perspectives of the age-old challenge of work motivation. *Nursing Forum, 31*(3), 29–36.

Rawlinson, H. (1988). Make awards count. *Personnel Journal, 67*(10), 139–146.

Reibstein, L. (1986 October 27). A finger on the pulse: Companies expand use of employee surveys. *The Wall Street Journal,* 27.

Rogers, E. F., Metlay, W., Kaplan, I. T., & Shapiro, T. (1995). Self-managing work teams: Do they really work? *Human Resources Planning, 18*(2), 53–57.

Rollins, T. (1987). Pay for performance: The pros and cons. *Personnel Journal, 66*(5), 104–107.

Schneider, B., & Alderfer, C. P. (1973). Three studies of measures of need satisfaction in organizations. *Administrative Science Quarterly, 18*(4), 489–505.

Schwarb, D. P., Devitt, W. H., & Cummings, L. L. (1971). A test of the adequacy of the two-factor theory as a predictor of self-report performance effects. *Personnel Psychology, 24,* 293–304.

Schwartz, H. S. (1983). Maslow and the hierarchial enactment of organizational reality. *Human Relations, 36*(10), 933–956.

Sherman, S. (1995). Stretch goals: The dark side of asking for miracles. *Fortune, 132*(10), 231–232.

Skinner, B. F. (1969). *Contingencies of reinforcement: A theoretical analysis.* New York: Appleton-Century-Crofts.

Stacy, A. W., Widaman, K. F., & Marlatt, G. A. (1990). Expectancy models of alcohol use. *Journal of Personality and Social Psychology, 58*(5), 918–928.

Steers, R. M., & Porter, L. W. (1987). *Motivation and work behavior.* New York: McGraw-Hill.

Steffen, T. M., Nystrom, P. C., & O'Connor, S. J. (1996). Satisfaction with nursing homes: The design of employees jobs can ultimately influence family members' perceptions. *Journal of Health Care Marketing, 16*(3), 34–38.

Taglinferri, L. E. (1988). Taking note of employee attitudes. *Personnel Administrator, 33*(4), 96–102.

Thomas, L. (1998). Maximizing the human resource asset. *The Health Care Supervisor, 16*(4), 35–39.

Tsui, A. S., Ashford, S. J., St. Clair, L., & Xin, K. R. (1995). Dealing with discrepant expectations: Response strategies and managerial effectiveness. *Academy of Management Journal, 38*(6), 1515–1543.

Tully, S. (1994). Why go for the stretch targets? *Fortune, 130*(10), 145–158.

Vance, A. (1997). Motivating the paraprofessional in long-term care. *The Health Care Supervisor, 15*(4), 57–64.

Vaughan, D. G., Fottler, M. D., Bamberg, R., & Blayney, K. (1991). Utilization and management of multiskilled health practitioners in U. S. hospitals. *Hospital and Health Services Administration, 36*(3), 347–419.

Vidaver-Cohen, D. (1998). Motivational appeal in normative theories of enterprise. *Business Ethics Quarterly, 8*(3), 385–407.

Vroom, V. (1964). *Work and motivation.* New York: Wiley.

Wahba, M. A., & Budwell, L. G. (1976). Maslow reconsidered: A review of research on the need hierarchy theory. *Organization Behavior and Human Performance, 15*(2), 317–333.

Wall, T. D., Kemp, N. J., Jackson, P. R., & Clegg, W. W. (1986). Outcomes of autonomous work groups: A long-term field experiment. *Academy of Management Journal, 29*(2), 280–304.

Wanous, J. P., Keon, T. L., & Latack, J. C. (1983). Expectancy theory and occupational/organizational choices: A review and test. *Organizational Behavior and Human Performance, 32*(1), 66–86.

Weiner, B. (1986). *An attributional theory of motivation and emotion.* New York: Springer-Verlag.

York, D. R. (1985). Attitude surveying. *Personnel Journal, 64*(5), 70–73.

Zigarelli, M. (1996). Human resources and the bottom line. *Academy of Management Executive, 10*(2), 63.

Zima, J. P. (1983). *Interviewing: Key to effective management.* Chicago: Science Research Associates, Inc.

Zimberg, S. E., & Clement, D. G. (1997). Physician motivation, satisfaction and survival. *Medical Group Management Journal, 44*(4), 19–20, 22, 24, 26, 63.

C H A P T E R

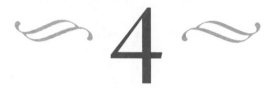

4

Leadership: A Framework for Thinking and Acting

Dennis D. Pointer, Ph.D.
Julianne P. Sanchez, M. A.

Chapter Outline

- Core Concepts
- Leadership Effectiveness and Success: What We Know
- Leadership: An Integrative Framework
- Several Distinctive Aspects of Leadership in Health Services Organizations

Learning Objectives

After completing this chapter, the reader should be able to:

1. Better appreciate why leadership skills are so important.
2. Understand what leadership is and what it is not.
3. Understand the distinction between management and leadership.
4. Understand the leadership role and how it is executed in health services organizations.
5. Understand the major leadership perspectives as well as some emerging theories and concepts.
6. Consider how different leadership perspectives can be combined into a more integrative framework.
7. Appreciate several distinctive challenges of leading in health services organizations.
8. Continue developing leadership knowledge and skills.

Key Terms

Attribution Theory
Authority
Behavioral Perspective
Charismatic Leadership
Clinical Mentality
Contingency Perspective
Gender Gap
Goal Accomplishment
Influence
Leadership Match Model
Leadership Role
Leadership Styles: S1, S2, S3, S4
LEAD Model
Managerial Office
Managerial Roles
Office
Path-Goal Model
Power
Trait Perspective
Transactional Leadership
Transformational Leadership

Chapter Purpose

We want to help you gain an understanding of one of the most fundamental concepts in organization and management theory: LEADERSHIP. Leadership is one of the most important things managers do. It is the means by which things are accomplished in organizations. A manager can establish goals, strategize, relate to others, communicate, collect information, make decisions, plan, organize, monitor, and control; but nothing happens without leadership.

In this chapter we will first explore the concept of leadership. As the "In the Real World" case demonstrates, leadership is very difficult to get a firm grip on. Second, we will describe what scholars working in the field have come to know about the factors related to leadership effectiveness and success. Third, we will develop an integrative model of leadership. Our objective is to blend together key features of the different perspectives that have been presented in the literature. Fourth, we will discuss

several distinctive aspects of leadership in health services organizations. Finally, we will offer some suggestions regarding how you can continue improving your leadership knowledge and skills.

CORE CONCEPTS

Can you imagine the following ad being run in the "Help Wanted" section of *Modern Healthcare?*

> Major nation-wide health care organization undergoing rapid expansion in every region of the country is seeking applicants for management positions at all levels, from executive to supervisory.
> *LEADERSHIP ABILITIES NOT REQUIRED*
> Send resume and salary history to:
>
> Modern Healthcare
> Box 554B
> 740 N. Rush Street
> Chicago, IL 60611

Of course not!

Leadership is one of the most highly valued management abilities. Health services organizations are presumed to thrive under great leadership and face considerable difficulty, or even fail, when it's poor. Everyone is on the lookout for individuals who have leadership ability. People who can convince others they are leaders generally get hired and promoted. Managers without the leadership "right stuff," no matter how good they are at performing other aspects of their jobs, often face career stagnation or, worse yet, find themselves looking for a different position and maybe even a new line of work. Think for a moment about yourself. How would you like to be tagged as a non-leader or someone who has no leadership potential? How would this label affect your ability to either get or keep a management position, irrespective of level, in a health services organization?

As important as leadership seems to be, when asked to define and describe it, people have trouble. Perhaps you experienced difficulty when attempting

IN THE REAL WORLD:
WE'RE SEARCHING FOR A LEADER BUT WE MAY NOT FULLY UNDERSTAND WHAT LEADERSHIP IS!

You are a board member of a 250-bed short-term general hospital that has just begun the process of working with an executive search consultant to recruit a new chief executive officer (CEO). The present occupant of the position will be voluntarily retiring in five months after 23 years of service. The headhunter has a unique background. She holds a Ph.D. in organization behavior and taught this subject in a health administration program for 10 years prior to starting her own executive search firm. In addition to all of the other types of experience, knowledge, and skills necessary for being a successful hospital CEO, the board wants to recruit someone who is an "exceptional leader." They have communicated this desire to the search consultant and selected her because they felt she could help them find such a person.

The consultant is meeting with board members, over dinner, for the first time since being retained. While coffee and dessert are being served, she begins talking with the board about why they feel leadership ability is so important in this search. She concludes by saying, "If we are going to locate someone with the type of leadership style and skills you want, we've got to have a shared notion of just what it is we are looking for. If you all define leadership in different ways and have varying ideas about what an exceptional leader is, we're in for some difficulties as this process unfolds. I have a few questions that I want you to think about. Take the next 10 minutes to jot down some notes on a piece of paper. Don't feel like you have to compose elegant prose; just go for substance. This exercise may seem a bit academic. Indeed, I asked these questions of students before we began the leadership module in my organization behavior and management course at the university. During the years I have taught this material, I've found that they're very helpful in getting people to begin thinking a bit more rigorously about leadership. Let me warn you up front that these are not easy questions to answer. After you're finished, we will spend the next half hour or so discussing your ideas."

Here are the questions.

- *What is leadership? Rough out a one- or two-sentence definition that captures the essence of the term.*
- *Is leadership synonymous with management, or is leading just one of many things that a manager does? In what ways are they different, or how are they the same?*
- *Think of some individuals whom you feel are really exceptional leaders. What, if anything, do they have in common?*
- *Think of some individuals who are truly lousy leaders. What, if anything, do they have in common?*
- *How does leadership affect the performance of what's being led (whether it's an individual, a group, or an entire organization)? That is, in what ways does leadership make a difference?*
- *Have you ever known people who were successful leaders in one situation and failures in others? Why is this so?*

To our readers: Pause a few moments, take out a piece of paper, and answer these questions. We realize that it's far easier not to expend the effort and just press ahead. However, prior to being exposed to our thinking about leadership, we feel it's important that you clarify your own. You might want to share your answers, and frustrations in composing them, with fellow students. One of the real benefits of this exercise is gaining an appreciation of how varied peoples' notions of leadership are. Save your responses to these questions. You will want to look at them again after you've completed this chapter.

to answer the first questions in the opening case. Leadership is an elusive management concept.

We want to begin by presenting a very stripped-down definition of leadership including only the essentials with which most scholars working in the field would have little disagreement.

> Leadership is the process through which an individual attempts to intentionally influence another individual or a group in order to accomplish a goal.

Simple enough, but the core concepts embedded in this seemingly simple sentence warrant some emphasis and elaboration. First, leadership is a process. It is a verb, an action word, not a noun. Leadership manifests itself in the doing; it is a performing art. Second, only individuals lead. The *locus of leadership* is in a person. Inanimate objects don't lead, groups don't lead, organizations don't lead; only people lead. When looking for and at leadership, our subject is the individual. Third, the *focus of leadership* is other individuals and groups. Leadership can't exist without this connection between someone who is leading and those who, for whatever reason, choose to follow. The follower might be just one other person, a group, members of an organization, or the population of a nation. Fourth, leadership entails influencing. **Influence** is leadership's center of gravity and most critical element. Who is influenced? Followers (individuals and groups), as just noted. What is influenced? The cognitive target of influence is their thoughts; the affective target is their feelings; and the behavioral target is their actions or deeds. For what purpose are followers influenced? This brings us to our fifth point; the objective of leadership is **goal accomplishment.** Leadership is instrumental; it is done for a purpose. Sixth, and last, leadership is intentional; it's not accidental. All of us unknowingly influence others hundreds of times each day. These, however, are not acts of leadership; they are just "happenings."

Leadership is exercised in a lot of different places and in a wide variety of situations. For example, you are engaged in leadership when attempting to persuade that person sitting next to you in accounting class to join you at the student center for lunch after

class. Keep in mind, all of the key elements are here—you, the locus of leadership; that person, the follower; and an act of intentional influence in order to accomplish a goal. However, the focus here is on a particular type of leadership—that engaged in by managers in organizations. To further develop our definition, we need to briefly explore this context.

Organizations exist to accomplish tasks that are so large or complex that they can't be undertaken by individuals and small groups. They do this by sequentially subdividing work over and over again. For example, the delivery of acute inpatient care in a community is a task that is so large and complex an organization must undertake it. A hospital assumes this task and proceeds to divide it up. Nursing services does some parts of it, ancillary services does other parts, professional services does others, and so on. For example, the delivery of nursing care is also such a large and complex task that it too must be subdivided. It is parceled out among different divisions (e.g., medicine, surgery, pediatrics, obstetrics/gynecology). Thus, organizations sequentially subdivide tasks until they are small and simple enough to be performed by an individual. In the process, the hospital is divided into a series of components, all of which must be managed.

Figure 4.1 presents a schematic organizational chart typical of a short-term general hospital. We've focused on one segment of a vertical slice that is composed of four components. In each component there is a **managerial office,** and associated with each are sets of expectations called **managerial roles.** Roles are constellations of things managers are expected to do because they hold the office (Katz & Kahn, 1966). Roles are attached to the office, not the particular person occupying it. Occupants of the office may come and go, but the roles remain, and they remain the same. There are a wide variety of ways to describe the roles of a manager; several models were presented in Chapter 2. The critical point is that leadership is only one of the many roles managers are expected to perform because of the office they hold in the organization. Leadership and management are not the same thing; they aren't synonyms. This is a terribly important notion. Keep the concepts of manager (an individual who holds an office attached to which are multiple roles) and leadership (one

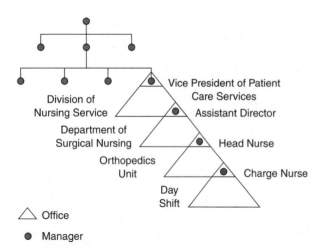

△ Office

● Manager

Figure 4.1. Organizational Components and Managerial Offices.

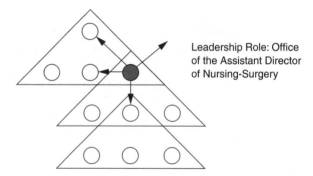

Leadership Role: Office of the Assistant Director of Nursing-Surgery

Figure 4.2. Directionality of the Manager's Leadership Role.

of these roles) straight. A lot of folks don't, and it leads to considerable confusion.

Execution of the **leadership role** is the way managers get things done. While leadership is not the only role of the manager, it is certainly the central one. Other roles such as information processing, decision making, and visioning are converted into tangible results by leading.

Put Figure 4.1 under a magnifying glass and you have Figure 4.2. It focuses on one managerial office in the hospital's chain of command, an assistant director of nursing service. This manager is a subordinate in one component of the organization (the division of nursing service), reports to a vice president, and is a peer of others having the same reporting relationship. Simultaneously, the manager holds a superordinate office in that component of the organization for which he is responsible, the department of surgical nursing. Reporting to the assistant director are other managers (head nurses), each of whom is responsible for a different unit.

This one office will be employed as an illustration to introduce several key points about leadership. First, leadership is multidirectional. The assistant director leads not only subordinates in the component of the organization of which he is the manager but also peers, his superior, and individuals or groups

outside of the organization. Only when we conceptualize leadership as intentional influence and when the proper distinction between managing and leadership is drawn does this notion become clear. For example, the assistant director of nursing intentionally influences or leads (but does not manage) his peers in chairing a departmental work group to implement a new scheduling system and his superior in providing direction prior to an upcoming budget review and negotiation session with the hospital's chief operating officer. Additionally, he might engage in the leadership role when working with individuals and groups outside of the organization such as suppliers, physician office staffs, and colleagues in other organizations. Not only does the assistant director lead in all directions, he is simultaneously led from these same directions—from above by his superior, from the side by peers, from below by subordinates, and from outside the organization. Leadership's arrows of influence point in two directions simultaneously.

Second, although leadership is multidirectional, it's the downward focus that has received the greatest amount of attention and study. When one thinks of leadership, the first thing that generally comes to mind is the relationship between managers and their subordinates. The vast majority of leadership research (which will be reviewed in the next section) has this focus. Most leadership is pointed downward, primarily toward one's direct reports (in the case of the assistant director, head nurses) and secondarily toward subordinates in lower and lower layers of the organization.

Third, when one engages in leadership, irrespective of its direction, the focus is generally on other managers. In our illustration, it's only at the level of the charge nurse that nonmanagers are led. For the most part, managers lead other managers.

Fourth, the extent to which leadership attempts are successful depends on the amount of **power** associated with a particular managerial office and the person holding it. The concept of power is addressed in Chapter 9.

LEADERSHIP EFFECTIVENESS AND SUCCESS: WHAT WE KNOW

We turn now to reviewing what is known about those factors that are related to leadership effectiveness and success. If you want to select an effective and potentially successful leader, what should you look for and at? If you want to improve your own leadership effectiveness and success, what factors should you focus upon?

As noted in Debate Time 4.1, there are several ways to go about answering these questions. The vast majority of the theorizing and research on leadership can be classified into three different perspectives—trait, behavioral, and contingency (Jago, 1982). These perspectives are described below along with the review of some of the major studies that have been undertaken in each. Additionally, several emerging leadership theories and concepts are introduced.

Readers should note that what follows is not an exhaustive review of the literature. The objective is to provide you with an introductory tour of the leadership terrain with key references provided for those who wish to explore the area further. Also, none of the basic work within these perspectives has been conducted in health services organizations.

The Trait Perspective

Because individuals lead, it's natural and reasonable to look for those characteristics of individuals that might separate successful from unsuccessful leaders or effective from ineffective leadership. And, indeed, this is where the search began. Early work on the **trait perspective** was biographical and focused almost ex-

clusively on military commanders and those holding political office. In the late 1930s psychologists became interested in the area and began investigating relationships between individual characteristics and leadership effectiveness in organizations. Even though critiques of this work in the 1940s suggested that such relationships were weak and not generalizable across different situations, the hunt continued (Jennings, 1947). Every attribute imaginable has been studied (Stodgill, 1948).

The most comprehensive review of this literature was conducted by Roger Stodgill (1974) in his classic work, *Handbook of Leadership*. Stodgill examined 287 studies undertaken from 1904 through 1970. He classified the hundreds of different traits that had been studied into six categories: physical (e.g., age, height, appearance); personality (e.g., self-confidence, independence, dominance); intelligence (e.g., fluency, decisiveness); social background (e.g., educational attainment, social status); social (e.g., cooperativeness, integrity); and task-related (e.g., initiative, persistence, need for achievement) (Bass, 1981).

Stodgill and others were able to identify a small number of traits that seemed to be present in leaders, as compared to followers, and good leaders as contrasted to poor ones (Sartle, 1956). Intelligence, dominance, self-confidence, high energy level, and task-relevant knowledge were on most lists. However, the findings were inconsistent, and relationships were weak; correlation coefficients generally ranged from 0.20 to 0.35. We could spend pages reviewing the different studies, describing their findings, and noting their limitations, but the bottom line is that there are no individual traits that predict leadership effectiveness or success, or that differentiate those who lead from those who follow (Lord, de Vader, & Alliger, 1986).

It is hard to argue that individual traits have no effect whatsoever on leadership effectiveness and success, as it is counter to experience, logic, and common sense. Researchers began to appreciate that traits had an impact, but not in the way originally imagined. First, traits are best thought of as predispositions. A particular trait, or set of them, tends to predispose (although does not cause) an individual to engage in certain behaviors which may or may not result in leadership

DEBATE TIME 4.1: WHAT DO YOU THINK

At this point you should have a fairly clear idea of what leadership is and what it is not in addition to possessing a better feel for the organizational context in which the role is performed by managers. It's clear that all managers are not equally effective or successful leaders. The question is, What sets of factors explain the variability? There has been a raging debate regarding this issue in the literature during the last 50 years or so. There are three very different points of view. What's yours?

The Nature Argument

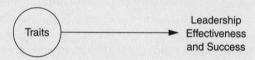

The greatest proportion of the variability in leadership effectiveness and success is due to traits and dispositions that individuals are endowed with at birth or that they develop very early in life. By the time a person assumes a management position, these characteristics are set and nearly impossible to change in any significant way. Some people have traits that predispose them to be successful leaders; others don't.

The Nurture Argument

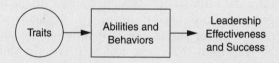

The greatest proportion of the variability in leadership effectiveness and success is due to abilities and behaviors that can be learned. Personal traits and dispositions provide the foundation upon which abilities are acquired and behaviors are developed, but they are only the foundation. Individuals who are exceptional leaders make themselves; they are not made.

The Situational Argument

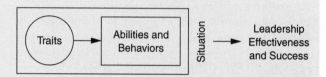

The greatest proportion of the variation in leadership effectiveness and success is due to the characteristics of the situation in which managers find themselves. Sets of traits, abilities, and behaviors are important, but they are very situation-specific. In one situation certain traits, abilities, and behaviors may predispose a manager to be an effective leader; in a different situation the result could be ineffectiveness and failure.

- If you agree with the nature argument, which personal traits and dispositions are most associated with leadership effectiveness and success?
- If you agree with the nurture argument, which abilities and behaviors are most associated with leadership effectiveness and success? What are the best ways to acquire these abilities and develop these behaviors?
- If you agree with the situational argument, which factors are most important?
- Think back for a moment to the opening case. Let's say that each of the three members of the board search committee agrees with a different argument. What would be the consequences?
- People often espouse a situational argument. However, their actual "theory in use" is generally a blend of the nature and nurture arguments. Do you find this to be the case, and if so why?

effectiveness. Traits and behaviors are only loosely coupled. Second, multiple traits are associated with a given behavior, and more than one behavior is linked to an individual trait. Third, it is one's behavior and not one's traits *per se* that is most related to leadership effectiveness and success. "What seems to be most important is not traits but rather how they are expressed in the behavior of the leader" (Van Vleet & Yukl, 1989). These three observations go a long way in explaining why a set of universal leadership traits has not been uncovered; yet research employing this perspective continues (Coska, 1984).

The Behavioral Perspective

Interest in leadership behaviors emerged due to the inability of traits to explain variations in effectiveness. Researchers reasoned that, if traits couldn't explain such variations, maybe the behaviors that flowed from them could. Most of the work has focused on identifying dimensions that could be employed to describe and categorize different leadership behaviors, developing models of leadership style (a style being defined by a combination of behaviors), and examining how specific leadership styles are related to effectiveness. Additionally, behaviorists began to develop more rigorous ways to conceptualize and measure leadership effectiveness.

The first study recognized as employing a **behavioral perspective** was conducted by Kurt Lewin, Ronald Lippitt, and their associates (1939) at the University of Iowa in the 1930s. They compared three styles of leadership—autocratic, democratic, and laissez-faire—in groups of preteen boys. Leaders of the groups were confederates of the researchers and instructed on how to perform the various styles. Democratic leaders coordinated activities of the group and facilitated majority-rule decision making on important decisions; autocratic leaders directed the activities of the group and made important decisions absent input from members; laissez-faire leaders (who accidentally emerged during the course of the study) provided neither facilitation nor direction. This work was significant because it focused on behavior rather than traits, identified and described different leadership styles, and found that variations in style had an impact on followers.

There were several major studies of leadership undertaken immediately after the conclusion of World War II; one of the most widely cited was conducted by a group of investigators at Ohio State University (Stodgill & Coons, 1957). The question addressed was, How does the behavior of a leader impact upon work group performance and satisfaction? Instruments were designed to measure leadership behavior as perceived by managers themselves, in addition to their peers, superiors, and subordinates. Two dimensions of leader behavior were identified: *initiating structure,* or the degree a manager defined and organized the work that was to be done and the extent attention was focused on accomplishing objectives established by the manager; and *consideration,* or the extent the manager exhibited concern for the welfare of the group and its members, stressed the importance of job satisfaction, expressed appreciation, and sought input from subordinates on major decisions. Initiating structure and consideration were not conceptualized as opposite ends of the same continuum, but rather separate and independent dimensions. A manager's behavior could range from high to low on both. As depicted in Figure 4.3, the two dimensions combine to form four distinct leadership styles. Researchers hypothesized that group performance would be maximized when a manager had a leadership style that was high on both consideration and initiating structure. However, numerous follow-up studies found little consistency between the type of leadership style and group satisfaction or performance (Fleishman, 1973; Halpin, 1954). As with the trait research, it appeared that some other factor was confounding results. One criticism of this work was that managers' perceptions of their own leadership style and those of peers, superiors, and subordinates were often dissimilar (Korman, 1966).

In related work, Rensis Likert (1961) and colleagues at the University of Michigan specified two leadership behaviors: job-centered and employee-centered. They were defined similar to consideration and initiating structure in the Ohio studies. Investigations conducted in a wide variety of industries found that

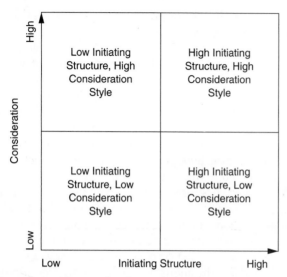

Figure 4.3. Ohio Leadership Study: Behaviors and Styles.

effective supervisors were employee-centered and focused on the needs of the group in addition to establishing high performance goals jointly determined by leaders and followers (Katz, 1950, 1951).

While the Ohio and Michigan studies provided the theoretical underpinning for the behavioral perspective, several other works are frequently referred to in most reviews of this literature.

Blake and Mouton (1978) drew upon previous research and formulated the *managerial grid* popularized in their book of the same name. Their model, originally developed as a consulting tool, was extensively employed in leadership development programs during the 1960s and 1970s. The grid has two dimensions: production orientation and people orientation. In expressing a production orientation, leadership behaviors are directive and focused on accomplishing assigned objectives and tasks. In expressing a people orientation, leadership behaviors focus on enhancing the quality of manager-follower and follower-follower interactions. The model suggests that a manager's behavior can range from low to high on both dimensions, resulting in five different leadership styles.

- *High production and low people orientation:* Leadership behavior focuses exclusively on goal and task ac-

complishment, and maximizing productivity through explicit direction and tight control.
- *High production and high people orientation:* Leadership behavior is goal and task centered but seeks a high degree of follower involvement.
- *Low production and high people orientation:* Leadership behavior focuses on creating fulfilling relationships even if goal and task accomplishment suffer.
- *Low production and low people orientation:* Leadership behavior is focused on neither goal and task accomplishment nor on fulfilling the needs of followers; minimal energy is expended on execution of the leadership role.
- *Moderate production and moderate people orientation:* Leadership behavior focuses on balancing goal and task accomplishment, and follower need fulfillment.

Blake and Mouton (1982) contended that the high production and high people oriented style was most effective and resulted in the best outcomes (group productivity and satisfaction) irrespective of the situation faced. Little research supports this assertion, but there is some evidence that this style is preferred by managers and perceived by them to be most effective.

Robert Tannenbaum and Warren Schmidt (1973) portrayed leadership behavior as a *continuum* that ranged from manager-centered to follower-centered. In the manager-centered style, considerable authority is exercised, and followers have little opportunity to participate in making decisions that affect them; leadership behavior is autocratic and directive. In the follower-centered style, the manager exercises a minimum amount of authority, and followers have considerable freedom to set their own goals and determine how tasks should be executed; leadership behavior is democratic and participative. Tannenbaum and Schmidt, contrary to previous models, conceptualized leadership behavior as bipolar. One was either manager-centered, follower-centered, or somewhere in between. The authors explicitly stated there was no one style that would be equally effective in all situations. Additionally, they noted that the effectiveness of a particular style depended upon three factors: characteristics of the manager (e.g., their traits or dispositions, skills, and values), characteristics of followers (e.g., their skills, knowledge, experience;

readiness to assume responsibility, understanding of goals and tasks), and characteristics of the situation (e.g., time availability, nature of the problem). This model underscored that leadership effectiveness depended on contingencies and suggested some important ones. However, it did not specifically indicate how a manager should go about selecting the most effective style in a specific circumstance.

The Contingency Perspective

In the early 1960s it became increasingly apparent that variations in leadership effectiveness and success could not be adequately explained by either traits or behaviors. Attention turned to incorporating situational characteristics, or **contingencies,** into leadership models. Recall that this notion was first forwarded in the 1940s. A number of leadership contingency models have been developed. We will introduce you to only three of them here: leadership match, path-goal, and leadership effectiveness and adaptability (LEAD). This selection is made because the leadership match and path-goal models have been the subject of considerable empirical research, and the LEAD model has been extensively employed as a teaching and leadership development tool. This section concludes with a discussion of attribution theory, which deals with the manager as a contingency.

Leadership Match Model

The first comprehensive contingency model of leadership, the **leadership match model,** was developed by Fred Fiedler. His model is complex, and only a highly simplified description of it is provided here. Readers interested in a more thorough treatment should refer to the original sources (Fiedler, 1967; Fiedler & Chemers, 1974; Fiedler, Chemers, & Mahar, 1976). The underlying notion of this model is that managers are unable to alter their style to any appreciable degree. Leadership effectiveness depends not on fitting one's style to the situation but rather on selecting a situation that is conducive to one's style (Hall & Norgaim, 1976).

Based on behavioral studies, two leadership styles were specified: task-oriented and employee-oriented.

Fiedler developed a unique and controversial way to measure them. After completing a 20-item questionnaire, a person was assigned a least preferred coworker (LPC) score. The score reflected the degree of regard a respondent held for that coworker she preferred least. Managers with low LPC scores (disregard for the least preferred worker) were classified as having a task-oriented leadership style. Managers with a high LPC score (favorable evaluations of the coworker they least preferred) were classified as possessing an employee-oriented style.

Fiedler identified three situational factors: manager-follower relationship, which could be good or poor; task structure, which could be either high or low; and manager position power, ranging from strong to weak. The combined effect of these three factors produce situations that are favorable, moderately favorable, or unfavorable to the manager.

Based upon studies conducted with hundreds of groups in a variety of organizations, it was determined that managers with a task-oriented leadership style were most effective in situations that were either favorable or unfavorable. Managers with an employee-oriented leadership style did better in situations that were moderately favorable. However, there have been a number of criticisms of this work, including questions regarding the validity of the LPC questionnaire and concerns that situational factors and leadership style may not be independent of one another (Nebeker, 1975; Stinson & Tracy, 1974).

Path-Goal Model

The **path-goal model** is based on the expectancy theory of motivation discussed in Chapter 3 (Porter & Lawler, 1968; Vroom, 1964). Expectancy theory is interested in the factors that affect an individual's choice of behavior, or why someone is motivated to do one thing rather than another. The focus is on effort, performance, rewards, motivation, and the relationships between them (expectancies, instrumentalities, and valences). While the expectancy theory of motivation focuses on describing such relationships, the path-goal model of leadership is interested in the factors that affect them. Initial formulation of this model was forwarded by Martin Evans (1970a, 1970b) in the early 1970s and then refined by Robert House (1971) and House and Terrance Mitchell (1974). It has undergone constant revision over the years.

From the perspective of the path-goal model, the manager exercises influence to increase the motivation of a follower attempting to accomplish a specific goal, in a particular context, during a finite period of time. As depicted in Figure 4.4, a follower's level of motivation is a result of her perceptions of expectancies, instrumentalities, and valences. Such perceptions are affected by three sets of contingencies: leadership behavior or style, features of the work environment, and characteristics of the follower.

In most leadership situations, follower characteristics and features of the work environment are not under the direct control of the manager; in the short run, they are fixed. Follower characteristics include such things as needs and motives (e.g., the degree to which achievement, power, and affiliation are important to the person), ability (knowledge, skills, and experience) to perform the task, and the extent to which individuals feel they have control over critical contingencies that affect their performance in a given situation. Features of the work environment include such things as the extent to which the task is structured or unstructured, amount of time available to complete the task, nature and degree of interdependence among work group members, and a host of organizational characteristics.

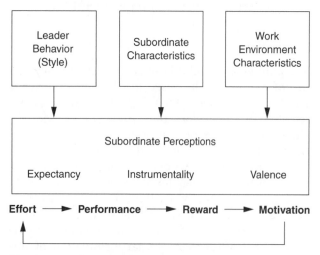

Figure 4.4. The Path-Goal Model.

The contingency most under a manager's control is his own leadership style. The dimensions that define leadership style are presently conceptualized as instrumental behavior (defining objectives and specifying the task to be performed), supportive behavior (providing support to and fulfilling needs of followers), participative behavior (seeking followers' input on decisions that affect them), and achievement-oriented behavior (establishing goals and setting expectations that challenge followers).

Given the number of contingencies and the numerous ways in which they can interact with one another, empirical tests have focused only on pieces of the model, and like most leadership research, the results have been conflicting (Schreisheim & von Glinow, 1977). Additionally, because of its complexity, the model is difficult to employ in real-life situations. However, several general observations and suggestions can be forwarded (House & Baetz, 1979).

- One of the most important aspects of leadership behavior is stimulating the release of and focusing follower effort on motivation.
- Often the path between effort, performance, and rewards is crooked, narrow, unpaved, and filled with barriers. The manager must do everything possible to turn what is often a cow path into a well-designed freeway.
- In leading, the manager should appreciate that individuals' valences are heterogeneous (i.e., people value various rewards differently). The manager should understand what a follower values and construct rewards accordingly.
- Leadership behavior should help followers define expectancies. Questions that need to be addressed include: How should a follower direct his/her effort so that it results in adequate, if not exemplary, performance? What additional knowledge, skills, and experiences does a follower need to perform assigned tasks?
- Leadership behavior should focus on clarifying instrumentalities. It is important that followers understand the specific type and amount of reward that will flow from a given level of performance.
- The manager should be mindful of how work environment characteristics affect follower expectan-

cies, instrumentalities, and valences and the implications of these effects for the selection of a leadership style. For example, when a task is very unstructured, a follower may not know how to perform the job successfully (e.g., instrumentality is low). In such instances, a higher level of instrumental leadership behavior may be required.

LEAD Model

The **LEAD model** was developed by Paul Hershey and Kenneth Blanchard (1977) while they were affiliated with the Center for Leadership Studies at Ohio University. Differing degrees of task- and relationship-oriented behavior (defined in a way similar to the Ohio, Michigan, and Blake and Mouton studies) produce four different **leadership styles: style 1,** high task and low relationship; **style 2,** high task and high relationship; **style 3,** low task and high relationship; and **style 4,** low task and low relationship.

Hershey and Blanchard argued that the single most important contingency in selecting an effective **leadership style** is follower task-relevant maturity. Maturity is a function of motivation, having energy and being willing to expend it in order to accomplish the assigned task; responsibility, being willing and able to assume responsibility for planning, organizing, and completing the task; and competence, possessing the necessary knowledge, skills, or experience to perform the task proficiently. A mature follower is highly motivated, willing and able to assume responsibility, and possesses the necessary competencies. An immature follower lacks motivation, is not willing or able to assume responsibility for the task, and doesn't have the necessary competencies. Maturity is situational and task-specific; a follower may be very mature performing one task and quite immature in executing another.

Hershey and Blanchard provide suggestions regarding which styles are most effective or successful with followers having varying degrees of task-relevant maturity. Here are two extreme examples.

- If the maturity of the follower is very low, the model suggests using a style that is high task-oriented and low relationship-oriented (style 1). The follower is unmotivated, not willing or able to as-

sume responsibility, and doesn't possess the competencies necessary to perform the task. Therefore, if the task is to get done, leadership must be very directive. A low degree of relationship-oriented behavior is recommended so as not to reinforce the follower's state of immaturity.

- If the maturity of the follower is exceedingly high, the model suggests using leadership style 4—low task- and relationship-oriented behavior. Here the follower is extremely motivated, is very responsible, and possesses all the competencies necessary to perform the task. The follower does not need and, in fact, would likely not appreciate task directiveness; she knows what to do and how to do it. High relationship-oriented behavior is not needed because followers get their "stokes" or reinforcement from each other and from performance of the task itself. In this case, task and relationship responsibilities are totally delegated to the follower.

This is a highly abbreviated and simplified description of a model that has many more features than can be discussed here. For example, the authors provide a dynamic interpretation that focuses on sequences of leadership behaviors to enhance follower maturity. They have designed a package of questionnaires that provide feedback regarding the extent to which individuals perceive themselves employing the four different leadership styles, how others (subordinates, peers, superiors) perceive a manager's leadership style, and how one's selection of different leadership behaviors aligns with the most appropriate style suggested by the model given the maturity of followers in a series of cases.

There has been virtually no research to confirm the linkage between follower maturity, execution of the "appropriate" style as suggested by the model, and leader effectiveness (Graeff, 1983). However, managers and students alike find the model simple to use, practical, and intuitively appealing.

Attribution Theory

One important leadership contingency factor is a manager's own frame of reference. **Attribution** (sometimes referred to as perceptual or cognitive) **theory** holds that a manager's selection of a leadership style depends on the way follower behavior is perceived and interpreted (Mitchell, Green, & Wood, 1981; Shaver, 1983). Managers notice some things and are totally unaware of others. Furthermore, what's noticed is always filtered through the manager's unique cognitive frame and reshaped by it. Based on these perceptions, a manager attributes causes to the follower's behavior. There are two general types of attributions: internal (e.g., lack of follower effort or ability) and external (e.g., bad luck, inadequate task design by others, poor supervision).

A manager's choice of leadership behavior is significantly influenced by such attributions. For example, a manager might employ one leadership style if she attributes a follower's poor performance to task overload and use a different one if she feels the cause is laziness. Attribution theorists argue that, in many cases, a manager's choice of leadership style might be due more to the manager's perceptual and cognitive frame than the "reality" of the situation itself; indeed, reality is only what one perceives it to be. The basic notion of attribution theory is a simple one. An important determinant of leadership style is the manager's perceptions and attributions (Lord, Soti, & de Vader, 1984). The resulting admonition is that managers need to be aware of these inherent biases and develop ways to minimize them (Mitchell, 1982).

The Contingency Perspective: Selected Implications

Noted below are several implications that transcend the specific models of leadership described in this section.

- The contingency perspective helps us appreciate that leadership effectiveness and success is situational. Leadership behaviors and styles focus on influencing specific followers, be they individuals or a group, in a specific context, performing a specific task in order to accomplish a specific objective at a particular point in time. All of these things—contingencies—vary from one situation to another. The most effective leadership style in one situation is not likely to be the most effective in another.
- Three sets of contingencies seem to be most closely related to leadership effectiveness or success: characteristics of the manager, characteristics of followers, and characteristics of the immediate context in which the manager and followers interact.
- Given the large number of contingency factors and the complex ways in which they are interrelated, it's highly unlikely that a "general theory" of leadership effectiveness or success will be formulated anytime soon.
- Much of leadership behavior has to do with stimulating and then focusing follower motivation.
- Leadership effectiveness depends, more than anything else, on a manager having a full and diverse repertoire of styles and being able to flexibly move among them; possessing the ability to diagnose the most critical contingencies of a given situation; based on the diagnosis, being able to select an effective leadership style for that situation; and having the ability to execute the chosen style well.
- The way in which a specific leadership situation is diagnosed depends, in no small measure, on the manager's perceptions and attribution of causes to follower behavior.
- Taken to the extreme, contingency-driven leadership—behaving differently toward the same followers in different situations or differently toward different followers in the same situation—may appear erratic and arbitrary. This can be confusing and frustrating for followers unless managers are very explicit about how they are behaving and the reasons why they are behaving in a particular way.

Emerging Theories and Concepts

The trait, behavioral, and contingency perspectives have traditionally been the basis of most leadership theory and research. There are, however, a variety of other perspectives, several of which are discussed below.

Transformational Leadership

James McGregor Burns, in his classic work *Leadership* (1978), identified two types of politicians: transactional and transformational. There is a growing body of literature that draws a distinction between these leadership orientations in organizations (Tishy & De-vanna, 1986). Whereas **transactional leadership** attempts to preserve and work within the constraints of the status quo, **transformational leadership** seeks to upset and replace it.

For the most part, the models of leader behavior that have been examined so far view managers as involved in exchange relationships with followers, the defining characteristic of which is, I'll provide what you want, if you'll give me what I want. Transactional leadership entails recognizing what followers want and giving it to them if their performance warrants. "In these exchanges transactional leaders clarify the roles followers must play and the task requirements followers must complete in order to reach their personal goals while fulfilling the mission of the organization (Kuhnert & Lewis, 1987). You'll note that this sounds very much like the path-goal model of leadership in which the manager attempts to influence follower expectancies, instrumentalities, and valences. The objective of leadership is to get followers to comply with the rules of the game as it is currently being played. The result of such transactions, contend proponents of the theory, is ordinary levels of performance (Liden & Dienesch, 1986). Performance improvements, if they occur at all, are marginal and achieved incrementally over a long period of time.

Transformational leaders, on the other hand, are more concerned with changes than exchanges. Seeking to alter both the objective and nature of manager-follower interactions, followers are motivated to take on difficult goals they normally would not have pursued and accept the value that work is far more than the performance of specific duties for specific rewards. The relationship between the manager and followers is not contractual, but empowering. Advocates of the transformational orientation suggest that it produces extraordinary levels of performance that flow from enrollment in a cause rather than compliance with a set of rules (Bass, 1985).

Transactional leadership and transformational leadership are differentiated by the type of goals pursued, the nature of manager-follower relations, and the values to which managers and followers adhere. Provided below is a comparison of these two orientations.

Dimension	Trans-actional	Trans-formational
Goal	Maintain status quo	Upset status quo
Activity	Play within the rules	Change the rules
Locus of reward	Self (maximize personal benefits)	System (optimize systemic benefits)
Nature of incentives	Tit for tat	The greater good
Manager-follower interaction	Mutual dependence	Interdependence
Needs fulfilled	Lower level (physical, economic, and safety)	Higher level (self-actualization)
Performance	Ordinary	Extraordinary

Presently, the transformational approach to leadership is little more than a rough framework. Foundational concepts have not been rigorously defined, a comprehensive model has not been developed, and there is virtually no empirical research supporting its primary assertions.

Charismatic Leadership

Charisma is derived from a Greek word meaning "divinely inspired gift or state of grace." It is a characteristic that has been attributed to those with truly exceptional leadership abilities for centuries. The concept was first introduced into the organizational literature by Max Weber, who defined *charismatic authority* as being based on "devotion to the specific and exceptional sanctity, heroism, or exemplary character of an individual person (Eisenstadt, 1986). The concept has received renewed interest by leadership scholars who have focused on a small subset of individuals able to exercise extraordinary levels of influence (Bass, 1985; House, 1977). **Charismatic leadership** is

. . . a distinct social relationship between the leader and follower, in which the leader presents a revolutionary idea, a transcendent image. . . . [T]he follower accepts this course of action not because of its rational likelihood of success, but because of an effective belief in the extraordinary qualities of the leader. (Dow, 1969)

It has been increasingly recognized that charisma is not a characteristic of the manager *per se,* but rather a result of the interaction of many factors—manager and follower traits, manager and follower behaviors, the relationship between the manager and followers, situational dynamics, and the nature of the goal being sought. The following characteristics have been identified in the literature (Berlew, 1974; Conger & Kanungo, 1987; Dow, 1969; Hummel, 1975; Oberg, 1972; Shils, 1965; Wilner, 1984):

- nature of the goal: revolutionary or transformational
- manager traits: self-confidence, dominance, need for influence or power, strong conviction in beliefs, creativity, high energy level, enthusiasm
- leadership behaviors: ability to conceptualize and convey transcendent vision or ideology, ability to inspire and build confidence, use of unconventional means, rhetorical fluency
- follower traits: dependence, need to transcend self and situation
- follower behaviors: dedication, commitment
- manager-follower interaction: projection of idealized traits and behaviors on the leader by followers, identification (psychological fusion) of followers with leader, empowerment of followers by leader
- nature of the context: crisis, uncertainty, transformation, deprivation.

As you can see, the present notion of charisma incorporates, and weaves together, concepts included in the trait, behavioral, and situational perspectives. Because charisma is (by definition) rare, and due to the complex dynamics involved, it is exceedingly difficult to study. As a result there has been little empirical research in this area, although sets of hypotheses have been suggested.

Toward a Broader Conceptualization of Leadership Effectiveness

There has been a discernible trend over the last decade to reconceptualize what constitutes leadership effectiveness or success and the factors that account for it

(Conger & Kanungo, 1987). The contention (although not always explicitly stated) is that past theorizing and research, in its quest for methodological rigor and empirically testable relationships, has been far too narrow. Writers such as Warren Bennis and B. I. Nanus (1985), James Kouzes and Barry Posner (1988), Gareth Morgan (1988), Tom Peters (1987), Peter Senge (1991), and Peter Vail (1989) suggest that high-performance leadership depends on such things as systems thinking, visioning, facilitating learning, and follower empowerment ("Management's new gurus," 1992).

Systems thinking (Kauffman, 1980)

Managers lead in systems. While their surface features may vary, all systems have a number of common attributes. Effective leaders possess a highly refined understanding of their form, operating dynamics, and the way in which they achieve stability and undergo change. Most of us like to believe that we are systemic thinkers when we're really not. Peter Senge (1991) notes that

> Since we are part of the lacework ourselves, it's doubly hard to see the whole pattern. . . . Instead we tend to focus on snapshots of isolated parts of the system and wonder why our deepest problems never get solved.

Systems thinking requires mastering a conceptual framework and associated set of analytical tools or techniques that allows us to understand these patterns and how they can be changed.

Visioning (Kouzes & Posner, 1988)

The most effective managers lead by pulling, not by pushing. They have the ability to formulate rich images of future states that are both possible to achieve and highly desirable. Such images, ranging from dreams to specific goals, may be the product of the manager, followers, or both. When communicated powerfully (often through symbols and metaphors) and shared by all members of a system, a vision releases and focuses a huge amount of energy; also, it fosters genuine commitment and enrollment, rather than just compliance. In order to lead, one must be going somewhere and accomplishing something that is worthy of a follower's effort—a vision is the target that beckons.

Facilitating Learning (Senge, 1991)

Organizations and the environments in which they operate are not static; they constantly undergo change. Increasingly such change is revolutionary rather than evolutionary. Change of the revolutionary variety has been characteristic of the health services industry during the last decade. In periods of revolutionary change, ways of thinking and doing that have been very successful in the past lose much of their value; they undergo rapid and significant depreciation. In such instances, organizations face two supreme challenges if they are to thrive. First, they must unlearn what is no longer relevant. Second, they must develop new mental maps, acquire new knowledge, and develop new sets of skills. Effective leaders facilitate follower unlearning and relearning.

Empowering Followers (Kelley, 1991; Peters, 1987)

Rosabeth Kanter observes that, "Powerlessness corrupts. Absolute powerlessness corrupts absolutely" (Kelley, 1991). The essence of leadership is getting things done. Yet there is pitifully little that managers can do by themselves. Effective leaders view followers as the primary source of organizational creativity, energy, and value added. They create a climate and the systems that empower followers so they are willing and able to make their maximum potential contribution. Followership is the reciprocal of leadership. Effective and successful leadership is dependent upon effective, successful, and empowered followers. Team-oriented approaches for providing patient care and programs to continuously improve quality, such as total quality management (TQM) and continuous quality improvement (CQI), have attracted increasing attention in health services organizations. Both require high levels of follower empowerment if they are to be successful.

LEADERSHIP: AN INTEGRATIVE FRAMEWORK

More than a half century of research has identified a number of factors that seem to be related to leadership effectiveness and success. Figure 4.5 provides a summary and interpretation of these findings. Given the concepts that have been covered in previous sec-

tions of this chapter, the model should be relatively self-explanatory. Accordingly, only selected aspects of it are highlighted here.

A manager's leadership style is the patterns of behavior in which that manager engages to intentionally influence followers in order to accomplish a specific goal in a particular situation. We suggest that leadership style can be defined by three sets of behavioral dimensions.

- Focus is the direction of a manager's influence attempts. External leadership focuses outside the boundary of the organizational component for which the manager is responsible (toward superiors, peers, or individuals and groups outside the organization). Internal leadership is directed downward toward subordinates.
- Objective is what a manager hopes to accomplish in exercising influence. Transformational leadership seeks to alter both the nature of goals sought and manager-follower interactions; the objective is to transcend the status quo. Transactional leadership attempts to optimize the outcome of manager-follower exchange relationships by achieving stated goals in the most efficient manner within the "rules" as presently defined.
- Approach is the way in which a manager influences followers. In exercising directive (initiating structure, job-centered) leadership, a manager defines the task and specifies how it is to be performed. The focus is on goal accomplishment, and little attention is paid to manager-follower or follower-follower relationships. In exercising facilitative (consideration, employee-centered) leadership, a manager involves followers in making decisions that affect them and pays considerable attention to fulfilling their needs.

A manager's behavior can vary between "high" and "low" on each of these three sets of dimensions, the specific combination of which defines one's leadership style in a given situation.

Selection of a leadership style is influenced by two sets of factors—the manager's traits and dispositions, knowledge, and skills—and the characteristics of followers and the situation, which are filtered through the manager's distinctive cognitive frame. The manager's

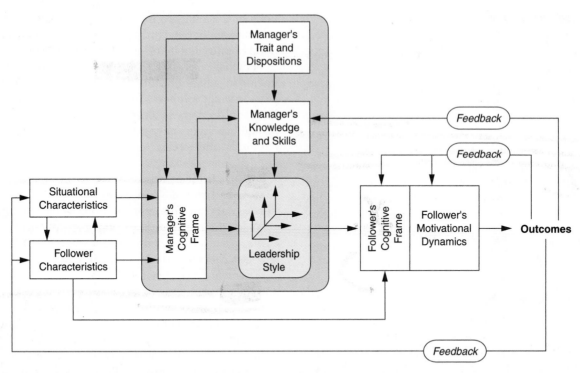

Figure 4.5. Leadership: An Integrative Framework.

leadership style affects the motivational dynamics (expectancies, instrumentalities, and valences) of followers mediated by their own cognitive frame. The outcomes of leadership attempts include follower efficiency, effectiveness, creativity, satisfaction, turnover, and absenteeism. The feedback loops depicted can be either positive (reinforcing a given characteristic) or negative (dampening or extinguishing it).

All models leave out more than they include in addition to overly simplifying complex relationships and dynamics. This one is no exception. The model is admittedly crude and incomplete, but we hope it will stimulate you to continue thinking about how pieces of the leadership "jigsaw puzzle" might fit together.

SEVERAL DISTINCTIVE ASPECTS OF LEADERSHIP IN HEALTH SERVICES ORGANIZATIONS

There are many distinctive aspects of leadership in health services organizations; we have chosen to address only two of them here, professionalism and

gender. First, health services organizations are populated by professionals who either perform or directly supervise most of the "real work" that gets done in them; they do patient care. Professionals control the organization's core input, transformation, and output processes. Second, managerial positions in health services organizations at all levels are being increasingly filled by women.

Leading Clinical Professionals

Professionals, because of the complexity and importance of the work they perform, are granted exceedingly high levels of autonomy regarding what they do and how they do it. Different occupations have varying degrees of autonomy, and hence, possess differing degrees of professionalism. The epitome in health services organizations is, of course, the physician. We will focus on physicians here as a prototypical example, although the notions forwarded can easily be applied to other categories of clinical professionals (e.g., nurses).

For a moment, entertain the notion that physicians possess a distinctly different mentality, cognitive frame, or paradigm than do managers. This mentality, of course, is not "hard wired." Rather, it is like mental operating system software programmed through a long and intensive education and socialization process. The programming begins in medical school, continues through residency training, and is reinforced every day by the nature of the work physicians do. Noted below are several critical aspects of this clinical mentality as contrasted to the mentality of managers (Freidson, 1972).

Aspect	Managerial Mentality	Clinical Mentality
Primary allegiance	To the organization	To their client
Responsibility	Shared	Personal
Authority relationships	Hierarchical (vertical)	Collegial (horizontal)
Time frame	Long/future	Short/present
Feedback	Delayed and vague	Immediate and concrete
Tolerance for ambiguity and uncertainty	High	Low

In general, the primary allegiance of physicians is to their individual patients for whom they must bear personal responsibility. They prefer, and are accustomed to, working in collegial-type relationships where power is symmetrical rather than in those where it flows primarily from the organizational office held. Physicians prefer mutual discussion with colleagues as the basis for decision making rather than formal rules. Through dealing with courses of illness that are generally time limited, physicians are trained to focus on the short run; the feedback they receive regarding their performance is generally very immediate and concrete (i.e., the patient either improves or gets worse, lives or dies), and their tolerance for ambiguity and uncertainty is quite low. Managers, on the other hand, owe their allegiance to the organization rather than to any one physician or set of patients. Because of the high degree of interdependence necessary for accomplishing managerial tasks, accountability is generally diffused or shared, and the power they exercise is often defined primarily by the office held. Managerial time frames are long (it takes forever to accomplish anything significant), and the feedback is often delayed and vague. As a consequence, managers have a high degree of tolerance for ambiguity and uncertainty. This is a highly stylized and exaggerated characterization, to be sure.

Two of the most frustrating and vexing aspects of leadership is when your behavior is misinterpreted by followers and followers do not respond at all like you expected, or hoped, they would. When the follower is a physician, the notion of **clinical mentality** helps explain why. Refer back to the integrative model of leadership (Figure 4.5) presented in the previous section. The cognitive frames of managers and physicians are quite different from one another. There are several important, and rather obvious, implications. First, physicians are likely to perceive and interpret a manager's leadership behavior in idiosyncratic ways and quite different than what might have been intended. Remember that the impact registered on physicians comes not from what you intended, or even your behavior, but rather is a result of what they perceive and the attributions they make. Second, physicians have distinctive motivational dynamics. Their expectancies, instrumentalities, and valences differ considerably from those of managers. Remember, to motivate physicians (exercise influence to release and focus energy) you have to do so on their terms, not your own. Third, managers, because of their mentality and distinctive cognitive frame, are prone to misinterpreting the intentions or behaviors of physicians and attributing negative cause to them (e.g., not in the best interest of the organization). "I just can't understand why Dr. _____ did that." What this generally means is the physician acted in a way differently than the manager would have in that situation. Our retort is, Why would you expect otherwise? Remember to interpret and attribute the causes of physician behavior from the perspective of the physician's mentality before attempting to understand it from your own.

Most of the writing in this area suggests that a style uniformly high in consideration, relationship orientation, and participation should be employed in leading professionals (Benveniste, 1987; Raelin, 1986; Shapiro, 1985). The degree of task orientation would then depend on the task-relevant maturity of the professional or professional group in that particular situation. If they understand the goal to be achieved, accept and are motivated to undertake it, and possess the competencies to do so (i.e., high maturity), task orientation should be low. When this is not the case, a greater degree of directiveness is warranted. It's important to re-

iterate that professional task-relevant maturity is situational. A professional might be very mature in one situation (e.g., doing her professional work) and quite immature in another (e.g., working on a hospital committee to design an independent practice association).

Leadership and Gender in Health Services Organizations

While issues related to gender and leadership are not necessarily distinctive to health services organizations, they are certainly very important. Several re-

 MANAGERIAL GUIDELINES

1. Identify and work with a mentor during the early stages of your career. Leadership is a performing art; becoming proficient requires continual and intensive coaching from an experienced practitioner who is invested in your development. There is a growing body of evidence that suggests that establishing an effective mentoring relationship is one of the most important things separating successful from unsuccessful leaders and managers (Dreher & Ash, 1990). If you would like to read more about how to work with a mentor, we recommend *Mentoring at Work: Developmental Relationships in Organizational Life* (Kram, 1985).

2. Become a reflective practitioner of leadership. Reflection is the key to really learning from experience. Just as a winning sports team reviews its game film, so should the manager. Get in the habit of replaying and analyzing the leadership situations in which you have been involved some time before each day ends. It's important that you look at both your successes and failures. What happened? Play the tape in your mind. Did you get the result anticipated? If so, why? If not, why not? What could/should you have done differently? What lesson have you learned from this experience? Such reflection requires considerable discipline; the effort, however, will pay handsome dividends.

3. Seek to better understand yourself. All accomplished artists have a very refined and rich feel for their tools. The primary (some would say only) tool of leadership is the self. One particularly efficient way to gain enhanced self-understanding is through the feedback provided by self-administered questionnaires, instruments, and inventories. There are a lot of different ones available, and we suggest that you seek the advice of a faculty member who teaches organization behavior regarding those that may be most useful.

4. Seek feedback from followers. Rest assured that your intentions and leadership behavior will be perceived by followers in idiosyncratic ways. Our perceptions of self are always somewhat at odds with how others perceive us. To be an effective and successful leader, you must understand the impact you have on others. The best way to gain such understanding is to ask and to do so constantly. How am I coming across? What am I doing that helps you to be as effective, creative, or satisfied as you can be? What types of things am I doing that create roadblocks and sap your energy or enthusiasm? Additionally, it's virtually impossible to lead if you don't have an in-depth understanding of who is following. Invest the time and energy in getting to know each follower upon whom your effectiveness and success depends. What

(continued)

views of the literature suggest that, while females may demonstrate different patterns of leadership behaviors than males, gender is not a particularly good predictor of leadership effectiveness and success (Morrison, White, & Van-Velsor, 1987; Rice, Instone, & Adams, 1984). This finding should not be surprising given problems associated with trait and behavioral theories of leadership, described previously. However, there does appear to be some evidence that individuals who ranked higher in male sex role orientation (describing themselves as having more masculine characteristics) were perceived to be better leaders than those with feminine, androgynous, or undifferentiated gender roles (Goktepe & Schneider, 1989). Keep this finding in mind as you read further.

The American College of Healthcare Executives (ACHE) (1991) in conjunction with the Graduate Program in Hospital and Health Administration at the University of Iowa, conducted a comparative study of female and male health care managers. The sample consisted of 1,108 College affiliates, about half women and half men. The study produced a number

 # MANAGERIAL GUIDELINES

are their aspirations? What are their wants and needs? What do they view as their most important competencies (knowledge, skills, experiences), and how could the organization make better use of them? What motivates them the most?

5. Keep reading and studying. Experience is, perhaps, the single best teacher of leadership. However, there are not enough hours in the day, days in the year, or years in life to acquire all the experience we need. Some of it has to be gained vicariously, and the best vicarious teacher is reading. Additionally, reading provides the essential models, concepts, and ideas that can help us to become much more effective and efficient experiential learners, avoiding the trap where years of experience is just one year's worth repeated many times over. We've included The Manager's Essential Leadership Bookshelf to get you started.

The Manager's Essential Leadership Bookshelf

There are thousands of books on leadership with hundreds of new ones published every year, all forwarding their own recipes for success. None of us have the time, energy, patience or money to consume even a small proportion of what is being written. Here's our picks, a handful of books that we have found to be the most sound, interesting, and useful. Although there are clearly many others that might warrant inclusion, we recommend these to you without reservation.

Bennis, W. (1989). *Why leaders can't lead: The unconscious conspiracy continues.* San Francisco: Jossey-Bass.

Covey, S. R. (1990). *Principle of centered leadership.* New York: Simon and Schuster.

Degeling et al. *Professional Subcultures and Hospital Reform.* Sydney, Australia: The Centre for Hospital Management and Information Systems Research, The University of New South Wales.

Gardner, J. (1990). *On leadership.* New York: The Free Press.

Hessesbein, F., Goldsmith, M., & Beckhard, R. (1996). *The leader of the future: New visions, strategies, and practices for the next era.* San Francisco: Jossey-Bass.

Kouzes, J. M., & Posner, B. Z. (1993). *Credibility: How leaders gain and lose it, why people demand it.* San Francisco: Jossey-Bass.

Kouzes, J. M., & Posner, B. Z. (1995). *The leadership challenge: How to keep getting extraordinary things done in organizations.* San Francisco: Jossey-Bass.

Senge, P. (1990). *The fifth discipline: The art and practice of the learning organization.* New York: Doubleday/Currency.

Vail, P. (1989). *Managing as a performing art.* San Francisco: Jossey-Bass.

of interesting findings regarding gender differences in career attainment, compensation, professional satisfaction, and work patterns.

With respect to general leadership qualities, the majority of respondents view males and females to be equal. Where differences in perceptions existed, both males and females overwhelmingly ranked males as being superior. The same general relationship emerged in other key factors associated with leadership effectiveness (e.g., support from those who are led—superiors, peers, and subordinates) and behaviors often associated with successful leaders (e.g., risk taking and competitiveness). Although not directly related to leadership, a striking disparity was perceived regarding chances for career advancement in health services organizations by both men and women. Fully 72% of the females and 46.4% of the males perceived men possessing significantly better advancement opportunities than women. These findings continue to be quite significant and have some important implications regarding gender differences and leadership in health services organizations.

Overall, there seems to be a stereotypical view of women possessing fewer of the qualities considered essential for exercising the leadership role of the manager in health services organizations. We underscore that this is a stereotypical perception, because evidence from other industries cited previously suggests that gender is a very poor predictor of leadership effectiveness or success. There is a **gender gap** in leadership in health services organizations, and it seems to be the result of a gender bias on the part of both women and men. The traditional solution is to close this gap by assimilation; helping women managers to think and act more like men. Many management educational and training programs, reinforced by organizational culture, implicitly embrace this approach. Elsie Cross (1992) notes, in addressing both gender and racial bias, that

> . . . white women and people of color cannot—nor should they attempt to—become like white men. The best I can hope for is that others will feel that I can "think like a man". . . . But I can never be more than an imitation white man. And in becoming an imitation, I give up the richness, the creativity, the strength that comes from who I really am.

Like Cross, we feel that assimilation is counterproductive. Irrespective of the trait focused upon (gender, race, ethnicity, sexual orientation), assimilation results in a reduction of diversity at a time when it is needed most in health services organizations. Managerial and leadership heterogeneity is essential for finding different ways to solve new problems and seize new opportunities in times of revolutionary change.

Discussion Questions

1. Reread the opening case and answer the questions again. Compare your answers written before and after reading this chapter. What are the differences? How have you altered your thinking about the nature of leadership and the factors that contribute to leadership effectiveness and success?

2. You are interviewing for a position, and your prospective superior asks you to describe your leadership style. How would you do so? This is a fairly typical question asked of candidates for management positions, irrespective of level, so it is a good idea to have a reasonably well thought-out and articulate answer. Draft a one- or two-paragraph statement. Share your statement with fellow students.

3. There are those who contend leadership is highly romanticized. That is, there's a tendency to ascribe far more to leadership as a cause than is actually warranted (Meindl, Ehrlich, & Dukeriok, 1985). While leadership certainly makes a difference, it may not make as much difference as either managers, followers, or onlookers generally think it does. Successful performance of a group, organization, or nation is the result of many factors interacting in complex ways. However, it is generally far easier and more reassuring to attribute such success to the leadership abilities of an individual. What do you think?

4. Several distinctive aspects of leading in health services organizations have been presented in this chapter. What are some other characteristics of health services organizations that pose challenges for effectively executing the leadership role of the manager? In thinking about this question,

consider distinctions between different types of health services organizations—acute care hospitals, long-term care hospitals, nursing homes, health maintenance organizations (HMOs), and group practices.

5. What do you *think* about the findings of the ACHE study presented in the section on gender and leadership? How do you *feel* about them? From your perspective, what are the implications? Discuss the differences between males and females in your class regarding cognitive and affective reactions to these findings and the nature of the implications they see as most significant. What are some specific approaches that health services organizations might employ to stimulate and capture the benefits of greater leadership diversity?

References

Bass, B. M. (1981). *Stodgill's handbook of leadership.* New York: Free Press.

Bass, B. M. (1985). *Leadership beyond expectations.* New York: Free Press.

Bennis, W. G., & Nanus, B. I. (1985). *Leaders.* New York: Harper and Row.

Benveniste, G. (1987). *Professionalizing the organization.* San Francisco: Jossey-Bass.

Berlew, D. E. (1974). Leadership and organizational excitement. *California Management Review, 17,* 21–30.

Blake, J., & Mouton, R. (1978). *The new managerial grid.* Houston, TX: Gulf Publishing.

Blake, R. R., & Mouton, J. S. (1982). Theory and research for developing a science of leadership. *Journal of Applied Behavioral Science, 18,* 275–291.

Bridging the leadership gap in healthcare. (1992). San Francisco: Healthcare Forum.

Burns, J. M. (1978). *Leadership.* New York: Harper and Row.

Conger, J. A., & Kanungo, R. N. (1987). Toward a behavioral theory of charismatic leadership in organizational settings. *Academy of Management Review, 12,* 637–647.

Coska, L. S. (1984). A relationship between leader intelligence and leader rated effectiveness. *Journal of Applied Psychology, 14,* 22–34.

Cross, E. Y. (1992, January–February). Making the invisible visible. *Healthcare Forum Journal, 29.*

Dow, T. E. (1969). The theory of charisma. *Sociological Quarterly, 10,* 315.

Dreher, G. F., & Ash, R. A. (1990). A comparative study of mentoring among men and women in managerial, professional and technical positions. *Journal of Applied Psychology, 75,* 539–546.

Eisenstadt, S. N. (1986). *Max Weber: On charisma and institution building.* Chicago, IL: University of Chicago Press, p. 46.

Evans, M. G. (1970a). The effects of supervisory behavior on the path-goal relationship. *Organizational Behavior in Human Performance, 5,* 277–298.

Evans, M. G. (1970b). Leadership and motivation: A core concept. *Academy of Management Journal, 13,* 91–102.

Fiedler, F. E. (1967). *A theory of leadership effectiveness.* New York: McGraw-Hill.

Fiedler, F. E., & Chemers, M. M. (1974). *Leadership and effective management.* Glenview, IL: Scott, Foresman.

Fiedler, F. E., Chemers, M. M., & Mahar, L. (1976). *Improving leadership effectiveness.* New York: John Wiley.

Fleishman, E. A. (1973). Twenty years of consideration and structure. In E. A. Fleishman, & J. G. Hunt (Eds.), *Current developments in the study of leadership* (pp. 1–37). Carbondale, IL: Southern Illinois University.

Freidson, E. (1972). The clinical mentality. In *Profession of medicine: A study of the sociology of applied knowledge* (pp. 158–184). New York: Dodd/Mead.

Gender and careers in healthcare management: Findings of a national study of healthcare executives (1991). (Research Series Number 3). Chicago: American College of Healthcare Executives.

Goktepe, J., & Schneider, C. (1989). Role of sex, gender roles and attraction in predicting emergent leaders. *Journal of Applied Psychology, 74,* 165–167.

Graeff, C. L. (1983). The situational leadership theory: A critical review. *Academy of Management Review, 8,* 271–294.

Hall, D. D., & Norgaim, K. E. (1976). The leadership match game: Matching the man to the situation. *Organizational Dynamics, 6–16.*

Halpin, A. W. (1954). The leadership behavior and combat performance of airplane commanders. *Journal of Abnormal and Social Psychology, 39,* 82–84.

Hershey, P., & Blanchard, K. H. (1977). *Management of organizational behavior: Utilizing human resources.* Englewood Cliffs, NJ: Prentice-Hall.

House, R. J. (1971). A path-goal theory of leader effectiveness. *Administrative Science Quarterly, 16,* 321–323.

House, R. J. (1977). A 1976 theory of charismatic leadership. In J. G. Hunt, &w L. L. Larson (Eds.), *Leadership: The cutting edge* (pp. 189–207). Carbondale, IL: Southern Illinois University Press.

House, R. J., & Baetz, M. L. (1979). Leadership: Some empirical generalizations and new directions. *Research in Organization Behavior, 1,* 385–386.

House, R. J., & Mitchell, T. R. (1974). Path-goal theory of leadership. *Journal of Contemporary Business, 3*(4), 81–98.

Hummel, R. P. (1975). Psychology of charismatic followers. *Psychological Reports, 37,* 759–770.

Jago, A. G. (1982). Leadership: Perspectives in theory and research. *Management Science, 28,* 315–336.

Jennings, W. O. (1947). A review of leadership studies with a particular reference to military problems. *Psychological Bulletin, 44,* 54–79.

Katz, D. (1950). *Productivity supervision and morale in an office situation.* Ann Arbor, MI: Institute for Social Research, University of Michigan.

Katz, D. (1951). *Productivity, supervision and morale among railroad workers.* Ann Arbor, MI: Institute for Social Research, University of Michigan.

Katz, D., & Kahn, R. L. (1966). The taking of organizational roles. In *The social psychology of organizations.* New York: John Wiley and Sons.

Kauffman, D. L., Jr. (1980). *Systems one: An introduction to systems thinking.* Minneapolis, MN: SA Carlton.

Kelley, R. E. (1991). *The power of followership: How to create leaders people want to follow and followers who lead themselves.* New York: Doubleday/Currency.

Korman, A. K. (1966). Consideration, initiating structure and organizational criteria: A review. *Personnel Psychology, 19,* 349–361.

Kouzes, I. M., & Posner, B. Z. (1988). *The leadership challenge: How to get extraordinary things done in organizations.* San Francisco: Jossey-Bass.

Kram, K. E. (1985). *Mentoring at work: Developmental relationships in organizational life.* Glenview, IL: Scott, Foresman.

Kuhnert, K. W., & Lewis, P. (1987, October). Transactional and transformational leadership: A constructive/developmental analysis. *Academy of Management Review, 12,* 649.

Lewin, K., Lippitt, R., & White, R. K. (1939). Patterns of aggressive behavior in experimentally created social climates. *Journal of Social Psychology, 10,* 271–276.

Liden, R. C., & Dienesch, R. M. (1986). Leader-member exchange model of leadership: A critique and further development. *Academy of Management Review, 11,* 618–634.

Likert, R. (1961). *New patterns of management.* New York: McGraw-Hill.

Lord, R. G., de Vader, C. L., & Alliger, G. M. (1986). A meta analysis of the relation between personality traits and leadership: An application of validity generalization procedures. *Journal of Applied Psychology, 71,* 402–410.

Lord, R. G., Soti, R. J., & de Vader, C. L. (1984, December). A test of leadership categorization theory: Internal structure, information processing and leadership perception. *Organizational Behavior and Human Performance, 34,* 343–378.

Management's new gurus. (1992, August 31). *Business Week,* 44–52.

Meindl, J. R., Ehrlich, S. B., & Dukeriok, J. M. (1985). The romance of leadership. *Administrative Science Quarterly, 30,* 78–102.

Mitchell, T. R. (1982). Attributions and actions: A note of caution. *Journal of Management, 8*(1), 65–74.

Mitchell, T. R., Green, S. G., & Wood, R. (1981). An attributional model of leadership and the poor performing subordinate: Development and validation. *Research in Organization Behavior, 3,* 197–234.

Morgan, G. (1988). *Riding the waves of change: Developing managerial competencies for a turbulent world.* San Francisco: Jossey-Bass.

Morrison, A. R., White, R. P., & Van-Velsor, E. (1987, August). Executive women: Substance plus style. *Psychology Today,* 18–21.

Nebeker, D. B. (1975). Situation favorability and perceived environmental uncertainty: An integrative approach. *Administrative Science Quarterly, 20,* 281–294.

Oberg, W. (1972). Charisma, commitment and contemporary organizational theory. *Business Topics, 20*(2), 18–32.

Peters, T. (1987). *Thriving on chaos: Handbook for a management revolution.* New York: Alfred A. Knopf.

Porter, I. W., & Lawler, E. E. (1968). *Managerial attitudes and performance.* Homewood, IL: Richard D. Irwin.

Raelin, J. A. (1986). *The clash of cultures: Managers and professionals.* Boston: Harvard Business School Press.

Rice, R. W., Instone, D., & Adams, J. (1984). Leader sex, leader success and leadership process. *Journal of Applied Psychology, 69,* 15–27.

Sartle, C. L. (1956). *Executive performance and leadership.* Englewood Cliffs, NJ: Prentice-Hall.

Schreisheim, C. A., & von Glinow, M. A. (1977). The path-goal theory of leadership: A theoretical and empirical analysis. *Academy of Management Journal, 20,* 398–405.

Senge, P. M. (1991). *The fifth discipline.* New York: Doubleday/Currency.

Shapiro, A. (1985). *Managing professional people.* New York: Free Press.

Shaver, K. G. (1983). *An introduction to attribution processes.* Hillsdale, NY: Erlbaum Books.

Shils, E. A. (1965). Charisma, order and status. *American Sociological Review, 30,* 199–213.

Stinson, J. E., & Tracy, L. (1974). Some disturbing characteristics of LPC scores. *Personnel Psychology, 27,* 77–485.

Stodgill, R. M. (1948). Personal factors associated with leadership: A survey of the literature. *Journal of Applied Psychology, 32,* 35–71.

Stodgill, R. M. (1974). *Handbook of leadership.* New York: Free Press.

Stodgill, R. M., & Coons, A. (Eds.). (1957). *Leader behavior: Its description and measurement.* Columbus, OH: Bureau of Business Research, Ohio State University.

Tannenbaum, R., & Schmidt, W. (1973). How to choose a leadership pattern. *Harvard Business Review, 51*(3), 162–180.

Tishy, N. M., & Devanna, M. A. (1986). *The transformational leader.* New York: John Wiley.

Vail, P. B. (1989). *Managing as a performing art: New ideas for a world of chaotic change.* San Francisco: Jossey-Bass.

Van Vleet, D. D., & Yukl, G. A. (1989). A century of leadership research. In W. E. Rosenbach, & R. L. Taylor (Eds.), *Contemporary issues in leadership* (p. 67). Boulder, CO: Westview Press.

Vroom, V. H. (1964). *Work and motivation.* New York: John Wiley.

Wilner, A. R. (1984). *The spellbinders: Charismatic and political leadership.* New Haven, CN: Yale University Press.

CHAPTER

5

Conflict Management and Negotiation

Jeffrey T. Polzer, Ph.D.
Margaret A. Neale, Ph.D.

Chapter Outline

Learning Objectives

After completing this chapter, the reader should be able to:

1. Identify reasons why conflict is prevalent in health care organizations.
2. Understand several different types of conflict and the levels at which conflict occurs.
3. Identify several different conflict-management techniques, based on various concerns of the disputants.
4. Identify the basic concepts and dimensions of negotiation.
5. Appreciate the importance of planning for a negotiation and know the key issues to consider when preparing to negotiate.
6. Identify and understand special types of conflict-management situations, such as multiparty negotiations and third-party intervention.

Key Terms

Accommodation
Administrative Conflict
Arbitrator
Aspiration Level
Avoidance
Bargaining Zone
Best Alternative to a Negotiated Agreement (BATNA)
Compatible Issues
Competition
Conflict
Distributive Dimension of Negotiation
Emotional Conflict
Equality Fairness Norm
Equity Fairness Norm
Inquisitor
Integrative Dimension of Negotiation
Intergroup Conflict
Interpersonal Conflict
Intragroup Conflict
Intrapersonal Conflict
Mediator
Need Fairness Norm
Negotiation
Pressing
Reservation Price
Task Content Conflict

Chapter Purpose

The parties involved in the Culpeper Medical Associates negotiations were able to reach a mutually satisfactory agreement despite their potentially conflicting interests. Other health services organizations have not fared so well in crafting good agreements among parties who disagree over how various issues should be resolved. **Conflict** is pervasive in health services organizations, as in all organizations. Conflict occurs every day in a wide variety of situations ranging from emotional disputes between two colleagues, to disputes between departments about lines of authority, to legal disputes involving several organizations. In this chapter, we will focus

primarily on the types of conflict that confront managers on a day-to-day basis.

THE IMPORTANCE OF CONFLICT MANAGEMENT

The field of conflict management has grown dramatically in the last decade, reflected both by the amount of research conducted on this topic and the increased importance placed on teaching conflict-management techniques. This increase in popularity, particularly concerning negotiation, has been fueled by several general environmental trends that are especially noticeable in the health services industry (Neale & Bazerman, 1991). First, the marketplace is growing increasingly global as firms face competition from foreign companies. For example, pharmaceutical firms such as Burroughs-Wellcome, Inc. increasingly find themselves conducting business in different countries as their current markets become more competitive. This increased diversity in potential business partners heightens the need for managers to be able to negotiate effectively with people who have different backgrounds, interests, and values.

Secondly, at the firm level, there has been a vast increase in corporate restructuring throughout the 1990s. Managers in corporations that are going through structural transformations need negotiation skills to ensure their position within the new organization. At an individual level, the workforce is growing increasingly mobile. Many employees proactively manage their career paths, often within multiple organizations. Increased mobility demands better negotiation skills of those changing jobs and those employing these people.

Finally, the shift from a manufacturing-based to a service-based economy means that typical negotiations are likely to be more difficult, because desired outcomes are more ambiguous and therefore harder to specify in negotiated agreements (Neale & Bazerman, 1991). For example, the primary care doctors who sold their practices to Culpeper Medical Associates agreed to use both historical earnings and current productivity to resolve the ambiguity inherent in calculating "fair" base salaries. Such ambiguity is clearly present in many areas of the health services field, increasing the importance of good negotiating skills as negotiations become more difficult.

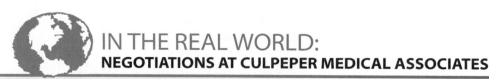

IN THE REAL WORLD:
NEGOTIATIONS AT CULPEPER MEDICAL ASSOCIATES

In the struggle between health care giants and small independent hospitals, Culpeper Memorial is proof that even the tiny can triumph. Located in rural Virginia about 60 miles from Washington, D.C., the 70-bed hospital recently staved off an attempted takeover of its doctor groups by the mighty University of Virginia. In the process, Culpeper has formed a partnership with its primary care doctors and is finalizing negotiations to bring in Health Care Partners, a for-profit affiliate of the university's foundation.

Culpeper focuses on basic acute care, so its 14 primary care doctors are an important asset, says CEO Lee Kirk. When he came to the hospital about a year ago, the doctors were being courted by outsiders. One internist decided to become an employee of the university's own physician group, and that worried Kirk and others. "We were concerned we'd face a divide-and-conquer strategy and what it might do to the community," he says. "So we decided to circle the wagons."

Culpeper called in Medimetrix, a consulting firm that had helped the hospital form its physician-hospital organization four years earlier. Over several months, the Cleveland company set up a series of sessions to help hospital executives and doctors mull over options to a takeover or merger. They eventually formed Culpeper Medical Associates, a tax-exempt, limited-liability company with a physician-chaired board made up of four doctors and four hospital representatives. Under the agreement, all 14 doctors sold their practices to Culpeper Medical Associates and became its employees, with base salaries calculated from historical earnings and current productivity. Incentives included a bonus tied to performance.

To buy the practices, Culpeper Medical Associates needed big money, so it put out feelers for an equity partner. Three hospital systems came forward, and Health Care Partners was chosen because of Culpeper's longtime relationship with the university, Kirk says. "We also send the majority of our tertiary referrals there," he adds. Two

representatives from Health Care Partners are to be added to the board, making the for-profit a minority partner with a 49% equity stake.

For John Ashley, M.D., associate vice president of the university's Health Sciences Foundation, the arrangement is better than an outright purchase. The doctors didn't want their practices acquired, and the university didn't really want to buy them. "We'd rather form partnerships because they require less investment," says Ashley. "Becoming the minority partner allows us to formalize a long-standing informal relationship in a more comfortable way than if we'd come in and played the heavy."

To boost referrals to the university, Culpeper Medical Associates has developed formal processes for the doctors to confer with specialists and use other resources. It also supports the university's mission by bringing in residents and other medical students more regularly. Morton Chiles, a doctor who heads the Culpeper Medical Associates board, sees several advantages. By sticking together, he says, doctors can pool resources, deliver care more efficiently, and negotiate contracts more competitively. And they keep their much-prized clinical autonomy. Finally, since the transition has been largely seamless, patients are ensured continuity of care. In fact, Medicare recipients now have better access to care because all of Culpeper's primary care doctors will take them.

Culpeper's solution may not be for everybody, Chiles warns. The new setup required delicate negotiating—and what with legal and consulting fees, it hasn't come cheap. Still, he's sure it's the right choice: "It eliminates the potential for fragmenting the local primary care market and devastating the hospital."

Reprinted from Nordhaus-Bike, A. M. (1997, August 20). Partnering: Unite and conquer. Hospitals & Health Networks, Vol. 71, No. 16, by permission, Copyright, 1997, American Hospital Publishing, Inc.**

We will explore negotiation in depth later in the chapter. Before we focus on ways to resolve conflict, though, we will discuss various types of conflict and some of the typical reasons conflict occurs in organizations.

THE CAUSES OF CONFLICT

The Role of Resource Scarcity

Conflict arises for many reasons and can be characterized in numerous ways. At a very basic level, most conflict occurs because of a fundamental problem inherent in every organization. Organizational members desire several types of resources, including power, money, information, advice, and praise (Homans, 1961). However, resource scarcity dictates that the members of an organization will not all be able to receive the level of resources they desire. Therefore, conflict arises between organizational members regarding the distribution of desired resources.

It is useful to distinguish conflict from **competition** because many people confuse the two concepts. While conflict is a typical result of resource scarcity, organizational members also compete for resources. However, conflict and competition are distinct concepts. In both cases, the goals of the parties are incompatible. In situations involving resources, this means that the parties cannot both acquire their desired level of resources. However, competition is characterized by parallel striving toward a goal that both parties cannot reach simultaneously, while conflict is characterized by mutual interference. Conflict occurs when a concern of one party is frustrated, or perceived to be frustrated, by another party (Thomas, 1976). Parties can compete and still remain relatively independent of each other. Conflict, on the other hand, requires some interaction or contact between the parties.

Conflict can also occur for reasons that are less tangible than resource acquisition. People may have conflicting perceptions, ideas, or beliefs as well as conflicting resource-allocation goals. For example, one subordinate may perceive that another subordinate receives more praise, even when both subordinates actually receive the same objective amount of praise; two administrators may have different ideas about what an employee dress code policy should entail,

and people may have different beliefs about the appropriateness of a certain medical treatment or procedure. A basic but important point to be drawn from these examples is that conflict always occurs because of the differences between people, even though these differences occur on a variety of dimensions.

Beneficial versus Detrimental Effects of Conflict

Because differences between people are unavoidable, conflict will always exist in organizations and groups. The question that must be addressed by successful managers is how to handle the conflicts that they will inevitably face. Should managers try to create a work environment in which there is as little conflict as possible or is some important purpose served by having certain levels of ambient conflict? This boils down to the question of whether conflict is good or bad, and therefore, whether it should be encouraged in work groups or discouraged and suppressed. This is the focus of Debate Time 5.1.

In trying to ascertain whether conflict is good or bad, functional or dysfunctional, something to be explored or suppressed, part of the puzzle may lie in differentiating various types of conflict. It may be that some types of conflict are important for successful organizational performance while other forms of conflict are associated with problematic organizational performance. In the next section, we will consider three different types of conflict—content conflict, emotional conflict, and administrative conflict—and their unique impact on organizational functioning.

Jehn's Typology of Conflict

Conflict within an organization can be characterized by type regardless of the level at which it occurs. Karen Jehn devised a typology that includes three types of conflict. **Task content conflict,** the first type, refers to disagreements about the actual task being performed by organizational members. The focus in this type of conflict is on differing opinions pertaining to the task, rather than the goals of the people involved (Jehn, 1995). For example, everyone in a group medical practice may agree that the group should have a marketing campaign, but members may disagree about

DEBATE TIME 5.1: WHAT DO YOU THINK?

POINT: Conflict is a necessary and useful part of organizational life. Not all conflict is unhealthy. Low levels of conflict can often stimulate the parties involved and heighten their attention. Novel or creative solutions frequently result from conflict when people search for ways to satisfy a diverse set of interests. In fact, the absence of conflict can be as indicative of problems as too much conflict. For example, Irving Janis (1982) originated the concept of groupthink, which occurs when too little conflict is expressed within decision-making groups. Very low levels of conflict may indicate that unavoidable differences are being suppressed or that the people involved do not have perspectives that differ enough to contribute to a well thought-out decision.

COUNTERPOINT: Conflict is dysfunctional. Especially in the United States, most people think of conflict as a negative phenomenon. They are usually correct. High conflict levels are typically detrimental and can be destructive. Instead of allocating resources to the production of the goods or services that are the mission of the organization, conflict requires that managers spend time and energy trying to resolve the conflict. In fact, one study discovered that managers spend almost 20% of their time in activities directly related to the resolution of disputes—time that could be much more productively applied directly to achieving the mission of the organization.

In addition, conflict is associated with higher levels of stress. Such an environment can reduce the psychological well-being of employees and make it difficult for them to develop trusting, supportive relationships within the organizational context. It is for this reason that managers spend so much of their time managing and resolving conflict.

---

the content of the advertisements and whether advertising should be run on radio, on television, or in newspapers.

Emotional conflict is an awareness of interpersonal incompatibilities among those working together on a task. It involves negative emotions and dislike of the other people involved in the conflict. The third type of conflict is **administrative conflict** and is defined as an awareness by the involved parties that there are controversies about how task accomplishment will proceed (Jehn, 1995). Disagreements about individual responsibilities and duties are examples of administrative conflict. For example, members of a group practice may disagree about who should decide what type of advertising to use or who should be responsible for working with an advertising agency.

In general, the research conducted by Jehn and others suggests that a moderate amount of task content conflict is critical to the effective functioning of groups. Groupthink, for example, is probably more likely to occur when there is an implicit avoidance of all conflict, but especially task content conflict. Administrative conflict and, to a greater extent, emotional conflict are likely to be the culprits when groups become dysfunctional or impaired because a high degree of conflict inhibits their ability to interact. All three of these types of conflict may occur between individuals, groups and individuals, or different groups as people perform the tasks that make up organizational life. These various levels at which conflict can occur are the focus of the next section.

LEVELS OF CONFLICT

It is useful to consider the level at which conflict occurs, along with the type of conflict, when trying to decide how to manage it. That is, conflict can occur within an individual (**intrapersonal conflict**), between individuals (**interpersonal conflict**), within a group (**intragroup conflict**), and between groups (**intergroup conflict**). The alternatives available for resolving the conflict may depend on the level in the organization at which it exists.

Individual Level

Individual conflict occurs when the locus of the dispute is the individual. Intrapersonal conflict may occur for a variety of reasons. People are often faced with a choice between two options that may vary in attractiveness. In characterizing conflict at this level, it is valuable to think about the relative attractiveness of each option. When two options are equally attractive, approach-approach conflict occurs within the person. This conflict results from the person's effort to differentiate between the two alternatives. For example, a health maintenance organization (HMO) executive may have two equally viable and attractive plans for expanding enrollment. It is difficult to choose either of the options because selecting one necessarily means the other must be turned down.

On the other side of the coin, avoidance-avoidance conflict occurs when a person has to choose between equally unattractive options. If a nursing home is trying to reduce costs, one of two good nurses may have to be laid off. The decision is made more difficult because the options are equally unattractive.

The most prevalent type of intrapersonal conflict is approach-avoidance conflict, which occurs when multiple options each have favorable and unfavorable features. Conflict that is initially approach-approach conflict often turns into approach-avoidance conflict when the person making the decision looks at the alternatives more critically in an attempt to differentiate them. Unattractive components of each option may be found that were overlooked initially, such as additional costs associated with each option for expanding HMO membership enrollment. A person may arrive at a different decision depending on which features of each option the person focuses. After the decision is made, postdecision regret frequently occurs, as the alternative that the person passed up looks increasingly better as more information is gathered about the chosen option.

Group Level

When most people think about conflict, the examples that first come to mind are at an interpersonal level, between two or more people. Conflict at this level typically occurs because of incompatible goals, ideas, feelings, beliefs, or behaviors, as illustrated by the examples in the first section of this chapter. This level of conflict is usually characterized by interdependence between the parties, whereby the choice of each party affects the outcome of the other party. The choice that is optimal for one party may result in a poor outcome for the other, leading to conflict. This is the most common level of conflict that comes to the surface in organizations.

Paralleling individual conflict, group conflict can occur between members of the same group (intragroup conflict) or between members of different groups (intergroup conflict). Intragroup conflict is similar in many ways to interpersonal conflict, with the former type being more complex because of the higher number of people involved. However, this is not the only difference. When a group is involved that has an identity above and beyond its individual members, several things can occur as a result of the influence of the group on its members. A formal definition of what we mean by a "group" may help to clarify the ideas that follow. In this context, a group is defined as

> an organized system of two or more individuals who are interrelated so that the system performs some function, has a standard set of role relationships among its members, and has a set of norms that regulate the function of the group and each of its members. (Northcraft & Neale, 1990)

As this definition of a group implies, the interactions of the group members are influenced by their roles within the group and by the norms of the group. Members of the group may not always be amenable to these influences, leading to conflict between the individual member and the group. Conflict between the members of a group may result in decreased coordination, communication, and productivity (Deutsch, 1949). Intragroup conflict will come up again later in this chapter in the section on multiparty negotiations.

Intergroup conflict can have a profound impact on the perceptions and behaviors of people. When acting as a member of a group, people tend to divide others into an ingroup and an outgroup. The ingroup consists of all the other members of the salient group. The outgroup consists of those outside the boundaries of the ingroup. Some examples of the characteristics people frequently use to divide people into in- and out groups include gender, race, religious preference, geographic location, organizational membership, departmental membership, and functional position within an organization. Most people are members of numerous groups based on demographic, organizational, or other demarcations. This creates abundant opportunities for intergroup conflict to arise. Intergroup conflict occurs whenever the disputants identify with or represent different groups that are relevant to the conflict during the conflict episode.

Intergroup conflict may have a variety of causes, many of which are the same as those that cause interpersonal conflict, such as resource scarcity, differing beliefs, or incompatible goals. The distinction is simply that the relevant unit from which the differences stem is the group rather than the individual. Intergroup conflict can have a variety of consequences both within and across the groups involved in the conflict. Within the groups, cohesiveness, task orientation, loyalty to the group, and acceptance of autocratic leadership may increase. Between the groups,

distorted perceptions, negative stereotypes of outgroup members, and reduced communication may result. A mentality of "us versus them" often forms and grows stronger as the conflict escalates (Sherif, 1977). As seen at Robbers Cave in "In the Real World," the strength of group affiliations as a contributing factor to conflict is often overlooked but should always be considered when trying to determine the causes of conflict.

MANAGING CONFLICT

It is clear that conflict is commonplace, and that for organizational members to function productively, they must manage conflict effectively. There are many strategies for managing conflict, including those that are planned as well as those that emerge as conflict is experienced. Some conflict-management techniques apply to conflict on all levels, while others are relevant for a limited number of types and levels of conflict. In this section, we will briefly introduce the dual-concern model as a typology of conflict-management techniques, focusing on four ways that people handle

IN THE (EXPERIMENTAL) REAL WORLD:
INTERGROUP CONFLICT AT ROBBER'S CAVE

Consider the experience of a group of young boys at the Robber's Cave Camp—a camp specifically set up to examine intergroup conflict. During the first days of camp, the boys—coming from different schools—were allowed to develop friends through a variety of campwide activities. The boys were then assigned to one of two cabins. The makeup of each cabin was such that about 60% of an individual's best friends were in the other cabin. Within a few days, however, the interaction patterns shifted dramatically. The boys tended to interact almost exclusively with others in their own cabins.

The boys were then involved in a series of competitive activities in which the two cabins were on opposite teams. To increase the conflict, the winners of each competition were awarded prizes. Quickly, the amount of hostility and stereotypes escalated. Raids and ambushes were

planned, and leaders emerged in each cabin who were effective at combat. There was a huge increase in intragroup solidarity.

The researchers then set up a party in which one cabin, the Red Devils, arrived considerably earlier than the other group, the Bulldogs. The food at the party was of two very different levels of attractiveness: half of the food was fresh and appealing; the other half was old and unappetizing. Because of the competition between the two groups, the Red Devils ate most of the good food and left the unattractive food for their competitors. When the Bulldogs arrived, they were so upset that the conflict quickly escalated from name-calling to a full-fledged food fight.

Adapted from Sherif M., and Sherif C. Groups in Harmony and Tension. *New York: Harper* **Brothers, 1953.**

conflict—accommodation, pressing, avoidance, and negotiation.

The Dual Concern Model

Kenneth Thomas (1976) has developed a two-dimensional model of conflict-management techniques that reflects a concern for both an individual's own outcomes as well as an opponent's outcomes. Depending on these two dimensions of concern, a negotiator might prefer one of five different strategies for handling conflict. If concern for both self and other's outcomes are low, this model predicts that one might prefer an **avoidance** strategy. If concern for one's own outcome is high and concern for the others' outcome is low, then one should prefer a competing, or **pressing,** strategy. If concern for one's own outcome is low and concern for the other's outcome is high, then **accommodation** or capitulation is probably the preferred strategy. If concern for both one's own outcome and the other's outcome is high, then collaboration is the appropriate strategy. Finally, if one has intermediate concern for both one's own and the other's outcomes, then one is likely to prefer a compromise strategy. The dual concern model is graphically represented in Figure 5.1.

If we think about how differing preferences for these five strategies might be expressed by an organizational actor in various situations, four different conflict-management techniques can be identified. Accommodation, pressing, avoiding, and **negotiation** (incorporating compromise and collaboration) are described in greater detail in the following sections.

Accommodation

Capitulating to or accommodating the other party is one popular way to deal with conflict. Accommodation does not necessarily require any interaction among the parties and can simply entail giving the other side what they want. It is one of the least confrontational methods for dealing with conflict. Capitulation has the advantage of being efficient in that, by giving the other party what he wants, the conflict ends quickly. Other advantages are that the relationship between the parties may be preserved and that

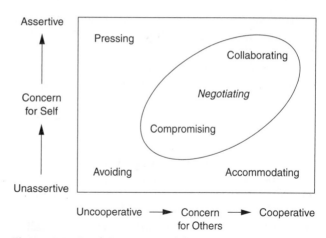

Figure 5.1. Dual Concern Model.
SOURCE: Adapted from Thomas, K. "Conflict and Conflict Management," in *Handbook of Industrial and Organizational Psychology*, ed. M.D. Dunnette (Chicago, IL: Rand-McNally, 1996), 900. Used by permission of Marvin D. Dunnette.

the other party may feel a sense of indebtedness, which may come into play in the future. The adage, it is better to give than to receive, seems to recommend accommodation, although it is not clear that this advice was meant for organizational members in an increasingly competitive environment. While capitulation may be recommended in some situations, people are unlikely to get what they want by relying on others accommodating them. They may rarely achieve outcomes that are good for them if they use capitulation too often. In most situations, there are better ways to manage conflict.

Pressing

When individuals have as their primary objective the achievement of their interests and are unconcerned about whether other parties get what they want (or even wish to "beat" the other side), they often rely on a series of strategies that are typically described as contentious. These strategies include a variety of tactics such as irrevocable commitments, threats or promises, and persuasive argumentation (Pruitt & Rubin, 1986).

Irrevocable commitments occur when one party credibly guarantees to continue behaving in a certain way that once begun will not be changed. An excellent example of an irrevocable commitment is the game of Chicken. The game involves two participants who are driving their cars at breakneck speed on a direct collision course with each other. The loser in this game is the one who first turns aside—the "chicken"—thereby avoiding a head-on collision and almost certain death for both players. In this game, each side tries to convince the other that they are committed to their course of action—driving straight toward the other car. More generally, irrevocable commitments occur when two parties engage in a test of wills in which neither side is willing to concede. A typical example of the risk of such games and tactics can be seen in the escalation of losses and acrimony that can occur when couples divorce.

Irrevocable commitments are useful because they do not require agreement of the other party to work nor do they require that the committing party be of equal or greater power. In the case of irrevocable commitments, weakness can become strength. Consider Gandhi's power, stemming from his weakness in the face of the other party's strength, to compel the British to modify their policies in India.

Threats and promises are both meant to convey intention. The typical promise is designed to induce some particular behavior by describing what will happen if such an action occurs. For example, one might promise to trade future support on issue A for current support on issue B. Promises do not give information about what will happen if compliance does not occur. Threats, on the other hand, convey what will happen if the preferred behavior does not happen. As such, one might threaten to vote against my interests unless I vote *for* her interests. Threats and promises are designed to have the same effect, but the mechanism by which the effects come about are different. Promises rely on the benefits of compliance while threats work because of the costs of noncompliance. In fact, compared with promises, threats provide more information because they describe how an individual intends to behave in response to a broader variety of actions. Promises tell me only what you will do if I take one particular action. They tell me nothing about what you would do if I take no action or another action.

Compared with threats and promises, persuasive argumentation is a less controlling tactic, although one that requires considerable skill. Through persuasive argumentation, I can influence you to give up something that you hold dear, change a situation you currently enjoy, or lower your aspirations. Consider the difficulty of persuading employees to work fewer hours rather than laying off other organizational members. When undertaking this tactic, one typically appeals to the unattractive alternatives that will ensue if the situation is left unchanged.

Avoidance

The most common response to conflict on any level is to avoid it. In many situations, people avoid conflict when both they and their organizations would benefit if they managed it more proactively. For example, issues involving quality of care are sometimes ignored because people fear the conflict associated with addressing them. However, avoidance does have its merits. If the issues involved in the conflict are trivial and the parties do not care much about their own outcome or the other party's outcome, avoidance may be the best strategy. The costs incurred by confronting the problem may be greater, at least in the short run, than the benefits that accrue from having the conflict resolved. Avoidance may also be the best way to deal with conflict when someone else can resolve the problem more effectively or when the problem would be better dealt with in the future after the involved parties have cooled down. If avoiding conflict becomes a habit, however, important issues, when they arise, may never get addressed.

Negotiation

Unlike other conflict-resolution tactics, negotiation is a process through which multiple parties work together on the outcome. People negotiate every day, although they do not always think of their activities as negotiations. This becomes clearer, however, when negotiation is defined as the process whereby two or more parties decide what each will give and take in an exchange between them (Rubin & Brown, 1975). This broad definition encompasses a preponderance of activities that people do every day, both within and outside organizations. Negotiations typically, but not always, involve some type of direct interaction between the parties, with the interaction being face to face, verbal, or written. The parties in a negotiation are interdependent in that they both desire something the other party has control over.

An interesting aspect of negotiation that distinguishes it from other forms of conflict resolution is the considerable amount of attention it has received in both applied and scholarly settings. One result of this trend is that we now know more about the behavior of negotiators and the structural factors that influence them than we did in the past. In the next section, we will provide a framework for thinking about negotiations that can be applied equally well to almost any negotiation situation, whether it involves a husband and wife or two nations. By analyzing the structure of a negotiation, negotiators should be able to improve their preparedness for, the process of, and the outcome of the negotiation.

NEGOTIATION

Basic Concepts

A negotiator never *has* to negotiate; there are always alternatives to reaching an agreement through a negotiation. Many were discussed above, such as avoiding the situation or giving the other party what they want. However, when a person in an interdependent situation (i.e., the person desires something the other party has control over and vice versa) does not reach a negotiated agreement with the other party, that person has to settle for another alternative regarding the desired resource controlled by the other party. For example, if a hospital is trying to hire a nurse but does not reach an agreement on an employment contract with a particular nurse, the hospital has to either accept the alternative of not having the position filled or choose the alternative of trying to hire another person for the job. From the nurse's point of view, if an agreement is not reached with the hospital, he will have to settle for another alternative, perhaps accepting a job with another hospital or continuing the job search.

Whether they have thought about them or not, the parties in a negotiation have alternatives that they will implement if the negotiation ends in an impasse. The negotiator will obviously choose her best alternative to an agreement if an impasse is reached, so this alternative will be our focus. Specifically, a negotiator's *Best Alternative To a Negotiated Agreement* (**BATNA**) is an important consideration because it is a source of power in the negotiation (Fisher & Ury, 1981). Being able to walk away from the negotiation if a satisfactory agreement does not appear to be forthcoming can be a valuable negotiating tool. Besides the opportunity to use this information strategically, it is also important to know when you actually should walk away. Knowing your best alternative allows a comparison to be made between the value of your best alternative and the value of various agreements that might be reached, which in turn allows you to know which agreements are desirable and which should be turned down.

A BATNA is put into action by determining a **reservation price.** A reservation price can be thought of as a bottom line, or the point at which you are indifferent between an impasse and an agreement (Raiffa, 1982). A reservation price should be stated in terms of whatever units are being negotiated. In many negotiations, the units of exchange are dollars so that, for example, a negotiator might have a reservation price of $18,000 when buying a car (i.e., the buyer will pay no more than $18,000). A BATNA and a reservation price, although closely related, are distinct concepts. The connection between the two is that a reservation price should equal the value placed on your best alternative *plus* whatever transaction costs you will incur to enact your best alternative (White & Neale, 1994). For example, the expenses that would be involved in hiring another nurse should be taken into consideration in determining a reservation price for a negotiation with a nurse candidate.

An **aspiration level** is what a negotiator would ideally like to achieve in the negotiation. It can also be referred to as a target or goal. An aspiration level should be challenging but attainable. A goal that is too challenging is not motivating because it is not within the realm of possibilities, while one that is too easy also loses its motivating potential once it is surpassed. Typically an aspiration level is stated in the same units as the reservation price (e.g., dollars).

The three concepts just discussed focus on one party rather than the constellation of parties involved in a negotiation. When the parties in a negotiation come together, additional structural features come into play. The most prominent feature is the **bargaining zone.** The bargaining zone is found by combining the reservation prices of each negotiator and determining whether they overlap, and if so, the extent of the overlap. A positive bargaining zone occurs if a set of agreements exists that both parties prefer over impasse (Neale & Bazerman, 1991). It is easier to understand this concept with the aid of a diagram. Imagine that a nurse and a hospital are negotiating over the nurse's salary. The nurse's reservation price is $30,000 and the hospital's reservation price is $35,000. This is outlined in Figure 5.2. The bargaining zone is the range of agreements between and including $30,000 and $35,000. If there is no overlap region between the reservation prices of the parties, then a negative bargaining zone exists. Because there are no agreements that are acceptable to both parties, no resolution is possible. It is important for a negotiator to gather information about the size of the bargaining zone during the course of the negotiation.

The Distributive Dimension of Negotiation

Of the two dimensions of negotiation, only the **distributive dimension** is necessarily part of every negotiation. The **integrative dimension,** on the other hand, is never applied in many negotiations. Negotiation always involves the allocation, or distribution, of some set of resources. The distributive dimension is often referred to as that part of negotiation in which value is claimed. In every negotiation, regardless of the amount of resources to be distributed, an integral task for the negotiators is to determine how much each party will take from the "pie" of resources. Single-issue negotiations are the most common example of purely distributive negotiations. The amount of resources is fixed, and whatever one party gains is always at the expense of the other party. Resolving negotiations that are distributive often entails compromise by both parties, as each party concedes a little at a time in a reciprocal manner until they reach an agreement. Negotiators should consider several strategies that may help them claim as large a share of the resources as possible. These strategies are outlined in Table 5.1.

Many negotiators presume that all negotiations are purely distributive and that their task as negotiators is to get as much as they can from the fixed amount of resources to be divided. A common assumption is that the interests of the other party are diametrically opposed to their own interests, and therefore a direct conflict arises over the resources in question. This is called the "fixed-pie bias" (Bazerman, Magliozzi, & Neale, 1985). Based on this assumption, they view ne-

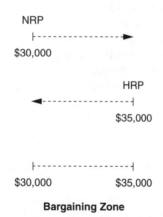

Figure 5.2. Bargaining Zones.

Table 5.1. Claiming Value: Distributive Bargaining Strategies

1. Know you BATNA.
2. Determine your bottom line or reservation price.
3. Set a goal or aspiration level that is (a) significantly better than your bottom line and (b) optimistically realistic.
4. Think of what objective standards might be acceptable to the other party.
5. Plan your opening. An initial offer should not be too extreme, but it should prevent the other party from "anchoring" the negotiation.
6. Develop reciprocity. Avoid making unilateral concessions.

gotiation as an adversarial process. The integrative dimension of negotiation is often overlooked because of this bias.

The Integrative Dimension of Negotiation

The most basic assumption underlying the integrative dimension of negotiation is that one party can gain without the other party necessarily having to lose. Another way to say this is that there are ways for the parties to mutually benefit. To do this, the parties need to take more of a problem-solving, cooperative approach rather than the contentious, competitive approach that typically characterizes purely distributive negotiations. In effect, the parties try to "expand the pie" of resources, or create value. A key element that should be present for a problem-solving orientation to work is trust between the parties. Trust is crucial because information sharing is at the heart of the negotiation process, and if information is not openly and accurately shared, albeit in a reciprocal manner, it is unlikely that integrative solutions can be found. Negotiating along the integrative dimension, or trying to find mutually beneficial solutions, can be difficult because it frequently requires finding creative or novel solutions that may not have been considered prior to the negotiation.

There are several ways to achieve integrative solutions. Most of them are based on differing interests underlying the conflict on the surface. Although this may sound strange because differences are the reason for the conflict, it is differences *in preferences* that allow integrative negotiation to occur. An example from the Culpeper Medical Associates case at the beginning of the chapter may help to clarify this point. Culpeper Memorial Hospital wanted to retain its 14 primary care doctors, but it did not have adequate financial resources to fend off rival employers. The University of Virginia wanted to formalize its relationships with more primary care doctors and had enough money to potentially acquire the practices of Culpeper's doctors. The doctors, on the other hand, did not want the University to acquire their practices and decrease their autonomy. The initial resolution to these conflicting interests was for the university to simply hire away one of Culpeper's internists, with the potential for more such hires to follow. However, a deeper analysis of the parties' interests revealed a better solution that made all parties better off. By forming Culpeper Medical Associates and then forming a partnership with Health Care Partners, the university formalized its relationship with the doctors while spending less money to do so, the hospital gained financial resources to retain its group of doctors, and the doctors retained their autonomy.

There are many techniques for finding integrative solutions. Logrolling entails trading issues that are of differing importance to the two parties (Pruitt & Rubin, 1986). Cost cutting occurs when one party finds a way to make the concessions of the other party less costly. This is often accomplished by one party offering the conceding party some sort of compensation that is related to the issues being negotiated. Cost cutting differs from nonspecific compensation, in which the party that concedes is paid by the other party in some currency that is unrelated to the negotiated issues. Obtaining added resources may sometimes be possible so that both parties can meet their goals. Frequently, the time and effort spent negotiating over a given set of resources may instead be spent finding ways to increase the amount of available resources (Pruitt, 1983). By undertaking one or more of these strategies, the parties in a negotiation may both be better off than if they simply compromised on the issues.

There are many obvious and some not-so-obvious benefits of finding integrative solutions in negotiations. Increasing the amount of resources to be distributed may be necessary for both parties to be able to reach their reservation prices. In these cases, an impasse is likely unless some integrative solution is found. An obvious benefit to finding integrative agreements is that a party's outcomes may be increased because a larger amount of resources is available to be distributed.

Less obviously, a party may also benefit from the opponent receiving a higher outcome. An opponent's satisfaction with the negotiation should increase as the outcome gets better. This should have a positive effect on the relationship between the two parties and should make the agreement more stable. If the other party is required to implement a decision that was reached as part of the negotiated agreement, successful implementation is more likely if the opponent is happy with the outcome, rather than disgruntled. Of course, the importance a party places on an opponent's outcome may vary with the expectation or probability of future interaction or with the types of issues that are being negotiated (e.g., some issues may require implementation, while others may not). The point here is that most people think only of their own outcome when they determine whether they were successful in a negotiation when several benefits, however indirect, may accrue to them if the other party also achieves a good outcome. Several specific strategies for reaching integrative agreements are outlined in Table 5.2.

The Mixed-Motive Nature of Negotiation

When thinking about the distributive and integrative dimensions of negotiation, it is crucial to keep in mind the mixed-motive nature of negotiations. Creating value by finding integrative solutions requires primarily cooperative behavior, while claiming value along the distributive dimension of the negotiation requires primarily competitive behavior. Many people make the mistake of thinking they can segment a negotiation into integrative and distributive components so that, for example, the parties can first integratively expand the pie and then negotiate the

Table 5.2 Creating Value: Integrative Bargaining Strategies

1. Know your BATNA. Try to ascertain the other side's BATNA.
2. Analyze your own and the other party's reservation prices to determine the bargaining zone.
3. Set priorities on your interests and those of the other party.
4. Construct multi-issue packages of offers that take into account differences between your own and the other party's priorities.

distribution of the enlarged pie. In fact, it is very unlikely for these to happen sequentially. Instead, the processes of integration and distribution occur simultaneously.

Negotiators must simultaneously balance cooperative and competitive behavior, so that they enlarge the pie *while* they claim an acceptable share of the enlarged pie. It is this "fundamental tension between cooperation and competition" that is the heart of negotiation, and that makes negotiation both an art and a science. The way that the value is created affects the way it is divided; the process of creating value is entwined with the process of claiming it (Lax & Sebenius, 1986). This is especially true if the motives and behaviors of the other party are unpredictable before the negotiation or are hard to read during the negotiation.

The Role of Information Sharing

Cooperative or competitive orientations are easy to talk about in general terms, but how do they manifest themselves in actual behavior during a negotiation? One of the core behavioral components of negotiation is information sharing. It is through the sharing of information that parties learn about their opponent's preferences on the issues, BATNA and reservation price, willingness to concede, interest in adding other issues to the negotiation, and in general, their opponent's overall orientation. Although the total amount of information that is shared during the negotiation is likely to affect the quality of the outcome reached by the parties, examining the subtleties of the parties' information-sharing patterns may be more revealing. First, if one party shares much more information than the other party, the party that receives the greater amount of information may have an advantage because they may know more about how far the other party can be pushed or what the chances are of finding an integrative solution. For example, if only one party knows the other's reservation price, the party with this information knows the size of the bargaining zone while the other does not. This could have a profound impact on the outcome of the negotiation.

One clarification here is that sharing information is not the same as talking. One side may talk more than the other party but share a lesser amount of important information. If negotiation is viewed solely as a persuasive process, then the party that talks more may be expected to do more persuading, and thus achieve a better outcome. However, persuasion is typically not included in what we refer to as information sharing. Information that is relevant in this analysis concerns the interests of the party, and thus the side that gives away less of this information may have an advantage.

Even if the amount of information shared by the parties is symmetric, the order in which it is shared may influence the outcomes of the parties. If one party gives away all of his information before the other party gives away any of her information, the party that delays sharing information may have an advantage, knowing more about the issues and the structure of the negotiation than the other party at an earlier point in the negotiation. Ideally, information should be shared in a reciprocal fashion so that one party gives away information incrementally while receiving equivalent amounts of information from the other party.

There are several strategies aimed at getting more information from the other party. Some of them, such as asking questions, are simple but often overlooked. These strategies include:

- building trust between the parties so that information is more likely to be shared
- asking questions
- giving away some information unilaterally in the hope that the other party will reciprocate
- making multiple offers simultaneously so the other party's interests can be inferred from the acceptability of each offer
- searching for post-settlement settlements (agreements that occur based on an extended search after an initial agreement is reached) (Raiffa, 1985).

Of course, the accuracy and specificity of information obtained by the other party is crucial. Discerning the accuracy of the information given by the other party is primarily a matter of trust, both on the part of the party giving information (trusting that the other party will not take advantage of true information) and on the part of the party receiving information (believing the information given by the other party).

Compatible Issues

There is one other type of issue we have not yet mentioned that is frequently overlooked when people think of negotiation. **Compatible issues** are those for which the parties have the same preferences. The parties have no conflict over these issues, perhaps making it seem odd that we include them in a chapter about conflict management. However, they are often included in negotiations because the negotiators do not know they have the same preferences on these issues and they make assumptions about the preferences of the other party.

Specifically, as mentioned earlier, many negotiators have a fixed-pie bias, meaning that they systematically assume their task in a negotiation is to split a fixed amount of resources (Bazerman, Magliozzi, & Neale, 1985; Thompson, 1991). The incompatibility bias inhibits negotiators in a related way, as they assume that the other party's preferences on the issues are necessarily in direct conflict with their own preferences and that they have no common interests (Thompson, 1991). Because of these biases, issues that are included in a negotiation for which the negotiators want the same outcome are often not identified as compatible, and a substantial number of negotiators settle for an outcome on these issues other than the one they both want.

Multiparty Negotiations

Most of the examples that are used to illustrate negotiations are dyadic, involving two parties. Although there are certainly many negotiations that involve only two parties, a substantial portion of negotiations involve three or more parties (which we refer to as multiparty). In health care, frequent examples involve negotiations among state or federal payment agencies, hospitals, and physicians. While many of the concepts of negotiation generalize from dyadic to multiparty negotiations, there are important differences between these types of negotiation.

The biggest difference is the increased complexity that occurs when parties are added to the negotiation. This complexity falls into two categories. First, interpersonal complexity increases as more people become involved in the interaction. For each person, there are more signals, gestures, and other types of communications from others to interpret. The second type of complexity involves the issues themselves. There are now multiple sets of preferences to be worked through rather than just two sets. For example, regarding the same subset of issues, two parties may have compatible preferences, two other parties may have opposite preferences but place a different amount of importance on these issues, while the preferences of two other parties may be diametrically opposed. Sharing the information to determine these preferences becomes much more difficult with multiple parties, and even if perfect information is shared, it is still a complex task to determine an optimal solution that is acceptable to everyone.

The bargaining zone in a negotiation with multiple parties is defined as the set of agreements that exceed every party's reservation price. It can be very difficult to determine whether a bargaining zone exists, much less the size of the bargaining zone. Furthermore, there may be people involved in the negotiation who would prefer that no agreement be reached, so that their purpose at the negotiation table (whether disguised or not) is to impede the process of the negotiation. Building trust may be more difficult between multiple parties, especially if coalitions form within the group of negotiators.

Coalition formation can have a major effect on the negotiation process and outcome. Coalitions may be based on long-standing relationships outside of the negotiation, or they may form during the negotiation based on similarity of preferences. They may form either to try to reach a specific agreement or to try to block a specific type of agreement. What is best for the coalition may not be what is best for the entire group. Negotiators in a multiparty situation should think about who they would like to form a coalition with, who might like to form a coalition with them, and who is unlikely to want to include them in a coalition.

Proactive behavior may be especially helpful in building a coalition because it should be easier to form a coalition initially than to break up an existing coalition and reform another one. However, coalitions, especially those formed around specific preferences in the negotiation, are likely to be unstable. When considering that the typical reason for joining a coalition is to increase your own outcomes, it is not surprising that people readily switch allegiances when they get better offers from other potential coalition partners. As such, coalitions may shift repeatedly during the course of a negotiation. A caveat to this reasoning is that social bonds between people may lend some stability to coalitions (Polzer, Mannix, & Neale, 1998). Whether it is based on an ongoing relationship or a shared group affiliation, such a bond may cause people to forego short-term gains from switching coalitions and instead opt for the longer-term benefits that flow from strong social connections.

Decision rules for reaching agreement may also be necessary in multiparty negotiations. Possible decision rules include unanimity, majority rule, or some other special rule detailing how many people must agree in order to reach a settlement. Some parties may also have veto power, which affects the power balance in the negotiation. These latter considerations may be influenced by the context within which the negotiation takes place. For example, if all the parties are working in the same organization (e.g., physicians employed by the same hospital), there may be hierarchical considerations, existing norms guiding the selection of a decision rule, or pressure from superiors to reach an agreement. Conversely, in a group negotiation in which the parties represent several different organizations (e.g., physicians having their own organizations), many of the parties may have more freedom to withdraw from the negotiation or force an impasse because they may have better alternatives with other sets of organizations. Also, few norms may exist if the negotiation itself is the first time the parties have been together in a group.

The above factors should be considered when preparing for and participating in a multiparty negotiation. If properly managed, the increased complexity inherent in this type of negotiation does not have to be an impediment and can in fact be used strategically if other parties are less prepared for or less able to cope with the complexity.

Fairness and Ethics in Negotiation

Negotiators often make claims about fairness to support their arguments. Fairness is not a unidimensional concept, however, and the application of different norms of fairness can lead to different outcomes. For this reason, it is important to think about which different norms of fairness can be applied in particular situations so that generalized claims for fairness are not used inappropriately. In a negotiation context, fairness will be discussed as it applies to the allocation of resources, which is the typical result of negotiation.

The most prevalent **fairness norm** in our society is **equality,** in which every party gets the same absolute amount of resources (Rawls, 1971). A second fairness norm that is used in most organizations to determine compensation is **equity,** whereby each person gets allocated an amount of resources proportional to his inputs (Adams, 1963; Homans, 1961). Defining what relevant inputs consist of and measuring these inputs can often lead to additional conflict, but once norms are in place in organizations regarding these issues, allocating resources equitably is often regarded as fair. Equity can be invoked in many negotiations other than organizational compensation situations as well. A third popular norm of fairness upon which allocations can be based is **need,** so that parties receive an amount of resources proportional to their need for them (Deutsch, 1975). As with inputs in the equity norm situation, determining the relative needs of each party can be tricky. Besides these three pure allocation norms of fairness, people may combine two or three of these norms to determine a fair allocation. Negotiators should consider which of these norms is applicable when they or one of their opponents claims that the negotiated outcome should be "fair."

Many people think of fairness and ethics in negotiation as somewhat entwined. Fairness may not always refer to the norm used for resource allocation, as discussed above, but instead may refer to the process by which people negotiate. For instance, people often say that if a negotiator is "unethical," she is not negotiating fairly. This triggers the same kind of problem that is triggered when determining fair allocations, in that people are not always in agreement about what

constitutes ethical behavior. This is especially relevant for negotiation because there are many typical negotiating strategies, such as bluffing or avoiding an answer to a specific question, that fall in a gray area concerning the ethicality of such behavior. Furthermore, many people believe that what is ethical is partially determined by context. For example, in some cultures, bribes are an accepted way of doing business when negotiating. Others adhere to a more absolute form of ethicality, believing that actions are either ethical or unethical regardless of the situation.

We are not going to state any rules about what is ethical or unethical. Instead, our purpose in discussing ethics is to increase the reader's awareness of several issues. First, however it is defined, unethical behavior is typically the result of self-interest (Murnighan, 1992). People act unethically because they benefit from it. When negotiating, regardless of your particular beliefs about ethics, it is important not to assume that the other party has the same beliefs you do or that they will behave (or restrict their behavior) in the same way you will. Also, unethical behavior can have consequences, especially regarding reputations, such that unethical behavior may help negotiators in the short run but may come back to haunt them in the long run. Negotiations can be full of ethical dilemmas. Thinking through and determining your own standards before you get into difficult situations is advised, as is being cautious, especially when making assumptions about the other party's ethical standards.

Preparing to Negotiate

Preparing for a negotiation often has as much to do with achieving a successful outcome as does the actual negotiation. But what exactly should a negotiator do to prepare for the negotiation? In this section, we offer several suggestions for how to increase the probability of a successful negotiation by preparing appropriately.

The least obvious, and perhaps most important, activity that should be worked on before the negotiation is to develop a BATNA, which was discussed earlier. If negotiators can develop a better and more certain alternative to a negotiated outcome, they will have more power in the negotiation and be likely to reach a better outcome. Determining a reservation price, based partially on the BATNA, is the next step to knowing in advance when you will be willing to walk away from the negotiation rather than reach agreement.

Concerning the negotiation more directly, a negotiator should think about what issues are likely to be included in the negotiation if they have not been specified in advance by either party. What additional issues could you bring to the negotiation? What issues might your opponent want to include? Whatever the set of issues includes, the negotiator should determine the importance of each issue relative to the other issues. This facilitates the process of comparing different offers made by the other party and trading low-priority issues for high-priority issues. Collecting information about the other party's alternatives and the importance that party places on each issue is a priority during a negotiation. It follows that negotiators can enhance their position if they can discover some or all of this information about their opponent before the negotiation. Sometimes this information can be

gathered directly from the other negotiator prior to negotiating, while in other situations it may be learned from other sources.

Another important piece of information to gather is how many negotiators the other party will be bringing to the table. This question, along with the determination of how many negotiators your party should bring to the negotiation, is the focus of Debate Time 5.2. A negotiator should also determine before the negotiation how important the relationship with the other party is. What future effects are likely to be caused by reputations that are developed in this negotiation? How much is the other party likely to be concerned about the relationship? The extent to which the decisions that are reached during the negotiation need to be implemented by either party after the negotiation is an important factor related to the relationship between the parties. If you have to rely on the other party to implement part of the deal, it is obviously not good to have the other party unhappy with the agreement or with you. Determining the

DEBATE TIME 5.2: WHAT DO YOU THINK?

*P*OINT: *The more people I can bring with me to the negotiation table, the better off I will be.* There are many benefits to be realized from including several people in a negotiation party. The more people that are at the negotiation, the more ideas they should be able to think of for ways to reach an integrative outcome. If expertise in different areas is helpful during the negotiation, it may be beneficial to have more "experts" on hand. Multiple roles, such as spokesperson, notekeeper, or financial analyst, can be performed more effectively at the table if a different person performs each function. A higher degree of critical thinking may occur when more people apply different perspectives to the problem being negotiated. Finally, if one party has more people at the negotiation than the other party, the bigger party may be perceived as having more power and may achieve better outcomes as a result.

COUNTERPOINT: I am better off negotiating by myself. The most obvious reason to negotiate alone

is that time is a valuable resource, and bringing other people to a negotiation that one person can handle is unnecessarily expensive. There are also more subtle reasons, stemming from intergroup conflict, that more people in each party may not result in better outcomes in a negotiation. When there is a team of negotiators on each side of the table, the intergroup boundaries between the parties may be much stronger than if each party consisted of just one person. When an "us against them" mentality occurs in a negotiation, which may be more likely with groups than with individuals, several negative consequences may result, including increased competitiveness, decreased trust, and a decreased level of information sharing. These may in turn result in outcomes that are inferior to those that may have been reached by individual negotiators bargaining in a more cooperative and trusting manner.

time constraints faced by each party can be useful, as the party who has the longer time before needing to reach an agreement has an advantage, if both parties know about the time constraints of the other.

Even the end of a negotiation requires preparation. If negotiators do not reveal all of their information during the negotiation, they should think about whether they want to share any of this information after the negotiation. It is usually advisable to keep some information confidential even after the negotiation so the other party does not grow concerned about whether she received a good outcome in the negotiation. The better-prepared party in a negotiation is often the most successful during the negotiation. As in school, doing your homework before the negotiation is half the battle when it is time to take the test.

MANAGING CONFLICT THROUGH THIRD-PARTY INTERVENTION

In many conflict situations, the disputants are unable to resolve the conflict. A third party that is not directly involved in the conflict can frequently intervene in one of several different ways to help resolve the conflict. There are many formal, institutional third parties that can be turned to outside of any particular organization. The court system in the United States is a very large example of a third party. Arbitrators are third parties that resolve differences between parties on many different issues, such as professional baseball salaries. The focus of this chapter, however, is on the manager's role as a third party in the day-to-day conflicts that occur in organizational life, rather than on formal third-party systems. To the extent that conflict is disruptive in organizations and hampers productivity, managers can increase the effectiveness of their organizations by intervening in conflict situations. Of course, the time the manager spends trying to resolve the disputes of other people is a cost to the organization, which needs to be balanced with the benefit derived from decreased conflict.

Dispute Intervention Goals

After making the decision to intervene in a conflict, the manager has a wide range of third-party intervention strategies from which to choose. The particular role the

manager plays in the dispute may depend on what he is trying to accomplish and on the constraints imposed by the situation. When intervening in a dispute between subordinates, a manager has a high level of authority, making any type of intervention an option. This is not the case when a manager intervenes in a dispute between two peers. The amount of conflict between the parties may also influence the manager's selection of intervention strategies. The importance of the issues in dispute, the amount of time pressure faced by the manager, the relative power of the disputants, and the relationships between the parties and between the manager and the parties may all affect the manager's choice of intervention strategies (Neale & Bazerman, 1991). The manager may also be concerned with how satisfied the disputants will be with the resolution and their perceptions of fairness regarding the intervention.

Types of Intervention Strategies

The types of intervention strategies a manager can undertake can be usefully categorized along two dimensions—the control the third party has over the process of the dispute and the control the third party has over the outcome of the dispute. Suppose a medical group practice manager is trying to manage the conflict between primary care physicians and specialists involving sharing revenue generated by the group practice. The control the manager desires over the process and outcome is likely to be affected by the factors discussed in the preceding paragraph. When the manager desires high control over both the process and outcome of the dispute, she may act as an **inquisitor**. In this type of intervention, the manager gathers information on the dispute by asking questions of the physicians, rather than letting them present the information as they would like. The manager then makes a decision about the outcome of the dispute and communicates this to the physicians. As in the court system, a manager acts as a judge or **arbitrator** when he controls the outcome but not the process of the dispute. The parties are free to present their sides of the dispute as they wish, after which the manager makes the decisions necessary to end the dispute. **Mediators** have control over the process of the dispute but have no authority, or do not use their

MANAGERIAL GUIDELINES

1. Managers need to analyze the amount and type of both beneficial and detrimental conflicts that currently exist in their organization so that they can focus on eliminating the detrimental conflict.

2. Health care managers should evaluate the level at which conflict usually occurs in their organization. Are there strong group boundaries (e.g., between departments or functional areas) that contribute to conflict, or is most conflict at the individual level?

3. When managers are involved in conflict, they should think explicitly about how much concern they have for the other party, as well as how concerned they are about their own outcomes for the issues involved in the conflict. This should help to determine what conflict-management strategy will be most appropriate.

4. When negotiating, managers need to determine the exact issues that are currently being negotiated and identify any other issues that might be included in the negotiation. Also, the importance of each issue to both the manager and the other party should be compared to determine where mutually beneficial trade-offs might occur.

5. Managers should think carefully about what ethical standards they feel comfortable with *before* they enter situations that involve ethical considerations.

6. Managers should not underestimate the importance of preparing for a negotiation. Failing to adequately prepare is probably the single biggest mistake made by negotiators.

7. If managers are going to intervene in a conflict as a third party, they need to consider how much control they want to have over both the process and the outcome of the dispute. Distinguishing between these types of control will facilitate effective intervention implementation.

authority, to control the outcome. Acting as mediator, the group practice manager may control the flow of information between the physician groups by separating them and acting as a go-between or may guide the discussion between them when they are together. The outcome, however, will ultimately be decided by the leaders of the respective physician groups.

The manager who chooses not to have high process or outcome control can choose from several options. The most efficient approach from the manager's perspective is to ignore the conflict and hope the disputants will resolve it by themselves. Managers can also delegate responsibility for getting the dispute resolved to someone else. Another option is to threaten the disputants to increase their motivation to resolve the conflict.

Managers have many choices in determining which third-party intervention strategies best fit their needs. It is possible that, for the same dispute situation, a manager may change intervention strategies if the previously chosen strategy does not work. When this happens, a manager will usually progress from strategies involving less control to strategies involving more control.

Although conflict is pervasive, it can be successfully managed through an understanding and application of various conflict-management techniques and negotiation skills. By managing conflict more effectively, health services executives make important contributions to organizational effectiveness while improving the productivity and satisfaction of the people with whom they work.

Discussion Questions

1. What types of skills do managers need to successfully manage conflict in their organizations? Which of these skills do you possess? What might be your greatest weakness as a conflict resolver? What can you do to strengthen your weak areas?

2. Related to Debate Time 5.1, what are some indications that a health services organization is experiencing dysfunctional levels of conflict? What systems can be put in place to monitor these indicators?

3. What third-party intervention strategies are likely to be favored by managers acting as third parties? What third-party intervention strategies are likely to be favored by the disputants? If these answers are different, what can a manager do to satisfy all the parties involved? What factors may affect your answers to these questions?

4. Regarding intergroup conflict, which groups do you most frequently represent or identify with in your interactions? How might this change depending on the type of health services organization with which you might be employed?

References

Adams, J. S. (1963). Toward an understanding of inequity. *Journal of Abnormal and Social Psychology, 67,* 422–436.

Bazerman, M. H., Magliozzi, T., & Neale, M.A. (1985). The acquisition of an integrative response in a competitive market. *Organizational Behavior and Human Decision Processes, 35,* 294–313.

Deutsch, M. (1949). An experimental study of the effects of cooperation and competition upon group process. *Human Relations, 2,* 199–232.

Deutsch, M. (1975). Equity, equality, and need: What determines which value will be used as the basis of distributive justice? *Journal of Social Issues, 31,* 137–149.

Fisher, R., & Ury, W. (1981). *Getting to yes.* Boston: Houghton-Mifflin.

Homans, G. (1961). *Social behavior: Its elementary forms.* New York: Harcourt, Brace.

Janis, I. (1982). *Groupthink: Psychological studies of policy decisions and fiascoes.* Boston: Houghton-Mifflin.

Jehn, K. A. (1995). A multimethod examination of the benefits and detriments of intragroup conflict. *Administrative Science Quarterly, 40,* 256–282.

Lax, D. A., & Sebenius, J. K. (1986). *The manager as negotiator.* New York: Free Press.

Murnighan, J. K. (1992). *Bargaining games.* New York: William Morrow and Company, Inc.

Neale, M. A., & Bazerman, M. H. (1991). *Cognition and rationality in negotiation.* New York: Free Press, p. 2.

Nordhaus-Bike, A. M. (1997, August 20). Partnering: Unite and Conquer. *Hospitals and Health Network 5,* 7(16).

Northcraft, G. B., & Neale, M. A. (1990). *Organizational behavior: The managerial challenge.* Homewood, IL: Dryden Press.

Polzer, J. T., Mannix, E. A., & Neale, M. A. (1998). Interest alignment and coalitions in multiparty negotiation. *Academy of Management Journal, 41,* 42–54.

Pruitt, D. G. (1983). Achieving integrative agreement. In M. H. Bazerman, & R. J. Lewicki (Eds.), *Negotiating in organizations.* Beverly Hills, CA: Sage.

Pruitt, D. G., & Rubin, J. Z. (1986). *Social conflict.* New York: Academic Press.

Raiffa, H. (1982). *The art and science of negotiation.* Cambridge, MA: Belknap.

Raiffa, H. (1985). Post settlement settlements. *Negotiation Journal, 1,* 9–12.

Rawls, J. (1971). *A theory of justice.* Cambridge, MA: Harvard University Press.

Rubin, J., & Brown, B. (1975). *The social psychology of bargaining and negotiation.* New York: Academic Press.

Sherif, M. (1977). *Intergroup conflict and cooperation.* Norman, OK: University Book Exchange.

Sherif, M., & Sherif, C. (1953). *Groups in Harmony and Tension.* New York; Harper and Row.

Thomas, K. (1976). Conflict and conflict management. In M. Dunnette (Ed.), *Handbook of industrial and organizational psychology.* Chicago: Rand-McNally.

Thompson, L. L. (1991). Information exchange in negotiation. *Journal of Experimental Social Psychology, 27*(2), 161–179.

White, S. B., & Neale, M. A. (1994). The role of negotiation aspiration and settlement expectancies on bargaining outcomes. *Organizational Behavior and Human Decision Processes, 57,* 303–317.

PART

3

Operating the Technical System

THE NATURE OF ORGANIZATIONS: FRAMEWORK FOR THE TEXT

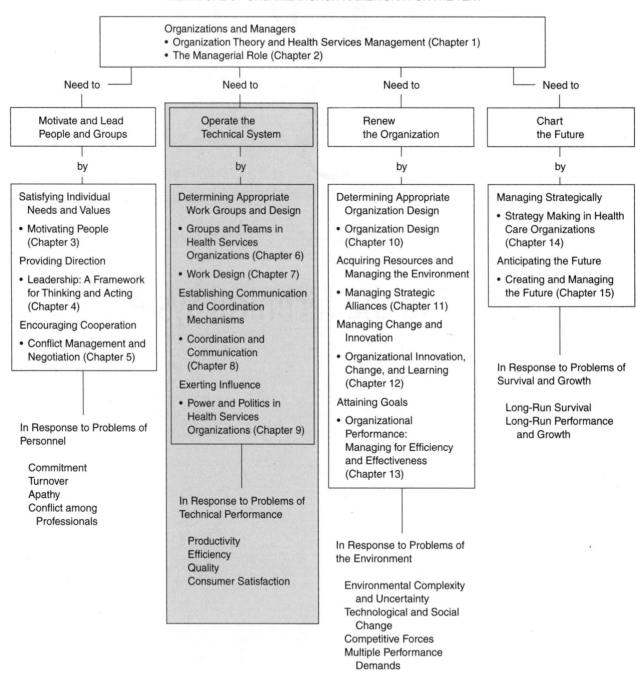

Organizations and Managers
- Organization Theory and Health Services Management (Chapter 1)
- The Managerial Role (Chapter 2)

Need to

Need to

Need to

Need to

Motivate and Lead People and Groups

Operate the Technical System

Renew the Organization

Chart the Future

by

by

by

by

Satisfying Individual Needs and Values

- Motivating People (Chapter 3)

Providing Direction

- Leadership: A Framework for Thinking and Acting (Chapter 4)

Encouraging Cooperation

- Conflict Management and Negotiation (Chapter 5)

In Response to Problems of Personnel

  Commitment
  Turnover
  Apathy
  Conflict among
    Professionals

Determining Appropriate Work Groups and Design

- Groups and Teams in Health Services Organizations (Chapter 6)
- Work Design (Chapter 7)

Establishing Communication and Coordination Mechanisms

- Coordination and Communication (Chapter 8)

Exerting Influence

- Power and Politics in Health Services Organizations (Chapter 9)

In Response to Problems of Technical Performance

  Productivity
  Efficiency
  Quality
  Consumer Satisfaction

Determining Appropriate Organization Design

- Organization Design (Chapter 10)

Acquiring Resources and Managing the Environment

- Managing Strategic Alliances (Chapter 11)

Managing Change and Innovation

- Organizational Innovation, Change, and Learning (Chapter 12)

Attaining Goals

- Organizational Performance: Managing for Efficiency and Effectiveness (Chapter 13)

In Response to Problems of the Environment

  Environmental Complexity
    and Uncertainty
  Technological and Social
    Change
  Competitive Forces
  Multiple Performance
    Demands

Managing Strategically

- Strategy Making in Health Care Organizations (Chapter 14)

Anticipating the Future

- Creating and Managing the Future (Chapter 15)

In Response to Problems of Survival and Growth

  Long-Run Survival
  Long-Run Performance
    and Growth

The four chapters of this section focus on operating critical components of the technical system within health care organizations. This involves determining the appropriate work design, establishing communication and coordination mechanisms, and ensuring and improving performance. The following chapters characterize these functions in order to enhance technical aspects of productivity, efficiency, quality, and consumer satisfaction.

Chapter 6, "Groups and Teams in Health Services Organizations," focuses on the effective management of groups and teams. The chapter addresses the following questions:

- Why are groups and teams important?
- How does group structure and process affect performance?
- What are the causes of intergroup conflict, and what strategies are available for its management?

Chapter 7, "Work Design," considers the design of work in organizations. The emphasis is on defining different types and components of work and assessing the interconnected nature of work within a variety of health services organizations. The chapter addresses the following questions:

- What is work? Is it different from working?
- How does work design affect individual motivation and productivity?
- How does the interconnectedness of work affect individuals and work groups?

Chapter 8, "Coordination and Communication," deals with the essential means through which managers link the various people and groups within the organization and link the organization to other organizations. The following questions provide the major focus of this chapter:

- What is the role of intraorganizational coordination? How is it similar or different from interorganizational coordination?
- What are the major components and barriers of effective communications?

The last chapter in this section, "Power and Politics in Health Services Organizations," discusses the means by which power distributions can be identified, the conditions under which conflict among groups may result, the uses of power to resolve conflict, and the strategies and tactics that are commonly employed to do so. The chapter addresses the following questions:

- What are the sources of power?
- What are the conditions that promote the use of power, politics, and informal influence?
- What approaches are available for consolidating and developing power by managers, physicians, and other groups of health care providers?

Upon completing these four chapters, the reader should be able to understand the nature of work and the processes affecting work within health services organizations.

CHAPTER
6

Groups and Teams in
Health Services Organizations

Bruce J. Fried, Ph.D.
Sharon Topping, Ph.D.
Thomas G. Rundall, Ph.D.

Chapter Outline

Learning Objectives

After completing this chapter, the reader should be able to:

1. Describe the importance and types of groups and teams in health services organizations.
2. Understand the dimensions of empowerment and why the bounding process is important.
3. Distinguish between different approaches to assessing team performance.
4. Understand the factors associated with high-performing teams.
5. Analyze the effects of a work group's composition and size on team performance.
6. Explain the relationship between work group norms and team productivity.
7. Identify the key roles assumed by individuals in work groups.
8. Understand the role that cohesiveness plays in determining team performance.
9. Describe key aspects of group process including leadership, the communication structure, decision making, and stages of group development.

10. Explain how the group task can have such a significant effect on team process and productivity.

11. Define the major causes and consequences of intergroup conflict and identify alternative strategies for managing conflict.

12. Explain how available resources, management support, and reward systems can affect teams.

Key Terms

Behavioral Masking
Behavior and Performance Norms
Building and Maintenance Roles
Communications Structure
Decision Making
Delphi Technique
Empowerment
Environmental Context
Formal and Informal Leadership
Formal Groups
Groupthink
Informal Groups
Intergroup Conflict
Management Teams
Nominal Group Technique
Performance Norm
Personal Roles
Role Differentiation
Stages of Team Development
Status Differences
Task Design Characteristics
Task Interdependence
Task-Oriented Roles
Team Cohesiveness
Team Composition
Team Productivity
Team Size

Chapter Purpose

As illustrated by the unfolding events involving multidisciplinary teams in the "In the Real World" case, groups are a mainstay of organizational life and will become more important in coming years. The work of health services organizations is increasingly being carried out by groups and teams, and we simply cannot escape the necessity of working in teams. Almost all clinical and managerial innovations are dependent to some degree on effective team performance. For example, as patient care technology becomes more specialized, there will be increasing need for team structure to coordinate the work of individual specialists. Quality improvement methods, such as continuous quality improvement, are highly dependent upon well-functioning cross-functional teams.

Teams are pervasive within health services organizations. When managed well, teams can be highly creative and productive and contribute in a positive way to organizational effectiveness. When poorly managed, the organization and its patients or clients can face disastrous consequences.

Most organizational members participate in a variety of teams such as:

- Boards of directors and their committees and sub-committees
- Nursing teams
- Operating room teams
- Strategic planning teams
- Treatment teams
- Interorganizational coordinating teams

Members of organizations may assume numerous roles depending on the team and their role in the group. An awareness of team concepts is key to organizational performance.

This chapter focuses on the effective management of groups and teams in organizations. It does this by building on Chapters 3–5, dealing with issues of motivation, leadership, and conflict management, respectively, and also touches on issues of work design, communication and coordination, and organization design, which are subsequently discussed in Chapters 7, 8, and 10, respectively. Following a discussion of the types of groups found in health services organizations, attention is given to issues of team cohesiveness, status differences, team size and composition, communication structure, and task characteristics, including task interdependence and complexity. The following section deals with the question of team productivity and why certain teams are more productive than others.

IN THE REAL WORLD:
MANAGING: ACROSS INTERORGANIZATIONAL BOUNDARIES: A CASE STUDY OF A MULTIDISCIPLINARY TEAM

As the late afternoon quiet descended over the office, Tom Landry, Orange County's Youth Initiative Coordinator, thought about the meeting tonight and its consequences. This was the first time that members of Anthony's Core Services Team would meet, and a lot depended on them being able to work together. Anthony, the focus of the team, was an intelligent 16 year old who had been diagnosed recently with schizophrenia. Although he had been in trouble at school, Anthony's future looked bright, if only he could obtain the necessary treatment. As the Youth Initiative Coordinator, it was up to Tom to make sure that the service providers worked together as a team. Would he be able to do that? How do you bring together such diverse members from totally different organizations and expect them to cooperate and coordinate with each other in the delivery of care to one teenager? Tom was worried.

Several years ago the state legislators appropriated funding for the Youth Initiative Program (YIP), an innovative program that provides individualized or "wraparound" services to children/youth with severe emotional disturbance and their families. In this program, services are tailored to the specific needs of the child and family and are based in the community where the youth resides. One of the critical elements of this program is the interdisciplinary services team that develops and coordinates the array of services. Members are those persons in the community, including the biological or adopted parents, who may be instrumental in delivery of effective services. Tom worked for YIP as one of the county case coordinators, and when assigned a client, like Anthony, it is his responsibility to manage the services team. As he was preparing for the meeting tonight, he considered the composition of Anthony's team:

Jean Nichols is Anthony's probation officer and is actively interested in his welfare. Until Anthony was 14 years old, he was a good student. Near the end of his ninth year in school, he started experimenting with alcohol and fighting in school. When he was found drunk during class with an open bottle of vodka in his backpack, he was placed on probation. Jean works for the county

Department of Juvenile Probation, where coordination with other agencies in the community is encouraged. The director is very interested in the Youth Initiative Program and serves on the statewide oversight committee. Jean and Tom have been on several teams together before, and the experience had always been positive.

Steve Hanks is Anthony's alcohol abuse counselor, who works for the regional Alcohol and Substance Abuse Center. Steve is a recovering alcoholic who believes that abstinence and the 12 "steps to recovery" program are the only effective treatment for alcoholism. He is the only counselor at the center who works with juveniles and is well liked and respected by his clients. However, the Department of Alcohol and Substance Abuse from the state level down discourages collaborative activity with other agencies. Consequently, employees prefer to work alone in a one-on-one relationship with their clients.

Mary Beth Powell is the psychological counselor from the local high school and knows Anthony's case well. She was instrumental in getting him diagnosed and treated for mental illness. During the time that Anthony started drinking, he also began to have hallucinations. He was terrified to tell his parents since his father had been abusive in the past. Eventually, he confided to Mary Beth.

Terri Morgan is the psychiatrist at the local mental health center treating Anthony for his psychotic symptoms. After one major psychotic episode, she admitted him to the state psychiatric hospital for a two-month stay. Anthony's father objected to his son's admission to the hospital and tried to change physicians. Since no other psychiatrists in town take Medicaid patients, Anthony had to continue his treatment at the mental health center under the care of Dr. Morgan. Since she is the sole psychiatrist at the center, Dr. Morgan is extremely busy and has little time for meetings outside of the clinic. Often, she picks the first person she sees to fill in for her.

Anthony's mother is nonassertive and unquestioning, willing to accept without comment or complaint whatever plans or actions others take in treating her son. However, she is committed to keeping Anthony in the YIP since she believes it is the only way to keep him out of trouble and out of the hospital.

Anthony's father is a brusque man who often drinks too much and gets into fights at neighborhood bars. He is a "know-it-all" who resents authority and as a result, has a problem holding a job. He was abusive to his older daughters when they were growing up and has continued this behavior with his son. When Anthony came to school with bruise marks and a black eye, the high school counselor, Ms. Powell, reported his father to the Department of Child Abuse and Protection. Consequently, he dislikes her intensely.

Bob Evans is a caseworker with the local office of the Department of Child Abuse and Protection and is actively involved with Anthony's case. Bob is a mild-mannered individual who is a respected member of the local community. Bob has been working with Anthony's family for over a year and has made substantial progress with his father. Known as a team player who gets things done, he is a valued member of any team.

Some of the questions and issues that Tom needs to address before his meeting are:

1. *Given the diversity of the team, who can he count on as allies and as troublemakers? Can he predict potential conflicts, and if so, how can he resolve them? (Don't forget the philosophical differences in approach to treatment between the medical, the Alcoholics Anonymous (AA), and psychosocial models.)*

2. *Since this is the first meeting of the team, what type of behavior should Tom expect? What can he do to prepare for the "forming" stage?*

3. *The goal of this YIP team is to develop a services plan and then coordinate the services that Anthony will need. How can Tom turn this team goal into one that every member wants to accomplish?*

4. *Given the diversity of the team and the complexity and interdependence of the task, how can Tom build cohesiveness among the team members?*

5. *It is important that this team maintains its relationship with other stakeholders, like the juvenile justice system, the Department of Alcohol and Substance Abuse, and the local mental health center. How can Tom make sure this is done? If conflict arises, how can the team resolve it?*

THE IMPORTANCE OF GROUPS AND TEAMS IN HEALTH SERVICES ORGANIZATIONS

As illustrated by the "In the Real World" involving a multidisciplinary group providing services to at-risk youth, teams are a mainstay of organizational life, and will become more important in coming years. The use of teams is not unique to health services organizations. It has been found, for example, that 82% of companies with 100 or more employees use teams (Gordon, 1992). The work of health services organizations is increasingly being carried out by teams, and we simply cannot escape the necessity of working in teams. In a study of 56,000 production workers, it was found that one of the most common skills required of employees is the ability to work in a team environment (Capelli &

Rogovsky, 1994). Almost all clinical and managerial innovations are dependent to some degree on effective group performance. For example, as patient care technology becomes more specialized, there will be increasing need for team structures to coordinate the work of individual specialists. Quality improvement methods, such as continuous quality improvement, are highly dependent upon well-functioning cross-functional teams (Fargason & Haddock, 1992). Given the importance of teams to organizational performance, it is surprising how little systematic attention organizations give to improving team performance, productivity, and efficiency, particularly when decades of research and experience have provided us with a clear understanding of the factors associated with high-performing teams (Cohen & Bailey, 1997).

Types of Groups and Teams

As discussed throughout this chapter, there are many different types of groups and teams in all organizations, and in health services organizations in particular. In this chapter, primary attention will be given to formally organized work groups and teams. However, in understanding organizations, it is essential that we understand informal as well as formal structures and processes (Mechanic, 1962). Thus, in addition to formally sanctioned teams, anyone working in an organization needs to be aware of informal groups and their influence on the organization. The importance of informal work group structure and group processes has been recognized for at least 50 years. The Hawthorne experiments firmly established the proposition that an individual's performance is determined in large part by informal relationship patterns that emerge within work groups (Roethlisberger & Dickson, 1939). The work group has a pervasive impact on individual behaviors and attitudes because it controls so many of the stimuli to which the individual is exposed in performing organizational tasks (Hasenfeld, 1983; Porter, Lawler, & Hackman, 1975).

Informal Groups

There are a variety of types of **informal groups** found in and between organizations. Informal groups can have high motivational value for individuals. A simple though valid example of an informal group is a car pool. Car pools meet individual needs by economizing on commuting costs and creating an opportunity for social interaction. They may also be viewed positively by the organization in that they may lead to decreased absenteeism and lateness as well as higher employee morale.

There are a number of circumstances under which informal groups can have a negative impact on an organization. Groups may become overly exclusionary and lead to interpersonal conflict. In other cases, informal groups can become so powerful so as to undermine the formal authority structure of the organization. Consider Etzioni's (1961) classic description of the role of informal groups in factories:

The workers constituted a cohesive group which had a well-developed normative system of its own. The norms specified, among other things, that a worker was not to work too hard, lest he become a "rate-buster"; nor was he to work too slowly, lest he become a "chiseler" who exploited the group (part of the wages were based on group performance). Under no condition was he to inform or "squeal." By means of informal social control, the group was able to direct the pace of work, the amount of daily and weekly production, the amount of work stoppage, and allocation of work among members.

In this instance, informal groups of employees were able to maintain social control as well as control over the pace of work through the imposition of informal, though well-enforced, rules of behavior.

Finally, informal groups can assume a change-agent role. Informal groups are often responsible for facilitating improvements in working conditions; such informal groups sometimes evolve into formal groups. A current example is the emergence of physician unions. These often begin informally, perhaps as a group focused on professional interests, but may evolve over time into union status (Erickson, 1997). Informal groups may also emerge to deal with a particular organizational problem or to work toward changes in organizational policies and procedures. Such groups may, in fact, initiate action against a corrupt manager or supervisor.

In sum, informal groups play a unique role in organizations. To the extent possible, managers should be aware of the roles informal groups play in the organization. Where they play a positive role, they may be encouraged by management; when they appear deleterious, managers might consider a variety of alternative options, such as developing a formal employee involvement process to ensure that such attitudes receive a fair hearing in the organizations. Negatively oriented informal groups may be a sign of dissatisfaction among employees.

Formal Groups

In the remainder of this chapter, we focus almost exclusively on **formal groups** and teams. Because of the difficulties involved in distinguishing between groups and teams, we use these terms interchangeably. We do, however, place certain boundaries on this construct. To distinguish organizational groups from large population-based groups (for example, an ethnic group in a city), we limit our attention to those groups or teams that are authentic organizational-based social systems. Such teams are intact social systems with boundaries, interdependence among members, and differentiated member roles. Organizationally based teams are task-centered: They have one or more tasks to perform and produce measurable outcomes. Finally, they operate within an organizational context and interact with a larger organization or organizational subunits (Hackman, 1990a). This approach is consistent with the following definitions:

> A group is defined as two or more persons who are interacting with one another in such a manner that each person influences and is influenced by each other person. (Shaw, 1976)
>
> A team is a collection of individuals who are interdependent in their tasks, who share responsibility for outcomes, who see themselves and who are seen by others as an intact social entity embedded in one or more larger social systems, and who manage their relationships across organizational boundaries. (Cohen & Bailey, 1997)

We include groups that are established for a relatively short period of time, such as project task forces, as well as more permanent groups. Cohen and Bailey (1997) provide a useful scheme for classifying teams in organizations. We adopt this scheme in this chapter, and provide health care examples of each type of team:

Work teams are continuing work units responsible for producing goods or providing services. These teams may be directed by supervisors or be self-managing. In the health care environment, these include treatment teams, emergency department personnel, research teams, and home care teams. They tend to be ongoing and relatively permanent in nature. As with other teams, membership may be stable or unstable over time, and may be multi- or unidisciplinary.

Parallel teams pull together people from different work units or jobs to perform functions that the regular organization is not equipped to perform. They usually have limited authority and generally make recommendations to individuals higher up in the hierarchy. These include quality improvement teams, employee involvement groups, and task forces. In the health care system, parallel teams may be involved in such activities as continuous quality improvement (CQI) and process improvement, community health needs assessment, and staff search committees. By their nature, they are often multidisciplinary. As suggested by the diversity of teams falling into this category, these teams may be temporary or permanent features of the organization.

Project teams are time-limited, producing one-time outputs such as a new product or service or a new information system. In health care, such teams may exist for purposes of planning a new hospital, developing a merger plan, or selecting a new human resources information system.

Management teams coordinate and provide direction to the subunits under their jurisdiction. Management teams may exist at the board level, senior management level, or departmental level.

From a personal perspective, it is important to understand that most people in organizations are members of a variety of formal and informal groups, and as such, may assume many different team roles. A surgeon, for example, may play a strong and influential leadership role in the operating room, but when working on a physician staff subcommittee with her peers, may have relatively little power or influence. Roles may vary dramatically with respect to power and normative and behavioral expectations. As team members, it is critical to understand where we fit within the context of a particular team. At times, the demands of multiple roles—particularly among professionals—may compete with one another for time and commitment, leading to feelings of role ambiguity, role conflict, and stress (Greene, 1978).

Notwithstanding the importance of teams in organizations, there is likely no other aspect of organizational life that causes as much ambivalence, and at times disdain and cynicism. Many teams achieve far less than their potential because of coordination, communication, or motivational problems among group members, collectively known as process losses (Steiner, 1972). While many of us enjoy the interactions and synergies associated with working on teams, groups may often create misunderstandings and bring out latent conflicts between individuals. Interprofessional rivalries and status differences are often played out in groups causing anger, dissatisfaction, lower productivity, and frequently, a sense that individuals' knowledge and skills are underutilized. Anyone who has spent time in teams is aware of the destructive potential of personality clashes; these are often severe in the relatively intimate environment of work groups and teams. Social loafing, a situation in which individuals may exert less effort when they work in a group than when they work alone (also known as "free-riding" and "shirking") is certainly not uncommon in many teams (George, 1992; Latane, Williams, & Harkins, 1979).

Teams and Empowerment

Teams can also be used as an extension of a general employee **empowerment** strategy. Empowering workers is typically achieved by providing them with information, knowledge, and power (Rundall, Starkweather, & Norrish, 1998). Empowerment techniques are often the management strategy of choice when traditional hierarchical management structure and command and control management techniques are no longer viable for an organization. In the context of empowerment management, teams fulfill a number of important functions. Teams tend to be "self-regulating," reducing if not eliminating the need for close supervision by senior managers. Individual behaviors of team members are visible to other team members, and the consequences of those behaviors for the team and the organization will similarly be visible to all members of the team. Further, the knowledge, skills, and experience that are present in teams far exceed those of any individual member, making teams more resourceful and effective in performing complex tasks with little direct supervision.

Dimensions of Empowerment

Empowered teams occur along four dimensions (Gordon, 1999; Kirkman & Rosen, 1997):

- Potency: Team members have a belief that they can be effective.
- Meaningfulness: Team members share beliefs and attitudes.
- Autonomy: Teams have freedom and discretion in deciding how to do their work.
- Consequences: A team knows that its work affects other parts of the organization.

In a hospital studied by one of the authors that implemented an employee empowerment strategy built around the creation of management and patient care teams, the effects on staff performance were striking. In this hospital, more authority for quality improvement, education programming, and staff scheduling was placed in patient care unit teams. The staff experienced empowerment with this sharing of decision making. One of the hospital's nurses summarized these effects:

> We've decreased the layers of management in the hospital. Problem solving is now at the unit level. Everybody has patient care in his or her title. Problems are brought to the table and discussed as a team. Through this group decision making process, staff has come to believe that 'I can make a difference; I can have a say in what's happening.' Now, everybody talks and walks team. Staff does not feel compelled to protect their turf. Employees feel okay to make decisions. We're not afraid to take on challenges such as starting up a new hospice. The nurses have become more assertive with the doctors. They are more willing to work collegially with doctors, and so are the doctors with them. The staff now sees this hospital as on the leading edge of rural health care, and this is exciting (Rundall, Starkweather, & Norrish, 1998).

The use of work teams is one important technique for ensuring that the work of empowered employees remains focused on improving organizational performance. However, even with the formation of work teams, the use of an employee empowerment management strategy typically requires additional efforts to focus the work of employees. Empowering employees without establishing the "boundaries" (Rundall et al., 1998) of that empowerment can have detrimental consequences. While empowerment develops the capacity of employees to improve their job and organizational performance, this strategy relies on the intrinsic motivation of individuals to demonstrate self-efficacy. While many employees are motivated to demonstrate self-efficacy at work, it is unrealistic to assume that every employee is so motivated. Many managers have found to their dismay that even when placed in work teams, many of their organization's empowered employees have taken advantage of the new management strategy to work fewer hours, work less productively, work on personal projects, or behave in other ways that do not contribute to improving organizational performance. However, it is important to note that even employees who have a strong desire to use their empowerment to improve organizational performance will be more effective if the boundaries of empowerment are established. For example, all employees must understand the mission of the organization in order to use their empowered status to improve organizational performance.

Bounding of Empowerment

The bounding of empowerment, then, is the process of defining the boundaries surrounding the actions of empowered employees in the context of the mission of the organization and its short- and long-term goals. The bounding of empowerment is primarily achieved through employees' internalizing the values and goals of the organization. In this way, employees become more self-reliant and self-regulating. Their work-related activities become more focused on improving job and organizational performance because their personal identity and self-esteem become more closely linked to the success of the organization. The bounding of empowerment is established in very different ways than are the constraints on the behavior of employees in a command management organiza-

tion. In a command management organization, employees are micromanaged by supervisors who direct their activities, limit their contributions to a narrow scope of work, and check on performance through close supervision. In an organization with empowered employees, controls on behavior are achieved through macromanagement techniques, such as encouraging the internalization of key values, setting team and organizational objectives, providing feedback, and giving rewards for successful team and organization performance.

UNDERSTANDING TEAM PERFORMANCE

In understanding team performance, it is important to disentangle two separate questions about performance. The first question, generally stated, is, Is a team approach (or a particular team approach) more effective than nonteam (or alternative team) approaches? In this question, we are asking, for example, if a team nursing approach produces better patient outcomes than traditional nonteam-based methods. The second question, however, assumes that a team approach will be used (for example, a basketball team), and the key question is, What factors account for different levels of team performance? In this chapter, the perspective generally taken is that teams are a mainstay of organizational life and that we need to seek ways of making them more effective. However, we need to be cognizant of the fact that novel team-based approaches are not necessarily superior to traditional methods (Cassard, Weisman, Gordon, & Wong, 1994).

We have all been members of many teams and have had the opportunity to observe other teams in action. From these observations, it is apparent that teams vary in their effectiveness and efficiency. Why is there such variation in the performance of teams? Some variation may be due to differences in the skills of individual members, an explanation that may be salient in certain types of teams, such as sports teams. On the other hand, there are many situations where individual team members may be highly talented, but produce poor decisions or other poor outcomes. Later in this chapter, we discuss the concept of "Groupthink" in which sometimes disastrously poor advice may be generated by a team of highly talented and skilled individuals because of dysfunctional group and communication processes.

A Model of Team Performance

What makes teams effective? What can leaders do to help teams become more productive and satisfying? To address these questions and others, we adopt the view that team performance is dependent upon a host of factors related to team characteristics, team processes, work characteristics, and the larger environment within which the group is embedded. A multidimensional model is necessary because team performance is not a simple phenomenon and is influenced by factors at a variety of levels. While we cannot always control these factors, an understanding of their potential impact on team performance should provide leaders with appropriate strategies for team management. Figure 6.1 provides an overview of these factors. At the team characteristic level, we include the following characteristics: composition and size, status differences, team norms, member roles, team roles, and team cohesiveness. At the team processes level, we include leadership, communication, decision making, and stages of group development. At the task level, we include a discussion of the nature of the task and the various characteristics that go into defining the task. Lastly, at the environmental level, we include intergroup relationships and conflict within the larger organization and environment and the availability of resources, support, and rewards. Taken together, these factors provide a useful diagnostic tool for understanding team performance.

Before embarking on a detailed discussion of these factors, several points are in order. First, our purpose in adopting a particular model of group performance is to provide a framework for organizing a large amount of research spanning several decades. Many other models are available, with varying strengths and drawbacks (Hackman, 1982; Kolodny & Kiggundu, 1980; Nieva, Fleishman, & Rieck, 1978; Steiner, 1972; Trist & Bamforth, 1951). The model developed here includes most of the variables considered in other models; further, the variables contained in this model have been subjected to empirical test with a large sample of work groups. The second point

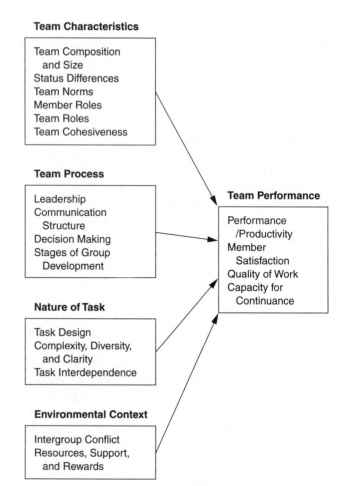

Figure 6.1. A Model of Team Performance.

concerns the nature of research that has led to our conclusions about group performance. Work group effectiveness research is frequently inconclusive, due in part to problems with generalizability, small sample sizes, as well as the general problems encountered in testing complex multivariate models. Conclusions and recommendations, therefore, are based on empirical research as well as the qualitative and cumulative experiences of managers.

Team Performance

What do we really mean when we talk about team performance? We distinguish between performance from *process* factors, such as team member satisfaction and the efficiency with which decisions are made (which may or may not be related to performance), and performance *outcomes.* We do not view such group process factors as ends in themselves, but as intermediate steps on the way toward effective group performance. This view is consistent with Hackman's (1982) perspective that team effectiveness should be viewed from three dimensions. First is the degree to which the group's productive output meets the standards of quantity, quality, and timeliness. Second is the degree to which the process of carrying out the work enhances the capability of members to work independently in the future. The third dimension is the degree to which the team experience contributes to the growth and personal well-being of team members. Thus, one can think about effectiveness on various interrelated levels. One level is related to the quality of team output and the efficiency with which these outputs are produced. The following types of questions represent quality indicators of performance:

- Does the cardiac surgery team produce successful surgeries?
- How much funding does the research center generate?
- How quickly is an operating room prepared for the next surgical procedure?
- Do self-managing nursing units have a positive impact on patient postdischarge outcomes?
- What is the level of satisfaction among patients seen by a physician group practice? On another level, we can think about member attitudes and satisfaction as a measure of performance.
- To what extent are members satisfied with the manner in which a team operates?
- Do team members feel the team is effective?
- Do team members trust each other?

We sometimes presume a positive relationship between these attitudinal measures and team performance, but this need not always be the case. For example, in a classic study that examined the relationship between group cohesiveness (a process measure) and productivity (an outcome measure), it was found that group cohesiveness is as often related to *low* produc-

tivity as to high productivity (Seashore, 1954). Similarly, researchers found that worker participation in decision making (again, a process measure) on teams improved satisfaction, but not productivity (Locke & Schweiger, 1979), while others concluded that participation had a positive but small relationship with performance (Wagner, 1994). Thus, team effectiveness is often confused with "good" group processes, such as communication, morale, and cohesiveness. In evaluating the work of a team, it is important to remember that the link between "process" and "outcome" is weak or poorly understood; however, a multidimensional perspective, in which both process and outcome measures are used, is recommended to obtain a comprehensive view of team performance.

As is the case with organizations as a whole, there is no universal way to define team effectiveness. Depending on the purposes of the team, effectiveness can be defined in a number of ways. A team can be assessed by measuring its **team productivity** or efficiency, which is essentially the amount of work produced with a given set of resources, such as time, people, money, and expertise. Steiner (1972) includes group process in the definition of productivity by defining group productivity as a group's *potential* productivity minus losses due to faulty group processes. Another method of assessing team effectiveness is suggested by the sociotechnical approach, which defines effective groups as those that not only fulfill the task requirements imposed on them by the organization but also the *social* needs and goals of group members (Cummings, 1978; Guzzo, 1990; Trist, 1981).

Assessing the *quality* of a team's work is even more difficult than assessing productivity. Shea and Guzzo (1987) suggest that effectiveness should be defined situationally; a team is effective to the extent that it fulfills its mission. Like an organization, a team can be *effective* in achieving its mission, but may do so in a highly inefficient manner. Sometimes, of course, efficiency and quality are inseparable. A strategic planning team may eventually produce a well-developed plan, but may take so long to complete the process that it is no longer relevant or useful to the organization. Alternatively, a team can be very efficient in its work, but produce ineffective decisions. In other situations, a team may be highly productive, but alienate members in the process and perhaps reduce its productivity in the future. Thus, group member satisfaction can have a substantial impact on current and future group functioning. When we consider team effectiveness, therefore, we usually consider (1) productivity; (2) quality of work; (3) team member satisfaction; and (4) the capacity of the group for continued cooperation (Nadler, Hackman, & Lawler, 1979).

TEAM CHARACTERISTICS

Teams are more than a collection of individuals. Every team has certain characteristics that influence and determine the way members interact with each other. These characteristics include team composition and size, status differences, team norms, member roles, team roles, and team cohesiveness. The manner in which these are understood and managed will affect the performance of a team. Remember that it is just as important to set the team up correctly as to run it correctly.

Team Composition and Size

Team membership is an important factor in understanding group performance. For certain types of teams, it is easier to control the membership of the group than in others. The CEO of a hospital can select from a wide variety of employees to sit on a strategic planning task force, while the director of nursing may be highly constrained in the nurses chosen for a self-managed nursing team in the pediatric oncology unit. In the latter situation, the director of nursing is limited by the pool of nurses in the unit or trained in such a specialty area. However, an awareness of likely problems related to membership helps, at least, to identify potential problems and to develop strategies to manage them. In our examination of **team composition,** we consider the following diagnostic questions (Hackman, 1990b):

- Is the team appropriately staffed? Is the diversity of members appropriate?
- Do members have the expertise required to perform team tasks well?

- Are the members so similar that there is little for them to learn from one another? Or, are they so heterogeneous that they risk having difficulty communicating and coordinating with one another?

Group composition may vary along a number of dimensions such as age, occupation, gender, tenure, abilities, personality, and experience of members and is an important factor affecting team process and effectiveness. Diversity or heterogeneity of membership is likely to affect the way individuals perceive each other in the group and how well they work together. This, in turn, affects team performance. Most research on group composition concludes that overall *heterogeneity* of group members is desirable when the task is complex and has a limited time span (Campion, Medsker, & Higgs, 1993; Nieva, Fleishman, & Rieck, 1978). This is especially true when members are heterogeneous in terms of abilities and experiences (Gist, Locke, & Taylor, 1987). On the other hand, when teams have long life spans, effectiveness may be related more to personal compatibility among members (Sundstrom, DeMeuse, & Futrell, 1990). Although diversity brings many advantages, it also comes with problems, such as an increase in conflict and a loss of cohesiveness (Bettenhausen, 1991). Researchers, finding a negative relationship between diversity and performance in new product development teams, suggest that group heterogeneity might prevent social integration and cohesion from occurring (Ancona & Caldwell, 1992b). As a result, conflict begins in the initial stages of group formation and affects performance throughout the team's existence.

Tenure diversity (i.e., the length of time members have been on the team) can be detrimental to member relations and team performance as well (Owens, Mannic, & Neale, 1998). New members coming into an already functioning team have to be socialized by the remaining members, taking valuable time away from the task at hand (Dyer, 1984; Moreland & Levine, 1988). Although continuity of staffing is important, boundaries of some groups are, by necessity, more permeable than others. For example, teams like the one described in "In the Real World" include parents and at-risk youth depending on the needs of the client or the team (Burchard, Burchard, Sewell, & VanDenBerg, 1993). Often, hospital teams include different physicians and nurses corresponding to the needs of the patients at certain points in their treatment and recovery. Having a clear mission and set of task priorities will decrease many problems associated with tenure diversity (Shaw, 1990), while the use of core and peripheral members and full-time and part-time members will increase team continuity and stabilize the process (Ancona & Caldwell, 1998; Walsh & Hewitt, 1996). Furthermore, the diversity liability can be alleviated to some extent if members have previous experience working in groups or have been given training in team-building techniques (Dailey, Young, & Barr, 1991; Horak, Guarino, Knight, & Kweder, 1991; Stoner & Hartman, 1993; Thyen, Theis, & Tebbitt, 1993). Katzenbach and Smith (1993) point out that successful teams don't just happen, but become effective when members have certain skills that permit them to function positively in a group situation. Training and previous group experience, especially if members have worked together before, provide these skills and reduce the potential for conflict.

Given the multidisciplinary nature of health care, heterogeneous groups are very common in health services organizations, and they present unique management challenges. Oncology treatment teams, for example, may include a variety of physician specialists (e.g., medical oncologists, radiation oncologists, surgical oncologists, pediatric oncologists, pathologists, surgeons, psychiatrists, hematologists, gynecologists, radiologists), physicists, nurses, social workers, psychologists, pharmacists, and nutritionists (Fried & Nelson, 1987). While these types of teams tend to be fluid (i.e., not all team members will be involved in all cases), the multidisciplinary nature of the team raises many questions about leadership, status differences, and the manner in which decisions are made. For example, a nurse who is present at all meetings may be the *formal* leader, but in all likelihood decisional power will reside with the physician most directly involved in treating the patient, even if he or she is an intern or resident. Thus, the role of formal leader may be reduced to that of coordinator rather than decision maker. We address these problems later in this section.

Perhaps no other aspect of group and organizational functioning has been studied as much as **team size.** In general, it is believed that size has a U-shaped relation to effectiveness so that too few or too many members reduce performance (Cohen & Bailey, 1997). As teams become larger, communication and coordination problems tend to increase, while cohesiveness decreases (McGrath, 1984); however, teams have to be large enough to accomplish the task assigned. In other words, groups need to be staffed to the smallest number to accomplish the work (Hackman, 1987). There is some indication that the U-shaped relationship may not hold for all situations or types of teams. In treatment teams, in which boundaries may be permeable, performance is negatively affected by size (Alexander, Jinnett, D'Aunno, & Ullman, 1996; Vinokur-Kaplan, 1995b). Probably, smaller groups are less cumbersome, having fewer social distractions. Smaller teams also have lower incidences of **behavioral masking,** known as "free riding" or "social loafing" (Fleishman, 1980; Jones, 1984). Individuals in large teams are able to maintain a sense of anonymity and gain from the work of the group without making a suitable contribution.

More often than not, team size is out of the control of the manager, particularly when democratic representational norms pervade an organization. In these situations, constituencies may demand to be represented, and the leader may need to design strategies to make the group more manageable (e.g., forming subcommittees). Otherwise, teams may be *overstaffed.* Overstaffed teams may tend to perform work in a perfunctory, lackadaisical manner. Large size may also lead to competition and jealousy among group members, with individuals guarding their particular domain. Some members may remain aloof from the team's efforts and be less willing to help others improve their performance (Wicker, 1979). On the other hand, breaking a team into subgroups (e.g., subcommittees) has its own set of problems. When large teams are divided into smaller ones, each subgroup may become cliquish, and while cohesive within themselves, they may become isolated from the rest of the team (Festinger, Schacter, & Back, 1950).

Although the empirical evidence on the relationship between the characteristics—team composition and size—and effectiveness is less than definitive, it still provides information that can be valuable in managing teams. It may be useful to keep in mind the potential problems and benefits that may emerge as a result of group size and diversity. On one hand, managers may have control over composition and size; conversely, they may not. In the former situation, the decision maker will want to consider the type of task and resources available for training before determining the size and heterogeneity of the team. In the latter, managers have many strategies and interventions to choose from that can help increase team's effectiveness.

Status Differences

Status is the measure of worth conferred on an individual by a group. **Status differences** are seen throughout organizations, and serve many useful purposes. Differences in status motivate people, provide them with a means of identification, and may be a force for stability in the organization (Scott, 1967). In teams, status differences can be a source of difficulty. Many groups develop democratic norms that may run counter to the formal or informal status of individual group members. Within a hospital, a physician may be very powerful. Within a CQI team, the same physician is expected to serve as an equal in analyzing problems and recommending solutions. This discrepancy between outside status and inside status may make management of these groups difficult.

Status differences have a profound effect on the functioning of multidisciplinary teams. Research findings are fairly consistent in showing that high-status members initiate communication more often, are provided more opportunities to participate, and have more influence over the decision-making process (Owens, Mannic, & Neale, 1998). Thus, an individual from a lower-status professional group may be intimidated or ignored by higher-status team members. The group, as a result, may not benefit from this person's expertise. This situation is very likely in health care, where status differences among the professions are well entrenched. Often, multidisciplinary teams are idealistically expected to operate as a company of equals, yet the reality of the situation makes this impossible. In a study of end-stage renal disease

teams, while the equal participation ideology was accepted by most team participants, it was clear that the physicians, who had higher professional status than other groups, had greater involvement in the actual decision-making process (Deber & Leatt, 1986). The mismatch between expectations and reality made many team members, particularly staff nurses, feel a sense of role deprivation, with accompanying implications for morale and job satisfaction.

If status inequality exists, it is advisable to build a trust-sensitive environment in which members can disagree with the leader and others on the team without repercussions. Often, CQI teams use training along with nonmember facilitators early in the team development process to cope with the problems brought about by status differences (LaPenta & Jacobs, 1996). In well-managed multidisciplinary groups, lower-status individuals should feel elevated by being part of such high-profile, effective teams.

Team Norms

A norm is defined as a standard that is shared by team members and regulates member behavior. **Behavior norms** are rules that standardize how people act at work on a day-to-day basis, while **performance norms** are rules that standardize employee output. Behavioral norms in teams are far reaching and may vary substantially from one group to another in the same organization. Norms may govern how much participation is required by each individual, how humor is to be used, the use of formal group procedures (e.g., Robert's Rules of Order), and rules related to absence and lateness. In their study of operating room nurses, Denison and Sutton (1990) describe their surprise at the behavioral norms present in the operating room:

> At first we were surprised by the norms of emotional expression in the operating rooms. The first time we entered the room where a coronary bypass operation was being done, for example, we were surprised by the loud rock music blaring from the speakers, the smiles on the faces of the surgical team, and the constant joking. Denison observed one surgeon who joked and told a series of funny

stories as he performed the complicated task of cutting the veins out of a patient's leg—veins that would be used to bypass clogged coronary arteries. Similarly, one reason that Sutton almost passed out during a tonsillectomy was that he became very upset when the surgeon laughed, joked, and talked about "what was on the tube last night" while blood from an unconscious child splattered about.

Performance norms, on the other hand, govern the amount and quality of work required of individuals, as well as the amount of time they are expected to work. Some performance norms require that workers not work *too hard* so that standards for the group as a whole are kept at a given level. Mullen and Baumeister (1987) use the term *diving* to describe situations in which norms play an important role in motivating individual team members to perform at less-than-optimum levels. One example of diving results from a team norm that discourages excellence in performance by any team member. Group members socialize other members as to the norm and will punish if violated (Cannon-Bowers, Oser, & Flanagan, 1992). Thus, "rate busters" would be subject to serious sanctions by the other team members. Researchers, in fact, have documented the practice of "pinging," which involved a periodical punch on the suspected rate buster's arm until he or she reduced the level of effort (Roethlisberger & Dickson, 1939).

Norms are powerful influences in organizations and teams, and the existence of norms is necessary for effective group functioning. Hackman (1976) suggests that norms have the following characteristics:

1. Norms summarize and simplify team influence processes. They denote the processes by which teams regulate member behavior.
2. Norms apply only to behavior, not to private thoughts and feelings. Private acceptance of norms is *not necessary*, only public compliance is required.
3. Norms are generally developed only for behaviors that are viewed as important by most team members.
4. Norms usually develop gradually, but members can quicken the process. Norms usually are developed by team members when the occasion arises,

such as when a situation occurs that requires new ground rules for members in order to protect team integrity.
5. All norms do not apply to all team members. Some norms apply only to newer members, while others may be applied to individuals based on seniority, sex, race, economic status, or profession.

Because of the significance of norms in effective group functioning, it is important to clarify norms publicly so members will know what is expected. This is especially the case for multidisciplinary teams in hospitals and other health care settings. If acceptable norms are established as part of the group process, there is less chance of a so-called interdisciplinary team functioning as cross-disciplinary, with one discipline dominating (Vinokur-Kaplan, 1995a).

Member Roles

To function effectively, teams differentiate the work activities of their members. This specialization of work activities is called **role differentiation.** Individuals assume both formal and informal roles in teams. Formal roles include that of leader as well as specific task-oriented functions, such as chairs and participants of subcommittees. However, individuals also assume informal roles that may positively or negatively affect work group productivity and effectiveness. A team leader should be cognizant of the existence of these roles and how they are carried out in the group setting. Benne and Sheats (1948) provide a clear distinction among these informal roles, distinguishing among **task-oriented roles,** which help accomplish team goals; **building and maintenance roles,** which help establish and maintain good relationships among team members; and (3) **personal roles,** or self-centered roles, which serve to satisfy individual needs unrelated to the team's goals or its maintenance (see Table 6.1).

Several points are in order with respect to these roles. First, members may simultaneously assume several roles in a particular group setting. Second, individual roles are not static; depending upon the team, an individual may assume different roles. Roles may even vary from one meeting of a team to another.

Table 6.1. Functional Roles of Group Members.

Category	Role Name	Description
Task-oriented roles are behaviors directed towards accomplishing the group's objectives, primarily through contributing to the problem-solving process.	Initiator	Proposes tasks, goals, or actions; defines group problems; and suggests work procedures.
	Informer	Offers facts, gives expression of feeling, gives opinions.
	Information seeker	Asks for opinions, facts, or interpretations.
	Clarifier	Interprets ideas or suggestions; defines terms; clarifies issues before the group.
	Summarizer/coordinator	Pulls together related ideas; restates suggestions; offers a decision or conclusion for group to consider.
	Reality tester	Makes a critical analysis of an idea; tests an idea against some data to see if the idea will work.
	Procedural technician	Records suggestions; distributes materials.
	Energizer	Attempts to increase the quality and quantity of task behavior.
	Elaborator	Expands on suggestions; offers examples; restates positions; offers rationales.
	Consensus tester	Asks to see if a group is nearing a decision; sends up a trial balloon to test a possible conclusion.
Building and maintenance roles are social-emotional behaviors aimed at helping the interpersonal functioning of group. Like the maintenance required to keep a car in good running condition, these behaviors are necessary to keep group members feeling good about the group and interacting effectively with one another.	Harmonizer	Attempts to reconcile disagreements; reduces tension; gets people to explore differences.
	Gatekeeper	Helps keep communication channels open; facilitates participation of others; suggests procedures that permit sharing remarks.
	Encourager	Friendly, warm, and responsive to others; indicates by facial expression or remark the acceptance of others' contributions.

(continues)

Table 6.1. *(Continued)*

Category	Role Name	Description
	Compromiser	When his/her own idea or status is involved in a conflict, offers a compromise that yields status; admits error; modifies an interest of group cohesion or growth.
	Observer/commentator	Comments on and interprets group's internal process.
	Follower	Serves as audience; passively goes along with ideas of others.
Personal roles are intended to satisfy individual needs rather than contribute to goals or maintenance of group. Although some personal-role behaviors do contribute to group's effectiveness, roles characteristic of this category are irrelevant to goals of group and not conducive to its functioning.	Aggressor	Deflates others' status; attacks the group or its values; jokes in a barbed or semiconcealed way.
	Blocker	Disagrees and opposes beyond reason; resists stubbornly the group's wishes for personal reasons; uses hidden agenda to thwart movement of group.
	Dominator	Asserts authority/superiority to manipulate group or certain group members; interrupts contributions of others; controls by means of flattery or other forms of patronizing behavior.
	Prince/princess	Makes a display of his/her lack of involvement; "abandons" the group while remaining with it physically: seeks recognition in ways not relevant to group task.
	Evader	Pursues special interests not related to tasks; stays off subject to avoid commitment; prevents group from facing up to controversy.
	Help seeker	Uses group to gain sympathy and solve personal problems unrelated to group's goal.
	Recognition seeker	Calls attention to self by boasting and referring to personal achievements; acts in appropriate ways to gain attention.
	Special-interest pleader	Speaks on behalf of represented group (e.g., "labor," "minorities," "management") in order to cloak own prejudices or biases in a stereotype that fits own personal needs rather than goals of the current group.

SOURCE: Adapted from: Benne, K., & Sheats, P. "Functional roles of group members." *Journal of Social Issues* 2, 42–47, 1948.

Finally, emphasis should be placed on the fact that these are informal roles that are not easily changed. Often, individuals assume roles because of their informal power within an organization. For example, a physician who dominates a strategic planning team may assume this role as a result of his or her status and power outside the group.

Team Roles

Many teams fail to achieve their mission simply because their roles were not clearly established. The output expected of a team may not be clear, which may lead to misunderstood expectations and decreased member morale and motivation. Similarly, the power or influence of a team may be misunderstood. A CQI team, for example, may assume that its recommendations will be fully implemented when in fact they are only advisory. This, too, can deflate the enthusiasm of team members. Managers can decrease the likelihood of these problems by clarifying the purpose of the team, the role of the team within the larger organization, and the authority of the team.

Team Cohesiveness

There are a variety of definitions for **team cohesiveness,** many of which focus on the degree to which members of a group are *attracted* to other members and, thereby, are motivated to stay in the group. Another, more narrow definition that may better fit the purpose of this chapter is used by Goodman, Ravlin, and Schminke (1987): "cohesiveness is the extent that members are committed to the group task." In this definition, the focus is on the decision to produce, and it acknowledges that members can be committed to a common task but not necessarily be attracted to each other. This is a much more realistic view of cohesiveness since we are concerned with managing teams in which members, like nurses, physicians, psychologists, and social workers, to name a few, are already highly committed to professional standards.

Cohesion is considered one of the most important components in understanding group process and effectiveness. Highly cohesive teams have higher performance, improved satisfaction, and lower levels of turnover (Bettenhausen, 1991; Gully, Devine, & Whitney, 1995). Moreover, the relationship between cohesion and effectiveness is stronger when the task requires coordination, communication, and mutual performance (Cannon-Bowers, Oser, & Flanagan, 1992). Specifically, research focusing on treatment teams in psychiatric hospitals, engaged in highly interdependent work, found that cohesive teams had higher performance levels than less cohesive ones (Vinokur-Kaplan, 1995a). Greater interdisciplinary collaboration between the team members was one of the principle reasons for this. Cohesiveness can also promote better enforcement of group norms and general control over group members; however, taken to extremes, this can lead to groupthink-like situations of undue conformity. For instance, there are circumstances under which high levels of cohesiveness can lead to *lower* levels of productivity. If a group's norms favor low productivity, then having a highly cohesive group will likely lead to high levels of conformity to the norm and, hence, lower not higher productivity. Similarly, a highly cohesive group may work against a manager's efforts to involve new members in a group, or to have the group interact with other groups. Cohesiveness, therefore, should be viewed in context. In most situations, it is a positive force, while in others, it can lead to conformity to counterproductive norms and practices (McGrath, 1984).

What are the sources of cohesiveness? A central tenet of social psychological theory is that individuals are attracted to others who are similar to them; therefore, homogeneous groups should be more cohesive than heterogeneous ones. Teams composed of all females, for instance, tend to be more cohesive than all-male and mixed sex groups (Bettenhausen, 1991). The lack of conflict and the presence of trust among members lead to increased cohesiveness as well (Bettenhausen, 1991; Pinto & Pinton, 1990). To complicate matters, some research suggests that conflict may be beneficial to group performance, particularly when a group is dealing with complex problem-solving tasks (Cosier, 1981; Janis, 1972; Schwenk, 1983). In this sense, multidisciplinary groups and groups composed of culturally diverse individuals, while likely to exhibit higher levels of conflict and less cohesiveness, may also be more creative and innovative in their approach to problem solving (Jackson, 1992).

Additionally, cohesiveness is influenced by the goal orientation or reward structure of the team. Let's consider two conditions. First is the situation of goal interdependence in which members are evaluated and rewarded (i.e., equal reward structure) as a group. Here, progress to each member's professional/personal goals is the same as progress to the group goals. Conversely, the second condition is one in which group members are judged and rewarded (i.e., unequal reward structure) as individuals. In essence, one member reaches his or her goal at the expense of another member. In general, the findings support the first or cooperative condition (Deutsch, 1949; Pennings, 1975; Sundstrom, DeMeuse, & Futrell, 1990). Team members in the second situation are more likely to be highly competitive, leading to lower cohesiveness due to (Deutsch, 1949):

1. Less intermember influence and acceptance of other's ideas,
2. Greater difficulty in communication and understanding, and
3. Less coordination effort, less division of labor, and less productivity.

Following from this, cohesive groups tend to have levels of interaction that are greater and more positive (Shaw, 1990). This is strengthened by conditions of high interdependency (Gully et al., 1995). That is, groups that have equal reward structures not only perform more efficiently, but also develop cooperative strategies such as teamwork and pooling of information that facilitate achievement of jointly shared goals (Okun & DiVesta, 1975).

TEAM PROCESSES

One of the most dominant views of groups historically has been the input-process-output perspective (McGrath, 1984). Many of the elements that have been discussed in the above section are group inputs. Process describes those things that go on *in* the team that affect performance. Specifically, it refers to the methods of interacting and performing work that emerge over the stages of team development and includes all interpersonal and intrapersonal actions by team members in the transformation of inputs into outputs. We include here issues related to the processes of leadership, communication, decision making, and stages of group development.

Leadership

Leadership in groups refers to the ability of individuals to influence other members toward the achievement of the team's goals. Because of its importance in determining team performance, leadership has been studied extensively using many different leadership styles. In one study, leadership in intensive care units (ICUs) was positively related to efficiency of operation, satisfaction, and lower turnover of nurses (Shortell, Zimmerman, Rousseau et al., 1994). Successful leaders adopted a supportive **formal** or **informal leadership** style, emphasizing standards of excellence, encouraging interaction, communicating clear goals and expectations, responding to changing needs, and providing support resources when possible.

There are times when teams have multiple leaders. There may be a formal leader as well as several informal ones. Examples of formal leaders are head nurses, department managers, and project committee chairs. Formal leaders have legitimate authority over the team (that is, the organization has granted these individuals power along with some ability to use formal rewards and sanctions to support that authority). The formal leader, of course, may not be the most *influential* person on the team. The extent to which team members will accept the formal leader's wishes is, in large part, determined by the reaction of the informal leader(s) to those wishes. Note that there is a difference between ad hoc groups, such as parallel and project teams, and formal work teams. In a parallel or project team, an informal leader may be selected as the group's formal leader. This is the rationale for appointing high-profile individuals to chair significant CQI teams or to serve as "honorary chairs" of important search committees. In work teams, however, there is no opportunity for choice. It may be that the formal leader is not the person on whom the teams depend, but it is the "informal leader who embodies the values of the group, aids it in accomplishing objectives, facilitates group maintenance, and usually serves as team spokesperson" (Hunsaker & Cook, 1986).

In deciding upon a leadership style, therefore, group leaders need to consider in realistic terms their formal and informal authority within the group. Use of a coercive or forceful style may backfire when the individual does not have the power to back up decisions. Such a leader may find that the informal leader is able to veto, modify, or sabotage demands. Webster et al. (1998), using case-management teams, found that "powerless leaders" were faced with the formation of cliques and competition from more influential members. It is best, therefore, for the formal leader not only to consider the views of informal leaders, but also to collaborate with them if possible. Related issues of leadership are discussed further in Chapter 4.

Communication Structure

A group cannot function effectively as a team unless members can exchange information. It is incumbent upon team leaders to manage communications within a team and between the team and external groups. Consider the case of a nurse in a neonatal intensive care unit who has just met with a patient's physician and must pass on vital information to the nurse on the next shift as well as the parents who will visit during the next shift. How does information get conveyed? Without a viable **communication structure,** important information may be lost or inaccurately communicated. In fact, the evaluation and design of communication structures are important components of many quality improvement projects.

Communication speed and accuracy in a team are influenced both by the nature of the group's communication network and by the complexity of the group's task. When a task is simple and communication networks are centralized (e.g., a wheel and spoke structure), both speed and accuracy are higher. When tasks are relatively complex, centralized communication networks lower both speed and accuracy, because people serving as network hubs (i.e., information disseminators) may suffer from information overload. In this situation, communication networks are best decentralized (e.g., a starlike structure), relieving a manager from the need to filter (and possibly distort) information before it is passed on. In the

example of the neonatal intensive care unit, it would be highly undesirable for the nurse at the earlier shift to first communicate the needed information to a head nurse and then have that individual pass it on to the next shift's nurse. Notwithstanding the need for the head nurse to have the information, timeliness and accuracy are likely to suffer if the information must first pass through the head nurse en route to the ICU nurse. It is obviously much more desirable to build a communication structure that encourages direct interaction between nurses on sequential shifts.

Although most of the focus in teams is on internal communications, those relationships maintained externally are significant determinants of performance as well, especially for ongoing teams (Gladstein, 1984). Nadler and Tushman's (1988) research found that successful groups matched information-processing capacity to the information-processing demands of the task environment. This points to the need for boundary-spanning activities and members to act in those roles. New product/technology teams, for example, use a diverse array of members—researchers from the marketing department, physicians from the medical staff, and administrators from the top management team—to serve in boundary-spanning roles. However, it is just not the amount of the external communication but also the type of communication activities that occur between a team and its outside boundaries. Ancona and Caldwell (1992a) use the following classification:

- Ambassador activities—Members carrying out these activities communicate frequently with those above them in the hierarchy. This set of activities is used to protect the team from outside pressures, to persuade others to support the team, and to lobby for resources.
- Task-coordinator activities—Members carrying out these activities communicate frequently with other groups and persons at lateral levels in the organization. These activities include discussing problems with others, obtaining feedback, and coordinating and negotiating with outsiders.
- Scout activities—Members carrying out these activities are involved in general scanning for ideas

and information about the external environment. These differ from the other two in that these activities relate to general scanning instead of specific coordination issues.

Generally, effective teams engage in high levels of ambassadorial and task-coordinator activities and low levels of prolonged scouting activities. The isolationist teams, neglecting external activity altogether, tend to do quite poorly, probably because they are out of touch with the environment within which they are embedded. The increasing reliance on teams and the expanding responsibilities placed on them require strong communication networks both within the team and between the team and other groups outside the boundaries.

Decision Making and Groupthink

Two aspects of team decision making are worthy of consideration by managers: the distinction between **decision making** and problem solving, and the processes by which decision-making groups make decisions.

Most teams are at some point involved in making decisions. However, not all team members are involved in actually making all decisions. For a particular decision, a hospital president may ask for the opinions of his or her senior management team, but retain the right to make the final decision. Similarly, a physician may obtain input from a variety of professionals, but make the final determination on treatment. Managers can decrease the probability of misunderstandings by clarifying the role of the team and the role of each member. Team members can generally deal with limitations on their influence as long as the boundaries of their influence are clear initially. Group leaders also need to clarify the difference between problem solving and decision making. Some groups, such as many CQI teams, are established to solve problems, or seek methods for improving a particular organizational process. They may not be given authority to implement decisions, however, particularly when substantial resources are required.

The second area of decision making regards the process by which information is exchanged and decisions made. Teams naturally attempt to make correct decisions, applying all available information to the problem at hand. One common problem that prevents complete sharing of information among members of a team is that of the "free rider." The term "free rider" refers to a member of a team who obtains the benefits of group membership but does not accept a proportional share of the costs of membership. "Cheap rider" (Stigler, 1974) is a more accurate term for such a team member because receiving benefits from group membership typically involves some minimal cost. Free rider, however, is the more generally used term (Albanese & Van Fleet, 1985). The free rider is seen as someone who promotes self-interest (the personal acquisition of benefits) over the public interest (the need to contribute to the activity that produces those benefits). It is often observed that the larger the group, the greater the free rider effect (Roberts & Hunt, 1991).

What can managers do to minimize free riding? Albanese and Van Fleet (1985) offer the following suggestions:

> Through effective use of power, design of organizations (including the size of the organizational units), and control of access to rewards and punishment, management influences the incentive system of group members. At a routine level, this influence may be achieved by offering financial incentives or special forms of recognition to particular group members.

In the longer run, it is also important for managers to deal with the free rider problem by attempting to broaden the individual's concept of self-interest and by creating, communicating, and maintaining a group culture that values effort expended on team processes.

Another problem that affects the decision-making process and may inhibit the effective use of information is polarization. When groups become highly cohesive over an issue, polarization occurs. There are two commonly accepted explanations for polarization (Cartwright & Zander, 1968). The social comparison explanation argues that as individuals compare their position on a matter with those of others on the team, pressures emerge toward accepting one position or another as the team position. In the persuasive argument explanation, it is argued that teams coalesce around a more forcefully argued alternative when initial discussion reveals no clearly favored argument.

Managers should be aware that team polarization does take place and that it often leads to a phenomenon known as **groupthink** (Janis, 1972). The concept emerged from Janis's studies of high-level policy decisions by government leaders including decisions about Vietnam, the Bay of Pigs, and the Korean War.

Groupthink occurs whenever the desire for harmony and consensus overrides members' efforts to appraise group judgments realistically. In other words, groupthink occurs when maintaining the pleasant atmosphere of the team becomes more important to members than coming up with good decisions. Signs that groupthink may be present include (Janis, 1972):

1. *The illusion of invulnerability.* Team members may reassure themselves about obvious dangers and become overly optimistic and willing to take extraordinary risks.
2. *Collective rationalization.* Victims of groupthink may overlook blind spots in their plans. When confronted with conflicting information, team members may spend considerable time and energy refuting the information and rationalizing a decision.
3. *Belief in the inherent morality of the team.* Highly cohesive teams may develop a sense of self-righteousness about their role and make them insensitive to the consequences of decisions.
4. *Stereotyping others.* Victims of groupthink hold biased, highly negative views of competing teams. They assume that they are unable to negotiate with other teams, and rule out compromise.
5. *Pressures to conform.* Group members face severe pressures to conform to team norms and to team decisions. Dissent is considered abnormal and may lead to formal or informal punishment.
6. *The use of mindguards.* Mindguards are members who protect the team from dissonant information that might interfere with the team's view of a problem. They may withhold or discount contrary information.
7. *Self-censorship.* Teams subject to groupthink pressure members to remain silent about possible misgivings and to minimize self-doubts about a decision.
8. *Illusion of unanimity.* A sense of unanimity emerges when members assume that silence and lack of protest signify agreement and consensus.

The consequences of groupthink are clear. Teams may limit themselves, often prematurely, to one or two possible solutions and fail to conduct a comprehensive analysis of a problem. When groupthink is well entrenched, members may fail to review their decisions in light of new information or changing events. The team becomes blinded to new information. Teams may also fail to consult adequately with experts within or outside the organization, and fail to develop contingency plans in the event that the decision turns out to be wrong.

Team leaders can avoid groupthink through a number of strategies. First, leaders can reduce groupthink by encouraging members to critically evaluate proposals and solutions. Where a leader is particularly powerful and influential (yet still wants to get unbiased views from team members), the leader may refrain from stating his or her own position until later in the decision-making process. Another strategy is to assign the same problem to two separate work teams. Most importantly, groupthink can be avoided by establishing norms of *critical appraisal* of ideas and solutions, and understanding the warning signs of groupthink. Managers might also consider alternative systematic methods of decision making that emphasize member participation. **Nominal group technique** and **Delphi technique** (Dalkey, 1969) elicit group members' opinions prior to judgments about those opinions. Through these and other approaches, help generate ideas, and facilitate objective debate (Delberg et al., 1975).

Stages of Group Development

Even though individuals may be designated as a team, they may remain independent of one another and never truly become a team. Thus, a key challenge is determining how to effectively build a team. To do this requires an understanding of the stages of team development and what opportunities and threats exist during each one. Recall the case at the beginning of this chapter when Tom, the Youth Initiative Coordinator, was anticipating the first meeting of Anthony's Core Services Team. It is important that Tom know that groups go through **stages of team development,** and that each stage is characterized by different group behaviors.

Although it is not possible to predict with certainty how a team will proceed through its various stages, the following sequence of development has been found to occur with striking similarity in many groups (Tuckman, 1965; Whetten & Cameron, 1998):

1. *Forming.* During the first stage of team development, members become acquainted with each other, the team purpose, and its boundaries. Members attempt to discover those behaviors that are acceptable and unacceptable, while trust and relationships are established. This early stage is characterized by polite interactions, frequent silence, and tentative interactions. Clarity of direction is needed from the team leader.

2. *Storming.* At this stage, the team is faced with disagreement, counterindependence, and the need to manage conflict. Members may attempt to influence the development of group norms, roles, and procedures; therefore, the stage has high potential for conflict and risk of groupthink. Team leaders need to focus on process improvements, recognizing team achievement, and fostering win/win relationships as much as possible.

3. *Norming.* During this stage, the team grows more cohesive and unified. There emerges agreement on rules and processes of decision making, roles and expectations of members, and commitment of members. Leaders need to provide supportive feedback and foster commitment to a vision or direction for the team.

4. *Performing.* Once team members agree on the purpose and norms of the group, they are able to move forward to the task of defining separate roles and establishing work plans. The team is faced with the need for continuous improvement, innovation, and speed. Leaders must be ready to sponsor new ideas, orchestrate their implementation, and foster extraordinary performance from members.

5. *Adjourning.* For temporary teams, the adjournment stage is characterized by a sense of task accomplishment, regret, and increased emotionality.

Several points are in order about these stages. First, not all teams pass through all stages. Some teams may begin at a norming or performing stage (e.g., members that have worked together before), while some may never move beyond the conflictual storming stage. Moreover, teams may not move in a linear fashion through the stages, but more like a "punctuated equilibrium" model (Gersick, 1989). Teams that follow this model exhibit long stable periods in which little occurs interspersed with relatively brief periods of drastic progress. Second, teams can revert to earlier stages of development. Regression can occur as a result of new tasks or responsibilities given the team, a change in formal or informal leadership, the addition of a new member, or the loss of a valuable member. Managers should consider the stage of team development in establishing expectations for the group.

NATURE OF THE TASK

One of the underlying themes throughout the research on teams and groups is the notion that group tasks can be classified according to their "critical demands" (Roby & Lanzetta, 1958) (that is, certain features of a task dictate the specific group behaviors critical to successful performance). These specific behaviors include not only individual effort but also cooperative and interdependent endeavors. This means that effective performance is a function of matching the team process to the task demands. In this section, we identify and discuss some of the critical demands—design characteristics, task complexity, diversity and clarity, and task interdependence.

Design Characteristics

Tasks can be distinguished using Hackman and Oldham's (1980) job design characteristics: autonomy, feedback, task significance, identity, and skill variety. These have been related to team commitment, satisfaction, and performance (Campion et al., 1993; Cohen & Bailey, 1997). One characteristic in this theme is self-management, which is analogous to group-level autonomy and is central in many definitions of work groups today. Self-management should enhance team performance since it increases members' sense of responsibility and ownership of the work. Member autonomy has consistently had a positive effect on performance, but the effect is stronger for self-directed work teams than parallel teams (Cohen & Bailey, 1997). Task variety, defined as giving each member the chance to perform a number of tasks, generally motivates team members since they can use different skills, thereby decreasing boredom. If members believe that their work has significant consequences either to the organization or its stakeholders, this should contribute to effectiveness as well. The last task design characteristic, task identity, or the degree to which a team completes a whole and separate piece of work, should also contribute to group motivation and effectiveness since it increases the group's sense of responsibility.

Task Complexity, Diversity, and Clarity

Team tasks can be categorized using several broad, yet related categories, such as task clarity, complexity, and diversity. A task, on one hand, may be fairly simple, requiring few operations and skills, or little knowledge, with a clear goal so that members understand exactly what has to be done. Usually, this is a fairly routine-type job having a single acceptable solution or outcome that is easily identified as correct. On the other hand, a task can be highly complex with goals that are unclear and requiring diverse operations, skills, or knowledge. Also, there may be many acceptable solutions, none of which are easily verifiable. Task clarity was a significant variable in determining performance of hospital treatment teams, allowing them to meet the hospital's standards of quality, quantity, and timeliness (Shaw, 1990; Vinokur-Kaplan, 1995a). Task complexity is related to team interaction (Shaw, 1976) (that is, the more complex the task, the greater the need for interaction, so that it is important that managers plan for enhanced communication among the team members in such situations). Others have found that an increase in task diversity, as defined by the number of different conditions treated within ICUs, challenges caregivers since their expertise and knowledge can be applied across a wider range of conditions, and leads to better outcomes (Shortell et al., 1994).

Task Interdependence

Another form of task diversity focuses on interdependence, which is generally the reason why teams form in the first place. **Task interdependence** refers to the interconnections between tasks, or more specifically, the degree to which team members must rely on one another to perform work effectively. A useful way of classifying this is to use a hierarchy of task interdependence based on exchange of information or resources (Thompson, 1967; Van de Ven, Delbecq, & Koenig, 1976):

Pooled interdependence. A situation in which each member makes a contribution to the group output without the need of interaction among members. Since each group member completes the whole task, team performance is the sum of the individual efforts. Standardized rules and procedures are needed to enhance coordination of team outputs.

Sequential interdependence. A situation in which one group member must act before another one can. Group members have different roles and perform different tasks in some prescribed order with the work flowing in only one direction. There is always an element of potential contingency since readjustment is necessary if any member fails to meet expectations. Coordination using schedules and plans is needed to keep the team on track.

Reciprocal interdependence. A situation in which the outputs of each member become inputs for the others; thereby, each member poses a contingency for the other. Group members often are specialists with different areas of expertise and have structured roles; therefore, they perform different parts of the task in a flexible, "back-and-forth" order. Leaders must provide for open communication between members and scheduled meetings as necessary.

Team interdependence. A situation in which team members diagnose, problem solve, and collaborate as a group while performing work or work-related activities. The workflow is simultaneous and multidirectional. Coordination requires mutual interactions with group autonomy to decide the sequencing of inputs and outputs among members. Leaders should plan frequent meetings, while also encouraging unscheduled ones.

Interdependence, by definition, increases uncertainty; therefore, as the degree of interdependence increases, so does the need for information processing along with the necessity of more coordination, communication, and cooperation. Implicit in this is the need for matching the information-processing requirements with interaction or coordination patterns that facilitate information exchange. If team members perceive low interdependence when high interdependence actually exists, then too little effort will go toward coordination. On the contrary, when interdependence is perceived as higher than it really is, too much effort will be expanded in coordination behavior at the expense of performance. For this reason, interdependence and coordination must be appropriately matched. Some researchers go so far as to suggest that successful teams are the ones that match interdependence in terms of task, goal, and feedback. That is, a successful team would be one in which reciprocal work is matched with group goals and group feedback. Group goals and feedback mean that rewards would be based on the group goal and feedback given on the group's performance as a whole. Conversely, pooled interdependence should be matched with a situation of individual goals and feedback (Salvedra, Earley, & Van Dyne, 1993).

Regardless of task characteristic—complexity, interdependence, and diversity—the important point for the manager to remember is the need to match team task with process and structure. One study, demonstrating this matching, described the reengineering effort in a large urban hospital system that used teams for the purpose of overcoming care delivery problems, particularly fragmentation and discontinuities in delivery (Schweikhart & Smith-Daniels, 1996). Focused teams, or relatively autonomous operating units, were formed by merging multidisciplinary clinicians into patient care units, so that pharmacists, respiratory therapists, nurses, and other caregivers were integrated through shared governance and cross-training. The teams were given high levels of autonomy and accountability, while sharing responsibility for both care production work, execution of patient's care plan, and care-management work, planning, and coordinating the care. In this case, high levels of task complexity and interdependence were matched with a team structure that allowed increased levels of communication and interaction.

THE ENVIRONMENTAL CONTEXT OF TEAMS

Teams do not exist and function in a vacuum. They are constantly affected by pressures and events from outside of the immediate team. In this section, we examine a range of external factors that may affect team performance.

Intergroup Relationships and Conflict

In many situations, effective team performance is dependent upon the team ability to interact with other teams in a positive and productive manner. There are many instances, in fact, where one of the central tasks of a team is to interact with other teams. Consider the myriad of intergroup interactions that need to occur in the merging of two hospitals. Teams may be assembled to deal with staffing issues, technology, finances, architectural concerns, and countless other factors. One could imagine the confusion if each team chose to work without the advice and input of other teams.

What happens when teams *have* to work together? What are the factors responsible for effective and ineffective intergroup relationships? How can intergroup relationships be improved? To begin to address these questions, the importance of intergroup, or lateral, relationships must be emphasized. As health care organizations have moved away from rigid hierarchical structures, and as they have become more specialized, there is increased need for coordination mechanisms. **Intergroup conflict** is *inevitable and unavoidable*. It is virtually impossible for work processes to be designed such that the work of groups meshes perfectly with the work of other groups. When conflicts or disagreements occur among groups, it is important that organizational leaders possess a repertoire of alternative conflict resolution strategies. In the best case, the interfaces among teams require only fine-tuning; in the worst situations, work processes need to be wholly overhauled to achieve functional intergroup relationships. Thus, we focus attention on (1) causes of intergroup conflict, (2) consequences of intergroup conflict, and (3) alternative strategies for resolving intergroup conflict.

Causes of Intergroup Conflict

While intergroup conflict can occasionally result from interpersonal differences or animosities, most conflict emerges because of factors related to the interdependence among work groups. Blake and Mouton (1984) stress that intergroup conflict cannot be addressed in the same manner as conflict between individuals.

> While obviously influenced by a variety of factors, individuals may choose to think or act in a given way simply because they want to or feel a need to. When differences or conflicts arise with another person, then an individual is free to react and to change his or her mind on the basis of new evidence and to give or withhold cooperation in keeping with personal desires.
>
> A group member is not free in the same sense as is an individual acting alone. Rules and standards of behavior—norms—are developed within the group that regulate the behavior of members through sometimes subtle but potent pressures. . . . Members who think or act differently are either punished, persuaded, or rejected. Seeking to solve interface disputes at the group level as though they were personal disputes between two individuals not only disregards these important dynamics but also may create new tensions that may provide short-term solutions and at the same time disrupt internal group cohesion, producing new and more serious problems in the future.

When individuals join a team, they tend to identify very strongly with the team; their reactions to and attitudes toward other teams may become highly biased and at times hostile (Ashforth & Mael, 1989). Thus, conflict between groups cannot usually be addressed at an individual level; one member of a group can rarely resolve an intergroup conflict in a unilateral manner. If intergroup conflict is viewed as resulting from problems in the *interface* between groups, then the analysis of the causes of conflict should examine the nature of intergroup relationships. The literature identifies several factors often seen as related to such conflict:

1. *Interdependence among groups.* For conflict to occur among groups, there is obviously a need for some type of interdependence. Teams that are isolated from each other are unlikely to have the opportunity to interact or to be in conflict. Because health services organizations are known for high levels of interaction, there are greater opportunities for the emergence of conflict.

2. *Group role and task ambiguity.* It is often the case that the roles and responsibilities of groups are unclear. Such lack of clarity may lead to conflict when there is lack of agreement on "who does what." Such is the situation in health services organizations when different groups may "lay claim" to the same patients or procedures. Conflict resolution procedures frequently focus on better articulating group roles and distinguishing between the responsibilities of similar groups.

3. *Intergroup differences in work orientation.* Every group has its own set of norms regarding the manner in which work is accomplished. A strategic planning team, for example, will by its nature have a long-term focus. Disagreements may occur when we attempt to intermingle the work of a strategic planning team with a team whose orientation is more immediate, such as a treatment team.

4. *Intergroup goal incompatibility.* Sometimes groups must work together whose goals are in conflict, or perceived to be in conflict. Such may be the case between groups whose orientation is primarily cost-containment and groups whose orientation is focused more on access concerns.

5. *Differences in group culture.* Each group develops its own unique norms, manner of communication, and values. Collectively, these are often referred to as a team culture. Where cultures are in conflict, effective intergroup relationships may be jeopardized.

6. *Competition for resources.* Groups may have much in common, be oriented toward the same goals, yet still be in conflict because they are competing for the same financial, human, or physical resources. This type of conflict assumes that group survival is of paramount importance. When group survival goals become so important so as to supplant organizational goals, the organization may truly suffer.

The organizational setting also influences the quality of intergroup relations. Organizations that encourage frequent interaction among teams and that have reward systems to encourage such interactions are likely to have relatively low levels of conflict (Nelson, 1989). Taking this perspective, conflict is most likely to occur when two teams are *dependent* upon each other to do their work. Consider the example of a medical group practice that needs to have laboratory results reported in a timely manner. Conflicts can easily result when information transfer procedures are ineffective or otherwise lacking. Cases of such "interface conflict" are pervasive in health care organizations.

Intergroup conflict is also more likely to occur when there is *ambiguity* about groups' respective responsibilities or roles. This situation in large part explains conflicts that occur between professional groups with overlapping practice domains (for example, between psychologists and psychiatrists). Role ambiguity is also common between groups located in different organizations, where there may be a lack of consensus over the domains of different organizations or where there are major differences in program or service philosophies. Finally, task ambiguity may lead to important job duties "falling between the cracks"; each team may be upset with the other for what it perceives to be the other's shortcomings (Arnold & Feldman, 1986). Task ambiguity may also be common in organizations undergoing rapid growth or change. In these situations, the substance or implications of change may be understood differently among different groups. Consider the different types of conflict that occur when an organization is in the midst of a merger process.

A third source of intergroup conflict is related to differences in groups' *work orientation.* In many organizations, teams have different perspectives on *time.* This difference in time orientation was identified and managed when strategic planning was attempted with a group of family physicians (Fried & Nelson, 1987):

> By its nature, the activity of planning is at odds with the role orientation of most physicians. Planning is a long-term process in which the results of strategic decisions appear over time. The outcomes of planning are often intangible in the short term. By contrast, physicians are trained to be action oriented.

It was discovered early in the planning process that physician attendance at meetings decreased when the pace of work lagged. Therefore, whenever possible, the pace of work was increased to a level more acceptable to physicians. A work plan with specific deadlines was followed.

Differences in work orientation may also be reflected in different *goals* among work teams. The finance department of a managed care organization, for example, may have a very different set of priorities from that unit of the organization concerned with quality assurance or quality improvement. Conflicts may emerge as each group works toward different, sometimes conflicting goals.

Differences in *culture* or interpersonal orientation among teams may also lead to conflict. Researchers, for example, may place great value on informality in dealing with colleagues. However, a principal investigator on a large research grant may need to interact with a highly formalized and bureaucratic human resources department to deal with employee issues, such as recruitment, hiring, and compensation. The researcher, accustomed to informality, may resist attempts by the human resources department to engage in formal interviews with job applicants or to write detailed job descriptions. Such conflicts are difficult to resolve unless there is at least recognition of the differences in work orientation as a primary cause of conflict.

Organizations under financial stress are more likely to exhibit intergroup conflict simply because groups may be competing for scarce organizational resources. Groups may find themselves competing for money, use of common support services, or the use of specialized organizational resources. In fact, the movement toward product or program management in hospitals would tend to increase the likelihood of intergroup conflict as product-line teams develop internal competitive thrusts. In such systems, teams may be involved in an incentive system related to team performance. This raises the issue of whether traditional modes of compensation that reward *individuals* and not *teams* are appropriate in the team-centered environment. Where teams compete with each other for scarce resources, a program manager must be able to compete with other programs and at times defend the relevance of the program. This type of competition may be healthy, but could also lead to dysfunctional intergroup conflict and inattention to broad organizational goals.

In sum, we would expect intergroup conflict to increase because of resource scarcity in the health care field. Organizational responses to resource scarcity will likely exacerbate tensions between teams.

Consequences of Intergroup Conflict

Through the years, researchers have observed the changes that occur within groups when faced with conflict with other groups (see Sherif & Sherif, 1953, for a classic study of these changes). Most important, when groups are faced with external threats, there is almost always a sense of increased team cohesiveness (Davis, 1964). Loyalty to the team becomes more important, and there is increased emphasis given to the accomplishment of group tasks. Members tend to be less concerned with individual need satisfaction, and may be more accepting of autocratic leadership (which often accompanies external threats). As loyalty to the team increases, work processes may become more rigid.

When intergroup conflict emerges, changes also occur in group members' perceptions. One's own group tends to look increasingly—and perhaps unrealistically—positive, and weaknesses may be denied. The perception of other groups and their accomplishments are likely to grow increasingly negative and become distorted. As a result of the hostility that develops between teams, intergroup communication decreases. This decreased interaction only increases the prevalence of negative stereotyping, and in turn, leads to further communication breakdown. Whatever communication occurs tends to be colored by a "we versus them" perspective. Each team acts on its assumptions about the other, automatically accepting the correctness of its own opinions and perceptions. They are likely to disregard contradictory facts or to reinterpret discrepancies to make them fit prevailing assumptions. The other group may be perceived as poorly managed, incompetent, devious, and inferior. These conditions do not enhance the probability of successful and productive intergroup relationships (Fried & Nelson, 1987).

Perhaps of greatest importance for the organization as a whole, as conflict emerges between groups, cooperative relationships are replaced by a win-lose mentality in which victory becomes more important than solving the problem that may have caused the conflict in the first place.

Strategies for Managing Intergroup Conflict

There are several types of approaches for dealing with intergroup conflict. Intergroup training is an organizational development approach that uses team-building techniques to improve the work interactions of different functions or divisions in an organization (George & Jones, 1999). Specific applications of intergroup training include organizational mirroring (French & Bell, 1990), organizational confrontation meetings (Beckhard, 1967), and a variety of organizational development methods developed by Blake and Mouton (1978). Each of these methods focuses on either preventing conflict or simply building strong intergroup relationships.

Once conflict has clearly emerged, the goal of management is to change the attitudes and behaviors of work groups and departments in conflict. In resolving existing conflict, managers can employ *tactical* approaches, which include specific strategies and managerial interventions. A common framework includes eight generic strategies (Arnold & Feldman, 1986). These range from avoidance strategies, such as ignoring the conflict or imposing a solution, to confrontational strategies. Table 6.2 summarizes these strategies and the circumstances under which each is most likely to be appropriate. The lesson here is that managers should be well equipped to employ each of these strategies. The particular circumstances of each situation determine the appropriateness of one strategy over another. These are also further discussed in Chapter 5.

Another tactical approach to conflict management involves restructuring the relationship between teams around *superordinate* goals. The emergence of concession bargaining, in which labor unions participate in "give-backs" is an example of using superordinate goals (i.e., survival of a company or industry) to overcome well-entrenched intergroup conflicts. Other strategies involve the use of buffer devices,

Table 6.2. Conflict-Management Strategies

Conflict-Resolution Strategy	Type of Strategy	Appropriate Situations
Ignoring the conflict	Avoidance	When the issue is trivial When the issue is symptomatic of more basic, pressing problems
Imposing a solution	Avoidance	When quick, decisive action is needed When unpopular decisions need to be made and consensus among the groups appears very unlikely
Smoothing	Diffusion	As a stop-gap measure to let people cool down and regain perspective When the conflict is over nonwork issues
Appealing to superordinate goals	Defusion	When there is a mutually important goal that neither group can achieve without the cooperation of the other When the survival or success of the overall organization is in jeopardy
Bargaining	Containment	When the two parties are of relatively equal power When there are several acceptable, alternative solutions that both parties would be willing to consider
Structuring the interaction	Containment	When previous attempts to openly discuss conflict issues led to conflict escalation rather than to problem solution When a respected third party is available to provide some structure and could serve as a mediator
Integrative problem solving	Confrontation	When there is a minimum level of trust between groups and there is no time pressure for a quick solution When the organization can benefit from merging the differing perspectives and insights of the groups in making key decisions
Redesigning the organization	Confrontation	When the sources of conflict come from the coordination of work When the work can be easily divided into clear project responsibilities (self-contained work groups), or when activities require a lot of interdepartmental coordination over time (lateral relations)

SOURCE: From Arnold, H. J., & Feldman, D. C. *Organizational Behavior.* New York: McGraw-Hill, 1986.

such as third-party negotiators, to help groups resolve conflicting interests. In labor-management negotiations, a mediator frequently assumes this role; in fact, we see increasing use of mediators outside of the union-management arena to help parties manage their relationships.

An alternative to tactical methods of conflict management is *strategic* approaches, which attempt to identify the underlying causes of conflict. Blake and Mouton (1978) caution against behavioral, or tactical, strategies because of their inability to have long-lasting effects. Their Interface Conflict-Solving Model attempts to build trust and cooperation among teams by examining the *interfaces* between teams. An interface is defined as any point of contact between groups at which interchanges are necessary to achieve a desired result.

Their conflict-solving model is highly structured and focuses on interface problems. They have had success with this model in a variety of situations, including union-management disputes, parent organization-subsidiary conflicts, and mergers. Specifically, this model of managing interface problems requires the participation of those individuals responsible for and capable of making the decisions necessary to bring about change. Participants in problem-solving sessions should also be familiar with the history of the relationship, current norms, and operating practices.

Perhaps the most innovative strategic approach to intergroup conflict is the establishment of *self-contained groups*. These are regroupings of conflicting groups into new groups that perform their work independently of other groups. These arrangements minimize coordination problems, since the individuals relevant to a particular task are grouped together. These groups are in some respects variants of matrix arrangements, except that self-contained groups are more permanent in nature. The use of focused teams in a large urban hospital system to overcome fragmentation and discontinuities in delivery of care illustrates the establishment of self-contained groups (Schweikhart & Smith-Daniels, 1996). Pharmacists, respiratory therapists, nurses, and other caregivers were assigned to individual care units instead of reporting to overall departments, such as pharmacy, as before.

Resources, Support, and Rewards

One of the most common complaints heard about teams in organizations is that they do not receive adequate support from the organization as a whole. While many organizations claim to want to move to a team-based organization, they often lack effective strategies for accomplishing this transition. What do managers need to do to implement the change to a team-based organization? A number of important points have been suggested. It is important for top management to ensure that a team culture is consistent with its overall strategy. Senior management needs (1) to believe that employees want to be responsible for their work; (2) to be able to demonstrate the team philosophy; (3) to articulate a coherent vision of the team environment; and (4) to have the creativity and authority to overcome obstacles as they surface (Moorhead & Griffin, 1998; Orsburn, Moran, Musselwhite, & Zenger, 1990).

As with other aspects of organizational life, teams require strong support from senior management to be effective. By support, we refer to philosophical backing and resource support. Resource support includes money, human resources, training, and time. Once senior management has made a commitment to teams, it may be necessary to develop a detailed implementation plan. This plan might include a clarification of the organization mission to focus on such things as continuous improvement, employee involvement, and customer satisfaction; selecting sites for teams; preparing a design team to assist with team staffing and operation; planning the transfer of authority from management to teams; and drafting a preliminary plan for implementation. Actual implementation of teams may also extend through various phases (Moorhead & Griffin, 1998). As with sports teams (with which many of us may be familiar), teams do not naturally flourish and improve; careful attention needs to be given to selecting, training, appraising, and compensating team members.

Training represents a key part of implementing and supporting teams. No one would ever consider the possibility of a soccer team being successful without substantial training or practice. Based on the experience of countless nonsports teams, the need for training—in fact, continuous training—is very apparent. There is a vast literature on selecting and training individuals to work in teams, and the knowledge, skills, and abilities necessary for effective teamwork. Such training may include cognitive concerns, such as the rationale or raison d'être of a team, through affective concerns such as the roles and responsibilities of team members and team norms, as well as logistical issues dealing with meeting management and compensation. Overall, for team training to be comprehensive, it optimally should include requisite technical, administrative, and interpersonal skills (Moorhead & Griffin, 1998).

A particular dilemma facing managers in team-oriented organizations is the question of reward systems. To what extent should the organization bestow team, as opposed to individual, rewards? Do team-based rewards improve team and/or individual performance? Despite the equivocal nature of the literature in this area, there seems to be a natural tendency for team-oriented organizations to at least consider the idea of team-based rewards. In a team-based environment, a variety of mechanisms may be employed to reward team member performance. In some situations, team members are rewarded for mastering a range of skills needed to meet team performance goals. In others, rewards are based on actual team performance. Skill-based pay may reward employees for acquiring specific skills needed by an employee's team. In these situations, team members may increase their compensation by acquiring value-added skill sets. Team bonus plans reward particular teams based on the performance of the team. Finally, gain-sharing plans (usually considered an organization-wide incentive system) typically reward all team members from all teams based on the performance of the organization as a whole (Moorhead & Griffin, 1998).

It should be stressed that while there are many options for rewarding team performance, the number of organizations that actually use team-based incentives is relatively small. A 1996–1997 survey of 2,500 corporations found that the number of companies with group incentives grew from 16% in 1995 to 19% in 1996 (Pascarella, 1997). While this growth is notable, the majority of organizations have yet to implement team-based incentive systems. Part of the reason for this lack of movement is the complexity of such schemes and the lack of agreement on the link between incentives and performance. While there is an intuitive appeal to performance-based compensation, there exists substantial dissent regarding the whole premise of pay-for-performance. Many managers and scholars believe that such schemes are highly destructive to individual, team, and organizational performance (Berwick, 1995). In addition, there are a number of critical questions that need to be resolved to ensure that a team payment system does not yield unintended negative consequences, including (Pascarella, 1997):

- Does the team as a whole receive rewards, or do individuals on the team receive rewards for outstanding team performance?

- If rewards are not uniformly distributed among team members, how does management assess the relative contributions of different team members?
- Should team members be compensated for results, behaviors, or both?
- How should people be rewarded when they have membership on multiple teams?

These are critical questions, the answers to which depend upon the particular manner in which teams are used in the organization as well as the culture of the organization.

CONCLUSIONS

One of the most important managerial tasks is the development and management of teams. It is now common wisdom that organizations as a whole, as well as individuals, are dependent upon strong and well functioning teams. As noted, however, teams do not naturally develop and improve. In fact, their level of performance may erode and become dysfunctional over time without deliberate and continuous supportive efforts. The successful manager—and the organization—will be rewarded with effective work teams that not only meet the needs of the organization, but also reward and support team members as well. McGregor's (1960) description of the characteristics of an effective work team, first published over 40 years ago, still stands as a useful statement of what managers should strive to achieve (Figure 6.2).

These characteristics are valid whether the team in question is a handful of people or a large division with hundreds of workers. Effective managers understand that improving a team's performance is a complex endeavor and that improvement strategies need to encompass team structure and process factors. In addition, while a team is obviously made up of individuals, each team develops its own existence and life cycle apart from its individual members and a personality all its own. The job of managers is to get things done not only through other people, but also through teams. Managers who learn well the concepts and techniques described in this chapter will help promote both greater organizational effectiveness and their own careers.

DEBATE TIME 6.1: DO WE REWARD INDIVIDUALS OR GROUPS?

Traditional methods of compensation reward individuals for individual performance. Theories of motivation focus on linking rewards to performance, facilitating individual performance through coaching and training, and setting challenging yet realistic goals. While there are some exceptions to this individualistic approach to rewards, such as gain-sharing plans where employees are rewarded for overall increased productivity, generations of managers have been inculcated with the need to reward individuals based on the merits of individual performance.

We are now in an era where groups and teams are becoming increasingly important. Teams are expected to work together to solve problems, care for patients, and engage in quality improvement and planning activities. Continuous quality improvement efforts, in fact, are based on effective team functioning. However, our reward systems are still almost entirely focused on the individual. Efforts to implement group reward systems are often met with hostility and suspicion. Many people fear the free-rider syndrome, where some members of the team do not perform up to standard yet receive the same reward as productive team members for group performance. Other people worry that group rewards dilute the motivational potential in rewards. With financial resources growing increasingly scarce, managers want to ensure that the impact of merit pay is maximized. There is therefore a reluctance to deviate from traditional merit pay systems. Finally, where employees are unionized, formally rewarding employees for team performance may be viewed as a breech of contract.

Is it possible to combine merit pay systems with team reward systems? If efforts continue to implement team rewards, will we eventually see a deterioration in individual motivation and commitment?

Figure 6.2. McGregor's Characteristics of an Effective Work Team

1. The "atmosphere" tends to be informal, comfortable, relaxed . . . It is a working atmosphere in which people are involved and interested . . .
2. There is a lot of discussion in which virtually everyone participates, but it remains pertinent to the task of the group.
3. The task or the objective of the group is well understood and accepted by its members. There will have been free discussion of the objective at some point, until it was formulated in such a way that the members of the group could commit themselves to it.
4. The members listen to each other. . . . Every idea is given a hearing . . .
5. There is disagreement. The group is comfortable with this and shows no signs of having to avoid conflict or to keep everything on the plane of sweetness and light . . .
6. Most decisions are reached by a kind of consensus in which it is clear that everybody is in general agreement and willing to go along. However, there is little tendency for individuals who oppose action to keep their opposition private and thus let an apparent consensus mask real disagreement . . .
7. Criticism is frequent, frank, and relatively comfortable . . .
8. People are free in expressing their feelings as well as their ideas both on the problem and on the group's operation.
9. When action is taken, clear assignments are made and accepted.
10. The chairman of the group does not dominate it, nor on the contrary, does the group defer unduly to him or her . . . [T]he leadership shifts from time to time, depending on the circumstances . . . The issue is not who controls, but how to get the job done.
11. The group is self-conscious about its own operations. Frequently, it will stop to examine how well it is doing or what may be interfering with its operation . . .

SOURCE: McGregor D. *The Human Side of Enterprise.* New York, NY: McGraw-Hill; 1960:232–235.

MANAGERIAL GUIDELINES

Managing teams is both an art and a science. In this chapter, we set forth several principles of group process and performance. The management of teams requires knowledge of these concepts as well as considerable skill and practice. The following managerial guidelines provide specific ideas for developing your skills as a group leader.

1. To increase the performance of a team, it is important for managers to ensure that the reward structure of the organization rewards team accomplishments as well as individual performance.
2. The manager should identify those group norms that are dysfunctional or obsolete and take steps to eliminate those norms.
3. The assignment of tasks among interdependent work groups should be clarified to avoid misunderstandings, conflict, and ambiguity.
4. Managers should be aware of their own conflict-management tendencies and seek to broaden their repertoire of conflict-management strategies.
5. Managers should be aware of how team members communicate with each other both inside and outside the team environment.
6. Managers should be aware of status differences among team members, and how these differences affect individual participation, group decision making, and productivity.
7. Managers should be able to apply a variety of structured group decision-making techniques, such as nominal group technique, brainstorming, and the Delphi technique, and understand when each is most appropriate.

8. Managers should be clear that group members understand the purpose and authority of the team, the role of the team in the organization, and the specific contributions expected of each individual.
9. Managers should be conscious of the symptoms of groupthink and develop strategies for preventing and dealing with groupthink.
10. Managers should be aware of the stage of group development and the limitations and strengths associated with each stage, and manage the group accordingly. Group leaders should also try to move group forward to more mature stages.
11. In managing meetings, group leaders should be aware of the following principles (Huber, 1980):
    a. At the beginning of the meeting, review the progress made to date and establish the task facing the group.
    b. Help group members feel comfortable with one another.
    c. Establish ground rules governing group discussions.
    d. As early in a meeting as possible, get a report from each member who has been preassigned a task.
    e. Sustain the flow of the meeting by using informational displays.
    f. Manage the discussion to achieve equitable participation.
    g. Close the meeting by summarizing what has been accomplished and reviewing assignments.

Discussion Questions

1. The recently hired director of a new ambulatory care center in a hospital has been instructed to begin holding weekly management team meetings. The management team is to consist of several physicians, nurses, physician assistants, and a social worker. What advice would you give the director to help promote the team's effectiveness?
2. An interorganizational community task force has been formed to identify obstacles facing the

elderly in obtaining needed health and social services. Given the large number of agencies involved in providing services to the elderly and the need for consumer representation, how would you balance the need for full representation with the need to keep group size at a manageable level?

3. Under what circumstances are noncohesive groups more productive than cohesive groups? What strategies can a group leader employ to increase the probability that a cohesive group will be productive?

4. What strategies can a team leader use to increase the commitment of team members? How does a team leader know if members are motivated and committed to the group?

5. If you were just appointed leader of a previously existing team of which you were not an original member, how would you determine its stage of development? Based on that stage, what strategies would you use to make the team effective?

References

Albanese, R., & Van Fleet, D. D. (1985). Rational behavior in groups: The free riding tendency. *Academy of Management Review, 10*, 244–255.

Alexander, J. A., Jinnett, K., D'Aunno, T. A., & Ullman, E. (1996). The effects of treatment team diversity and sex on assessments of team functioning. *Hospital & Health Services Administration, 41*, 37–53.

Ancona, D. G., & Caldwell, D. F. (1992a). Bridging the boundary: External activity and performance in organizational teams. *Administrative Science Quarterly, 37*, 634–665.

Ancona, D. G., & Caldwell, D. F. (1992b). Demography and design: Predictors of a new product team performance. *Organization Science, 3*, 321–341.

Ancona, D. G., & Caldwell, D. F. (1998). Rethinking team composition from the outside in. In D. H. Gruenfeld (Ed.), *Research on managing groups and teams* (pp. 21–37). Stamford, CN: MAI Press.

Arnold, H. J., & Feldman, D. C. (1986). *Organizational behavior.* New York: McGraw-Hill.

Ashforth, B. E., & Mael, F. (1989). Social identity theory and the organization. *Academy of Management Journal, 32*, 20–39.

Beckhard, R. (1967). The confrontation meeting. *Harvard Business Review, 43*, 159–165.

Benne, K., & Sheats, P. (1948). Functional roles of group members. *Journal of Social Issues, 2*, 42–47.

Berwick, D. M. (1995). The toxicity of pay for performance. *Quality Management in Health Care, 4*(1), 27–33.

Bettenhausen, K. L. (1991). Five years of group research: What we have learned and what needs to be addressed. *Journal of Management, 17*, 345–381.

Blake, R. R., & Mouton, J. S. (1978). *The new managerial grid.* Houston, TX: Gulf.

Blake, R. R., & Mouton, J. S. (1984). *Solving costly organizational conflicts.* San Francisco: Jossey-Bass.

Burchard, J. D., Burchard, S. N., Sewell, R., & VanDenBerg, J. (1993). *One kid at a time.* Juneau, AK: State of Alaska Division of Mental Health and Mental Retardation.

Campion, M. A., Medsker, G. J., & Higgs, A. C. (1993). Relations between work group characteristics and effectiveness: Implications for designing effective work groups. *Personnel Psychology, 46*, 823–850.

Cannon-Bowers, J. A., Oser, R., & Flanagan, D. L. (1992). Work teams in industry: A selected review and proposed framework. In R. W. Swezey, & E. Salas (Eds.), *Teams: Their training and performance.* Norwood, NJ: Ablex Publishing.

Capelli, P., & Rogovsky, N. (1994). New work systems and skills requirements. *International Labour Review, 133*(2), 205–220.

Cartwright, D., & Zander, A. (1968). *Group dynamics: Research and theory* (3rd ed.). New York: Harper & Row.

Cassard, S. D., Weisman, C. S., Gordon, D. L., & Wong, R. (1994). The impact of unit-based self-management by nurses on patient outcomes. *Health Services Research, 29*, 415–433.

Cohen, S. G., & Bailey, D. E. (1997). What makes teams work: Group effectiveness research from the shop floor to the executive suite. *Journal of Management, 23*, 239–290.

Cosier, R. A. (1981). Dialectical inquiry in strategic planning: A case of premature acceptance? *Academy of Management Review, 6*, 643–648.

Cummings, T. (1978). Self-regulating work groups: A socio-technical synthesis. *Academy of Management Review, 3*, 625–634.

Dailey, R., Young, F., & Barr, C. (1991). Empowering middle managers in hospitals with team-based problem solving. *Health Care Management Review, 16*, 55–63.

Dalkey, N. (1969). *The delphi method: An experimental study of group opinion.* Santa Monica, CA: The Rand Corporation.

Davis, J. H. (1964). *Group performance.* Reading, MA: Addison-Wesley.

Deber, R. B., & Leatt, P. (1986). The multidisciplinary renal team: Who makes the decisions? *Health Matrix, 4*(3), 3–9.

Delbecq, A., Van de Ven, A., & Gustafson, D. (1975). *Group techniques for program planning.* Glenview, IL: Scott, Foresman.

Denison, D. R., & Sutton, R. I. (1990). Operating room nurses. In J. R. Hackman (Ed.), *Groups that work (and those that don't): Creating conditions for effective teamwork.* San Francisco: Jossey-Bass.

Deutsch, M. (1949). An experimental study of the effects of co-operation and competition upon group process. *Human Relations, 2*, 199–232.

Dyer, J. L. (1984). Team research and team training: A state-of-the-art review. In F. A. Muckler (Ed.), *Human factors review: 1984* (pp. 285–323). Santa Monica, CA: Human Factors Society.

Erickson, J. (1997). Turmoil in Tuscon. *American Medical News, 40*(34), 1, 23.

Etzioni, A. (1961). *A comparative analysis of complex organizations.* New York: Free Press, p. 114.

Fargason, C. A., & Haddock, C. C. (1992). Cross-functional, integrative team decision making: Essential for effective QI in health care. *Quality Review Bulletin, 7*, 157–163.

Festinger, L., Schacter, S., & Back, K. (1950). *Social pressures in informal groups.* Stanford, CA: Stanford University Press.

Fleishman, J. (1980). Collective action as helping behavior: Effects of responsibility diffusion on contributions to a public good. *Journal of Personality and Social Psychology, 38*, 629–637.

French, W. L., & Bell, C. H. (1990). *Organizational development.* Englewood Cliffs, NJ: Prentice-Hall.

Fried, B., & Nelson, W. (1987). Strategic planning with family physicians. *Canadian Family Physician, 33*, 1309–1312.

George, J. F., & Jones, G. R. (1999). *Understanding and managing organizational behavior* (2nd ed.). Reading, MA: Addison-Wesley.

George, J. M. (1992). Extrinsic and intrinsic origins of perceived social loafing in organizations. *Academy of Management Journal, 35*, 191–202.

Gersick, C. J. G. (1989). Marking time: Predictable transitions in task groups. *Academy of Management, 32*, 274–309.

Gist, M. E., Locke, E. A., & Taylor, M. S. (1987). Organizational behavior: Group structure, process, and effectiveness. *Journal of Management, 13*, 237–257.

Gladstein, D. (1984). Groups in context: A model of task group effectiveness. *Administrative Science Quarterly, 29*, 499–517.

Goodman, P. S., Ravlin, E., & Schminke, M. (1987). Understanding groups in organizations. *Research in Organizational Behavior, 9*, 121–173.

Gordon, J. (1992, October). Work teams: How far have they come? *Training*, 59–65.

Gordon, J. R. (1999). *Organizational behavior: A diagnostic approach.* Upper Saddle River, NJ: Prentice-Hall.

Greene, C. N. (1978). Identification modes of professionals: Relationship with formalization, role strain and alienation. *Academy of Management Journal, 21*, 486–92.

Gully, S. M., Devine, D. J., & Whitney, D. J. (1995). A meta-analysis of cohesion and performance. *Small Group Research, 26*, 497–520.

Guzzo, R. A. (1990). Group decision making and group effectiveness in organizations. In P. S. Goodman (Ed.), *Designing effective work groups.* San Francisco: Jossey-Bass.

Hackman, J. R. (1976). Work design. In J. R. Hackman, & J. L. Suttle (Eds.), *Improving life at work.* Santa Monica, CA: Goodyear.

Hackman, J. R. (1982). *A set of methods for research on work teams* (Technical Report No. 1). School of

Organization and Management. New Haven, CT: Yale University.

Hackman, J. R. (1987). The design of work teams. In J. Lorsch (Ed.), *Handbook of organizational behavior.* New York: Prentice-Hall.

Hackman, J. R. (1990a). *Groups that work (and those that don't).* San Francisco: Jossey-Bass.

Hackman, J. R. (1990b). Introduction. Work teams in organizations: An orienting framework. In J. R. Hackman (Ed.), *Groups that work (and those that don't): Creating conditions for effectiveness teamwork.* San Francisco: Jossey-Bass.

Hackman, J. R., & Oldham, G. R. (1980). *Work redesign.* Reading, MA: Addison-Wesley.

Hasenfeld, Y. (1983). *Human service organizations.* Englewood Cliffs, NJ: Prentice-Hall.

Horak, B. J., Guarino, J. H., Knight, C. C., & Kweder, S. L. (1991). Building a team on a medical floor. *Health Care Management Review, 16*, 65–71.

Huber, G. (1980). *Managerial decision making.* Glenview, IL: Scott, Foresman.

Hunsaker, P. L., & Cook, C. W. (1986). *Managing organizational behavior.* Reading, MA: Addison-Wesley.

Jackson, S. E. (1992). Team composition in organizational settings: Issues in managing an increasingly diverse work force. In S. Worchel, W. Wood, & J. A. Simpson (Eds.), *Group process and productivity.* Newbury Park, CA: Sage.

Janis, I. L. (1972). *Victims of groupthink.* Boston: Houghton-Mifflin.

Jones, G. R. (1984). Task visibility, freeriding, and shirking: Explaining the effect of structure and technology on employee behavior. *Academy of Management Review, 9*, 684–695.

Katzenbach, J. R., & Smith, D. K. (1993). The discipline of teams. *Harvard Business Review, 71*, 111–120.

Kirkman, B. L., & Rosen, B. (1997). A model of work team empowerment. In R. Woodman, & W. Pasmore (Eds.), *Research in organizational change and development* (pp. 131–167). Greenwich, CT: Jai Press.

Kolodny, H., & Kiggundu, M. (1980). Towards the development of a sociotechnical systems model in woodlands mechanical harvesting. *Human Relations, 33*, 623–645.

LaPenta, C., & Jacobs, G. M. (1996). Application of group process model to performance appraisal development in a CQI environment. *Health Care Management Review, 21*, 45–60.

Latane, B., Williams, K. D., & Harkins, S. (1979). Many hands make light the work: The causes and consequences of social loafing. *Journal of Personality and Social Psychology, 37*, 822–832.

Locke, E., & Schweiger, D. M. (1979). Participation in decision-making: One more look. In B. M. Staw, & L. L. Cummings (Eds.), *Research in organizational behavior* (p. 2). Greenwich, CT: Jai Press.

McGrath, J. E. (1984). *Groups: Interaction and performance.* Englewood Cliffs, NJ: Prentice-Hall.

McGregor, D. (1960). *The human side of enterprise.* New York: McGraw-Hill.

Mechanic, D. (1962). Sources of power of lower participants in complex organizations. *Administrative Science Quarterly, 7*(4), 349–364.

Moorhead, G., & Griffin, R. W. (1998). *Organizational behavior: Managing people and organizations.* Boston: Houghton Mifflin.

Moreland, R. L., & Levine, J. M. (1988). Group dynamics over time: Development and socialization in small groups. In J. E. McGrath (Ed.), *The social psychology of groups* (pp. 151–181). Beverly Hills, CA: Sage.

Mullen, B., & Baumeister, R. F. (1987). Group effects on self-attention and performance: Social loafing, social facilitation, and social impairment. In C. Hendrick (Ed.), *Review of personality and social psychology.* Beverly Hills, CA: Sage.

Nadler, D. A., Hackman, J. R., & Lawler, E. E., III. (1979). *Managing organizational behavior.* Boston: Little, Brown.

Nadler, D. A., & Tushman, M. L. (1988). *Strategic organization design: Concepts, tools, and processes.* Glenview, IL: Scott, Foresman.

Nelson, R. E. (1989). The strength of strong ties: Social networks and intergroup conflict in organizations. *Academy of Management Journal, 32*, 377–401.

Nieva, V. F., Fleishman, E. A., & Rieck, A. (1978). *Team dimensions: Their identity, their measurement, and their relationships* (Final Technical Report for Contract No. DAHC19-78-C-0001). Washington, DC: Advanced Research Resources Organizations.

Okun, M. A., & DiVesta, F. J. (1975). Cooperation and competition in coacting groups. *Journal of Personality and Social Psychology, 31,* 615–620.

Orsburn, J. D., Moran, L., Musselwhite, E., & Zenger, J. (1990). *Self-directed work teams: The new American challenge.* Homewood, IL: Business One Irwin.

Owens, D. A., Mannic, E. A., & Neale, M. A. (1998). Strategic formation of groups: Issues in task performancer and team member selection. In D. H. Gruenfeld (Ed.), *Research on managing groups and teams* (pp. 149–165). Stamford, CN: MAI Press.

Pascarella, P. (1997, February). Compensating teams. *Across the Board,* 16–22.

Pennings, J. M. (1975). Interdependence and complementarity—the case of a brokerage office. *Human Relations, 28,* 825–840.

Pinto, M. B., & Pinton, J. K. (1990). Project team communication and cross-functional cooperation in new program development. *Journal of Product Innovation Management, 7,* 200–212.

Porter, L. W., Lawler, E. E., III, & Hackman, J. R. (1975). *Behavior in organizations.* New York: McGraw-Hill.

Roberts, K. H., & Hunt, D. M. (1991). *Organizational behavior.* Boston: PWS-Kent Publishing Co.

Roby, T. B., & Lanzetta, J. T. (1958). Considerations in the analysis of group tasks. *Psychological Bulletin, 55,* 88–101.

Roethlisberger, F. J., & Dickson, W. J. (1939). *Management and the worker.* Cambridge, MA: Harvard University Press.

Rundall, T. G., Starkweather, D. B., & Norrish, B. A. (1998). *After restructuring: Empowerment strategies at work in America's hospitals.* San Francisco: Jossey-Bass.

Salvedra, R., Earley, P. C., & Van Dyne, L. (1993). Complex interdependence in task-performing groups. *Journal of Applied Psychology, 78,* 61–72.

Schweikhart, S. B., & Smith-Daniels, V. (1996). Reengineering the work of caregivers: Role redefinition, team structures, and organizational redesign. *Health Care Management Review, 41,* 19–36.

Schwenk, C. R. (1983). Laboratory research on ill-structured decision aids: The case of dialectical inquiry. *Decision Sciences, 14,* 140–144.

Scott, W. G. (1967). *Organization theory.* Homewood, IL: Irwin.

Seashore, S. (1954). *Group cohesiveness in the industrial work group.* Ann Arbor, MI: Institute for Social Research, University of Michigan.

Shaw, M. E. (1976). *Group dynamics: The psychology of small group behavior.* New York: McGraw-Hill.

Shaw, R. B. (1990). Mental health treatment teams. In J. R. Hackman (Ed.), *Groups that work (and those that don't)* (pp. 320–348). San Francisco: Jossey Bass.

Shea, G. P., & Guzzo, R. A. (1987). Group effectiveness: What really matters? *Sloan Management Review, 28,* 25–31.

Sherif, M., & Sherif, C. W. (1953). *Groups in harmony and tension.* New York: Harper.

Shortell, S. M., Zimmerman, J. E., Rousseau, D. M., Gillies, R. R., Wagner, D. P., Draper, E. A., Knaus, W. A., & Duffy, J. (1994). The performance of intensive care units: Does good management make a difference? *Medical Care, 32,* 508–525.

Steiner, I. D. (1972). *Group process and productivity.* New York: Academic Press.

Stigler, G. J. (1974). Free riders and collective action: An appendix to theories of economic regulation. *Bell Journal of Economics and Management Science, 5,* 359–365.

Stoner, C. R., & Hartman, R. I. (1993). Team building: Answering the tough questions. *Business Horizons, 36,* 70–78.

Sundstrom, E., DeMeuse, K. P., & Futrell, D. (1990). Work teams: Applications and effectiveness. *American Psychologist, 45*(2), 120–133.

Thompson, J. D. (1967). *Organizations in action.* New York: McGraw-Hill.

Thyen, M. N., Theis, R., & Tebbitt, B. V. (1993). Organizational empowerment through self-governed teams. *Journal of Nursing Administration, 23,* 24–26.

Trist, E. (1981). *The evolution of socio-technical systems: A conceptual framework and an action research program.* Toronto, Canada: Ontario Quality of Working Life Centre.

Trist, E., & Bamforth, K. (1951). Some social and psychological consequences of the Longwall method of goal-setting. *Human Relations, 4,* 1–38.

Tuckman, B. W. (1965). Developmental sequences in small groups. *Psychological Bulletin, 63,* 384–399.

Van de Ven, A. H., Delbecq, A. L., & Koenig, R. (1976). Determinants of coordination modes within organizations. *American Sociological Review, 41,* 322–338.

Vinokur-Kaplan, D. (1995a). Enhancing the effectiveness of interdisciplinary mental health treatment teams. *Administration and Policy in Mental Health, 22*(5), 521–530.

Vinokur-Kaplan, D. (1995b). Treatment teams that work (and those that don't): An application of Hackman's group effectiveness model to interdisciplinary teams in psychiatric hospitals. *Journal of Applied Behavioral Science, 31,* 303–327.

Wagner, J. A. (1994). Participation's effects on performance and satisfaction: A reconsideration of research evidence. *Academy of Management Review, 19,* 312–330.

Walsh, J., & Hewitt, H. (1996). Facilitating an effective process in treatment groups with persons having serious mental illness. *Social Work with Groups, 19,* 5–18.

Webster, C. M., Grusky, O., Young, A., & Podus, D. (1998). Leadership structures in case management teams: An application of social network analysis. *Research in Community and Mental Health, 9,* 11–28.

Whetten, D. A., & Cameron, K. S. (1998). *Developing management skills* (4th ed.). Reading, MA: Addison-Wesley.

Wicker, A. W. (1979). *An introduction to ecological psychology.* Monterey, CA: Brooks/Cole.

CHAPTER

Work Design

Martin P. Charns, D.B.A.
Jody Hoffer Gittell, Ph.D.

Chapter Outline

Learning Objectives

After completing this chapter, the reader should be able to:

1. Identify the range of approaches to work design, including the psychological and technical approaches.
2. Understand the relationships between work design and individuals' motivation and productivity.
3. Discuss the differences between work and working.
4. Identify tasks, their characteristics, and their performance requirements.
5. Analyze the interconnectedness of tasks among individuals and among work groups.
6. Understand how to approach the design of individual jobs and of work units.

Key Terms

Analyzing Work
Approaches to Work Design
Coordinating Mechanisms
Designing Individual Jobs
Designing Work Groups to Address Coordination Needs
Direct Work
Feedback Approaches to Coordination
Horizontal Division of Labor
Interconnectedness of Work
Job Skill and Knowledge Requirements
Management Work
Motivating Potential of a Job
Multiskilled Employees
Programming Approaches to Coordination
Psychological Approach to Work Design
Scientific Management
Support Work
Task Inventory Approach to Work Design
Technical Approach to Work Design
Uncertainty Inherent in Work
Vertical Division of Labor
Work Requirements

Chapter Purpose

Differences between the effectively functioning Unit B and the chaotic Unit A are seen by many administrators and health care professionals as arising from differences in leadership or staff competence. Others attribute the differences in unit performance to differences in work design. But they disagree whether Unit B's work design is more effective because it leads to more job satisfaction and a more motivated staff, or because it better supports the flow of information across interconnected jobs. Is Unit B's superior performance due to the psychological or technical benefits of its work design?

The purpose of this chapter is to provide a framework for the design of individual jobs and organizational work groups, and to describe the relationships between work design, motivation,

and information flow. Two major approaches to job design are discussed along with their inherent assumptions, strengths, and limitations. An integration of the concepts and a framework for their managerial application are then presented.

Work design concepts can be applied at several levels in an organization. In fact, they can be applied to analyze and design the work of two or more related organizations, such as integrated delivery systems, an organization and its suppliers, or referral networks. In this chapter, the concepts are applied in a single organization. Attention is directed to the design of work contained within single jobs (i.e., job design) and the design of work within organizational units consisting of several jobs (i.e., work unit design).

CHANGES IN THE DESIGN OF HEALTH CARE WORK

Health care has undergone major transitions in the past 10 years. Work arrangements that made half-hearted attempts at efficiency in the fee-for-service health care system are no longer viable. Coordination and the management of care have become primary tools for controlling health care costs. The caregiver—physician, nurse, or other provider—cannot choose the course of treatment, or the equipment or supplies used to provide that treatment without considering the cost implications of these decisions on the patient, themselves, or their related organization. Where once a provider's convenience in scheduling a procedure was dominant, patient-centered services in today's leading organizations often dictate care be given at a time and location preferred by the patient and the insurer. No longer do we assume without question that providers always know or do what is "right" for their patients. Patients, health care organizations, and the benefits provided a patient through their insurance are limiting the discretion of physicians and other providers.

The force of the changes occurring in the health care system is reflected in shifts in power between physicians and managers (also see Chapter 9). There has been a relative increase in power and control ex-

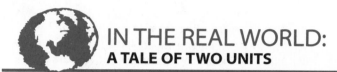

IN THE REAL WORLD:
A TALE OF TWO UNITS

Unit A, an orthopedics unit in a major Eastern teaching hospital, is characterized by high dissatisfaction among the nursing staff and is the target of frequent complaints from residents and attending physicians. Communication among the nurses, therapists, social workers, residents, and attending physicians regarding patient care is poor, and relationships among them are strained.

The unit generally appears to be in a state of chaos. Patients and their families seek information about their status from physicians, nurses, and other staff, and frequently complain that they receive conflicting information from the medical and nursing staffs. At the same time, lengths of stay are unacceptably long due to poor communication among the staff rather than due to unique patient needs.

The organization of the hospital is similar to that of most major teaching facilities, with the major departments representing professional (nursing, social service, dietary) and nonprofessional (housekeeping, security, transportation) functions. Nursing staff members are assigned to patient care units. Unit A offers primary nursing care, an approach to care delivery where each RN is responsible for the total nursing needs of a number of patients. Each primary nurse on Unit A has primary responsibility for six to seven patients at a time. The nursing staff reports to a nurse manager, who is responsible for 155 nurses on Unit A and another unit.

Unit A has two case managers, RNs by training, whose case loads are typically 32 patients each. They are responsible for reviewing resource utilization, for ensuring that all staff members adhere to care paths, and for planning patient discharges. Care paths—protocols specifying the sequence and timing of tasks for patients with particular routine conditions—have been introduced over the past five years to streamline communication among the staff. Unit A staff stopped holding interdisciplinary rounds several years ago on the belief that these meetings consume too much valuable staff time, and have chosen to manage care primarily through care paths instead.

Unit B is an orthopedics unit in a different Eastern teaching hospital. It has a reputation for quality care and responsiveness to both patients and their families. Nurses and other staff express high satisfaction about their work. Communication between nurses, therapists, social workers, residents, and attending physicians is said to be frequent, timely, and accurate, and relationships among them appear to be strong. In general, the unit runs smoothly and responds well to routine situations as well as unusual cases. Patients are routinely discharged on the anticipated day, except when their health status dictates a longer stay.

Unit B differs organizationally from Unit A in several ways. Unit B also uses primary nursing, but its nurses have primary responsibility for four to five patients at a time, permitting them to more closely manage the care of their patients with physicians and other staff members. The orthopedics nurse manager is responsible for 36 nurses in all. Unit B also has two nonprofessional staff members who are cross-trained to assist and feed patients, draw blood, stock supplies, and perform other technical tasks.

Case managers work in four teams made up of one RN and one social worker. Each team has a case load of 16 patients, giving each team member an effective case load of only eight patients. Along with their smaller case loads and their broader set of skills, Unit B case managers have a broader range of tasks than their counterparts on Unit A. Like Unit A's case managers, they are responsible for monitoring resource utilization and adherence to care paths and for planning discharge, but they are also responsible for attending and leading interdisciplinary patient rounds, for attending physician rounds, and for coordinating clinical care. Case managers also follow patients after discharge, to assess any follow-up needs they might have.

Each case-management team is assigned to a small number of orthopedic surgeons, and follows the patients of those surgeons exclusively. The dedication of case managers to a small number of physicians allows them to attend physician rounds and report the physician *perspective back to the rest of the staff through interdisciplinary rounds. As a result of their multiple roles and assignment to physicians, case managers on Unit B are the nexus of communication regarding orthopedic patients.*

Unit B patients with routine conditions are assigned to care paths, as on Unit A, but their care is still actively managed through interdisciplinary rounds. Interdisciplin- *ary rounds are held twice weekly on Unit B, and are attended by a broad range of functions—the nurse manager, the nurse and social work case managers, primary nurses, physical therapists, and a radiologist. Also attending patient rounds are representatives from the rehab facilities and home care agencies to which patients are referred for follow-up care, facilitating communication and continuity of care across settings.*

ercised by management and a relative decrease in the power of physicians. These changes have been fueled by a surplus of physicians and a lessening of demand for their services as managed patient care, health maintenance organizations (HMOs), and other capitated payment arrangements constrain the volume of services used. Capitated arrangements have also given administrators increased influence over physicians' incomes. Previously, managers had limited means by which to control practitioners in their institutions or organizations. Now, however, they can decide whether the productivity and practice style of these practitioners are consistent with the economic survival of the organization. If it is not, physicians and others are being denied contracts, receiving reduced payments from HMOs and preferred provider organizations (PPOs), and facing an array of sanctions never before encountered. The impact of such controls has only begun to be felt.

Through direct efforts, such as utilization management and tying financial considerations to patient care practices, as well as more indirect efforts, such as creating a cost-conscious culture for the organization, managers are influencing physician decision making. The combination of organizational pressures and national efforts to define practice guidelines and outcomes of care are working together to force change. Although it is difficult for physicians to change practice styles developed over many years, to varying degrees they are changing their behavior. Whether the changes will improve or reduce the quality of care or the risk associated with it is still uncertain, but it is a question that will accompany the

health care system over the next decade and help drive the quest for quality improvement, as further discussed in Chapter 13.

Like physicians, nurses are facing challenges to their practice. In the 1980s, health care organizations experienced a severe shortage of nurses and other health professionals. This was caused by many factors including increased acuity of hospitalized patients, increased numbers of jobs in ambulatory settings and case review for insurance approval, women's increased professional opportunities outside of health care, and the drop in the number of nurses needing to work when other family income earners are doing well in a strong economy. The shortage led many hospitals to rethink the design of professional and nonprofessional jobs both to match the availability of lower skilled workers in the labor force and to create more stimulating jobs that workers would not leave. In addition, some organizations used this as an opportunity to redesign their patient care delivery systems to emphasize the patient as the raison d'etre. Even though the nursing shortage ameliorated with the downturn in the world economy in the late 1980s, many organizations continued their redesign efforts (Donnelly, 1989; "Strengthening hospital nursing," 1992; Tonges, 1989). Many rural hospitals, characterized by a highly variable patient census, have found **multiskilled workers** and cross-trained staff to be effective ways to meet their highly fluctuating demand. It has become a critical element to their survival and is increasingly seen as important in the efforts to efficiently manage larger urban hospitals (Brider, 1992).

CONTRASTING APPROACHES TO WORK DESIGN

The individual job is the basic element of any organization. As such, job design has been a focus of attention in the literatures of organizational behavior and health management. Contrasting **approaches to work design,** however, are found both in the literature and in practice. The **technical approach to work design** emerges from the tradition of scientific management, which recommends extracting maximum efficiency from workers by designing narrow, repetitive jobs. This approach has broadened beyond its roots in scientific management but still focuses on how job design affects skill and information requirements. The **psychological approach to work design** focuses instead on how job design affects worker motivation. This approach recommends motivating workers by designing jobs that are broad and relatively autonomous from supervisors and other workers. Both approaches argue that job design affects organizational performance, but they disagree about whether job design does so primarily through its effect on technical or psychological factors.

In many health care organizations, jobs that are designed and managed from these differing perspectives exist side by side. For example, professionals (e.g., physicians, nurses, social workers) generally determine for themselves both what work to do and how to do it. Technical workers often have more narrowly defined jobs. The psychological approach suggests that professionals should therefore be more highly motivated than technical workers. Yet problems of low productivity, low morale, and dysfunctional individual behaviors, such as alcoholism and drug abuse, exist among both professional and technical workers. The technical approach suggests that information flow should be more problematic among those with narrowly defined jobs, but that the benefits of specialization override these costs of coordination. Yet complaints about the lack of timely, accurate communication are endemic in health care organizations. To solve problems of motivation and information flow, it is necessary to address both the technical and psychological elements of jobs.

One of the prime reasons for poor management and less than optimal performance in health care and other organizations is that managers confuse "work" and "working" (Charns & Shaefer, 1983; Drucker, 1973) and inappropriately manage the relationship between them. Work is objective and impersonal. It is energy directed at organizational goals, identifiable separately from the person who does it. It is analyzable. Working, on the other hand, is a worker's affective response to work. Far from totally analyzable, it is individual, personal, and subjective.

Managers of technical, nonprofessional workers tend to follow the technical approach to job design. They focus on work and largely ignore working. The workers' affective responses are seen as extraneous elements to be controlled so that they do not interfere with work. In contrast, managers of professional workers tend to follow the psychological approach. Their attention is almost exclusively on working, to the neglect of work. The result is that work is directed at goals chosen by the professional, which may or may not be organizational goals. Similarly, managerial efforts to improve working conditions or to humanize work are often pursued with working in mind and with insufficient and inappropriate consideration for the work requirements. Yet work affects working, and working affects work. Both are important elements in efforts to manage patient care in a way that produces high quality and efficient outcomes.

In the next two sections, we lay the groundwork for exploring the technical and psychological approaches in greater depth. Regardless of which approach one takes, one must address how work is to be divided into jobs, and what qualities are required of the people who perform them.

DIVIDING WORK INTO JOBS

Work is divided into jobs along two dimensions—horizontal and vertical. The horizontal dimension determines how broad a particular job is—how many related tasks are included in that job. The vertical dimension determines how deep a particular job is—whether that job includes direct work, managerial work, and support work, or just one of the above. (See Figure 7.1 for a depiction of job breadth and depth.) These dimensions are relevant to both the technical

DEBATE TIME 7.1: WHAT DO YOU THINK?

The technical and psychological approaches to work design were developed by different groups of scholars based on different sets of premises. When applied to the design of any particular job, the two approaches yield very different outcomes.

The **scientific management** school as one technical approach prescribes breaking down work into discrete, repetitive components, and training workers to be expert in their narrow areas of responsibility. Proponents of this approach argue that simplifying work allows development of expertise, and through repetition of tasks, workers become highly proficient. Developed through this form of job engineering, highly skilled workers contribute to organizational productivity.

The psychological school argues that people should be provided with work that represents whole tasks with which they can identify. This provides the opportunity for people to feel that their work is meaningful, and they are more highly motivated to do it well. Workers' high motivation, in turn, is critical to organizational productivity. From the perspective of the psychological school, repetitive tasks are not rewarding to individuals. Without interest in their work, workers' motivation is low, and so is productivity.

How do you reconcile these different perspectives? What different assumptions form the underpinnings of the two different approaches? What situational factors have to be considered in applying the different theories?

and psychological approaches to job design. The two approaches suggest different criteria, however—skill and information requirements rather than motivational requirements—for determining how broad or deep a particular job should be.

Vertical Division of Labor

All organizations perform three different types of work in the **vertical division of labor: management**

work, direct work, and support work. Direct work is effort that directly contributes to the accomplishment of an organization's goals. In health care organizations, clinical work performed by doctors, nurses, and other care providers is direct work. In organizations that have multiple goals, such as teaching hospitals, there is a set of direct work activities for each goal (e.g., teaching, research, and patient care). Although an individual may perform more than one type of direct work, the work itself is identifiable and analyzable separate from the person performing it (Charns & Schaefer, 1983; Stoelwinder & Charns, 1981).

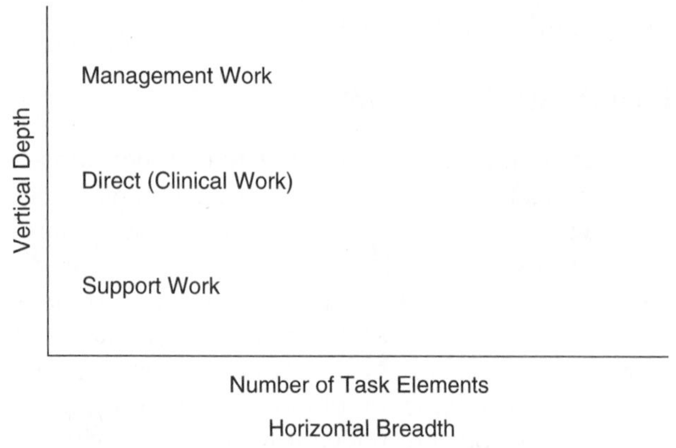

Management work includes providing the resources and context within which direct work can be performed effectively and maintaining an alignment between an organization and its external environment. Management work is decision making about the organizational context within which other work is performed (Charns & Schaefer, 1983). For example, it includes determining what services to provide, what services to develop or reduce, what resources to make available to whom, and what systems will perform various functions. Since the primary method of influencing decision making is to influence its premises—the information that is considered in making a decision—management work affects

Figure 7.1. Dimensions of Work

all other work because it influences the premises on which other decisions are made (Simon, 1976).

Support work does not directly result in achievement of an organizational goal, but it is needed for effective accomplishment of other work. For example, support work for clinical work includes such things as maintaining medical records, transporting patients, maintaining the physical surroundings in which care is delivered, and performing laboratory tests. Support work for management work includes providing legal counsel, clerical assistance, data on both internal operations and the external environment, and planning and analytical assistance, as well as personnel support.

These three types of work can be divided into distinct jobs, or combined in the same job. Jobs that encompass two or more of these types of work are considered to have more depth than jobs that encompass only one type of work.

Horizontal Division of Labor

The best approach for identifying tasks in the **horizontal division of labor** is to assess the natural boundaries in work that occur along the dimensions of time, technology, and territory (Miller, 1959). When different work is or can be performed at different points in time, such as on different days or at different times of the day, distinct tasks can be identified. For example, patient care given during one office visit is distinguishable from that given during another visit, as is patient care delivered to a patient during different hospital admissions. Similarly, discrete tasks can often be identified by the fact that they are performed in different places (territories), such as in hospital, ambulatory, and home care settings. Finally, tasks can be identified by the technology involved.

Technology should be considered broadly to include not only hardware, but also skills and training, personality characteristics and interpersonal orientations, and different practices associated with performing different work. Such different practices may result from tradition, from regulation of government, licensing agencies, or accrediting bodies, or from professional norms of accepted practice. Thus, for example, the work performed by different professional groups is a natural place to look for inherent boundaries (Charns & Schae-

fer, 1983). In doing so, however, analysis must determine whether differences are real and inherent in the work or are maintained only by tradition.

By taking a broad perspective of technology, we can also ask what differences in work are associated with different parts of an organization's environment. For example, do different patients represent different types of work? Do treating different diseases, preventing illness in contrast to treating it, or interacting with people from different ethnic or socioeconomic backgrounds represent the use of different technologies and therefore different work? Often differences in technology overlap with differences in time or territory, but together they help identify discrete tasks.

The more discrete tasks included in a particular job, the broader that job is considered to be. Health care professionals have typically performed broad jobs. Physicians, nurses, and physical therapists have traditionally been responsible for determining a plan of care, as well as delivering that care; but increasingly, these tasks are being carried out by others in the division of labor. Physicians, nurses, and therapists are still responsible for determining the plan of care, while physician assistants, nursing aides, and therapy assistants are increasingly employed for carrying out the plan of care. Where possible, however, broader jobs such as primary nursing have been designed to encompass more interrelated tasks, to decrease the number of providers in contact with the patient, and to simplify coordination.

JOB REQUIREMENTS

Once a job has been defined as a set of tasks in the horizontal and vertical divisions of labor, several approaches exist for determining the personal attributes needed to perform well in that job. Galbraith (1977) has provided a set of categories for determining the behaviors required for effective task performance. Galbraith's five categories in cumulative order are:

1. decisions to join and remain in an organization
2. dependable role performance
3. effort above minimum levels
4. spontaneous and innovative behavior
5. cooperative behavior

In general, all jobs require the first two categories of behavior. Organizations require that people join and remain employed in their jobs and that they perform dependably. These two minimum levels of behavior, however, are often not completely met. Where the work itself or the working conditions do not provide a worker with an acceptable level of rewards—including satisfaction—turnover and absenteeism result. Dependable role performance also does not occur when people do not know what is expected of them or they feel that the work that is expected of them is not equitably balanced with the rewards of the job.

When jobs require more than the first two minimum categories of behavior, the design of the job itself becomes a greater concern. When all elements of the work cannot be anticipated, spontaneous and innovative behavior is required. This requirement can be distinguished from behavior above minimum levels by the frequency with which unanticipated events occur and the degree of innovative behavior required. It is characterized by an individual needing to recognize that spontaneous and innovative behavior is required and having the skills and willingness to act. When, in addition, the work requires an individual to recognize and be willing and able to work with others to achieve the desired outcome, it requires cooperative behavior.

The five categories of behavior are cumulative and form a scale directly related to the inherent uncertainty of the work. Thus, work that is highly certain and predictable generally requires only the first two categories of behavior. Work that is highly uncertain and unpredictable requires cooperative behavior in addition to all four other categories of behavior.

Regardless of whether one takes the psychological or technical approach, one must address how work is to be divided into jobs, and what qualities are required of the people who perform them. Each approach suggests a different criterion, however—motivation versus information—for thinking about these job design issues.

PSYCHOLOGICAL APPROACH

The psychological approach, rooted in psychology and organizational behavior, focuses on worker motivation. This approach assumes that, when individuals perform work that meets their needs for growth, and jobs themselves are intrinsically rewarding, substantial motivation results (also see Chapter 3). Professional jobs, in which there generally is a strong relationship between an individual's self-concept and her work, are examples. On the other hand, routine, repetitive jobs that encompass only a small portion of a larger task or jobs that are strictly and narrowly delineated are difficult for anyone to identify with. Such jobs limit the extent of an individual's involvement in the work and the motivation to perform well; therefore, productivity suffers. The psychological approach therefore argues that well-designed jobs are broad rather than narrow.

Sometimes, however, when individuals have total discretion over the way they do their work and what work they perform, their motivation may be directed toward other than organizational goals. In fact, they may work against the organization's goals. The assumption that motivation will result in organizationally desirable productivity does not necessarily hold. Even so, professional workers are often given complete discretion over what they do and how they do it. This, in fact, is one of the attributes of a profession. In medicine, generally regarded as the prime example of a profession, professional work is typically off limits to organizational job design analysis.

The autonomy of health care professionals, however, is being challenged. The issues of cost control, quality, competition, and responsiveness to customers have come to dominate the health care system of the 1990s. Health care managers have responded to these issues and to the challenges of a market-driven health care system by moving to make their organizations more price sensitive; cost effective; and patient, family, and client centered.

Assumptions Underlying the Psychological Approach

Underlying the design of any job are assumptions about individuals and the relationship between individuals and their work. These assumptions may be formally stated (as in a labor contract) or not, and they may be recognized by managers or not. The psychological job design approach is based upon the general assumptions that people work to satisfy a broad range of needs and that the design of a job affects the person's ability to meet those needs. Two perspectives can be taken to consider in greater detail the relationship between job design and motivation.

First, consider that people are motivated by unfulfilled needs and that they exert effort to satisfy those needs. If opportunities for meeting a person's needs are provided by the work itself, the person will be motivated to perform the work. Where work itself does not provide opportunities to satisfy individual needs, the person will seek other outlets and may not be motivated to perform the work. Thus, it is important to match people and their needs to jobs and their inherent **work requirements.** For example, if work requires an individual only to join and remain in the organization and to perform dependably, these behaviors can often be obtained by matching the job to people with economic needs and rewarding them monetarily. When such jobs are held instead by people whose needs are for achievement or other forms of personal growth, the individuals most likely will not respond only to monetary rewards and will direct their efforts away from the dependable role performance required by the organization (McClelland, 1975). These people are better matched to jobs that require spontaneous and innovative behavior.

A second perspective on individual motivation is based upon the assumption that people evaluate courses of action for the purpose of choosing among them. The expectancy model of motivation posits that individuals exhibit behavior that they perceive will result in outcomes that yield valued rewards (Porter & Lawler, 1968; Vroom, 1961). In its simplest form, the model indicates that people subjectively evaluate possible behaviors in terms of three elements: the probability that a behavior will yield a desired outcome, the probability that the outcome will yield rewards, and the value of those rewards to the individual. These three elements combine multiplicatively in a person's assessment so that, if any one element is low, it is unlikely that the person will choose the associated behavior. Where that behavior is required to perform work effectively, we must ask how the elements of the model of motivation are affected by the job.

When work is intrinsically rewarding to individuals—that is, when effectively performing the work itself is inherently rewarding—we can see that there is a direct connection between behavior and rewards. This is likely to occur with the following psychological conditions (Hackman, Janson, Oldham, & Purdy, 1975):

* *Experienced meaningfulness.* The job is seen as important, valuable, and worthwhile.
* *Experienced responsibility.* Individuals feel personally responsible and accountable for the results of their efforts.
* *Knowledge of results.* Individuals understand how effectively they are performing the job.

These three aspects of working have a major impact on a person's motivation and are themselves affected both by characteristics of the individual and by the content of the work itself.

Three characteristics of a job contribute to its experienced meaningfulness: skill variety, task identity, and task significance. Skill variety refers to the variety of different skills and talents required of an individual in performing a job. A job that has task identity represents an identifiable piece of work that an individual can perform from beginning to end and that has a visible outcome. Task significance refers to the impact a job has on the lives of other people. In general, because health care organizations perform work that directly affects other people, great potential exists for designing jobs with high task significance. Yet by designing isolated jobs in which people cannot see how their work is an important part of a whole effort that helps other people, one can create jobs low in all three core dimensions.

Experienced responsibility for work outcomes is directly affected by the degree of autonomy in a job. The components of autonomy are freedom and discretion in scheduling work and in determining procedures to be used in performing it. A considerable degree of autonomy is present in jobs falling into Galbraith's (1977) categories of "effort above minimum levels," "spontaneous and innovative behavior," and "cooperative behavior."

Feedback on work performance provides an individual with the third psychological dimension, knowledge of results. The most direct feedback is from the work itself, available primarily in situations in which an individual has responsibility for a whole and identifiable element of work. Where job design itself cannot provide direct feedback, it is important to obtain feedback from supervisors or peers.

An additional potential source of feedback is an organization's performance evaluation system. In some organizations, performance evaluation is based solely on the subjective appraisal of an employee's supervisor. In others, however, it is based upon achievement of measurable goals. To the extent the goals for assessment of an individual align with the organization's goals, the individual's efforts can be directed at achievement of the organization's goals, in addition to serving as a feedback mechanism. In some organizations, the goals used for performance evaluation are goals of the program or department for which the individual has a major share of responsibility (Kotch et al., 1986).

To some degree, skill variety, task identity, and task significance can substitute for one another because they all contribute additively to experienced meaningfulness. Together they combine multiplicatively with autonomy (experienced responsibility) and feedback (knowledge of results) in contributing to the overall **motivating potential of a job.** A job's motivating potential score (MPS) can be expressed as follows (Hackman et al., 1975):

$$MPS = 1/3 \text{ (Skill Variety + Task Identity} + \text{Task Significance)} \times \text{Autonomy} \times \text{Feedback}$$

Whether a job with a high MPS will actually result in high individual motivation depends upon the characteristics of the jobholder. People with high growth needs—strong needs for achievement, self-actualization, and personal development—will be most motivated by jobs with high motivating potential. It is also possible for people who do not have high growth needs to find their growth needs stimulated by jobs with a high MPS. On the other hand, not all people react positively to challenging jobs, and the autonomy and challenge may result instead in anxiety and low performance. Individuals also differ in their preferences for working individually versus

working in groups, or for routine versus innovative work. Fit between an individual's preferences for work and the organization's preferred mode of working results in greater job satisfaction (Chatman, 1991).

When people successfully accomplish work that satisfies their needs, job satisfaction is experienced. This in turn contributes to the expectation that future performance will result in satisfaction, and high levels of motivation generally result. Satisfaction, however, can result from meeting other needs, either within or outside of the workplace, but without contributing to motivation or to job performance. For example, satisfaction results from meeting one's social needs in the work setting. Although meeting the social needs of one's staff may increase satisfaction and even reduce turnover, it will not necessarily result in high motivation or performance.

TECHNICAL APPROACH

The technical approach is based on the scientific management school of thought developed by Taylor (1911) and Gilbreth (1911). Scientific management had its genesis in manufacturing organizations and led to the development of industrial engineering. Through examination of job activities in time-and-motion studies, industrial engineers design jobs to most efficiently utilize technology and to minimize wasted human effort. Within a technologically driven work setting, workers most suitable to the jobs are selected and trained. Through experience, workers become more proficient at their jobs, and thus specialization and routinization of work activities attempt to take advantage of the individual's learning curve. Since an objective of this approach is elimination of extraneous activities, its success depends on ensuring that people perform the job as designed.

Scientific management has made important contributions to management, especially in heavy industries such as the U.S. automobile industry. Scientific-management approaches have gone beyond manufacturing settings, however, and have made contributions to both inpatient and ambulatory health care settings.

There are three assumptions underlying the scientific-management approach to job design:

1. Work can be divided into repetitive routine elements.
2. Workers can be trained and motivated to perform dependably.
3. Workers' motivation derives primarily from economic rewards that can be associated with reliable performance of the work, rather than from job design itself.

Although these assumptions have face validity in many situations, they are also inherently limiting. Often the work cannot be divided into elements that can be repetitively performed. In addition, workers frequently seek more than economic rewards from their work and react to routine repetitive jobs by not performing dependably or by quitting the job. From a purely economic perspective, the cost of repeated recruiting and training often exceeds the benefits believed to be gained from technological efficiency. In human terms, the inefficiency and potential for errors that might harm patients are increased.

The routine nature of many jobs in support services in hospitals and other care settings, such as transport, laboratory, laundry, and radiology, allows job activities to be studied from a scientific-management perspective. However, systems designed in this manner are tailored to meet specific conditions and are inherently unresponsive to change or uncertainty. Since patient needs and emergencies are not always subject to specification, employees at *all* levels of a health care organization are frequently required to use their own judgment, which limits the usefulness of scientific-management principles.

The **task inventory approach to work design is** a more flexible version of the technical approach and is often used in studies of jobs of health professionals, especially nurses, physicians, and physician assistants. In the mid-1960s, a shortage of health workers was predicted in the United States. In response, the task inventory methodology was developed in order to categorize job activities and determine whether parts of a professional's job might be performed by other workers (Braun, Howard, & Pond, 1972; Nelson, Jacobs, & Breer, 1975; *The utilization of man power*, 1975). Kane and Jacoby (1973), for example, demonstrated the feasibility of using physician assistants

(Medex) for job activities not requiring a fully trained physician. The same methodology is currently the basis for studies seeking to determine the costs of nursing and other care activities in response to hospital prospective payment, managed care, and continuing changes in health care financing.

In this tradition Gilpatrick (1977), for example, conducted the Health Services Mobility Study, identifying and analyzing tasks of health care workers and determining skills and knowledge needed to perform each task. This approach specified the required skills and knowledge of health care workers, thereby providing a basis for defining their educational needs. Common educational needs for various jobs and career ladders were developed by which individuals could advance not only upward but also across traditional disciplines. Curricula in many schools of allied health have been modified to produce multicompetent health professionals to work in health care settings (Beachey, 1988; Blayney, Wilson, Bamberg, & Vaughn, 1989; Hedrick, 1987; Russell, Richardson, & Escamilla, 1989).

In applying the task inventory approach, it is helpful to develop a table similar to that in Figure 7.2. Elements of work, or tasks, are listed in the first column. Then for each task, who currently performs the task is (are) listed in column 2, the knowledge and skills required are listed in column 3, and other individuals who perform the task or other jobs in which the task could be incorporated are listed in column 4. Additionally, the training required for the individuals is noted in column 4. The task inventory method provides a helpful approach to identifying tasks. When using this method, it is important not to overlook significant but difficult to observe aspects of work. Furthermore, this approach starts with a description of the status quo. To the extent that a set of jobs does not include important aspects of work that should be present, the analysis will be incomplete.

Unlike scientific management, the task inventory methodology does not assume that jobs are better if narrowly defined. The methodology could yield the recommendation that a given job should be either more narrowly or more broadly defined, based on skill and information requirements.

(1)	(2)	(3)	(4)
Task	Who Now Performs Task	Knowledge and Skills Required	Alternative Performers and Their Training Needs
1.			
2.			
3.			
4.			
5.			

Continue as needed.

Figure 7.2. Task Inventory.

The Interconnectedness of Work

Once tasks have been identified, it is necessary to determine how they fit together to form a coherent whole. While the psychological approach considers how tasks should be combined to improve worker motivation, the technical approach is to determine for each task the other tasks essential to its effective performance. Some tasks are more interconnected than others. At one extreme are tasks that can be performed independently of each other. For example, feeding one patient and performing laboratory tests on a specimen from another patient are independent tasks. In contrast, successful performance of other types of work requires that different tasks occur in sequence or that one element affects a second task that, in turn, acts upon the first task. For example, in medical diagnosis, initial diagnosis determines what laboratory and radiologic procedures are required. The results of those studies refine the original diagnosis. At the most complex level, tasks affect each other simultaneously. Van

de Ven, Dethecq, and Koenig (1976) have called this "team interdependence," while Thompson (1967) called it "reciprocal interdependence," exemplified by the administration of anesthesia and the performance of surgery on a patient.

The concept of **interconnectedness of work** is critical to effective work design. When interconnected elements of work are performed by different people, components must be coordinated to ensure effective performance. Coordination requires resources from the organization, such as development and use of plans and protocols, supervision of people responsible for interconnected elements, or discussion among those people. Where possible, therefore, it is most effective to design jobs to minimize spreading interconnected elements over several people. This model is not always feasible because elements are often too numerous for a one-person assignment; because elements are so different from one another that no one individual has the skills, training, desire, or inclination to do them all; or because technological advantages outweigh costs of coordination. When the interconnected elements cannot reside within one single job, it is best to organize work to contain the interconnected elements within a single work group (Charns & Schaefer, 1983; Thompson, 1967).

It is often the interconnectedness of work that health care organizations fail to address as they attempt to respond to the pressures of a competitive health care system. Efforts to improve institutional responsiveness through reorganization, continuous quality improvement, and other measures must address how the elements of work fit together and how they influence job design and performance.

Coordinating Interconnected Work within Units

Coordination of work has been the subject of considerable research. How to achieve coordination among interconnected tasks within a single unit is the subject of this section. Additional aspects of coordination are considered in Chapter 8.

Much research has shown, in health care and other settings, that coordination affects organizational performance (Argote, 1982; Duncan, 1973; Georgopoulis & Mann, 1962; Shortell et al., 1994; Van de Ven et al.,

1976). Knaus, Draper, Wagner, and Zimmerman (1986) found that variations in mortality in critical care units were related to the level of coordination in the units. With the development of more refined measurement tools, this line of work continues to be advanced (Shortell, Rousseau, Gillies, Devers, & Simons, 1991). Recently Young et al. (1998) found the pattern of coordination among nurses, surgeons, and anesthesiologists to be related to risk-adjusted rates of postsurgical complications. In addition to clinical outcomes, some studies have found a link between coordination and outcomes such as greater patient satisfaction and shorter lengths of stay (Gittell, 1998). These performance outcomes are increasingly relevant in a more cost-conscious, patient-centered health care environment.

But research also shows that the most effective way of achieving coordination varies with the characteristics of the work performed. Duncan (1973), for example, provided one of the first empirical studies of variation in coordination within work units, finding that work units change their patterns of interaction in response to differing levels of task uncertainty. Building upon the theoretical work of March and Simon (1958) and Van de Ven et al. (1976) found variations in patterns of coordination among units facing different levels of task uncertainty.

Charns, Stoelwinder, Miller, and Schaefer (1981) and Charns and Schaefer (1983) extended the findings of Van de Ven et al. (1976) and the theoretical writings of Mintzberg (1979) to suggest that work groups use two primary approaches to coordination—programming and feedback—and that the use of these approaches is related to the effectiveness of patient care units. Charns and Strayer (1981) replicated these findings in a residential school for severely emotionally disturbed children.

The set of **programming approaches to coordination** includes three ways of standardizing the performance of work that are most effective when the work is well understood and programmable.

- Standardization of work processes is the use of rules, regulations, schedules, plans, procedures, policies, and protocols to specify the activities to be performed. Included are care plans and multidisciplinary clinical critical paths, which specify

for a particular patient condition the interventions required and anticipated results at various times.

- Standardization of skills is the specification of the training or skills required to perform work. Often this is achieved through specification of minimum levels and types of education, certification as evidence of meeting minimum qualifications, or on-the-job training.
- Standardization of output specifies the form of intermediate outcomes of work as they are passed from one job to another.

In situations of high uncertainty, programming approaches alone cannot provide the needed coordination. Exchange of information and feedback is needed. **Feedback approaches to coordination,** which facilitate the transfer of information in unfamiliar situations, include the following:

- Supervision is the basis for coordination through an organization's hierarchy. It is the exchange of information between two people, one of whom is responsible for the work of the other.
- Mutual adjustment is the exchange of information about work performance between two people who are not in a hierarchical relationship, such as between two nurses, between a nurse and a physician, or between a case manager and other care providers.
- Group coordination is the exchange of information among more than two people, such as through meetings, rounds, and conferences.

Feedback approaches to coordination are more time consuming and require more effort than programming approaches. However, they are needed in situations characterized by high levels of uncertainty. Evidence indicates that higher-performing patient care units in teaching hospitals differ from lower-performing units in their greater use of all six types of **coordinating mechanisms** (Charns et al., 1981). High-performing units utilize plans, rules, procedures, and protocols not as constraints and organizational red tape but as guidelines for routine work. Contrary to previous research findings, effective use of programming approaches actually allows staff—especially nurses—greater discretion in their work.

In addition, when faced with unfamiliar situations, the higher-performing units increase their use of feedback approaches to a greater extent than the lower-performing ones. This result is consistent with findings from an earlier study of emergency rooms that nonprogrammed approaches to coordination were more effective under conditions of high uncertainty. A more recent study shows, however, that even for relatively straightforward procedures such as joint replacements, greater use of feedback approaches significantly improves coordination (Gittell, 1998). Programmed mechanisms such as care paths appeared to be effective only when used in the context of feedback mechanisms.

Feedback mechanisms in particular rely on strong relationships among physicians, nurses, and other health care providers who must coordinate their efforts; but such relationships are not often achieved in health care organizations. Nursing staff turnover and rotation, house staff rotation, and limited physicians' and other professionals' involvement in a unit or a remote care setting greatly hinder the development of such relationships and can prevent full use of feedback approaches to coordination. But other aspects of organization design can strengthen these relationships. One study found that staff relationships are better in hospitals where staff are selected for their teamwork skills, and where processes are established for resolving conflicts among staff members involved in the care of a given patient population (Gittell, 1998).

To summarize, coordination affects both the quality and efficiency of organizational performance. Second, the types of coordinating approaches that can be used effectively depend somewhat upon the nature of the work of the unit. Greater advantage can be taken of programming approaches when the work of the unit is limited in scope and uncertainty, though even then programming appears to work better in tandem with feedback approaches. It should be noted that people with greater experience in a particular job will encounter fewer unfamiliar situations than people with less experience. The people with less experience, therefore, need to use feedback approaches to a greater extent than do highly experienced people. This is typically reflected in their greater reliance on discussions with their manager or peers. Finally, feed-

back approaches require trust and understanding among people, which in turn requires organizational practices such as consistency in working together, conflict-resolution processes, or selection of staff members who are skilled at teamwork.

SUMMARY OF CONTRASTING APPROACHES

Both approaches to job design explored in this chapter—psychological and technical—reflect the belief that job design affects organizational performance; but they have different views on how job design affects organizational performance. According to the psychological approach, design can improve organizational performance by increasing worker motivation. According to the technical approach, job design can improve organizational performance by improving the flow of information among interconnected jobs. Figure 7.3 depicts this essential difference between the two approaches.

In reality, job design may improve performance through both paths. When coordination is not fully achieved, work performance is hindered due to both technical and psychological factors. In addition to having a direct negative effect on patient care, the failure to coordinate precludes people who perform the work from attaining the levels of achievement or obtaining the sense of competence that would satisfy their needs. Professionals often feel that they are prevented from effectively carrying out their professional work by the ineffective way their organization func-

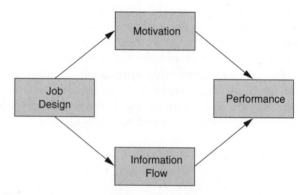

Figure 7.3. Assumptions of Causality in Psychological and Technical Approaches to Work Design

tions. Where organizational factors hinder work accomplishment, people come to believe that hard work will not result in the desired outcome of good patient care. Using the expectancy model of motivation, the probability that effort will result in the desired outcome is low, and thus the motivation to work hard is reduced. Despite the satisfaction derived from their broadly defined, autonomous jobs, professionals may be dissatisfied by the difficulty of coordinating their work with others to achieve good patient care.

Effective work design therefore requires taking multiple perspectives based upon the analysis of work itself. In **designing individual jobs,** the work requirements should be matched to each workers' needs. To the extent possible, interconnected elements of work should be combined into individual jobs that possess high levels of skill variety, task identity, task significance, autonomy, and feedback. The design of individual jobs must be done within a framework that considers other related jobs, including that of the supervisor.

Given the pressure to achieve both efficient and high-quality health care, it is more important than ever for managers to examine work design. How a health care manager chooses to do this is influenced by the range of approaches to work design and their conflicting underlying assumptions. But the failures of job redesign too often have been caused by taking too narrow and restrictive a focus. When managers become believers in one or another approach to job design, they limit their effectiveness and the opportunity to integrate a variety of approaches for maximum advantage. In the multifaceted health care system of today, no one approach can guarantee success.

APPLYING THE FRAMEWORK

Work design concepts introduced in this chapter provide a framework for analyzing Units A and B (described in "In the Real World") and determining options for change. Both units changed from a functional nursing organization to primary nursing. In the functional organization, each nurse performed one or at most a few related functions, such as administering medications, providing physical care, or taking vital signs, to a large number of patients. Following the traditions of scientific management, this approach attempted to use the personnel efficiently and in line with their education.

DEBATE TIME 7.2: WHAT DO YOU THINK?

In applying the work design concepts to the redesign of patient care delivery systems, two conflicting perspectives typically are raised. On the one hand, heads of existing support departments such as dietary, environmental services, and patient transport argue that staff efficiency can be maximized when staff performing similar activities are organized into separate functional departments. The staff can then be assigned to different patient care units in response to the varying needs of those units. This provides both the most efficient utilization of staff and responsiveness to fluctuations in need for services among patient care units. In addition, when organized in this manner, staff can best maintain proficiency in their particular skill area, thereby assuring the quality of their services.

On the other hand, nurse managers and directors of clinical units argue that multiskilled employees, cross-trained in several functional areas, should be permanently assigned to individual units. Having a broad range of skills reduces fragmentation of delivery of care and allows for flexibility in meeting the varying needs of each unit. By working consistently with the same group of other employees, the multiskilled workers can become part of the patient care team and be most responsive to the unique needs of their units.

Which of these perspectives is correct? If you choose to implement one of these approaches, how do you address the needs expressed by proponents of the other approach? Can you incorporate both perspectives in another creative work design? If so, how?

Primary nursing, used on both units, provides staff more responsibility and broader professional roles. Jobs of primary nurses inherently have greater skill variety, task identity, autonomy, and feedback than functional nursing and, therefore, have higher motivational potential. While a primary nurse is at work, most of the interconnected elements of nursing work reside within his or her job. These benefits often outweigh the costs of having highly skilled nurses do routine tasks. Primary nursing thus has both psychological and technical advantages over the traditional approach to nursing job design.

Components of patient care performed by different staff on a unit are highly interconnected. In different ways and with different success, both units used coordinating mechanisms to address these interconnections. Both utilized patient care paths, although on Unit B they were used in conjunction with, rather than as substitutes for, feedback mechanisms such as interdisciplinary rounds. Unit A had eliminated interdisciplinary rounds on the belief that they consumed too much staff time, but more staff and patient time was wasted as a result. Exceptions to the care path were not addressed and resolved in a timely, systematic way, requiring staff to spend much unnecessary time resolving these issues on the unit. Meanwhile, patients were left wondering about their status, and target discharge dates were missed.

Unit B continued to hold interdisciplinary rounds even after adopting care paths, on the belief that exceptions would arise even for patients underdoing routine treatments, and would require a dependable forum for their resolution. Holding rounds twice weekly and involving a broad range of staff members was costly in staff time, but was believed to save more staff time on balance. Unit B administrators also felt patients were better informed as a result of interdisciplinary rounds, therefore reducing patient complaints about conflicting information, and were more likely to be discharged on their target date, therefore satisfying payor needs for efficient resource utilization.

On Unit A, the administration thought that, since primary nurses had total responsibility for their patients, case managers could handle larger patient loads. On Unit B, both the primary nursing patient load and the case-management patient load were significantly smaller, allowing primary nurses and case managers to allocate more of their time to coordinating information flow on a personal basis with physicians and other members of the hospital staff. In addition, the broad range of responsibilities included in the Unit B case manager's job, and the combination of nursing and social work skills achieved through team staffing, made Unit B case managers the lynchpin for coordination of patient care on the unit.

Hospital administrators for Unit A also believed that supervision could be reduced as a result of primary nursing and case management. Thus, the head nurse's responsibilities were expanded to cover several units. Physically removed from the unit, the head nurse gave insufficient attention to professional development of new and junior staff. The head nurse did not effectively orient new nursing and medical staff to the unit's routines, and standardized approaches to coordination broke down. Due to her wide span of control, the head nurse was also unable to effectively coach Unit A nurses on coordinating exceptions to the care path with other staff members.

It was expected that primary nurses would coordinate their work with other members of the nursing and medical staffs, but Unit A's organizational arrangements hindered coordination. Nursing assignments were arranged almost randomly, so that a consistent pattern of interactions among staff members that would encourage strong working relationships did not develop. This hindered use of personal approaches to coordination among nurses. It also made it difficult for a nurse providing care for another's patient to be involved or to identify with the patient, thereby limiting the motivating potential inherent in those efforts. Interactions with house staff also did not follow any consistent pattern, and each house officer had patients cared for by many different primary nurses. Whereas before implementation of primary nursing many house officers depended upon the head nurse to function as the coordinating link between themselves and the staff nurses caring for their patients, under the new arrangement they had to seek out several different primary nurses. Usually they did not bother to do so. Over time the trust between the nursing and medical staff members on Unit A deteriorated.

On Unit B, the internal organization of nursing into two groups provided a basis for facilitating coordination both among nurses and between nurses and physicians. The small size of each nursing group and the arrangement for associates to cover for primary nurses within their group allowed nurses to identify with their group's patients. This contributed to the motivating potential of their jobs. Furthermore, the work interconnections among nurses were contained within each group. This facilitated management of these interconnections and contributed to development of trust needed among nursing staff for effective personal coordination. Each group included a mix of experienced and less experienced nurses, and together with the head nurse, the formally designated group leader had responsibility for staff development. By aligning teams of house staff and case managers with the nursing groups, the organization facilitated coordination.

As physicians, nurses, and case managers worked together on Unit B, trust among the groups developed, adding to their ability to use mutual adjustment to coordinate their efforts. All of the staff experienced a greater sense of accomplishment, contributing to their satisfaction and motivation. Because of the closeness and commitment of the personnel to other members of their group, they felt a sense of responsibility for the unit. Absenteeism was therefore low, and the more stable staffing in turn contributed to the unit's smooth functioning. The head nurse considered house staff orientation to be a critical responsibility, and this further contributed to the unit's ability to coordinate its work. Staff and physicians were chosen explicitly for their willingness to work as part of a team, and conflicts were regularly addressed in a weekly problem-solving meeting involving all key disciplines.

In the late 1980s, Unit B introduced multiskilled employees to perform routine work that had been done by staff from several departments. To utilize these staff efficiently, they cared for patients of both teams, which did not allow them to be fully integrated into the teams. By being assigned to a single unit, however, they did feel a part of that unit. Performing many tasks for each patient, the multiskilled employees were responsive to patient needs. They saw the results of their efforts and gained much greater satisfaction from their work than had been the case when many people from different departments did those tasks. Multiskilled workers also contributed to patient satisfaction by reducing the number of staff going into each patient's room. Overall, Unit B addressed its work requirements more effectively than Unit A.

As the examples demonstrate, several factors must be considered to design productive work units consisting of inherently motivating and rewarding jobs. The basis for this design is **analyzing the work** itself. The content of individual jobs, the organization of work units, and the coordination of work both within and between units can be designed effectively only when the work requirements are understood. Just as the framework presented in this chapter was used to analyze the jobs of health professionals on two different patient care units, it can be used to design work in other settings.

Discussion Questions

1. Under what conditions does a job with a high motivating potential lead to high jobholder motivation? To high satisfaction? To frustration?
2. What are the potential pitfalls in job redesign?
3. Give examples of highly motivated people who do not contribute greatly to organizational outcomes.
4. What is the relationship among individual motivation and satisfaction and an organization's ability to coordinate work?
5. Give examples of situations in which dependable role performance is required in a job, but effort above minimum levels is not. What happens when individuals in such jobs innovate? Give examples of jobs requiring cooperative behavior. What happens when people in such jobs are willing to give only dependable role performance?
6. Under what conditions are programming approaches to coordination constraints to effective performance? Under what conditions are they facilitating? When are feedback approaches to coordination inappropriate?

MANAGERIAL GUIDELINES

1. Jobs should be designed with both technical (information) and psychological (motivation) considerations in mind, taking account of the work itself as well as the subjective experience of working. These design considerations are relevant for both technical and professional jobs, and for jobs involving high or low uncertainty.

2. To enhance motivation, individual jobs should be designed to provide opportunities to satisfy the needs of the person performing a given job. People with high growth needs are more highly motivated by jobs providing experienced meaningfulness, experienced responsibility, and knowledge of results.

3. Work should be designed so that the most highly interconnected elements are contained within individual jobs to the extent that is possible, given considerations of size, limitations imposed by technology, and separation of job elements in time and space. Interconnected work elements that cannot be self-contained within single jobs should to the extent possible be placed within single work groups.

4. Coordination of interconnected work elements that are not contained within a single job directly affects work performance. This coordination generally can be facilitated most effectively through a combination of programming (standardization) and feedback (personal) approaches. Feedback approaches require strong relationships among those who use them.

References

Argote, L. (1982). Input uncertainty and organizational coordination in hospital emergency units. *Administrative Science Quarterly, 27,* 420–434.

Beachey, H. W. (1988, November). Multi-competent health professionals: Needs, combinations, and curriculum development. *Journal of Allied Health,* 319–329.

Blayney, K. D., Wilson, B. R., Bamberg, R., & Vaughn, D. (1989, Winter). The multiskilled health practitioner movement: Where are we and how did we get here? *Journal of Allied Health,* 215–226.

Braun, J. A., Howard, D. R., & Pond, L. R. (1972). The physician's associate: A task analysis. *Physician's Associate, 2*(3), 77–82.

Brider, P. (1992). The move to patient-focused care. *American Journal of Nursing, 9,* 26–33.

Charns, M. P., & Schaefer, M. J. (1983). *Health care. organizations: A model for management.* Englewood Cliffs, NJ: Prentice-Hall.

Charns, M. P., Stoelwinder, J. U., Miller, R. A., & Schaefer, M. J. (1981, August). Coordination and patient unit effectiveness. Presented at the Academy of Management Annual Meetings, San Diego, CA.

Charns, M. P., & Strayer, R. G. (1981, August). A socio-structural approach to organization development. Presented at the Academy of Management Annual Meetings, San Diego, CA.

Chatman, J. A. (1991). Matching people and organizations: Selection and socialization in public accounting firms. *Administrative Science Quarterly, 36,* (459–484).

Donnelly, L. (1989, March/April). NME's caregiver system: 21st century patient care delivery. *Healthcare Executive, 4*(2), 25–27.

Drucker, P. F. (1973). *Management: Tasks, responsibilities, practices.* New York: Harper & Row.

Duncan, R. B. (1973). Multiple decision-making structures in adapting to environmental uncertainty: The impact on organizational effectiveness. *Human Relations, 26*(3), 273–291.

Galbraith, J. R. (1977). *Organization design.* Reading, MA: Addison-Wesley.

Georgopoulis, B. S., & Mann, F. C. (1962). *The community general hospital.* New York: Macmillan.

Gilbreth, F. B. (1911). *Motion study.* New York: Van Nostrand.

Gilpatrick, E. (1977). *The health services mobility study.* Springfield, VA; National Technical Information Service.

Gittell, J. H. (1998). Organization design, networks and outcomes: A study of patient care coordination, Harvard Business School working paper, Cambridge, MA.

Hackman, J. R., Janson, R., Oldham, G. R., & Purdy, K. (1975). A new strategy for job enrichment. *California Management Review, 17*(4), 57–71.

Hedrick, H. L. (1987, August). Closing in on cross-training. *Journal of Allied Health,* 265–275.

Kane, R., & Jacoby, I. (1973, November). Alterations in tasks in the physicians office as a result of adding a Medex. Presented at American Public Health Associates Meeting, San Francisco, CA.

Knaus, W. A., Draper, E. A., Wagner, D. P., & Zimmerman, J. E. (1986). An evaluation of outcome from intensive care in major medical centers. *Annals of Internal Medicine, 104,* 416–418.

Kotch, J. B., Burr, C., Toal, S., Brown, W., Abrantes, A., & Kaluzny, A. (1986). A performance-based management system to reduce prematurity and low birth weight. *Journal of Medical Systems, 10*(4), 375–390.

March, J. G., & Simon, H. A. (1958). *Organizations.* New York: John Wiley & Sons.

McClelland, D. C. (1975). *The achievement months* (2nd ed.). New York: Halsted Press.

Miller, E. J. (1959). Technology, territory and time: The internal differentiation of complex production systems. *Human Relations, 12*(3), 243–272.

Mintzberg, H. (1979). *The structuring of organizations.* Englewood Cliffs, NJ: Prentice-Hall.

Nelson, E., Jacobs, A., & Breer, D. (1975). A study of the validity of the task inventory method of job analysis. *Medical Care, 13*(2), 104–113.

Porter, I. W., & Lawler E. E., III. (1968). *Managerial attitudes and performance.* Homewood, IL: Irwin-Dolsey.

Russell, D. D., Richardson, R. F., & Escamilla, B. (1989, Spring). Multicompetency education in radiologic education. *Journal of Allied Health,* 281–289.

Shortell, S. M., Rousseau, D. M., Gilles, R. R., Devers, K. J., & Simons, T. L. (1991). Organizational assessment in intensive care units (ICUs): Construct development, reliability, and validity of the ICU nurse-physician questionnaire. *Medical Care, 29*(8), 709–727.

Shortell, S. M., Zimmerman, J., Rousseau, D., Gillies, R., Wagner, D., Draper, E., Knaus, W., & Duffy, J. (1994). The performance of intensive care units: Does good management make a difference? *Medical Care, 32*(5).

Simon, H. A. (1976). *Administrative behavior* (3rd ed.). New York: Free Press.

Stoelwinder, J. U., & Charns, M. P. (1981). A task field model of organization design and analysis. *Human Relations, 34*(9), 743–762.

Strengthening hospital nursing. A program to improve patient care—gaining momentum: A progress report. (1992). St. Petersburg, FL: National Program Office of the Strengthening Hospital Nursing Program.

Taylor, F. W. (1911). *The principles of scientific management.* New York: Harper & Row.

Thompson, J. D. (1967). *Organizations in action.* New York: McGraw-Hill.

Tonges, M. C. (1989). Redesigning hospital nursing practice: The professionally advanced care team (ProACT) model, Part 1. *Journal of Nursing Administration, 19*(7), 31–38.

The utilization of man power in ambulatory care: Development of a study methodology. (1975). Bureau of Health Manpower Education. Report of a Cooperative Study.

Van de Ven, A. H., Dethecq, A. L., & Koenig R., Jr. (1976). Determinants of coordination modes within organizations. *American Sociological Review, 41,* 322–338.

Vroom, V. H. (1961). *Work and motivation.* New York: John Wiley & Sons.

Young, G., Charns, M., Desai, K., Khuri, S., Forbes, M., Henderson, W., & Daley, J. (1998, December, Part I). Patterns of coordination and clinical outcomes: A study of surgical services. *Health Services Research, 33*(5), 1211–1236.

C H A P T E R

8

Coordination and Communication

Beaufort B. Longest, Jr., Ph.D.
Gary J. Young, J.D., Ph.D.

Chapter Outline

- Interdependence
- Coordination
- Communication

Learning Objectives

After completing this chapter the reader should be able to:

1. Differentiate between pooled, sequential, and reciprocal interdependence.
2. Differentiate between intraorganizational and interorganizational coordination.
3. Know a variety of coordination mechanisms used in intraorganizational and interorganizational settings.
4. Understand the importance of applying various coordinating mechanisms to a given situation using a contingency approach.
5. Know how to diagram the communication process and discuss its components.
6. Know ways to make communication more effective.
7. Know the environmental and personal barriers to communication, and ways to overcome them.
8. Understand the flows of intraorganizational communication, and know their uses.
9. Understand important aspects of communicating with two external stakeholders: the public sector and the community.
10. Understand the relationship between conducting stakeholder analysis and effective communication with external stakeholders.

Key Terms

Communication
Communication Channels
Communication Networks
Contingency View of Coordination
Coordination
Clinical Guidelines or Protocols
Critical Pathways
Direct Supervision
Environmental Barriers to Communication
Feedback
Informal Communication
Interdependence
Integrators
Linking Pins
Mutual Adjustment
Outcomes Assessments
Personal Barriers to Communication
Pooled Interdependence
Programming
Project-Management Design
Reciprocal Interdependence
Sequential Interdependence
Standardization of Work Outputs
Standardization of Work Processes
Standardization of Worker Skills

Chapter Purpose

Coordination and **communication** are closely related strategies through which managers link together the various people and units within their organization and link their organization to other organizations and agencies. Central to understanding the importance of communication and coordination strategies is an appreciation of the high level of interdependence exhibited by health care organizations. Interdependencies exist in both their internal structure and external relationships. Because health care organizations have become increasingly complex internally and have established a wide variety of external relationships, the establishment and maintenance of effective linkages are significant managerial challenges. If linkages are not effective, organizations may become

fragmented, fractionated, and isolated with concomitant declines in performance.

The purpose of this chapter is to explore the managerial challenges associated with coordination and communication and to examine effective strategies for meeting these challenges. As demonstrated by Advocate Health Care, (see In the Real World on following page) a number of approaches are available to achieve effective communication and coordination.

INTERDEPENDENCE

The need for both coordination and communication arises from interdependencies among the people and units within an organization or among organizations pursuing a common goal. Such interdependencies exist within and among organizations whenever work activities are interconnected in some manner physically or intellectually (Charns & Tewksbury, 1993). The degree of **interdependence** varies with the nature of the work requirements as well as the relative roles, responsibilities, and contributions of those performing the work itself (Van de Ven, Delbecq, & Koenig, 1976). Thompson (1967) has identified three forms of interdependence: pooled, sequential, and reciprocal.

Pooled interdependence occurs when individuals and units are related but do not bear a close connection; they simply contribute separately in some way to the larger whole. For example, a group of geographically dispersed nursing homes owned by a single corporation may be viewed as linked largely in the sense that each contributes to the overall success of the corporation, but they have very little direct interdependence. Their activities are pooled to make the corporation more effective.

Sequential interdependence occurs when individuals and units bear a close, but sequential, connection. For example, patients admitted to an acute care hospital become the focal points for extended chains of sequentially interdependent activities. The admitting office checks them in and schedules them in the operating room or other diagnostic and treatment units, notifies the dietary department of special needs, notifies the laboratory of the need for tests, and so on. Most of what is done for the patients until they are discharged occurs in a sequential manner.

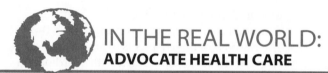

IN THE REAL WORLD:
ADVOCATE HEALTH CARE

Advocate Health Care in Park Ridge, Illinois, is the product of a 1995 merger between Evangelical Health System (EHS) and Lutheran General Health System (LGHS). This system was identified in a major longitudinal study of integrated health care systems as one that demonstrated significant progress in achieving functional integration, which is defined as "the extent to which key support functions such as financial management, human resources, information systems, strategic planning, and total quality management are coordinated across the operating units of a given system so as to add the greatest overall value to the system" (Shortell, Gillies, Anderson, Erickson-Morgan, & Mitchell, 1996, p. 30).

The efforts of this system to achieve functional integration have been described by Marjorie A. Satinsky (1998, pp. 151–152) as follows:

Before the merger, EHS looked carefully at the way in which its separate operating components functioned as a system and identified opportunities for improvement. These included development of a system culture, clear communication of the goals and processes of integration, introduction of financial incentives based on system performance, and use of programs on diversity in the workplace. The CQI/TQM [con-

tinuous quality improvement/total quality management] process was an important part of the effort. Using CQI/TQM methods, EHS developed training programs on system mission, values, and standards. These programs were targeted at all levels of employees and permitted people in different operational units to participate in shared learning experiences. Eventually, these educational programs were formalized into EHS University, enabling employees to earn continuing education unit credits. At a senior level, financial incentives were related to systemwide performance.

Since the merger of EHS and LGHS, Advocate has continued to focus on functional integration, addressing conceptual, economic, and cultural factors. To some extent it has had to go backward before it moves forward. Features of the Advocate approach to functional integration are regional management teams located at corporate headquarters, programs directed toward development of physician executives, asset merger and consolidation of financials, creation of a single board, and creation of a "super" PHO [physician-hospital organization] to which local PHOs relate.

Reciprocal interdependence occurs when individuals and units bear a close relationship, and the interdependence goes in both directions. For example, a vertically integrated health care system with acute care and long-term care capacity exhibits reciprocal interdependence. The long-term care beds are occupied by patients referred from the acute care beds. The acute care unit releases certain patients to the long-term care unit and suffers if long-term care cannot accept a patient. Conversely, the long-term care unit suffers if patients are not discharged to it from the acute unit. Further, the long-term care unit may need to transfer patients back to the hospital when acute episodes of illness occur. The interdependence between these units is reciprocal.

The level of interdependence intensifies as its form moves from pooled to sequential to reciprocal. In general, the higher the level of interdependence, the greater the need for managerial attention to effective linkages. Health care organizations generally exhibit very high levels of interdependence among their component parts, usually of the sequential or reciprocal forms. In highly interdependent health care organizations, coordination and communication are critical tasks for managers. These tasks are examined in depth below.

COORDINATION

Coordination is a means of dealing with interdependencies by effectively linking together the various parts of an organization or by linking together two or more organizations pursuing a common goal. This conscious activity is aimed at achieving unity and harmony of effort in pursuit of shared objectives, either within an organization or among organizations participating in a multiorganizational arrangement.

Coordination has long been viewed as one of the most important functions of management. One study found that "coordinating interdependent groups" was rated highly important by middle managers and executives and increased in importance as one moved into higher management positions (Kraut, Pedigo, McKenna, & Dunnette, 1989). Lawrence and Lorsch (1967), in a seminal study carried out more than 30 years ago with manufacturing firms, found that the effective coordination of interdependent units contributed substantially to better firm performance.

Much research also indicates that coordination plays an important role in the performance of health care organizations. Specifically, several studies of intensive care units have demonstrated that effective communication and coordination among clinical staff results in more efficient and better quality of care (Baggs, Ryan, Phelps, Richeson, & Johnson, 1992; Knaus, Draper, Wagner, & Zimmerman, 1986; Shortell et al., 1994). Recent studies of other health care delivery settings also indicate that effective coordination of staff leads to better clinical outcomes (Gittell & Wimbush, 1998; Young et al., 1997; Young et al., 1998). Additionally, research suggests that ineffective coordination and communication among hospital staff contributes substantially to adverse events. For example, one study of the care of 1,047 patients in a large tertiary care hospital found that approximately 15% of the 480 adverse events identified (e.g., failure to order indicated tests, misplaced test results) had causes related to the interaction of staff, such as the failure of a consultant team to communicate adequately with the requesting team (Andrews et al., 1997).

For many types of health care organizations, staff coordination is also relevant to their ability to comply with the requirements of regulatory bodies. The Joint Commission on the Accreditation of Health Care Organizations (JCAHO) (1997), which is the dominant accrediting body for hospitals in the United States, has accreditation standards that specifically address staff coordination. Other accrediting bodies, such as the National Committee on Quality Assurance, which accredits managed care organizations, also have standards addressing staff coordination.

Much of the general literature on coordination pertains to coordination within an organization, an intraorganizational perspective. An interorganizational perspective has become increasingly important within the health care industry with the rise of a wide variety of multiorganizational arrangements for providing patient care (also see Chapter 11). While much of what is known about intraorganizational coordination also applies to interorganizational coordination, there are important differences, and these will be discussed in a subsequent section.

Intraorganizational Coordination

From an intraorganizational perspective, coordination is a necessary response to the internal differentiation of organizations. Differentiation, in this context, is defined as "the state of segmentation of the organizational system into subsystems, each of which tends to develop particular attributes in relation to the requirements posed by its relevant environment (Scott, 1982). Organizational units are typically differentiated based on functions or disciplines relative to the organization's overall work activities. Organizations differentiate their units in these ways to handle the complexity of the work itself (Charns & Tewksbury, 1993). That is, through internal differentiation, staff can focus on a particular set of work activities for which they develop expertise. Thus health care organizations create specialized units for dealing with, for example, finance and human resources on the administrative side, and medicine, surgery, pediatrics, and so forth on the clinical side.

Within health care organizations, the degree of differentiation is particularly great, often reflecting the structure (discipline-based) of American medicine as a whole (Charns & Tewksbury, 1993). For instance, in a hospital there are the primary clinical departments of medicine, surgery, and neurology, each of which may be further differentiated into various subspecialities (e.g., cardiology within the department of medicine). Nursing homes and other institutional providers also tend to be differentiated based on either traditional clinical disciplines or functions.

However, the internal differentiation of health care organizations has also been undergoing some change to accommodate economic pressures and new developments in medical technology. For example, some managed care organizations, such as HMOs, are differentiated in part based on the practice setting of staff physicians (Diamond, Goldberg, & Janosky, 1998). Physicians are either based in a hospital and thus responsible for managing inpatient care services for HMO patients (sometimes called hospitalists) or based in ambulatory settings and thus responsible for managing outpatient care services for HMO patients. This type of inpatient/outpatient specialization for physician services, a relatively new concept in health care, reflects a growing need for health care organizations to manage inpatient care efficiently and at the same time maintain strong outpatient capabilities.

Clearly, the internal differentiation of an organization leads to substantial coordination requirements. For example, consider a hospital that is differentiated based on traditional clinical disciplines. If a patient's needs fit within a single clinical specialty (e.g., cardiology), this form of differentiation does not generate coordination requirements. However, when a patient's needs span two or more clinical specialties and the needs are interrelated (e.g., cardiology and pulmonary medicine), effective coordination between clinical specialties becomes necessary.

Similarly, consider the example of a managed care organization where physicians have specialized roles in relation to practice setting—inpatient or outpatient. To the extent that a patient requires only outpatient care, this form of differentiation does not in and of itself entail coordination requirements. But if a patient should require hospitalization, mechanisms for coordinating inpatient and outpatient care must be in place. These mechanisms are necessary to manage the hospital admission process and to ensure the effective and efficient exchange of clinical information between the physician responsible for the patient's inpatient care and the physician responsible for the patient's outpatient care.

It is thus important to recognize the interaction between the need for differentiated units and require-

ments for coordination. The more differentiation and specialization of labor, the greater the need for coordination.

Intraorganizational Mechanisms of Coordination

Managers use a variety of mechanisms to coordinate work activities. Several different conceptual frameworks have been developed for classifying these mechanisms. March and Simon (1958) identified two primary types of coordination: **programming** and **feedback.** Programming approaches to coordination seek to clarify work responsibilities and activities in advance of the performance of work, as well as to specify outputs of the work process and skills required. Programming approaches essentially standardize work activities for all expected requirements. By contrast, feedback approaches to coordination entail the exchange of information among staff, usually while the work is being carried out. These approaches permit staff to change or modify work activities in response to unexpected requirements and rely extensively on effective communication, which is discussed in the second half of this chapter.

Mintzberg (1983) elaborates on the March and Simon framework by identifying five coordination mechanisms. They are mutual adjustment, direct supervision, standardization of work processes, standardization of work outputs, and standardization of worker skills. Mutual adjustment and supervision are forms of feedback, while standardization of work processes, standardization of work outputs, and standardization skills are forms of programming. Figure 8.1 illustrates these coordinating mechanisms, which can be summarized as follows:

1. **Mutual adjustment** provides coordination by informal communications among individuals who are not in a hierarchical relationship to one another. Two physicians sharing information about a patient's clinical condition is an example of mutual adjustment.
2. **Direct supervision** is a way of coordinating work that occurs when someone takes responsibility for the work of others, including issuing them instructions and monitoring their actions. Direct supervi-

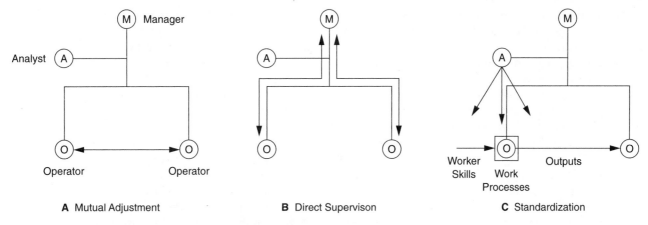

Figure 8.1. Mintzberg's Five Coordinating Mechanisms.
SOURCE: *Structure in Fives: Designing Effective Organizations* by Mintzberg, Henry, © 1993. Reprinted by permission of Prentice-Hall, Inc. Upper Saddle River, NJ.

sion entails some form of hierarchy within the organization. An example of direct supervision would be a nurse manager providing patient care instructions to a staff nurse.

3. **Standardization of work processes** is an alternative coordinating mechanism that programs or specifies the contents of work. Health care organizations standardize work processes when possible, such as standard admission and discharge procedures or standard methods of performing laboratory tests.

4. **Standardization of work outputs** specifies the product or expected performance, with the process of how to perform the work left to the worker.

5. **Standardization of worker skills** occurs when neither work processes nor output can be standardized. If standardization is to occur in such situations, it must be through worker training. This form is often found in health care organizations where the complexity of much of the work does not allow standardization of work processes or outputs. In such situations, standardization of worker skills and knowledge is an excellent coordinating mechanism. "When an anesthesiologist and a surgeon meet in the operating room to remove an appendix, they need hardly communicate; by virtue of their respective training, they know exactly what to expect of each other. Their

standardized skills take care of most of the coordination" (Mintzberg, 1979, pp. 6–7).

Other conceptual frameworks for coordination are similar to Mintzberg's, though some offer additional perspectives as well. For example, Hage (1980) has developed a framework that includes customs as a co-ordination mechanism. Many managers rely heavily upon the history and customs of their organizations as coordination mechanisms. For example, it may be customary in a particular nursing home to use the holiday season as an occasion to invite the families of residents into the facility for a meal and social interaction. Knowing this custom permits the various departments to begin their preparations for this event well in advance and facilitates the coordination of their various contributions to its success.

While organizations typically have some combination of these various coordination mechanisms in place, a critically important question for managers is which combination of mechanisms to use or emphasize in a given situation. Indeed, a particular mechanism or combination of mechanisms will achieve different levels of success depending upon characteristics of specific situations. This **contingency view of coordination** is very important for the reader to keep in mind; no single approach to coordination is best for all situations. A contingency approach to intraorganizational coordination requires that managers match the most appropriate coordinating mechanism or mechanisms to a given situation.

In general, programming approaches are relatively efficient to use, as they require little time for personal interaction. However, several factors reduce the utility of programming approaches in favor of greater emphasis on feedback approaches. *Task uncertainty* is perhaps the most important factor to consider. Task uncertainty refers to the variability of the work. As noted by Charns and Schaeffer (1983), if the work methods or processes are largely the same from day to day, most things can be planned for in advance. Different units can perform their work with only a few exceptions that require changes in the methods or processes. For example, the methods by which laboratory tests are ordered and carried out can be largely standardized. However, if work requirements are unpredictable, there will be greater need to establish feedback mechanisms to enable staff to modify or change methods as necessary.

The *degree of interdependency* among organizational units is also a relevant factor. Some research suggests that as interdependencies among units move from pooled to reciprocal, the ability of programming approaches to coordinate work becomes increasingly strained (Van de Ven et al., 1976). This limitation of programming approaches reflects the difficulty of anticipating and specifying all of the work activities in advance in situations of reciprocal interdependence. Accordingly, effective coordination may require a relatively heavy emphasis on feedback approaches.

Managers also need to consider the *size* of the organization. Larger organizations tend to be more differentiated internally; thus, the interdependencies among units are also likely to be greater. To the extent this is the case, coordination may require a substantial emphasis on feedback approaches (Van de Ven et al., 1976).

In recent years, health care organizations have been moving toward increased standardization of direct patient care activities. While health care managers have long relied heavily on the standardized skills of their staff, historically, they have not attempted to standardize the processes or outputs of direct patient care. This orientation to coordination reflects a long-standing sentiment that patient care is not amenable to such standardization (Flood, 1994; Kapp, 1990). Several considerations underlie this sentiment. First, task uncertainty in patient care is considered to be relatively high due to variability among patients' responses to medical interventions. Second, patient care also entails high levels of interdependencies because it requires input from a variety of clinical disciplines. Third, standardizing the outputs of patient care is difficult because the outputs themselves are not easily defined. Is the output, for example, the treatment of a patient's clinical condition? the prevention of a reoccurrence of the condition? or an improvement in the patient's quality of life?

This orientation to coordinating direct patient care appears to be changing. Today, efforts are being put forth to standardize work activities and outputs of direct patient care. This change in orientation is in large part a response to growing pressures on health care organizations to reduce resource utilization and to demonstrate the value of their services.

There are several approaches to standardizing the processes and outputs of patient care activities. One important approach is the use of **critical pathways.** Critical pathways, also known in health care circles as *clinical pathways, care maps,* and *critical paths,* originated in the manufacturing sector, where they have been used for identifying and managing steps in production processes. Applied to health care settings, "[c]ritical pathways are management plans that display goals for patients and provide the corresponding ideal sequence and timing of staff actions to achieve those goals with optimal efficiency" (Pearson, Goulart-Fischer, & Lee, 1995). Thus for a given diagnosis or condition, a critical pathway specifies the work activities in advance. Critical pathways are most often used for high-volume, high-cost conditions, such as coronary bypass graft procedures and dementia. The development of critical pathways (an example of which is shown in Figure 8.2) may entail a comprehensive review of the scientific literature to identify best practices for managing a clinical condition.

Clinical guidelines or protocols are also being used to standardize patient care processes. Clinical guidelines address the appropriateness of care by specifying the indications for either tests or treat-

M – Met
U – Unmet
N – Not applicable   Expected LOS: _____   DRG: _____   Date: _____

Shift/Day/Week	Days 5-8	M	U	N	Days 9-12	M	U	N	D/C Outcomes	M	U	N
Consults	• Psych test complete with verbal report (MD) • OT cognitive testing complete (AT)				• Psych test written report back				• Pt/Family will verbalize understanding of results of consult evaluations (T)			
Measurements/ Treatments					• Assessments for depression Possible psychosis, substance abuse Medical status, elimination pattern ADLs & Nutritional status complete (T)							
Tests					• Tests to R/O reversible cause complete (MD) • Appropriate lab work complete (MD)							
Activity/ Safety					• Sleep pattern stable (RN)				• Pt/Family will demonstrate knowledge of patient needs regarding mobility, self-care, and safety factors (T)			
Diet/ Hydration					• Nutrition/Hydration stable (RN)				• Pt/Family able to demonstrate knowledge of patient's nutritional needs (T)			
Medication					• Medication education complete • Establish D/C pharmacy needs				• Pt has stabilized on meds (T) • Pt is compliant w/ meds (T)			
Discharge Planning (Education, Psych/Soc, Homecare, etc.)					• Disposition finalized (SW) • Guardian eval complete (SW) • Support agency referrals complete (HHC, MOW) (T) • Output f/u in place (T) • D/C instructions given (T)				• Pt/Family demonstrates knowledge of f/w plan (T) • Pt/Family demonstrates knowledge of financial coverage (T)			
Special Needs: TX of conc med probs	• Problematic behaviors stable (T)								• Pt/Family demonstrates knowledge of advanced directive (T)			
Variance Facts/ Analysts												
Plan												
Signatures & initials												

Suicide Attempts: _____   Transfer to/from a med/surg unit _____   Re-admits: _____

Patient Falls: _____   Treatment of concurrent medical problems/diagnoses _____

Figure 8.2. Dementia Critical Path—Excerpt.
SOURCE: Medical Center Hospital of Vermont.

ments (Pearson et al., 1995). Thus, whereas critical pathways standardize the treatment approach for a given clinical condition, clinical guidelines standardize the decision process for adopting a treatment approach. Various government agencies and professional associations have been involved in the development of guidelines. These developmental efforts always involve a comprehensive review of relevant literature.

Another effort to standardize direct patient care is **outcomes assessments.** This is an effort to standardize the outputs of patient care through systematically collecting, monitoring, and reporting performance results. Through such assessments, managers from different organizations or units can detect and attend to undesirable variation in outputs (over time or relative to competitors) by changing or modifying work activities as needed. The selected outcomes essentially define the outputs. Thus, for example, outcomes assessments for inpatient care may focus on mortality and complication rates. For managed care organizations, outcomes assessments may include the percentage of enrollees who receive basic preventive services such as cholesterol screening. Outcomes assessments can also focus on the larger community for which a health care organization is considered accountable. Such outcomes might include the general health status of the population or the incidence of specific clinical conditions such as heart disease. Some regulatory bodies have developed profiles of the outcomes of health care organizations that are commonly called report cards (General Accounting Office, 1994).

How will these efforts to standardize direct patient care affect the quality of services health care organizations provide? Certainly there are concerns that efforts to standardize patient care will compromise quality by limiting the flexibility of providers to adapt to unexpected patient care requirements (Kapp, 1990). However, a recent study by Young et al. (1997) suggests that standardization efforts can improve patient care if they are accompanied by well-developed feedback mechanisms. They studied 44 surgical departments and found that departments that combined a relatively high emphasis on standardizing patient care activities with a relatively high emphasis on

feedback-type approaches had better surgical outcomes than their counterparts. Better-performing surgical departments standardized patient care activities when work requirements were well understood. For example, one surgical department developed and implemented a protocol to assist nurses in identifying patients at risk for pressure sores. Nurses would then hold a conference with the attending surgeon and a consulting physician from the department of medicine to consider appropriate prevention strategies. The protocol is a form of standardization of work, while the conference is a feedback mechanism.

Organizations can also establish various structural arrangements for facilitating coordination. For example, Lawrence and Lorsch (1967) found that well-coordinated organizations often rely upon individuals, whom they term **integrators,** to achieve coordination. Successfully playing an integrator role depends more on having professional competence than occupying a particular formal position. People are successful integrators because of specialized knowledge and because they represent a central source of information. Examples of effective integrators are found among all health professionals. In most health care organizations, individual nurses, regardless of formal position, often function as integrators linking physicians to the organization's formal administrative structure. These integrators often provide significant coordination among various departments and subunits, particularly as they relate to patient care.

Along similar lines, organizations may have people serve formally as "**linking pins**" between various units in the organization (Likert, 1967, p. 156). Horizontally, there are certain organizational participants who are members of two separate groups and serve as coordinating agents between the groups. On the vertical axis, individuals serve as linking pins between their level and those above and below. Thus, through this system of linking pins, the coordination necessary to make the dynamic system operate effectively is achieved. This forms a multiple overlapping group structure in the organization. Likert (1967, p. 167) notes:

> To perform the intended coordination well, a fundamental requirement must be met. The entire

organization must consist of a multiple, overlapping group structure with every work group using group decision-making processes skillfully. This requirement applies to the functional, product, and service departments. An organization meeting this requirement will have an effective interaction-influence system through which the relevant communications flow readily, the required influence is exerted laterally, upward, and downward, and the motivational forces needed for coordination are created.

The use of a **project-management design** is a structural means for coordinating a large amount of talent and resources for a given period on a specific project (Cleland & King, 1997). For example, a health care organization may wish to organize services into a comprehensive home health care program for the chronically ill by establishing a team organized around the focus of the program—home services for the chronically ill. Team members would be drawn from nursing, social services, respiratory therapy, occupational therapy, pharmacy, and physicians specializing in chronic disease. To market the program and to handle finance and reimbursement issues, expertise would be provided by team members drawn from the organization's administration. A project manager would be responsible for coordinating the activities of team members. In this situation, project organization would permit flexibility and facilitate coordination.

Health care organizations can use the project-management design by superimposing it on an existing functional departmental design. This can be done in a few selected areas or for the whole organization. As discussed in Chapter 10, when the entire organization is structured in this way, it is called a *matrix design.* Figure 10.6 is a matrix design for a psychiatric hospital in which functional managers head departments, and program or product line managers head major clinical programs or product lines. Notice that the individual worker depicted is a member of nursing *and* the Alzheimer's program. This coordination mechanism is very important when health care organizations move toward a product-line management orientation.

Health care organizations can also move completely to a program or product-line design for some or all of their activities (Charns & Tewksbury, 1993).

This design replaces the traditional functional departmental design with differentiated departments or specialized units according to program or product (sometimes referred to as "centers of excellence"). For example, a cancer center will bring together organizationally oncologists, surgeons, social workers, and other professional and technical staff whose roles and responsibilities focus on the care of cancer patients. Although this type of design potentially reduces some of the coordination requirements associated with a functional- or discipline-based design, it has problems and limitations that should be carefully considered. These issues are further considered in Chapter 7.

Other management approaches such as quality circles and cross-functional quality improvement teams also promote coordination. They rely on nominal group process, multicriteria decision making, cause-and-effect diagrams, and related problem-identification and problem-solving tools to improve communication, coordination, and ultimately the quality of work.

Interorganizational Coordination

As noted, interdependence is not limited to situations *within* organizations. Increasingly, health care organizations experience interdependencies with other health care organizations, as in the case of vertically integrated delivery systems (Longest, 1998b; Shortell et al., 1996). Such organizations require patient care to be coordinated across different settings and among health care providers with different educational backgrounds and training. Health care organizations also experience interdependencies with other elements in their external environments, such as various regulatory bodies, suppliers, third-party payors, and so on.

While many of the mechanisms discussed for managing intraorganizational coordination requirements also can be used to manage interorganizational coordination requirements as well, interorganizational coordination does raise special circumstances that must be considered. First, interorganizational arrangements bring together organizations that do not operate, at least not initially, under common ownership. Accordingly, a structural hierarchy (supervision in the previously discussed Mintzberg framework) for

DEBATE TIME 8.1: WHAT DO YOU THINK?

As we have seen, there are a number of intra-organizational coordination mechanisms, including supervision, standardization of work, customs, integrators, linking pins, and matrix organization. Utilizing a contingency approach, managers in health care organizations use various combinations of these mechanisms to achieve coordination; usually a number of them are used concurrently. Depending upon situations, various packages of these mechanisms might be appropriate.

Assume you are the president of a large teaching hospital and are concerned about coordinating the responsibilities and roles of the hospital's departments. Choose several coordination mechanisms

discussed above that you would emphasize in ensuring good coordination among the departments in your hospital. Be prepared to explain and defend why you think these are the most appropriate mechanisms.

Now, assume that you are the vice president for nursing services in the same hospital and are concerned about the level of coordination *within* nursing service. Again, choose several coordination mechanisms that have been discussed thus far that you would emphasize in ensuring good coordination within the nursing service. Be prepared to explain and defend why you think these are the most appropriate mechanisms for this purpose.

---

coordinating activities is not readily available. This presents a potentially significant barrier to effective coordination and, at a minimum, requires careful consideration of other available coordination mechanisms. Second, the interorganizational arrangement itself by design may be temporary, anticipating that the participating organizations will separate once a specific, mutual goal has been achieved. Kanter (1990) refers to such arrangements as opportunistic alliances and observes that they are often used as a means for the participating organizations to access new markets or develop new technological capabilities. But the ephemeral nature of these arrangements may be relevant to the types of coordination mechanisms that are appropriate.

Given these distinctions, it is important to consider the types of linkages and coordination mechanisms for managing interorganizational interdependencies specifically. These can range from straightforward buying and selling of goods and services between organizations as they seek to manage their interdependencies through market transactions, to the buying and selling of organizations themselves. In between is a number of more subtle strategies for managing interorganizational interdependencies. For example, Thompson (1967) developed a categorization of in-

terorganizational linkages including contracting, coopting, and coalescing. Pointer, Begun, and Luke (1988) have applied the concept of the quasifirm to the health care sector. Zuckerman and Kaluzny (1991) have examined interorganizational linkages from the construct of strategic alliances. Longest (1990) incorporates many of these categorizations into a typology of three general classes as summarized below.

Market Transactions

Market transactions involve focal organizations entering into relationships with other organizations in order to access product markets or obtain operational resources. This is perhaps the simplest form of linkage between organizations. It may entail nothing more than establishing an acceptable contract to purchase some needed item of supply or service or to provide services to a defined population as in an agreement with an HMO. At the more complex level, contracts permit a health care organization to establish stable and predictable (albeit interdependent) relationships with the federal government for reimbursement for Medicare patients, with state governments for reimbursement for Medicaid patients, and with commercial insurers and health plans for their subscribers or members. Contracts are formal agreements, usually negotiated, which define parameters of exchanges between two or more parties. Thus, they are widely used as a mechanism of coordination in a great variety of interorganizational relationships. Negotiation ability as discussed in Chapter 5 is the most important managerial skill for market transactions.

Voluntary Interorganizational Relationship Transactions

A second category of interorganizational linkages is distinguished by the voluntary dimension of the transactions. Horizontal and vertical systems, joint ventures, partnerships, various affiliations, consortia, and confederations are examples of voluntary interorganizational relationships. They can be further categorized as follows:

Co-opting

This form of linkage involves the absorption of leadership elements from other organizations into the focal organizations. In the health care industry, this coordination mechanism often takes one of two forms: management contracts and the placing of representatives of interdependent organizations on the focal organization's governing body.

Management contracts permit one organization to supply to another day-to-day management by agreement (Starkweather, 1981). Management includes at least the CEO, who reports to the governing body of the managed organization and to the managing organization. This is in contrast to the practice prevalent in many health care organizations of using outside contractors to manage individual departments and programs such as housekeeping, food service, or respiratory therapy.

The second co-opting mechanism for achieving interorganizational coordination is by appointment of significant representatives from external organizations to positions in the focal organization, usually the governing body. For example, a hospital system interested in access to capital may find considerable advantage in placing a banker on its governing body. Similarly, an HMO may find it advantageous to place members of its medical group on its board.

Coalescing

This linkage mechanism includes such forms as joint ventures, partnerships, consortia, and federations that occur when two or more organizations *partially* pool resources to pursue defined goals. This is often referred to as "loose coupling" and is characterized by interorganizational relationships in which interdependent and mutually responsive organizations are linked while preserving their legal identities and autonomies and much of their functional autonomy (Weick, 1976). Such linkages are stronger than those in market transactions, but less binding and less extensive than in a merger or acquisition.

Joint ventures, increasingly common among health care organizations, "can be predicted by considerations of resource interdependence, competitive uncertainty, and conditions that make various forms of interdependence more or less problematic (Pfeffer & Salanick, 1978). Shortell (1991) has described primary care group practices sponsored jointly by hospitals and physicians as one form of joint venture activity. A physician-hospital organization (PHO) is another common joint venture involving hospitals and physicians (Gorey, 1994). A PHO is typically jointly sponsored by a hospital and members of its medical staff for the purpose of securing managed care contracts. Major health care networks such as the Voluntary Hospitals of America and the American Health Care System explore joint venture relationships with health insurance providers to develop a range of new alternative delivery system products.

Trade associations are a particularly prevalent form of loosely coupled or coalesced structure in the health care industry. For example, the American Hospital Association has over 5,000 member organizations and has developed a sophisticated political/lobbying activity on behalf of its member hospitals. Similarly, there are regional and state hospital associations that base affiliation on a geographical or state community of interests. As states have become increasingly involved in regulation of the health care sector and in its reform, state hospital associations have increasingly undertaken important lobbying efforts. Associations serve other functions that help member organizations deal with their interdependencies; centralized information, research, and product definition are examples.

Quasifirm

Defined as "a loosely coupled, enduring set of interorganizational relationships that are designed to achieve purposes of substantial importance to the viability of participating members" (Luke, Begun, & Pointer, 1989), the quasifirm lies between market transactions and ownership arrangements. Quasifirms are similar to a true firm in relation to shared goals, mutual dependency, task subdivision and specialization, bureaucratic structures, and formal coordinating and control mechanisms. However, they are critically distinguished by their absence of ownership linkages.

The collaboration of an acute care general hospital, a large multispecialty group practice, a skilled nursing facility, and an insurance carrier for the purpose of designing, producing, and marketing a managed care product is an example of a quasifirm configuration. This arrangement, which might also be thought of as a virtual integrated delivery system, may be strategically important to the survival of the participants, but allows each to pursue independently other objectives as well (Pointer et al., 1988, p. 171).

Ownership

Critical to this category of interorganizational relationships is the voluntary nature of the ownership transaction. In recent years, there has been a growing number of cases when hospitals *voluntarily* engage in mergers or acquisitions. Although hostile acquisitions and takeovers are also possible and foreseeable in the future, even under conditions of bankruptcy, most ownership transactions involving health care organizations to date have been voluntary.

One form of ownership transaction is to create a new organization, sometimes called an "umbrella" organization, to span but not to replace the original organizations. Starkweather (1981, pp. 37–38) describes two important subtypes of the umbrella corporation in regard to hospitals. One subtype gives the umbrella corporation limited authority within which its decisions are final. In the other, the umbrella corporation has more general authority that is usually exercised through unified management, policy, and fiscal control.

Another organizational response to interdependence is merger or consolidation. Consolidation is a formal combination of two or more organizations into a single new legal entity that has an identity separate from any of the preexisting institutions. Merger is a formal combination of two or more institutions into a single new legal entity that has the identity of one of the preexisting organizations. Both forms of consumption, as interorganizational coordinating mechanisms, involve an essential restructuring of organizational interdependence. The restructuring can be in the form of vertical integration (a nursing home merges with a hospital in which the hospital gains the ability to discharge patients to a less intensive level of care, and the nursing home gains a source of referrals), horizontal expansion (two hospitals merge with a resulting larger capacity), or diversification (a hospital absorbs a retail pharmacy chain, gaining a new source of revenue).

Involuntary Interorganizational Transactions

Market transactions and voluntary interorganizational transactions are not sufficient to manage all organizational interdependencies found in the health care sector. Examples include relationships with regulatory agencies, fiscal intermediaries, and utilization-management companies. Regulated organizations have an interdependent relationship with the organizations that regulate them. Such interdependence cannot be legally managed through market transactions, which, by definition, involve economic exchanges. Furthermore, the nature of the interdependent relationship between a regulated health care organization and its regulator means that the relationship is not subject to the voluntary types of interorganizational transactions described above.

These involuntary relationships lead to unique ways of managing interdependence. Many ingenious strategies have evolved (Altman, Greene, & Sapolsky, 1981). While these strategies are specific to an individual organization's interactions with regulatory bodies, but they can be modified for use in other involuntary interorganizational transactions as well. Perhaps the most common approach, and always available to organizations in dealing with their regulators, is litigation. Most regulatory decisions can be appealed in the courts, which are sensitive to procedural errors or infringement of due process rights. Regulators who overlook requirements for

MANAGERIAL GUIDELINES

The development of effective coordination mechanisms is one of the most difficult tasks managers face. This activity is especially difficult in health care organizations owing to their high degree of internal differentiation. Managing interdependencies among health care organizations can be even more complicated. To assist such endeavors, we offer the following suggestions:

1. Within health care organizations, managers must be aware of the relationship between functional specialization and the need for coordination. The establishment of additional organizational units may improve the coordination *within* such units, but the added units may make it more difficult to coordinate activities *among* all units within the organization or the multiorganizational system.

2. In their efforts to manage interdependencies among organizational units, managers select coordination mechanisms that best match the situation at hand. Factors to consider include task uncertainty, degree of interdependencies among units, and size of the organization.

3. In relationships with other interdependent organizations, health care managers should choose from a variety of interorganizational mechanisms for coordination. In making their selection, managers should carefully consider the relative benefits and costs inherent in available mechanisms.

---

notice, public hearings, or the opportunity for full consideration of issues invite litigation. While distasteful to many, another strategy organizations use to deal with their regulators involves cultivating supportive relationships with the executive and legislative branches and with state and federal regulatory agencies. Such political intervention strategies can afford effective protection against overly enthusiastic or even dutiful regulators. It is no accident that hospitals routinely place prominent public officials and politically connected private citizens on their governing bodies, that physicians are among the most generous political campaign contributors, or that well-connected consultants flourish in and around Washington, D.C., and state capitals.

Other strategies, unethical and/or illegal though they may be, are sometimes used by regulated organizations to attempt to manage relationships with their regulators. For example, one advantage regulated organizations often have over their regulators is their technical expertise and the ability to assemble and manipulate large volumes of data. When challenged, regulated organizations may flood their regulators with technical data seeking to justify their position, or simply obscure the issues as part of a data overload strategy intended to foster ambiguity. Although it is

clearly illegal and unethical, outright deception is possible in relationships between organizations and their regulatory stakeholders. The cost and scope of projects can be understated; pertinent data can be fabricated or falsified; projects or protocols can be altered after approval. The complexity of projects, long lead times, turnover of regulatory staff, and the difficulty government agencies have in coordinating their programs can prevent close scrutiny of regulated organizations and encourage cheating.

Managing Interorganizational Linkages

As with intraorganizational coordination, it is important for a manager to use a contingency approach when establishing and maintaining relationships with interdependent organizations. The manager must do this both when selecting the interdependent organizations with which linkages should be established and when determining the most appropriate forms of linkages from the available menu. Chapter 11 elaborates on this process.

It is important to note here that interorganizational coordination is not achieved without costs. The obvious costs are time, personnel, and money needed to support the various forms of linkages. The less obvious, but very important, costs include what Porter (1985) has termed the cost of compromise and the cost of inflexibility. The cost of compromise arises in the context that effectively coordinating across organizational boundaries may require that an activity be performed in a consistent way that may not be optimal for any of the participants in the interorganizational relationship. From the manager's perspective, the cost of compromise can be reduced if an activity is *designed* for sharing. For example, two merger participants may find that a new management information system that is designed to accommodate the needs of the new organization is better than applying—either separately or linked—the previously existing management information systems.

The cost of inflexibility is not an ongoing expense of interorganizational coordination mechanisms, but arises with the need for flexibility, usually in the form of responding to a competitor's move or to a new market opportunity. It is simply a matter that linkages developed to manage interorganizational interdependencies involve added complexity and often greater inflexibility.

COMMUNICATION*

As noted, both coordination and communication present significant challenges to managers as they seek to effectively manage interdependencies by establishing linkages within and outside their organizations. As with coordination, communication becomes more important as interdependence moves from pooled to sequential to reciprocal forms.

Following the paradigm established by March and Simon (1958) in which they identified two primary types of coordination—programming and feedback—this section discusses the role communication plays in both approaches. Remember, as was discussed earlier in the chapter, that programming approaches to coordination seek to clarify work responsibilities and activities in advance of the performance of work, as well as specify the outputs of the work process and the skills required. In essence, programming approaches seek to

*This section is adapted with permission from Rakich, J. S., Longest, B. B. Jr., and Darr, K. *Managing Health Services Organizations*, 3rd ed. Baltimore, MD: Health Professions Press, 1992, Chapter 15.

standardize work activities. By contrast, feedback approaches to coordination entail the exchange of information among staff while the work is being carried out, which permits staff to change or modify work activities in response to unexpected requirements. Both programming and feedback approaches to coordination rely extensively on effective communication.

Communication, which is *the creation or exchange of understanding between sender(s) and receiver(s),* plays a vital role in both programming and feedback coordination mechanisms. It also serves other purposes as well. When managers communicate effectively, one of four things or some combination of them is accomplished: information transmission, motivation, control, and emotive expression (Scott, Mitchell, & Birmbaum, 1981).

Information about operating activities, resources, alternatives, and the plans and activities of others in the organization—information people need if they are to make good decisions or take appropriate actions—is routinely transmitted within health care organizations. Managers also provide information to their organizations' external stakeholders such as its potential customers, health plans, and regulators. *Information transmission* is essential if organizations are to function effectively within their environments.

Although *motivation* is a process internal to the person experiencing it (see Chapter 3), managers have an effect on motivation in others by informing them about rewards that will result from their performance, by giving them information that builds commitment to the organization and its objectives, and by using communication skills to help people understand and learn how to fulfill their personal needs. Managers also communicate with external stakeholders to influence and motivate them to act in ways that benefit the health care organization, such as selecting the organization as a provider of medical services, offering favorable reimbursement levels for services, or establishing favorable regulatory policies.

Many kinds of communications help *control* the performance of health care organizations and those who work in them: activity reports, policies to establish standard operating procedures, budgets, and face-to-face directives are examples. Such communications enhance control when they clarify duties, authorities, and responsibilities. These communications play a central part in coordination.

A final function of communication results from the fact that it permits people to express their emotions and feelings, such as satisfaction, happiness, sadness, and anger. *Emotive communication* permits necessary venting of feelings to occur among people within organizations. It also permits the health care organization to increase acceptance of the organization and its actions, both internally and with external stakeholders. Whether the purpose of communication is transmitting information, motivating, controlling, or emoting, and whether it pertains to programming or feedback approaches to coordinating, it is accomplished through a specific process.

The Communication Process

All effective communication, whether intraorganizational or communication with external stakeholders, involves the creation or exchange of understanding between sender(s) and receiver(s) through a process diagramed in Figure 8.3. In this model, the *sender*—which can be one or more individuals, departments, or units of an organization, or a system of organizations—has ideas, intentions, and information that

they wish to convey. A sender uses words and symbols to *encode* ideas and information into a *message* for the intended *receiver.*

Because words may have different meanings for different people, or people may not understand certain words, it is often useful to augment the words in a message with other symbols to make communication more effective. In health care organizations, many kinds of symbols, which may be physical things, pictures, or actions, play a role in communication. Consider how many words would be needed to explain a hospital's complex organization design in lieu of information displayed in an organization chart. Or, imagine the difficulty of trying to communicate all the information in a PET scan using only words. A smile or a hearty handshake has meaning. A promotion or pay increase conveys a great deal to the recipient, as well as to others. Lack of action can also have symbolic meaning. As has been noted,

> Failure to act is an important way of communicating. A manager who fails to praise an employee for a job well done or fails to provide promised resources is sending a message to that person. Since we send messages both by action and inaction, we communicate almost all the time at work, regardless of our intentions. (Newstrom & Davis, 1993)

The **communication channels** or methods of communication are the means by which messages are transmitted. Channels include face-to-face or telephone conversations involving an individual and/or groups of senders and receivers, E-mail, facsimile messages, letters, memos, policy statements, operating room schedules, reports, electronic message boards, web pages, video teleconferences, newspapers, television and radio commercial spots, and newsletters for internal or external distribution.

The selection of channels is an important part of the communication process. Effective communication often involves using multiple channels to transmit a message. For example, a major change in an organization's human resources policy, such as changing the benefit package, might be announced in a letter from the vice president for human resources to all

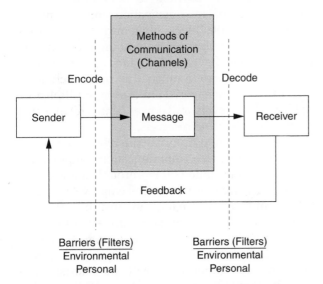

Figure 8.3. The Basic Mechanism of Communication.
SOURCE: Rakich, J. S., Longest, B. B. Jr., and Darr, K. *Managing Health Services Organizations,* 3rd ed. Baltimore, MD: Health Professions Press, 1992, p. 562. Reprinted by permission.

employees, graphically illustrated by posters in key locations, and then reinforced in group meetings where managers explain the policy and answer questions. A decision to lobby the state legislature for more generous Medicaid reimbursement might result in messages transmitted through channels such as letters to legislators, direct contact between the organization's managers and trustees and legislators, and newspaper advertisements stating the organization's position. If other organizations would benefit from the legislation, they might participate, perhaps through an association, to produce and distribute television commercials or use other channels to increase support for their position.

Messages transmitted over any channel must be *decoded* by the receiver. Decoding means interpreting the words and symbols in the message. Because decoding is done by the receivers of messages, it is affected by their prior experiences and frames of reference. Decoding involves the receiver's perceptual assessment of both the content of the message *and* the sender, and the context in which the message is transmitted. The fact that messages must be decoded (interpreted) by the receiver raises the possibility that the message the sender intends is not the message the receiver gets. The closer the decoded message is to the one intended by the sender, the more effective the communication.

The most effective way to determine if messages are received as intended is through *feedback*. "Without feedback, you have a one-way communication process. Feedback makes possible a two-way process, reversing the sender and receiver roles so that information can be shared, recycled, and fine-tuned to achieve an unambiguous mutual understanding" (Holt, 1992).

In intraorganizational communication, where interdependencies among individuals and units of an organization are significant, the feedback loop is very important in assuring that enough information is exchanged to effectively manage these interdependencies. Similarly, communication with external stakeholders is greatly improved if receivers provide feedback to senders, who can then adjust the message if it is not received as intended. Effective two-way communication occurs when a sender encodes and transmits a message to a receiver, who decodes the message and indicates understanding by giving feedback.

Feedback can be direct or indirect. Direct feedback is the receiver's response to the sender regarding a specific message. Indirect feedback is more subtle and involves consequences that result from a particular message. Internally, indirect feedback on a policy to change the organization's benefit package might include higher levels of employee satisfaction if the change is liked or increased turnover if the change is disliked. Externally, indirect feedback on attempts to change Medicaid reimbursement might include an increase in rates if the legislature agrees with the organization, no action if they disagree, or even hostile action if they disagree with the message or are upset by the methods used to communicate it.

Whether communication is within organizations or between them and external stakeholders, there are almost always barriers that must be overcome if communication is to be most effective. The environmental and personal barriers illustrated in Figure 8.3 are ubiquitous in the communication process, and can block, filter, or distort messages as they are encoded and sent and when they are decoded and received.

Environmental barriers to communication are characteristics of an organization and its environmental context that block, filter, or distort communications. Such barriers can be nothing more than the fact that people have too little time to communicate carefully. Other environmental barriers include the organization's managerial philosophy, multiplicity of its hierarchical levels, and power/status relationships between senders and receivers.

Managerial philosophy can directly inhibit, as well as promote, effective communication. Requirements that all communication "flow through channels," inaccessibility, lack of interest in employees' frustrations, complaints, or feelings, and insufficient time allotted to receiving information are symptoms of a philosophy that retards communication. Managerial philosophy also has a significant impact on an organization's communications with its external stakeholders. This topic is addressed more fully in a later section.

Multiple levels in an organization's hierarchy, and other organizational complexities such as size or scope of activity, present barriers that tend to cause message distortion. For example, a message sent from the CEO to employees through several layers of an organization might be received in quite a different form than that originally sent. Or, a report prepared for the CEO that passes through the hierarchy may not reach its destination because it is lying on a desk and is, in essence, blocked.

Power/status relationships can also present barriers to effective communication by distorting or inhibiting transmission of messages. How often does the nurse with 20 years of experience tell a new medical resident that a procedure or treatment thought to be appropriate and about to be ordered is not efficacious? How is the nurse's message encoded—bluntly or obliquely?

Another environmental barrier stems from the fact that managers in health care organizations may use terminology that is very different from that used by those responsible for direct care. Both may use terminology unfamiliar to external stakeholders. This barrier is widespread in communication within health care organizations; it is almost universal in communications between them and many of their external stakeholders.

Another set of barriers—**personal barriers to communication**—are always potentially present when people communicate. These barriers arise from the nature of people, especially in their interaction with others and apply equally to communication within organizations and between them and their external stakeholders. Examples of personal barriers to effective communication include people distorting the encoding or decoding of their messages according to their frames of reference or their beliefs and values. People may also consciously or unconsciously engage in selective perception, or permit their emotions—such as fear or jealousy—to influence their communications.

Unless one has had the same experiences as others, it is difficult to completely understand messages from them or to construct messages that others completely understand. The wealthy may have difficulty understanding the concerns of people without health insurance. Because personalities and backgrounds differ, people have idiosyncratic opinions and prejudices in areas such as politics, ethics, religion, equity in the workplace, sex, race, and lifestyle. These biases, beliefs, and values filter and distort communication. Selective perception means that people tend to filter out the "bad" of a message and retain the "good," usually because it makes them feel better or helps them protect their status quo.

Awareness that environmental and personal barriers to effective communication exist is the first step in minimizing their impact, but positive actions are needed to overcome them. Although the specific steps necessary to overcome the barriers depend on circumstances, several general guidelines can be suggested.

Environmental barriers are reduced if receivers and senders ensure that attention is given to their messages and that adequate time is devoted to listening to what is being communicated. In addition, a management philosophy that encourages open and free flow of communications is constructive. Reducing the number of links (levels in the organizational hierarchy or steps between the organization as a sender and external stakeholders as receivers) through which messages pass reduces opportunities for distortion. The power/status barrier is more difficult to eliminate because it is affected by interpersonal and interprofessional relationships. However, consciously tailoring words and symbols so messages are understandable and reinforcing words with actions significantly improves communications among different power/status levels. Finally, using multiple channels to reinforce complex messages decreases the likelihood of misunderstanding.

Personal barriers to effective communication are reduced by conscious efforts of sender and receiver to understand each other's frame of reference and beliefs. Recognizing that people engage in selective perception and are prone to jealousy and fear is a first step toward eliminating or at least diminishing these barriers. Empathy with those to whom messages are directed may be the surest way to increase the likelihood that the messages will be received and understood as intended.

Effectively communicating among component organizations in a health system can be especially demanding. Barriers resulting from organizational complexity in systems can be quite formidable. Adapting

Porter's (1985) approach to achieving effective linkages among business units in a diversified corporation suggests ways for managers to overcome some of these barriers to effective communication within a system.

- Use devices or techniques that cross organizational lines, such as partial centralization and interorganization task forces or committees, to actively facilitate communication. At the governance level, systems can enhance communication through interlocking boards, which are defined as boards with overlapping membership.
- Use management processes that include cross-organizational dimensions in areas such as planning, control, incentives, capital budgeting, and management information systems to enhance communication.
- Use human resource practices that facilitate cooperation among the organizations in a system, such as cross-organizational job rotation, management forums, and training because these increase the likelihood that managers in one part of the system will understand their counterparts elsewhere in the system and that they will communicate more effectively.
- Use management processes that effectively and fairly resolve conflicts among organizations in a system to enhance communication. The key to such processes is that corporate management installs and operates a process that fairly settles disputes among component organizations in the system. Equitable settlement of disputes facilitates effective communication.

Making the Communication Process Effective

Managers use the process outlined in Figure 8.3 when they communicate. Their success in achieving understanding when they communicate depends upon a number of variables. Shortell (1991, pp. 70–92) identifies several key elements of effective communication in a model developed for physicians and hospitals to improve their communications. The following summarizes these elements, and Figure 8.4 illustrates their interrelationships.

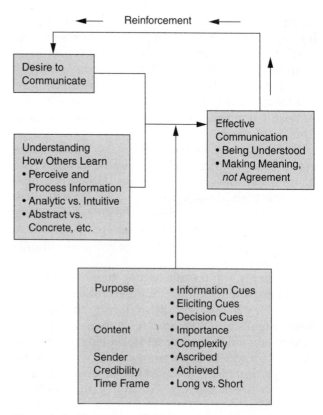

Figure 8.4. Elements of Effective Communication: A Guiding Framework.
SOURCE: Shortell, S. M. *Effective Hospital-Physician Relationships.* Chicago: Health Administration Press, 1991; p. 87. Reprinted by permission.

1. An effective communicator must have a *desire to communicate,* which is influenced both by one's personal values and the expectation that the communication will be received in a meaningful way.
2. An effective communicator must have an *understanding of how others learn,* which includes consideration of differences in how others perceive and process information. For example, is the receiver analytic or intuitive? Does the receiver prefer abstract versus concrete information? Is the receiver better able to interpret verbal or written information?
3. The receiver of the message should be cued as to the *purpose* of the message. That is, whether the message is to provide information, elicit a response or reaction, or to arrive at a decision.

4. The *content, importance, and complexity* of the message should be considered in determining the channels through which the message is communicated.

5. The achieved or ascribed *credibility of the sender* affects how the message will be received—"trust" (an achieved credibility) being most significant.

6. The *time frame* associated with the content of the message (long versus short) needs to be considered in choosing the channels through which and the manner in which the message is communicated. That is, faster channels and more precise cues are needed with shorter time frames.

The application of these elements of effective communication can improve a manager's communications, especially if they are considered in conjunction with the process model described in Figure 8.3. The elements of effective communication, and the process itself, apply whether communication is the intraorganizational communication that takes place within a health care organization or the communication between an organization and its external stakeholders.

Intraorganizational Communication

Intraorganizational communication flows downward, upward, horizontally, and diagonally within organizations, with each direction of flow having its appropriate uses and unique characteristics. Typically, downward flow is communication between superiors and subordinates in organizations; upward communication uses the same channels but in the opposite direction. Horizontal flow is manager to manager or worker to worker. Diagonal flow cuts across functions and levels. While this violates an organization's hierarchical chain of command, it may be permitted in situations where speed and efficiency of communication are particularly important.

Downward Flow

Downward communication flow primarily involves passing on information from superiors to subordinates in organizations. It commonly consists of information, verbal orders, or instructions from organiza-

tional superior to subordinate on a one-to-one basis. It may also include speeches to groups of employees or meetings. The myriad of written methods such as handbooks, procedure manuals, newsletters, bulletin boards, and the ubiquitous memorandum are also channels of downward communication. Computerized information systems contribute greatly to downward flow in many health care organizations.

Upward Flow

Upward communication flow serves to provide managers with decision-making information, reveal problem areas, provide data for performance evaluation, indicate the status of morale, and generally underscore the thinking of subordinates. Upward flow becomes more important with increased organizational complexity and scale. This is especially emphasized with the organizational growth of health care organizations and their increasing participation in systems. Managers rely on effective upward communication, and they encourage it by creating a climate of trust and respect as integral parts of the organizational culture (Robbins & Coulter, 1998).

In addition to being directly useful to managers, upward communication flow helps employees satisfy personal needs. It permits those in positions of lesser organizational authority to express opinions and perceptions to those with higher authority; as a result, they feel a greater sense of participation. The hierarchical chain of command is the main channel for upward communication in health care organizations, but this may be supplemented by grievance procedures, open-door policies, counseling, employee questionnaires, exit interviews, participative decision-making techniques, and the use of ombudspeople (Luthans, 1997).

Horizontal and Diagonal Flows

Unhindered downward and upward communication are insufficient for effective organizational performance. In complex organizations, which are frequently subject to abrupt demands for action and reaction, horizontal flow must also occur. For example, the work of interdependent patient care units must be coordinated. Health care organizations using matrix designs, as described in Chapters 7 and 10, illustrate the value of horizontal communication and coordination in these organizations. Committees, task forces, and cross-functional project teams are all useful mechanisms of horizontal communication.

The least common flows of communication in health care organizations are diagonal flows, although they are growing in importance. For example, diagonal communication occurs when the director of a hospital pharmacy alerts a nurse in medical intensive care about a potential adverse reaction between two medications ordered for a patient. Diagonal flows violate the usual pattern of upward and downward communication flows by cutting across departments, and they violate the usual pattern of horizontal communication because the communicators are at different levels in the organization. Yet, such communication is extremely important in health care organi-

zations. Committees, task forces, quality circles, and cross-functional project teams made up of members from different levels of the organization or system can each serve as useful mechanisms of diagonal communication.

Communication Networks within Organizations

Downward, upward, horizontal, and diagonal communication flows within organizations can be combined into patterns called **communication networks,** which are communicators interconnected by communication channels (Scott et al., 1981, p. 168). Figure 8.5 illustrates the five common networks: chain, Y, wheel, circle, and all-channel. The *chain network* is the standard format for communicating upward and downward and follows line authority relationships. An example is a staff nurse who reports to a nurse manager, who reports to a nursing supervisor, who reports to

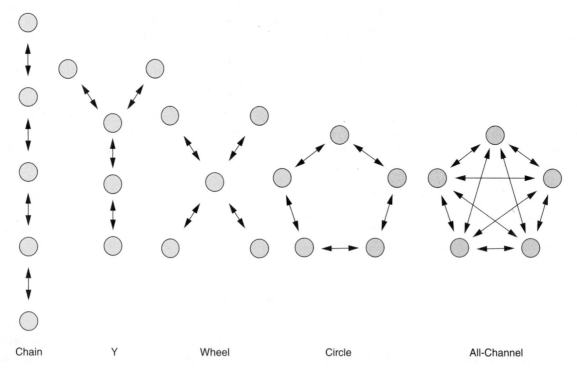

Chain   Y   Wheel   Circle   All-Channel

Figure 8.5. Common Communication Networks.
SOURCE: Rakich, J. S., Longest, B. B. Jr., and Darr, K. *Managing Health Services Organizations,* 3rd ed. Baltimore, MD: Health Professions Press, 1992, p. 568. Reprinted by permission.

the vice president for nursing, who reports to the president.

The *Y pattern* (turned upside down) shows two people reporting to a superior who reports to two others. An example is two staff pharmacists who report to the pharmacy director, who reports to the vice president for professional affairs, who reports to the president. The *wheel pattern* shows a situation in which four subordinates report to one superior. There is no interaction among subordinates, and all communications are channeled through the manager at the center of the wheel. This pattern is rare in health care organizations, although elements of it can be found in the situation in which four vice presidents report to a president if the vice presidents have little interaction among themselves. Even though this network pattern is not used routinely, it may be used in circumstances in which urgency or secrecy is required. For example, the president with an emergency might communicate with vice presidents in a wheel pattern because time does not permit using other modes. Similarly, if secrecy is important, such as during an investigation of possible embezzlement, the president may require that all relevant communication with the vice presidents be kept confidential for a period of time.

The *circle pattern* allows communicators in the network to communicate directly only with two others, but since each communicates with another communicator in the network, the effect is that everyone communicates with everyone and there is no central authority or leader. The *all-channel network* is a circle pattern except that each communicator may interact with every other communicator in the network.

Communication networks vary along several dimensions. The most appropriate pattern depends upon the situation in which it is used. The wheel and all-channel networks tend to be fast and accurate compared with the chain or Y-pattern networks, but the chain or Y patterns promote clear-cut lines of authority and responsibility. The circle and all-channel networks enhance morale among those in the networks better than other patterns because everyone is equal in the communication activity, but these patterns result in relatively slow communication. This is a serious problem if an immediate decision or response is needed.

Managers must construct communication networks to fit the various communication situations they face.

Informal Communication

Coexisting with formal communication flows and networks within organizations are **informal communication** flows, which have their own networks. Like informal organization structures, informal communication flows and networks result from the interpersonal relationships of people in organizations. The common name for informal communication flows is *grapevine*, a term that arose during the Civil War, when telegraph lines were strung between trees much like a grapevine (Newstrom & Davis, 1993, p. 441). Messages transmitted over those flimsy lines were often garbled. As a result, any rumor was said to come from the grapevine.

By definition, the grapevine, or informal flow of communication, consists of channels that result from the interpersonal relationships in organizations. Informal communication flows in an organization are as natural as the patterns of social interaction that develop in all organizational settings. Like the informal organization structure, informal communication flows coexist with the formal flows established by management. There is no doubt that informal communication channels can be and routinely are misused in health care organizations, especially in transmitting rumors. For example, in times of crisis, organizations are rife with rumors; frequently, the rumors are wrong. Yet, properly managed, informal communication flows can be useful. Downward flows move through the grapevine much faster than through formal channels. In a health care organization, much of the coordination among units occurs through informal give-and-take in informal horizontal and diagonal flows. In the case of upward flow, informal communication can be a rich source of information about performance, ideas, feelings, and attitudes. Because of their potential usefulness and pervasiveness, managers should try to understand informal communication flows and use them to advantage.

The multidirectional communication flows and the networks they form within organizations each have a purpose, and each is an important tool for managers.

To the extent these flows are planned and designed into the organization, they are part of its formal design, and they represent formal communication channels and networks. To the extent they are natural communication between and among people arising outside the formal design, they are informal communication channels and networks. Figure 8.6 summarizes the key uses of downward, upward, horizontal, and diagonal communication flows in health care organizations.

Communicating with External Stakeholders

Health care organizations typically maintain relationships with a large and diverse set of external stakeholders (Longest, 1990), which can be shown in a *stakeholder map*, such as the one for the Indiana State Health Department shown in Figure 8.7. Effective communication between a health care organization and its external stakeholders is necessary because these organizations are affected, sometimes quite dramatically, by what the external stakeholders think or do. A health care organization's external stakeholders include the individuals, groups, or organizations outside the organization that have a stake in its decisions and actions and attempt to influence those decisions and actions (Blair & Fottler, 1998). The sheer number and variety of external stakeholders complicate communication with them. Communication is further complicated by the nature of the relationships. Positive relations with external stakeholders usually makes it easier to manage the relationships, and communication flows tend to be more effective than when relations are negative.

Boundary spanning is another name for the process through which organizations communicate with their external stakeholders, and *boundary spanners* are the people who carry out this process. On the one hand,

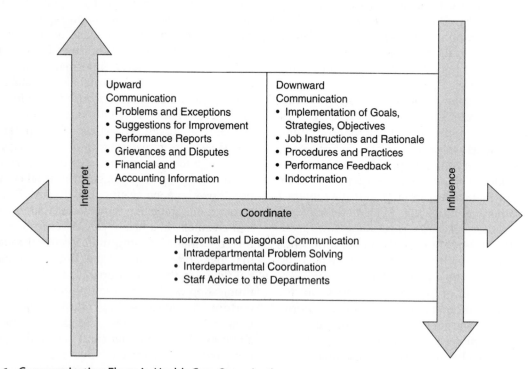

Figure 8.6. Communication Flows in Health Care Organizations.
SOURCE: Draft, R. L. & Steers, R. M. *Organizations: A Micro/Macro Approach,* 538. Reading, MA: Addison-Wesley Educational Publishers, Inc., 1986. Reprinted by permission.

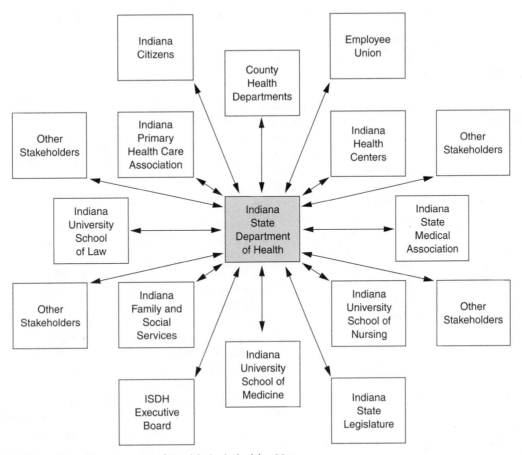

Figure 8.7. Indiana State Department of Health Stakeholder Map.
SOURCE: Ginter, P. M., Swayne, L. M., and Duncan W. J. *Strategic Management of Health Care Organizations,* 3rd ed., 458. Malden, MA: Blackwell Publishers Inc., 1998. Reprinted by permission.

boundary spanners obtain critical information from external stakeholders that can be useful to the organization. Strategic planning and marketing departments or functions are examples of such boundary spanning. On the other hand, boundary spanners also represent the organization to external stakeholders. This activity takes many forms, including marketing, public relations, guest or patient relations, government relations, or community relations. Because information is the object of these boundary-spanning activities, communication is critical to their success. An organization's ability to glean necessary or useful information from its external stakeholders or to be effectively represented to them depends upon effective communication.

While the communication process with all external stakeholders is essentially the creation of understanding between sender and receiver utilizing the process outlined in Figure 8.3, each stakeholder must be considered in terms of its unique dimensions if effective communication is to occur. This is especially true of two important sets of external stakeholders in the typical health care organization: the public sector with which the organization interacts and the geographical community in which the organization is located.

Communicating with the Public Sector

Health care organizations, perhaps as much or more than any organizations in American society, are affected by public policies—the formal decisions made in the public sector. The fact that they are affected by so much public policy stems from the fundamental contributions health care organizations make to the physical and psychological condition of the American people, as well as the role these organizations play in the nation's economy. In view of these very important contributions, it should not surprise anyone that government, at all levels, is keenly interested in the performance of health care organizations. Nor should there be surprise that this intense interest results in numerous public policies—including policies affecting the provision and financing of health care services as well as the production of inputs (e.g., the education of health professionals and the development of health technology) to those services (Longest, 1998a, Chapter 1). The importance of public policies to health care organizations makes effective communication with the public sector vital to the well-being of these organizations.

Managers have two important categories of communication responsibilities regarding the public sector environments of health care organizations (Longest, 1997). First, they are responsible for *analyzing* this environment. Done properly, this analysis permits them to acquire sufficient information and data to understand the strategic consequences of events and forces in their organization's public policy environment. Such analysis yields an accurate assessment of the impacts—both in terms of opportunities and threats—of public policies on the organization. Furthermore, such analysis permits managers to position their organizations to make strategic adjustments that reflect planned responses to these opportunities and threats.

Second, managers of health care organizations are responsible for *influencing* the formulation and implementation of public policies. This responsibility derives from the fact that effective managers seek to make their organization's external environment, including the public policy component of that environment, as favorable to the organization as possible. Inherent in this responsibility are requirements to identify public policy objectives that are consistent with their organization's values, mission, and objectives and to seek through appropriate and ethical means, such as lobbying and joining with associations, to help shape public policies accordingly.

Communicating with the Community*

Health care organizations almost always consider the communities in which they are physically located to be among their most important external stakeholders, and view them as requiring extensive communication. Perhaps more than with other external stakeholders, the basis for effective communications between health care organizations and their communities is a clear understanding and acceptance of the expectations each has of the other. By establishing and clearly communicating what the community can expect from it, an organization establishes the best possible foundation for all communication with its community.

In establishing what the community can expect from it, a health care organization must think systematically about all that it can do for its community. As Figure 8.8 illustrates, health care organizations can do much for their communities, although many do not play their fullest possible role nor make clear the extent of what the community can expect from them. This means that the relationship between the organization and its community is not as clearly established as it could be. This, in turn, impairs communication between the organization and its community.

As shown in Figure 8.8, the most fundamental contribution a health care organization can make to its community is fulfillment of the health-enhancing purpose for which the organization was established. The mission-related activities of health care organizations, especially when broadly conceived and pursued across the range of determinants of human health—physical, social, and economic environments; lifestyles and behaviors; genetics; and health services (Blum, 1983; Evans, Barer, & Marmor, 1994)—are vital aspects of what communities can expect. However, as Figure

*This section is adapted from Longest, B. B., Jr. "The Civic Roles of Healthcare Organizations," *Health Forum Journal*, Vol. 41, No. 5 (September/October 1998), pp. 40–42.

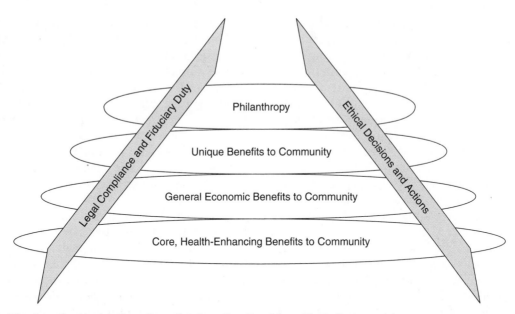

Figure 8.8. The Benefits Health Care Organizations Can Provide to Their Communities.
SOURCE: Longest, B. B., Jr., and Rakich, J. S. *Managing Health Services Organizations and Systems,* 4th ed. Baltimore, MD: Health Professions Press, forthcoming. Used with permission.

8.8 illustrates, health care organizations can do much more for their communities.

They provide significant—in some cases extraordinarily significant—general economic benefits to their communities. In many communities, they are among the largest and most stable employers. The economic contributions organizations can make to their communities go well beyond their role as employers, and even beyond the economic ripples that paychecks spread across communities. Financially sound health care organizations can share the burden of community infrastructure such as paying for municipal services, whether through the taxes paid if they operate as for-profit entities or by payments in lieu of taxes from not-for-profit organizations.

In addition to providing mission-related and economic benefits, health care organizations provide a set of unique benefits to their communities (see Figure 8.8) because of *how* and *for whom* they choose to pursue their core, health-enhancing missions. These benefits have been identified along a number of dimensions (Claxton, Feder, Shactman, & Altman, 1997; Gray, 1997; Schlesinger, Gray, & Bradley, 1996), but

the most important ones include making some of their services available on a charitable basis, and subsidizing costly but unprofitable services such as burn units or primary care clinics in neighborhoods with high poverty rates.

Health care organizations can also voluntarily assume commitments of corporate social responsibility in their communities, which may extend into the realm of philanthropy (Carroll, 1991). In these endeavors, which are a completely discretionary aspect of any organization's relationship to its community, the organization adopts a set of essentially philanthropic responsibilities and activities. It seeks to share in helping relieve some of the burdens of poverty, violence, and ignorance in the community. The organization, through philanthropy, seeks to advance the overall well-being of the community by embracing charitable acts, by contributing philanthropic resources to the community, and by seeking generally to improve the quality of life in the community.

As can be seen in Figure 8.8, the relationships between health care organizations and their communities include other important elements that are vital in establishing the foundation upon which the organization communicates with its community. Health care organizations have obligations of legal compliance, fiduciary duty, and ethically sound decision making and actions, as well as all the other benefits they provide to their communities. As legal entities, the manner in which health care organizations fulfill their legal obligations affects their relationships with their communities. Beyond their legal obligations and the potential inherent in their fulfillment for community good, if organizations choose to operate ethically, they bind themselves to ethical responsibilities that add yet another, higher dimension to their relationships to their communities.

Law establishes a minimum standard of performance that is expected from all members of a community. However, certain members of communities—including health care organizations—while expected to abide by the law like all members generally, are expected to do more. These organizations have well-established fiduciary obligations of trust, confidence, and integrity, which if met permit members of communities to explicitly trust that their health care organizations will act in their best interest.

Beyond these legal and fiduciary requirements, however, lie the even more demanding obligations inherent in the assumption of a commitment to ethical behavior toward the community. An ethical health care organization voluntarily seeks to embody and perhaps raise the standard of community moral values. In pursuing this element of relationship to community, the organization assiduously applies the principles of ethical behavior to all of its decision making and actions, including:

- Respecting the autonomy and individual dignity of members of the community through such actions as ensuring the confidentiality of medical information about them, or fully honoring *their* wishes for and directives about their health care;
- Ensuring justice, honesty, and fairness in all interactions, whether with patients, employees, competitors, suppliers, regulators, or the community at large;
- Making beneficence and nonmaleficence hallmarks of the organization's decisions and actions through such beneficent steps as establishing a full-

service hospice program to meet the needs of terminally ill patients in the community *and* developing associated policies to enable and encourage physicians to utilize the program, or through such nonmaleficent actions as disposing of medical waste in the safest possible way; and
- Valuing *and* practicing economic efficiency through such actions as building for technical quality, patient comfort, and reasonable amenity, but not ostentation; or seeking, always, to provide true value in all economic exchanges.

Health care organizations make maximum contributions to the communities in which they are located by attention to all of the elements contained in Figure 8.8. How well these elements are pursued—synergistically and in collaboration with others in the community when appropriate—determines the nature of what a community can expect from a health care organization. It also serves as the foundation for the organization's communication with its community. All communication with the community is enhanced when a solid basis for the relationship between the organization and its community is first clearly established and effectively communicated to the community.

Listening to External Stakeholders

When managers in health care organizations want to effectively listen to their external stakeholders, they approach the task in a systematic, analytical way called *stakeholder analysis* (Fottler et al., 1989). By doing so, the chances increase of acquiring useful or necessary information from external stakeholders—whether they be the public sector, the community, or any of its other external stakeholders.

Although specific approaches for systematically listening to external stakeholders vary widely, these efforts generally include a set of interrelated activities akin to the environmental assessments organizations make in the context of their strategic management. In conducting environmental assessments, health care organizations *scan* their environments to identify strategically important issues, *monitor* the issues, *forecast* trends in the issues, *assess* the importance of the issues for the organization, and *diffuse* information obtained to those in the organization or system who need it (Fahey & Narayaman, 1986; Ginter, Swayne, & Duncan, 1998, pp. 53–58; Longest, 1997, pp. 63–79). In conducting stakeholder analyses, they also *scan* to identify important stakeholders, *forecast* or project the trends in stakeholders' views or positions, *assess* the implications of the stakeholders' views and positions for the organization, and *diffuse* the results of the first four steps to those in the organization who need to know the views and positions of external stakeholders.

Scanning activities involve acquiring and organizing important information about who are the organization's external stakeholders. In most instances, this is rather straightforward to determine and can readily lead to the development of a stakeholder map, such as the one shown in Figure 8.9.

Considerations about who are an organization's external stakeholders are frequently judgmental. In order to ensure quality in these judgments, it is useful to use ad hoc task forces or committees of people from within the organization, perhaps with the aid of outside consultants. Any of several formal expert-based techniques of assistance help determine who are the stakeholders. The most useful among these are the Delphi technique, the nominal group technique, brainstorming, focus groups, and dialectic inquiry (Ginter, Swayne, & Duncan, 1998, pp. 60–64).

Scanning to identify external stakeholders must be followed by the next step, monitoring the identified stakeholders by tracking or following closely their views and positions on matters of importance. Monitoring is especially important when the views and positions are dynamic, not well structured, or are ambiguous as to strategic importance. Monitoring stakeholder views and positions permits clarification of the degree to which they are strategically important. As with scanning, techniques that feature the acquisition of expert opinions can help managers determine which stakeholders should be monitored.

Effective scanning and monitoring cannot provide managers with all the information they need about the frequently quite dynamic views and positions of their organization's external stakeholders. Managers need forecasts of stakeholders' emerging views and perceptions. Such forecasts, if accurate, can give managers ample time to factor these views and preferences into their decisions and actions.

Scanning and comprehensively monitoring the views and positions of an organization's external stakeholders, and even accurately forecasting trends in their views and positions, are not enough to ensure good stakeholder analysis. Managers must also concern themselves about the specific and relative importance of the information they are receiving. That is, they must be concerned with an assessment or interpretation of the strategic importance and implications of this information.

Minimally, this involves characterizing stakeholders as negative, positive, or neutral, as in Figure 8.9. While the determination of these positions is relatively easy to make, based on past experience if nothing more, careful assessments of stakeholders' importance is far from an exact science. Intuition, common sense, and best guesses all play a role in this determination. Aside from the difficulties encountered in collecting and properly analyzing enough information to fully inform the assessment, there sometimes are problems derived from the influence of personal prejudices and biases of those making judgments. This can force assessments that fit some preconceived notions about which stakeholders are strategically important rather than the realities of a particular situation (Thomas & McDaniel, 1990).

The final step in the process of conducting useful stakeholder analyses involves diffusing or spreading the results of the effort to all those in the organization who need to have access to this information. This step is frequently undervalued as part of the process and, in extreme cases, even overlooked. Unless it is effectively carried out, however, it really does not matter how well the other steps in the stakeholder analysis are performed. Thus, attention must be given to the task of diffusing the results of these analyses if the analytical process is to have its desired useful effect.

There are two basic ways that those who have produced information about the external stakeholders of an organization can diffuse this information into the organization or system. They can rely upon the *power* of senior-level managers to dictate diffusion and use of the information, including using coercion or sanctions to see that the information is diffused, and even

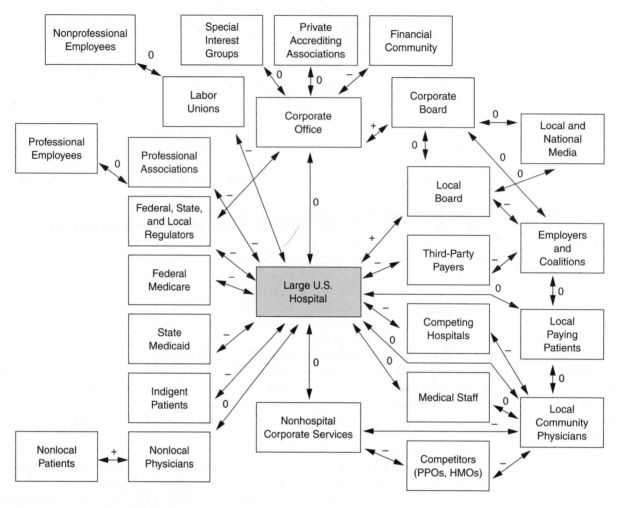

Key: + = Generally Positive Relationship
0 = Generally Neutral Relationship
− = Generally Negative Relationship

Figure 8.9. Stakeholders in a Large Hospital.
SOURCE: Fottler, M. D., Blair, J. D., Whitehead, C. J., Laus, M. D., and Savage, G. T. "Assessing Key Stakeholders: Who Matters to Hospitals and Why?" *Hospital & Health Services Administration,* Vol. 34, No. 4 (Winter, 1989), p. 530. Copyright 1989, Foundation of the American College of Healthcare Executives.

used, in the organization or system. Or they can use *reason* to persuade or educate those involved in the organization's decision making to utilize the information. Combinations of power or reason-based approaches to stimulation use of this information tend to work best.

Diffusion of strategically important information obtained from or about the organization's external stakeholders brings the process of stakeholder analysis to completion. The ability of any organization's managers to effectively listen to the organization's external stakeholders depends very heavily on the quality with which this process is conducted. In fact, today, given the vital linkage between health care organizations and their external stakeholders such as customers, payers, and regulators, it is unlikely that any organization can succeed in the absence of a reasonably effective process through which its managers effectively listen to the external stakeholders and respond to what is received in communication with them.

Communicating When Things Go Badly

Occasionally things go very badly, even in a well-managed health care organization. A hospital, for example, may lose its accreditation by the Joint Commission on Accreditation of Healthcare Organizations or lose a state certification because of code violations; serious clinical errors occur, perhaps causing a patient's death; infections break out; or serious financial difficulties arise, perhaps raising the specter of major layoffs or closure. As in other large, complex organizations, things can—and do—go wrong in health care organizations. When they do, communication within the organization as well as communication between it and its external stakeholders takes on intensified importance. How managers communicate in such circumstances is significant in resolving the problems and in the perception of the organization held by those within it and by its external stakeholders *after* the problems are resolved.

An example of communication in a bad situation arises if a diabetic patient being treated for complications of that disease dies unexpectedly in a hospital, with results of blood tests on a sample taken 6 hours before his death showing insulin levels 200 times too high. There are several possible explanations, but none of them is good. The possibilities include a fatal overdose of insulin given by accident or on purpose in a criminal act committed by any of several people. How should the hospital handle communication about this situation? Whose interests are to be protected? What information is to be communicated? To whom? By whom? There are few hard-and-fast rules to guide managers in communicating under circumstances such as these, either within the hospital or with external stakeholders.

The range of approaches that health care organizations can take in response to serious problems such as the one described above, as well as communications made about the actions, can be characterized along a continuum of *reactive* to *proactive* (Carroll, 1979). At one end of the continuum depicted in Figure 8.10, reactive responses include concealing a problem—do and say nothing. Less extreme, but highly reactive, is to admit that a problem may exist (perhaps in response to a reporter's query), but deny any wrongdoing and take no action to find the cause of the problem or resolve it. An obstructionist position could be taken by the health care organization's managers regarding further communication about the problem.

A similar reaction is one labeled defensive. The organization's managers and spokespersons act and communicate about a problem in a way that complies

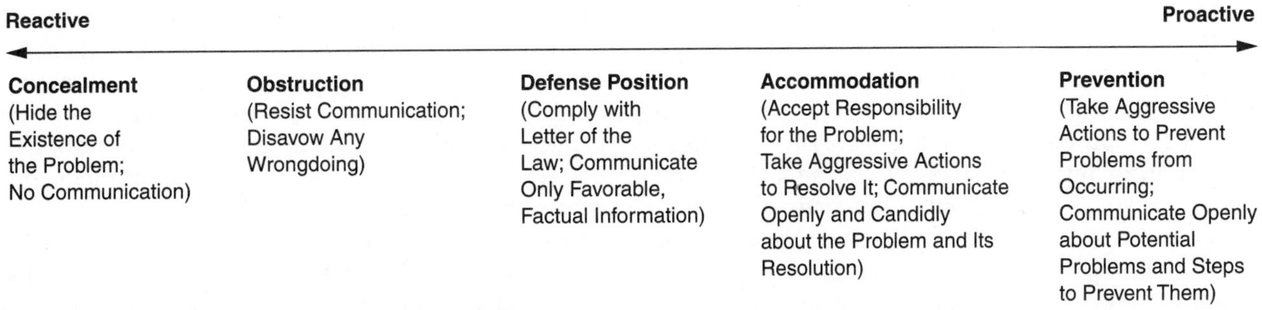

Reactive				Proactive
Concealment (Hide the Existence of the Problem; No Communication)	**Obstruction** (Resist Communication; Disavow Any Wrongdoing)	**Defense Position** (Comply with Letter of the Law; Communicate Only Favorable, Factual Information)	**Accommodation** (Accept Responsibility for the Problem; Take Aggressive Actions to Resolve It; Communicate Openly and Candidly about the Problem and Its Resolution)	**Prevention** (Take Aggressive Actions to Prevent Problems from Occurring; Communicate Openly about Potential Problems and Steps to Prevent Them)

Figure 8.10. Continuum of Actions and Communications to Stakeholders in Difficult Times.
SOURCE: Rakich, J. S., Longest, B. B. Jr., and Darr, K. *Managing Health Services Organizations*, 3rd ed. Baltimore, MD: Health Professions Press, 1992, p. 575. Reprinted by permission.

MANAGERIAL GUIDELINES

1. A key to assigning the proper managerial priority to coordination and communication efforts is the degree to which *interdependence* exists between or among people and units within an organization, and between the organization and its external environment. Assessing the degree and nature of interdependence is the first step toward effective coordination and communication strategies.

2. Managers should pay careful attention to selecting and implementing compatible and, whenever possible, mutually reinforcing mechanisms of coordination and communication if they are to successfully link together the people and units within their organizations and link their organizations to its external stakeholders.

3. The predominance of professionals in health care organizations both facilitates and complicates coordination and communication. Their presence facilitates because professional education prepares these people to link their efforts with those of others as part of the normal course of their work. But their presence also requires careful attention to maintaining collegial and consultative relationships, which, in turn, should guide managers' choices about coordination and communication.

4. Coordination and communication, while treated separately in this chapter for ease of presentation, are in fact highly interrelated and interactive phenomena. Managers should always consider the communication implications and opportunities when seeking to coordinate, and vice versa.

with the letter of the law. Such actions and communications are frequently intended to minimize legal liability, reflecting in part how expensive liability for serious problems involving human health and life can be. However, when difficult problems or issues arise, some health care organizations prefer to take defensive positions in communicating with people inside the organization and with external stakeholders. They prefer this approach even when the issues are layoffs, mergers, or closures in which many inside and outside the affected organization have a legitimate interest.

Figure 8.10 illustrates these reactive responses and two that are more proactive: accommodation and prevention. Accommodation involves accepting responsibility for a problem and taking aggressive actions to resolve it. In this type of response, the actions and communications about them are proactive. Communications are characterized by openness and candor about the problem, its causes, and the actions being taken to resolve it. Prevention is further along the continuum and focuses on taking aggressive and concerted actions to prevent problems from occurring. Continuous quality improvement (CQI) is an impor-

tant approach in prevention, as are risk management and quality assessment and improvement programs. Communications are characterized by openness and candor, as in accommodation, but they focus on the existence and probabilities of potential problems and the steps that have been taken to prevent them.

Health care organizations are far better served in managing difficult situations by actions and communications that are proactive rather than reactive. Reactive responses (concealment, obstruction, and, to a large extent, defense positions) imply crisis management and invite the scrutiny of those affected by the problem, including external stakeholders. Technically, managers who choose accommodation are reacting to a problem, too, but their response is positive and proactive in that they take responsibility, aggressively seek to resolve the problem, and communicate openly and candidly about the problem and their actions regarding it. Prevention involves aggressive proaction to avoid problems. Here, managers communicate to interested parties that problems might occur, but that actions have been taken to prevent them and minimize their impact. No level of effort will prevent all problems from occurring in health care organizations, but many can be prevented by careful actions. Furthermore, their consequences can be managed far more effectively if managers have laid a foundation of understanding and trust (Whitener, Brodt, Korsgaard, & Werner, 1998) within the organization as well as with its external stakeholders by communicating about potential problems and their actions to prevent them or prepare for them.

Discussion Questions

1. Distinguish between intra- and interorganizational coordination in health care organizations. What are the key mechanisms available to managers to achieve each type of coordination?
2. Define *communication* and draw a model of the basic technical process. How can managers overcome the barriers to effective communication?
3. Discuss the various types of communication flows in organizations and the uses of each. Discuss the various types of communication networks and describe the advantages and disadvantages of each.
4. You have just been appointed manager of a joint venture between the hospital where you work and some members of its medical staff to operate an ambulatory surgery center. One of your initial concerns is the establishment of effective linkages to the hospital. Drawing upon the material in this chapter, develop your approach to this task and indicate the reasons for your plan.
5. Think of a situation in which a health care organization receives bad press. How might the organization respond along the reactive-proactive continuum? How should it respond?

References

Altman, D., Greene, R., & Sapolsky, H. M. (1981). *Health planning and regulation: The decision-making process.* Ann Arbor, MI: Association of University Programs in Health Administration Press.

Andrews, L. B., Stocking, C. T., Krizek, T., Gottlieb, L., Krizek, C., Vargish, T., & Siegler, M. (1997, February). An alternative strategy for studying adverse events in medical care. *Lancet, 349,* 309–313.

Baggs, J. G., Ryan, S. A., Phelps, C. E., Richeson, J. F., & Johnson, J. E. (1992). The association between interdisciplinary collaboration and patient outcomes in a medical intensive care unit. *Heart and Lung, 21*(1), 18–24.

Blair, J. D., & Fottler, M. D. (1998). Effective stakeholder management: Challenges, opportunities and strategies. In W. J. Duncan, P. M. Ginter, & L. E. Swayne (Eds.), *Handbook of health care management* (pp. 19–48). Malden, MA: Blackwell.

Blum, H. K. (1983). *Expanding healthcare horizons: From a general systems concept of health to a national health policy* (2nd ed.). Oakland, CA: Third Party Publishing.

Carroll, A. B. (1979). A three-dimensional conceptual model of corporate performance. *Academy of Management Review, 4,* 497–505.

Carroll, A. B. (1991, July-August). The pyramid of corporate social responsibility: Towards a moral management of organizational stakeholders. *Business Horizons, 34*(4), 39–48.

Charns, M. P., & Schaefer, M. J. (1983). *Health care organizations: A model for management.* Englewood Cliffs, NJ: Prentice-Hall.

Charns, M. P., & Tewksbury, L. J. (1993). *Collaborative management in health care.* San Francisco: Jossey Bass.

Claxton, G., Feder, J., Shactman, D., & Altman, S. (1997, March/April). Public policy issues in nonprofit conversions: An overview. *Health Affairs, 16*(2), 9–28.

Cleland, D., & King, W. R. (1997). *Project management handbook.* New York: John Wiley & Sons.

Diamond, H. S., Goldberg, E., & Janosky, J. E. (1998). The effect of full-time faculty hospitalists on the efficiency of care at a community teaching hospital. *Annals of Internal Medicine, 129*(3), 197–203.

Draft, R. L., & Steers, R. M. (1986). *Organizations: A micro/macro approach.* Reading, MA: Addison-Wesley Educational Publishers, Inc.

Evans, R. G., Barer, M. L., & Marmor, T. R. (1994). *Why are some people healthy and others not? The determinants of health of populations.* New York: Aldine De Gruyter.

Fahey, L., & Narayaman, V. K. (1986). *Macroenvironmental analysis for strategic management.* St. Paul, MN: West Publishing.

Flood, A. B. (1994). The impact of organizational and managerial factors on the quality of care in health care organizations. *Medical Care Review, 51*(4), 381–428.

Fottler, M. D., Blair, J. D., Whitehead, C. J., Laus, M. D., & Savage, G. T. (1989, Winter). Assessing key stakeholders: Who matters to hospitals and why? *Hospital and Health Services Administration, 34*(4), 525–546.

General Accounting Office. (1994, September). *Health care reform: Report cards are useful but significant issues need to be addressed.* (GAO/HEHS-94-219). Report to the Chairman, Committee on Labor and Human Resources, U.S. Senate.

Ginter, P. M., Swayne, L. M., & Duncan, W. J. (1998). *Strategic management of health care organizations* (3rd ed.). Malden, MA: Blackwell.

Gittell, J. H., & Wimbush, J. (1998, July). *Improving care coordination and patient outcomes: Initial report to participants in the care coordination study.* Cambridge, MA: Harvard Business School.

Gorey, T. (1994, August). PHOs enhance health care delivery through physician-hospital cooperation. *Wisconsin Medical Journal,* 461–465.

Gray, B. H. (1997, March/April). Conversion of HMOs and hospitals: What's at stake? *Health Affairs, 16*(2), 29–47.

Hage, J. (1980). *Theories of organizations: Forms, processes, and transformations.* New York: Wiley-Interscience.

Holt, D. H. (1992). *Management: Principles and practices* (3rd ed.). Englewood Cliffs, NJ: Prentice-Hall.

Joint Commission on Accreditation of Healthcare Organizations. (1997). *Accreditation manual for hospitals,* Continuum of Care (cc5). Chicago: Author.

Kanter, E. M. (1990). *When giants learn to dance.* New York: Simon and Schuster.

Kapp, M. B. (1990, March). Cookbook medicine: A legal perspective. *Archives of Internal Medicine, 150,* 496–500.

Knaus, W. A., Draper, E. A., Wagner, D. P., & Zimmerman, J. E. (1986). An evaluation of outcome from intensive care in major medical centers. *Annals of Internal Medicine, 104*(3), 410–418.

Kraut, A. I., Pedigo, P. R., McKenna, D. D., & Dunnette, M. D. (1989, November). The role of manager: What's really important in different management jobs. *The Academy of Management EXECUTIVE, 3*(4), 286–293.

Lawrence, P. R., & Lorsch, J. W. (1967, June). Differentiation and integration in complex organizations. *Administrative Science Quarterly, 11*(3), 1–47.

Likert, R. (1967). *The human organization.* New York: McGraw-Hill.

Longest, B. B., Jr. (1990, Winter). Interorganizational linkages in the health sector. *Health Care Management Review, 15,* 17–28.

Longest, B. B., Jr. (1997). *Seeking strategic advantage through health policy analysis.* Chicago: Health Administration Press.

Longest, B. B., Jr. (1998a). *Health policymaking in the United States* (2nd ed.). Chicago: Health Administration Press.

Longest, B. B., Jr. (1998b, March/April). Managerial competence at senior levels of integrated delivery systems. *Journal of Healthcare Management, 43*(2), 115–135.

Longest, B. B., Jr., & Rakich, J. S. *Managing Health Services, Organizations and Systems,* 4th ed. Baltimore, MD: Health Professions Press, forthcoming.

Luke, R. D., Begun, J. W., & Pointer, D. D. (1989). Quasi firms: Strategic interorganizational forms in the health care industry. *The Academy of Management Review, 14*(1), 13.

Luthans, F. (1997). *Organizational behavior* (8th ed.). New York: The McGraw-Hill Companies.

March, J., & Simon, H. (1958). *Organizations.* New York: John Wiley & Sons.

Mintzberg, H. (1979). *The structuring of organizations.* Englewood Cliffs, NJ: Prentice-Hall.

Mintzberg, H. (1983). *Structure in fives: Designing effective organizations.* Englewood Cliffs, NJ: Prentice-Hall.

Newstrom, J. W., & Davis, K. (1993). *Organizational behavior: Human behavior at work* (9th ed.). New York: McGraw-Hill, p. 102.

Pearson, S. D., Goulart-Fischer, R. N., & Lee, T. H. (1995). Critical pathways as a strategy for improving care: Problems and potential. *Annals of Internal Medicine, 123*(12), 941–948.

Pfeffer, J., & Salanick, G. R. (1978). *The external control of organizations: A resource dependence perspective.* New York: Harper & Row.

Pointer, D. D., Begun, J. W., & Luke, R. D. (1988, Summer). Managing interorganizational dependencies in the new health care marketplace. *Hospital and Health Service Administration, 33*(2), 167–177.

Porter, M. E. (1985). *Competitive advantage: Creating and sustaining superior performance.* New York: The Free Press.

Rakich, J. S., Longest, B. B. Jr., & Darr, K. (1992). *Managing Health Services Organizations, 3rd ed.* Baltimore, MD: Health Professions Press.

Robbins, S. P., & Coulter, M. K. (1998). *Management* (6th ed.). Englewood Cliffs, NJ: Prentice-Hall.

Satinsky, M. A. (1998). *The foundations of integrated care.* Chicago: American Hospital Publishing.

Schlesinger, M., Gray, B. H., & Bradley, E. (1996, Winter). Charity and community: The role of nonprofit ownership in a managed healthcare system. *Journal of Health Politics, Policy and Law, 21*(4), 697–751.

Scott, W. R. (1982, Fall). Managing professional work: Three models of control for health organizations. *Health Services Research, 17*(3), 213–240.

Scott, W. R., Mitchell, T. R., & Birmbaum, P. H. (1981). *Organization theory: A structural and behavioral analysis* (4th ed.). Homewood, IL: Richard D. Irwin.

Shortell, S. M. (1991). *Effective hospital-physician relationships.* Chicago: Health Administration Press.

Shortell, S. M., Gillies, R. R., Anderson, D. A., Erickson-Morgan, K., & Mitchell, J. B. (1996). *Remaking healthcare in America: Building organized delivery systems.* San Francisco: Jossey-Bass.

Shortell, S. M., Zimmerman, J. E., Rousseau, D. M., Gillies, R. R., Wagner, D. P., Draper, E. A., Knaus,

W. A., & Duffy, J. (1994). The performance of intensive care units: Does good management make a difference? *Medical Care, 32*(5), 508–525.

Starkweather, D. B. (1981). *Hospital mergers in the making.* Ann Arbor, MI: Health Administration Press.

Thomas, J. B., & McDaniel, R. R., Jr. (1990). Interpreting strategic issues: Effects of strategy and the information-processing structure of top management teams. *Academy of Management Journal, 33*(2), 288–298.

Thompson, J. D. (1967). *Organizations in action.* New York: McGraw Hill.

Van de Ven, A., Delbecq, A., & Koenig, R. (1976, April). Determinants of coordination modes within organizations. *American Sociological Review, 41,* 322–338.

Weick, K. (1976). Educational organizations as loosely coupled systems. *Administrative Science Quarterly, 21*(1), 1–19.

Whitener, E. M., Brodt, S. E. M., Korsgaard, A., & Werner, J. M. (1998, July). Managers as initiators of trust: An exchange relationship framework for understanding managerial trustworthy behavior. *The Academy of Management Review, 23*(3), 513–530.

Young, G. J., Charns, M. P., Daley, J., Forbes, M. G., Henderson, W., & Khuri, S. F. (1997). Best practices for managing surgical services: The role of coordination. *Health Care Management Review, 22*(4), 72–81.

Young, G. J., Charns, M. P., Desai, K., Khuri, S. F., Forbes, M. G., Henderson, W., & Daley, J. (1998). Patterns of coordination and surgical outcomes: A study of surgical services. *Health Services Research, 33*(5).

Zuckerman, H. S., & Kaluzny, A. D. (1991, Spring). Strategic alliances in health care: The challenges of cooperation. *Frontiers of Health Services Management, 7*(3), 3–23.

CHAPTER

9

Power and Politics in Health Services Organizations

Jeffrey A. Alexander, Ph.D.
Laura L. Morlock, Ph.D.

Chapter Outline

- The Role of Power and Politics in Health Services Organizations
- Power, Influence, and Politics—Definitions
- Why Systems of Power and Politics Arise
- Rational versus Political Perspectives on Management
- Power Use Conditions
- Sources of Power
- Developing and Using Power—Domains of Political Activity
- Consolidation of Power
- The Structure of Political Activity in Organizations
- Power Strategies and Tactics
- Power, Politics, and Organizational Performance

Learning Objectives

After completing this chapter, the reader should be able to:

1. Distinguish between rational and political models of organization and their appropriateness to health services organizations.
2. Know the practical, managerial implications of the effective use of power in health services organizations.
3. Identify the conditions that promote the use of power, politics, and informal influence in health services organizations.
4. Understand the range of political strategies and tactics employed by members of health services organizations.
5. Understand the sources of power in health services organizations.
6. Know the key approaches for consolidating and developing power by managers, physicians, and other groups in health services organizations.

Key Terms

Alliances
Authority
Coalitions
Co-optation
Cope with Uncertainties
Formal Authority System
Influence
Influence Systems
Interdependency
Interests
Political Games
Political Model of Organizations
Politics
Power
Rational Model of Organizations
Sources of Power
Uncertainty

Chapter Purpose

Whether at hospitals, health maintenance organizations (HMOs), group practices, or preferred provider organizations (PPOs), the conflicts presented at Suburban Healthcare System are not unique. Managers of health care organizations are continually required to balance the rational, or task-oriented, with the social reality of organizational life (Buck, 1966; Cyert & March, 1963; MacMillan, 1978; March & Olsen, 1976). This chapter will discuss the means by which power distributions in health care organizations can be identified, the conditions under which conflict between groups may result, the use of power to resolve conflict, and the strategies and tactics that are commonly employed in the effective use of power.

THE ROLE OF POWER AND POLITICS IN HEALTH SERVICES ORGANIZATIONS

Health care managers continually strive to improve efficiencies and productivity in the delivery of clinical care as well as meeting established organizational goals. Yet the reality is that these goals are not easily defined or universally accepted by organizational members. As we see at Suburban Healthcare System, interests within a given organization vary widely across departments, occupational groups, and individuals; and the role of management is to achieve a sense of balance. Success requires that managers must be cognizant of the distribution of power in their organization, the circumstances under which power is utilized, and tactics and strategies associated with the effective use of such power (Pfeffer, 1981, 1992).

If asked, most health services managers would acknowledge the existence and importance of informal power and politics as central forces in their organizations. However, these same managers are often reluctant to legitimize power and politics as acceptable bases of the management process (Pfeffer, 1992). Official de-emphasis of the use of informal power in organizations stems from a number of sources. First, such power is viewed as illegitimate by many managers because it often operates outside the formal authority system of the organization (Kanter, 1979; Kotter, 1985). Any casual examination of the organization chart of a large tertiary hospital would reveal a complex system of reporting relationships and authority channels. This official system of accountabilities, control, and influence, however, does not fully represent what transpires between managers, physicians, and other groups of health care providers (Young & Saltman, 1985). What gets done, how it gets done, and even the establishment of organizational goals themselves may be determined largely through a process of coalition building and influence that operates outside of, and sometimes in spite of, the formal authority structure expressed on the organizational chart (Perrow, 1961, 1963).

Secondly, many view the use of informal power as leading to subversion of organizational goals. Anything that occurs outside the formal authority structure of the organization is potentially motivated by self-serving interests on the part of individuals or groups. Such behavior is often assumed to run counter to the attainment of officially sanctioned organizational goals (Pfeffer, 1992).

Because health care has been subject to a rapid pace of technological, financing, social and market

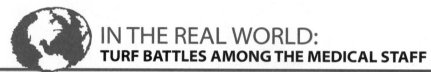

IN THE REAL WORLD:
TURF BATTLES AMONG THE MEDICAL STAFF

Terry Johnson leaned back in her chair feeling over-whelmed by the stacks of memos and reports piled on the desk before her. As the new administrative resident at Suburban Healthcare System, she had been delighted when Sandy Shulman, the chief operating officer, sug-gested that Terry assist her and the finance director to pre-pare for a series of meetings with clinical chiefs that would help develop the next three-year capital budget.

Sandy had handed over a thick folder filled with budget requests and then explained that Terry's role would be to help track down any additional patient volume and market-area data that could help determine both the need for and the desirability of each of the major proposals for equipment or renovations. Delight had quickly faded into dismay, however, as Terry wondered what types of infor-mation could possibly be helpful to senior management and the governing board as they tried to evaluate the ar-ray of proposals with their competing priorities and some-times contradictory assumptions.

A good example was the proposal from the Department of Surgery for renovation funds and equipment to create their own capability within the department for perform-ing coronary angiographies. Currently this procedure

was performed in laboratories within the Department of Radiology, but according to the Surgery Department pro-posal, the limited space and equipment available could no longer accommodate the growing demand. Terry noted that the budget request from the Department of Radiology included funds to purchase an additional image intensi-fier as well as other equipment needed to increase the ca-pacity of radiology for performing angiographies and other interventional radiological procedures.

At Sandy's suggestion, Terry had met with the man-ager in Radiology responsible for scheduling these proce-dures. It appeared that afternoon time slots were almost always available without a long waiting period for an ap-pointment. Competition was severe, however, among physicians trying to schedule patients in the early morn-ing, particularly during the 7 A.M.–9 A.M. periods. In addition, during the past few months a number of com-plaints had resulted from emergency cases "bumping" patients undergoing elective procedures from the sched-ule. Perhaps additional capacity was needed, but in which department?

There also seemed to be several other duplicate propos-als with requests for similar equipment purchases. It ap-

change, there has been a corresponding need for health care organizations of all types to make deci-sions rapidly, respond quickly to competitors' ac-tions, develop new services and enter new markets in a timely fashion. Under such time-related pressures, health care organizations can no longer depend on traditional, cumbersome vertical channels of author-ity and reporting relationships to make decisions and implement them quickly. Less hierarchical methods of getting things done are becoming the norm, and these methods often rely more on power and influ-ence, negotiation and network positioning than for-mal authority, or position in the organizational hier-archy (Pfeffer, 1997).

Jeffrey Pfeffer (1981, 1992), for example, has re-cently argued that this is a short-sighted view of the

use of power and politics in organizations and that informal power can be used within the framework of organizational goals and objectives. His argument rests on the premise that making decisions is a rela-tively easy job for managers. It is the implementa-tion of these decisions that brings into play various constituencies, interests, and potential resistance. The use of power provides a means through which good managers can manage the consequences of their decisions.

The importance of power and its use is reinforced if one considers that, in most health care organiza-tions, ambiguity and uncertainty surround both the establishment of organizational goals and the means to achieve these goals. The pervasiveness of ambiguity and uncertainty in health delivery or-

peared, for example, that both the Department of Radiology and the Obstetrics and Gynecology Service were planning to double their capacity to perform pelvic ultrasounds and mammography. Terry was aware that a large freestanding diagnostic imaging center recently had opened nearby and wondered whether the utilization projections of either proposal would be likely to materialize.

In a subsequent meeting with Sandy to go over detailed population projections by gender and age group for their market area, Terry voiced her confusion regarding the duplication in requests for new equipment. Could it be cost-effective for the same types of procedures to be performed by multiple specialties in different clinical services within the health system?

Sandy commented that this question was being pondered throughout the country as technological advances continued to create important new devices and techniques that are not clearly the domain of any one specialty. In some hospitals, for example, general surgeons and gastroenterologists argued over who should be credentialed to perform laparoscopic cholecystectomies—a surgical procedure that allows a patient's gallbladder to be removed through small incisions in the abdomen. In other medical centers, disputes waged over whether obstetricians-gynecologists or radiologists were better trained to perform and interpret pelvic ultrasounds and mammograms; and whether radiologists or gastroen-

terologists should perform gastrointestinal endoscopy. In some hospitals, heated discussions were occurring regarding whether general surgeons or otolaryngologists were more appropriately trained to conduct head and neck surgery; whether ears, nose and throat specialists or plastic surgeons should perform facial reconstructive surgery; and whether carotid endarterectomies were more appropriately performed by vascular surgeons or neurosurgeons.

Sandy emphasized that such "turf disputes" were only likely to intensify as technological advances continued to outstrip the development of medical standards and guidelines for designating the credentials appropriate for performing specific procedures and utilizing specialized medical equipment. These uncertainties were often compounded by the difficulties in obtaining adequate data on patient outcomes and costs in order to compare alternatives. Terry realized that these controversies were likely to have important economic consequences as physicians attempted to retain and further expand their patient bases. But how, she wondered, could these types of conflicts be resolved?

Adapted by permission from Stephanie Lin Bloom, "Hospital Turf Battles: The Manager's Role," Hospital and Health Services Administration 36:4 (Winter 1991):590–599. Health Administration Press, © 1991, Foundation of the American College of Healthcare Executives.

ganizations suggests that problems, particularly important problems, are typically not solved exclusively by logical analysis and sound reasoning. The existence of disagreements about what organizational goals should be, how they should be measured, how they should be prioritized, and the means by which they should be achieved creates situations where different perspectives and interests come into play (Kotter, 1977; Kouzes & Posner, 1988; Salancik & Pfeffer, 1977). Managerial success in organizations is frequently a matter of working with and through other people (Pfeffer, 1992). Organizational success is often a function of how well individuals can coordinate their activities (Bennis & Nanus, 1985; Kotter, 1978). These functions are often a direct outcome of the effective use of power by

managers. Informal power, although frequently operating outside the boundaries of the formal authority system of health care organizations, is not necessarily antithetical to the achievement of organizational goals. To acknowledge power and its utility in organizations is simply to acknowledge the diversity of interests and goals within the organization, the existence and normalcy of conflict, and that organizational results may stem from the political behavior of participants with different preferences (Morgan, 1986). Power can be analyzed systematically so as to make management more effective. An underlying theme is that politics is a means to resolve disagreements and that an appropriate role for politics is to resolve conflicts in order to achieve ends that benefit the organization.

POWER, INFLUENCE, AND POLITICS—DEFINITIONS

Power has been a notoriously elusive term to define and identify within organizations (Bacharach, 1980; Mintzberg, 1983). It cannot be seen, it is not wholly captured in formal organizational charts, and it is not well operationalized or researched in the organizational literature. Indeed, terms such as *power, influence,* and *authority* have been used in a variety of ways in the literature on organizations and management. To facilitate our discussion, we will define power as the ability (or potential) to exert actions that either directly or indirectly cause a change in the behavior and/or attitudes of another individual or group. Put another way, power may be defined as the probability that one actor within a social relationship will be in a position to carry out his own will despite resistance, regardless of the basis on which this probability rests (Morgan, 1986). The term **influence** has been used most often to indicate actions that, either directly or indirectly, cause a change in the behavior and/or attitudes of another individual or group. Influence might be thought of as power translated into action (Cialdini, 1984; Mintzberg, 1983). Finally, **politics** is a domain of activity in which participants attempt to influence organizational decisions and activities in ways that are not sanctioned by either the formal authority system of the organization, its accepted ideology, or certified expertise (March & Olsen, 1976).

WHY SYSTEMS OF POWER AND POLITICS ARISE

Most writers agree that the use of power and politics in organizations occurs most frequently in situations in which goals are in conflict, where power is decentralized or diffused throughout the organization, where information is ambiguous, and where cause-and-effect relationships between actions and outcomes are uncertain or unknown (high task or strategic uncertainty) (Mintzberg, 1983; Morgan, 1986; Perrow, 1961, 1963; Pfeffer, 1981). Although health services organizations are far too varied to claim that they all meet these conditions, one could easily see how, for certain decisions and domains of activity, these characteristics might easily apply to organizations as diverse as hospitals, HMOs, nursing homes, and group practice organiza-

tions. It is often the case, for example, that governing boards and senior management have difficulty expressing clear, unconflicting goals and objectives capable of being operationalized by the formal structure and control systems of the organization (Crozier, 1964; Young & Saltman, 1985). Many argue that political activity and informal influence systems arise because of inherent failings in the formal system of authority. This logic is based on the notion that an important function of the formal control system is to articulate and operationalize organizational goals and to direct the behavior of organizational members toward the achievement of those goals (Mintzberg, 1983; O'Donnell, 1952). In many organizations, particularly health care organizations, this is at best an imperfect process since many goals are operationalized quite imperfectly, and some, such as the quality of medical care and service, are difficult to operationalize at all. In addition, most health services organizations have multiple goals such as providing high-quality and accessible care and maintaining financial viability. However, organizational participants are rarely provided with the means to weigh the importance of different goals in order to direct their activities.

The ambiguity and uncertainty in how to operationalize and prioritize organizational objectives creates an arena for potential conflict among even the most dedicated, well-intentioned participants (Morgan, 1986). As the opening example illustrates, this situation may be reinforced by the complex division of labor and differentiation that occurs in many health care organizations. This pattern may be due to the assignment of different tasks and sometimes different organizational goals to different units or occupational groups. The tendency is for each unit or subgroup to emphasize the importance of its own activities and sometimes to treat its own tasks as ends in themselves rather than focusing on larger organizational goals (Lourenco & Glidewell, 1975; Perrow, 1970). Such differentiation creates group pressures that promote solidarity within the group and mistrust or misunderstanding of other groups—a we–they relationship (Morgan, 1986; Pfeffer, 1992). Table 9.1, for example, illustrates the differences in principal orientations of managers and physicians that often foster conflict between the two groups.

Table 9.1. Cultural Differences between Health Care Executives and Physicians

Attribute	Health Care Executives	Physicians
Basis of knowledge	Primarily social and management sciences	Primarily biomedical sciences
Exposure to relevant others while in training	Relatively little exposure to physicians, nurses, other health care professionals, or patients	Great deal of exposure to nurses, other health care professionals, and patients; little exposure to broader business or economic world of health care
Patient focus	Broad: all patients in the organization and the larger community	Narrow: one's individual patients
Time frame of action	Middle to long run; emphasis on positioning the organization for the future	Generally short run; meet immediate needs of patients
View of resources	Always limited; challenge lies in allocating scarce resources efficiently and effectively	More limited view emphasizing resources needed for one's own patients; resources should be available to maximize the quality of care
Professional identity	Less cohesive; less well developed	More cohesive; highly developed

SOURCE: From S. Shortell, *Effective Hospital-Physician Relationships.* Ann Arbor, MI: Health Administration Press, 1992. Reprinted with permission from the Hospital Research and Educational Trust.

Together, these types of organizational factors generate attempts to influence decisions and activities outside of the formal system of authority in organizations. Of primary importance here is that such systems of power and influence outside the formal authority system are naturally occurring phenomena in organizations and must be acknowledged and used by managers to effectively render some decisions and to implement those decisions in such a way as to benefit the organization as a whole.

RATIONAL VERSUS POLITICAL PERSPECTIVES ON MANAGEMENT

The acknowledgment and effective use of power, influence, and politics in organizations requires a fundamentally different outlook on organizational life than that prescribed in many graduate programs of health administration. The key differences between the **rational** and **political models** of organizations are displayed in Table 9.2. Rational models imply that the managers of health care organizations are orchestrating the activities of a team whose members all subscribe to a common set of goals and objectives. Organizational members—whether physicians, nurses, ancillary care personnel, or others—are expected to perform the roles for which they have been appointed. Their behavior should be consistent with the achievement of commonly agreed upon organizational goals. Conflict in this context is seen as a source of trouble and an unwanted intrusion. Formal authority or professional expertise are the only legitimate sources of power, and all others are viewed as antithetical to the attainment of organizational goals.

By contrast, managers who acknowledge the existence of power and influence other than that vested in the formal authority system or professional expertise have a fundamentally different view of organizational life. These managers recognize that individuals and groups have different **interests,** aims, and objectives and that organizational membership is often a platform for pursuing their own ends. The central task of management is to balance and coordinate the various interests of organizational members so that concerted

Table 9.2. Rational vs. Political Models of Organizations

Organizational Characteristic	Rational Model	Political Model
Goals, preferences	Consistent across members	Inconsistent, pluralistic within the organization
Power and control	Centralized	Diffuse, shifting coalitions and interest groups
Decision process	Logical, orderly, sequential	Disorderly, give and take of competing interests
Information	Extensive, systematic, accurate	Ambiguous, selectively available, used as a power resource
Cause-and-effect relationships	Predictable	Uncertain
Decisions	Based on outcome maximizing choice	Results from bargaining and interplay among interests
Ideology	Efficiency and effectiveness	Struggle, conflict, winners and losers

effort can be achieved to work within the constraints set by the organization's formal goals. Perhaps most importantly, the power-oriented manager often uses uncomfortable situations involving disagreements and conflicts and turns them into positive aspects of organizational life. Conflict, for example, can energize an organization, keep it from becoming lethargic, stale, and subject to inertia (Hannan & Freeman, 1984). Conflict can form the basis for self-evaluation that challenges conventional wisdom and theories in use (Tushman, Newman, & Romanelli, 1986). Indeed, organizations themselves are viewed from this perspective not as unified systems but as loosely coupled systems where semiautonomous parts strive to maintain a degree of independence while working under the same name and framework provided by the organization. To be successful, managers must have the ability to read developing situations, analyze the interests that affect or are affected by these situations, understand conflicts, and explore power relations.

To put these claims in perspective, consider the various means by which things get done in health services organizations. The most commonly considered mechanism through which decisions are implemented and action is developed is through the hierarchical authority system, reflected in the organizational chart. But as an effective means for accomplishing organizational goals or implementing decisions, the formal au-

thority structure suffers from several shortcomings. First, it is somewhat out of fashion in an era in which cooperation, teamwork, and cross-disciplinary integration are emphasized. Second, in most health services organizations, to accomplish objectives requires the cooperation of others outside the formal chain of command. Finally, the use of the hierarchical authority system assumes that those decision makers at the apex of this system are infallible, or at least most knowledgeable, in their judgments. It does not allow for poor judgment or bad decisions on the part of top level managers (Pfeffer, 1981, 1992).

A second means for marshaling concerted action to meet organizational goals is through a shared vision or organizational culture. Whereas this perspective has been gaining wide currency recently, it also suffers from several shortcomings. First, it takes considerable time and effort to fashion an effective organizational culture that is consistent with the overarching vision or mission of the organization. Second, the culture, once established, tends to be relatively impervious to new ideas or paradigms and thus may become a significant obstacle to organizational change (Pfeffer, 1981, 1992).

This leaves power and influence as a primary means by which change is accomplished in organizations. Here the emphasis is not so much on the structure established by hierarchical authority or the system of norms and values subsumed under the organization's culture but on the methods by which political support and resources are marshaled to get things done (Pfeffer, 1981, 1992).

Although important, power is not used indiscriminately in health services organizations, nor can it be used as the only means by which organizational change is achieved. This is true largely because converting power into influence requires expenditure of time, energy, or other limited resources and may also demand utilization of interpersonal or political skills that are not equally distributed among organizational members. One might think of power itself as a finite resource that must be selectively utilized to preserve that resource (Mintzberg, 1983; Morgan, 1986).

POWER USE CONDITIONS

To effectively use power, it is important to recognize the conditions under which it is most appropriately used. First, because power is a finite resource, organizational members are more apt to employ it for decisions they consider to be important such as those made at higher organizational levels and those that involve crucial issues like reorganization and budget allocations (Pfeffer & Salancik, 1974). Second, power is more likely to be a factor for those domains of activity in which performance is more difficult to assess (e.g., staff activity rather than line production) and in situations in which there are likely to be uncertainties and disagreement (e.g., goals, priorities, and the means to achieve them) (MacMillan, 1978; Salancik & Pfeffer, 1974).

It is interesting to note that *all* of these conditions are evident in the description of turf battles among medical staff members at Suburban Healthcare System. The decisions to be made involve critical resource allocations across departments that will determine what major equipment purchases and renovations will be made during the next three years. These decisions are likely to have important economic consequences for the departments involved as well as for individual physicians. Moreover, the major disagreements described are in new areas of activity in which performance is difficult to assess due to the lag time involved in developing medical standards, including appropriate certification and credentialing requirements for innovative diagnostic and

IN THE REAL WORLD:
BUILDING EXTERNAL COALITIONS RESULTS IN INTERNAL SUCCESS

John O'Conner has been successful as CEO of Urbanwide Health Plan largely because of the external base of influence that he has developed. To ensure that his Atlanta-based company provides cutting-edge insurance products in his market, O'Conner realized that he must take specific steps to find out how other businesses run, develop a broader knowledge of political behaviors within organizations, and establish coalitions of external stakeholders. He became involved with the Atlanta Chamber of Commerce, and as a result of informal ties to local executives, was asked to join a number of boards of directors. He was elected president of both the local trade association of health insurance executives and later served as an officer in the national association of the same or-

ganization. He testifies frequently before Congress on matters of health insurance and writes guest columns in several widely read health and business periodicals. These and similar activities have enabled O'Conner to become a more effective manager by positioning him to scan the external environment for both opportunities and threats that might affect Urbanwide and provide him with tremendous informal authority and leverage among potential purchasers of his firms' products. Although some of his vice presidents joke that he is rarely around the office, they all acknowledge that his wide array of activities conducted outside the formal chain of command of Urbanwide are what maintains the firm's leadership position in its market.

therapeutic procedures. The situation is also characterized by disagreements regarding which specialties are more competent to perform specific procedures and who should have priority in scheduling patients and accessing equipment and support staff. In addition, there are uncertainties regarding future demand for the new technologies and the likely impact of increased competition in the market area. These circumstances in combination are highly likely to stimulate attempts to influence decisions and events through the exercise of political power.

The conditions described above are created by **interdependencies** among organizational members or units. Interdependence exists whenever one actor does not entirely control all the conditions necessary for the achievement of an action or for obtaining the outcomes desired from the action. When interdependence exists, our ability to get things done requires us to develop power and the capacity to influence those on whom we depend (Pfeffer, 1981, 1992). The development and use of power is particularly important when the people or groups with whom we are interdependent differ in their point of view from ours and thus cannot be relied upon to do what we would want. Even where there is clear agreement on these goals, different perspectives have a way of presenting problems. Consider the challenges facing a multispecialty group practice.

Given the multifaceted and reciprocal nature of patient care activity, there is often a high need for interdepartmental coordination. Further, there tends to be higher degrees of interdependence at higher levels of the organization, where tasks are less likely to be either simple or self-contained (e.g., strategic planning, restructuring).

It is important to note, however, that *very* high degrees of interdependence do not promote political or power activity because failure to cooperate under such conditions would assuredly mean the demise of the organization or the organizational unit. For example, very little political maneuvering occurs in the operating room or in intensive care units where interdependence is extremely high and where strong incentives to work together and coordinate activities are tantamount to organizational success. Taking the opposite perspective, we would expect power and political activity to be relatively low in those organizational settings that are characterized by simple or self-contained tasks (Hinings, Hickson, Pennings, & Schneck, 1974). In the hospital setting, for example, housekeeping and security might be examples of functional units that reflect a low degree of interdependence and, thus, limited political activity. These ideas are easy to illustrate with respect to medical staff turf battles. For example, conflict can be decreased and the resulting political activity dampened if resources

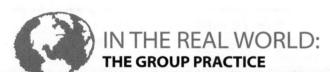

IN THE REAL WORLD:
THE GROUP PRACTICE

In a medium-sized midwestern city, a multispecialty group practice wanted to recruit a new board-certified cardiologist. The group presently had only one cardiologist, and several of the primary care physicians felt the patients they referred to the cardiologist were not being seen on a timely basis. The cardiologist who was currently a member of the group was extremely busy, and due to the contractual mechanisms by which she was compensated, quite satisfied with her income. However, being the only board-certified cardiologist in the group gave her consid-

erable influence in decisions such as capital acquisition and in her contract negotiations. Thus she was not in favor of recruiting a new cardiologist and was able to stall the process. This resulted in some of the primary care physicians losing patients who went to see cardiologists associated with other group practices. Eventually, the group practice threatened to risk terminating the cardiologist's contract and recruit two new cardiologists rather than lose patients.

are plentiful enough to decrease departmental interdependence by providing duplicate equipment, space, and support staff. Bloom (1991) describes a hospital where an intense dispute arose between radiologists and cardiologists regarding the most effective size for the lens on an image intensifier—a piece of equipment used during catheterizations and angiographies. Although both groups of specialists performed the same procedures and used the same type of equipment, the radiologists preferred a 14-inch lens, while the cardiologists had a strong preference for a 9-inch lens. To satisfy both groups, hospital management purchased image intensifiers with lenses of each size and established separate catheterization and angiography laboratories with their own distinct support staffs. If patient volumes and financial resources are not adequate to support such duplication, however, it is likely that conflicts of this type will be resolved through the political process.

The degree of interdependence in organizations is, in part, determined by the amount of resources available to the organization (Pfeffer & Salancik, 1978). Slack resources reduce interdependence, while scarcity increases it. When resources are plentiful, individual and departmental interests are more easily satisfied (Pfeffer, 1992). Organizational members and units tend to depend less on each other for the achievement of their personal or subunit interests, and thus interdependence is decreased. However, when resources are scarce, interdependencies are increased. The allocation of scarce resources means that some organizational units will benefit while others will lose.

Interdependence as a catalyst for the use of power and politics in organizations is only applicable if the players in the interdependent situation possess different points of view. If everyone has the same goals and shares the same assumptions about how to achieve those goals, there will be minimal conflict and thus little room for power and influence. Such differences in points of view are more likely to emerge where there is a higher degree of task specialization or differentiation in the organization (Hinings et al., 1974). Simply put, when work is divided into different specialties and units, it is more likely that these units will be staffed by people with different backgrounds and training, which will cause them to take different views

of similar situations. Table 9.1, for example, illustrates some of the fundamental differences in orientations between managers and physicians that may promote different perspectives on organizational goals, "best practices," and legitimate authority.

It is important to note that, even if the above conditions are met, power and influence will not be used indiscriminately. As mentioned previously, power is a valuable resource, and it is typically conserved for important issues. Thus, power is more likely to be exerted in situations involving major capital outlays, budget allocations, or strategic change as opposed to decisions on dress codes or changes in reporting forms. However, even minor decisions can sometimes hold significant symbolic importance in their ability to convey the appearance of power. For example, decisions regarding the relative location of the offices or parking spaces of the vice president for planning and marketing and the vice president for finance may be bitterly disputed since locations are often symbolic of an individual's or department's power within the organization (Edelman, 1964).

SOURCES OF POWER

Understanding the conditions under which power is used can help health care managers determine when power and influence are appropriate as methods for achieving organizational objectives. However, effectively using power in these domains assumes that one has the requisite amount of power to influence the outcomes of organizational decisions. Thus, understanding the **sources of power** is an important step in acquiring such power. Although some power is derived from personal attributes such as sensitivity, articulateness, self-confidence, and aggressiveness, an alternative perspective suggests that structural sources of power are more important (Brass, 1984; Hickson, Hinings, Lee, Schneck, & Penning, 1971; Mechanic, 1962; Pfeffer, 1992). From this perspective, power is derived from where individuals stand in the division of labor and the communications system of the organization. One's placement in these structures fosters power from a control over resources, the ties one has to other influentials in the organization, the formal authority system of the organization, or the ability to deal with important uncertainties or contingencies that face the organization.

Jurisdiction over resources is an important source of power within the structural framework but only to the extent that one actually controls the resource and its use. Further, resources that serve as a basis of power must be critical for the organization. That is, the resource must be essential to the functioning of the organization, in short supply (or concentrated in terms of the number of people who possess it), and nonsubstitutable. These three attributes make the resource critical and thus create organizational dependency on those individuals or groups who control its availability and use. Power is created by the dependence of others, and that dependence is a function of how much others need what we control, as well as how many alternative sources for that resource there are (Blau, 1964; Jacobs, 1974; Pfeffer & Davis-Blake, 1987). For example, many physicians in health services organizations will emphasize the revenue-generating capabilities of their clinical departments as the basis for further capital acquisition or the purchase of new medical technology. One hospital physician noted, "Of course, our argument about our financial contribution to the hospital is primarily useful with the administration and the board. It should also have some meaning to other physicians, however, if our work conditions become so intolerable that we are unable to continue to generate revenue for the hospital, and we are unable to continue maintaining our quality of service, there will be financial ramifications for everyone associated with the hospital (Young & Saltman, 1985). Access to and control over critical resources can occur at lower as well as higher levels in health services organizations (Mechanic, 1962). For instance, a purchasing agent often has considerable latitude regarding negotiating contracts for equipment and supplies. She can seriously inconvenience a surgical suite by dragging her feet on ordering replacement equipment or by refusing to expedite a request without approval from a department's administrator.

The acquisition of power through access to and discretionary control over resources is often accomplished through the formation of **alliances** and **coalitions** (Gamson, 1961; McNeil, 1978). The literature attaches considerable significance to the importance of finding others with common interests and building long-term relationships with them. Such coalitions differ from ad hoc arrangements insofar as they imply future as well as present commitment. Alliances and coalitions are developed through several different mechanisms, including helping people to obtain positions of power through appointments and promotions and doing favors for those whose support is needed (Pfeffer, 1992). Although both these strategies would appear to some to be decidedly antirational, and even illegitimate, they are often necessary in complex, interdependent systems with many actors and points of view. In health service organizations, alliances often emerge among the chiefs of clinical services in their requests for capital improvements. For example, the chief of radiology and the chief of orthopedic surgery may support each other in their respective requests for a portable fluoroscope and for renovations to departmental facilities. Frequently, such alliances may be used to mount a campaign against capital requests by other services or service chiefs.

A second major strategy for acquiring and developing new sources of power is control over or access to information. Power accrues as a function of one's position in the network of communications and social relations within organizations (Hackman, 1985; Izraeli, 1975; Pfeffer, 1992). How central one is in this network is dependent on one's location within the communication pathways that link individuals within the organization, the number of others with whom one has contact, and the distance between one's own location and all other individuals in the communication network.

A second source of power based on access to information derives from claims to special knowledge or skills that are critical to the organization. The primary power base of the hospital medical staff, for example, is usually perceived to be its control over a specialized body of knowledge and technical skills used to diagnose and treat patients (Burns et al., 1989; Scott, 1982; Shortell, 1992). Because patients are vital to the hospital's continued viability and survival, physicians' expertise gives them a strong power base within the organization. However, it has recently been recognized that the expertise required to deal effectively with increasing financial and legal complexities of health care organizations has accrued to management and that that expertise has increased the power of management in their relationships with physicians over the past several decades (Moore & Wood, 1979).

The third and most obvious source of power in organizations is that which is vested by formal authority, often expressed in the role or position of an individual in the organizational hierarchy (Tannenbaum, 1968; Weber, 1947). When observing an organizational chart, such as that depicted in Figure 9.1, it is relatively easy to discern what positions have **authority** over others and what positions are subordinate to higher positions. The **formal authority system** of the

organization is usually defined in terms of rights and obligations that create a field of influence within which an individual or department can legitimately operate with the formal support of those with whom one works. In other words, the organizational structure codifies official control over resources, information, and interaction with potential sources of uncertainty. Typically, those in higher positions are vested with the power to direct and influence those in lower positions. However, this should not be taken as a given by managers. Power vested in the formal authority structure of the organization holds only so long as those who are subject to this kind of authority

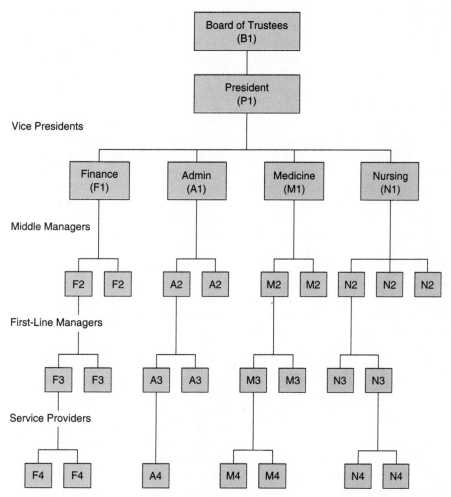

Figure 9.1. Formal Authority Structure: Acute Care General Hospital

respect and accept the nature of that authority. If formal power is not legitimated by those who fall under its purview, the source of power itself will be weakened. This sometimes occurs in situations where a tyrannical boss will so alienate the workers of an organization that they will refuse to further acknowledge his authority and will delegitimate his power by refusing to carry out his orders or by quitting the organization.

The ability to cope with uncertainties that influence the day-to-day operations of an organization is yet another source of power for individuals and groups (Brass, 1984; Fligstein, 1987; Hickson et al., 1971; Pfeffer, 1992). Much organizational **uncertainty** stems from interdependencies that occur within organizations—expressed by relationships between departments, occupational groups, or subunits—interdependencies that are defined in terms of the organizations' relationship to external organizations or actors upon which the focal organization depends for critical resources. With respect to the latter, the ability to deal with the vagaries of markets, sources of raw materials, or financing and capital can provide opportunities for those with the skills to tackle these critical elements and minimize their effects on the organization as a whole. Thus, managers in health care organizations who are equipped with the skills to deal with regulatory, accrediting, and legal forces affecting the viability of their organizations are in a position to cope with the critical uncertainties that these external forces create (Alexander, Morrisey, & Shortell, 1986; Glandon & Morrisey, 1986; Roemer & Friedman, 1971). From an internal uncertainty perspective, it may be argued that physicians are particularly skilled at dealing with the complex and uncertain situations presented by certain types of patients. Indeed, some have argued that the use of professionals in organizational settings is an administrative mechanism to deal with critical uncertainties that would be too costly to handle through the use of bureaucratic means (Scott, 1982). It should be noted, finally, that the power derived from an individual's or group's ability to deal with organizational uncertainties is directly related to the centrality of their functions to the organization and inversely related to the degree to which their skills are substitutable. For example, a political analyst in the health care organization whose responsibility is to interface with state regulatory agencies may lose some of his power if such functions can be performed equally well by a member of the hospital's marketing department. In health services organizations, physicians are viewed as a central source of unpredictability vis-à-vis the organization's production of patient-care services. Physicians admit patients, diagnose them, order tests and procedures, decide on levels of care, and make the discharge decision. Through their exclusive control over patient care, physicians control three of health services organizations critical resources: admissions, length of stay, and demand for ancillary services (Young & Saltman, 1985). The centrality of physicians to the organization is a major source of power to this occupational group. However, this power is increased by virtue of monopolistic control over a specialized body of knowledge. Physicians' monopoly over technical expertise frees them from most supervisory controls by hospital management and further weakens any attempts to reduce the unpredictability of patient care in most health services organizations. Finally, physicians maximize their control over the uncertainties in health care production through implicit or explicit threats to send their patients to other hospitals or facilities (Burns et al., 1989; Heydebrand, 1973). The use of these and other strategies are illustrative of the use of present power advantages by an occupational group to ensure and expand their prerogatives in the future.

Health services managers, despite having to deal with the uncertainties created by physician control over the production of health care delivery, are not without their own sources of power. The first of these are represented in procedural checks upon hospital activities imposed by external agencies such as certificate of need programs, PPOs, prospective payment systems, utilization review, and others. Such programs represent yet another source of uncertainty for health care organizations, which managers are well positioned to deal with. Also reducing the power base of physicians are changes in the numbers and employment patterns of other physicians within the organization's market or region. This has the effect of diluting explicit or implicit threats to deprive health care organizations of critical resources (e.g., patients, admissions). Finally, new competitive pressures facing health services organizations often compel trustees to take a more proactive stance toward limiting the prerogatives of physicians so as to increase the competitive viability of the organizations they govern.

DEVELOPING AND USING POWER—DOMAINS OF POLITICAL ACTIVITY

Power is a latent force until the possessor of such power chooses to utilize it in the form of influence or political action. In general, the use of influence and political tactics to reach decisions or to assist in the implementation of decisions is highest under conditions of high uncertainty. In its most extreme form, some view organizations themselves as consisting of nothing more than a variety of political interests or coalitions that disagree about goals and have poor information about alternatives for action (see Table 9.2). Because of the existence of groups that have separate interests, goals, and values, disagreement and conflict are normal and expected, and the exercise of power through influence and political processes are needed to reach and to implement decisions. It is unlikely that most health care organizations are as totally politicized as these models would suggest. However, there are certainly conditions within many health care organizations that promote the use of power and politics as a means for accomplishing the ends of certain groups or coalitions.

There are four domains of activity, in particular, that tend to be linked most strongly with the use of power and politics in organizations. These are structural change, interdepartmental coordination, management succession, and resource allocation and budgeting. Structural change is important because it potentially reallocates formal authority on the organizational chart. If, for example, a hospital is considering shifting from a functional to a divisional design, change in responsibility and tasks attendant to such design changes will also affect the underlying power base of various departments and individuals within the organization. Because of the potential effect on increasing and decreasing power among certain groups or individuals, political activity is often needed to initiate and implement such a change (Eisenhardt & Bourgeois, 1988).

One of the primary conditions for the use of power is interdependencies between different groups or departments within organizations. Such interdependencies often compel coordination among departments with different goals, strategies, and cognitive orientations. Because formal rules, policies, and procedures with respect to conducting tasks are often department-specific, there are few rules to guide the way in which departments should deal with one another. Perhaps more important, coordination often has implications for the responsibility and prerogatives of departments involved in a particular task. Hence, it is often the case that political processes and influence help define respective authority and task boundaries (Morgan, 1986). For instance, in some institutions medical staff turf battles have resulted in the clear delineation of practice domains. To cite one example, it may be determined that radiology should have the authority to control cardiac catheterization laboratories with their associated technology, technicians, and policies, while other specialists may request use of the facilities. Task boundaries also may be established and turf battles reduced through a negotiation process in which strict performance-based credentialing criteria are determined that must be met by any medical staff members seeking to expand their scope of practice.

In many health care organizations today, there is a great deal of instability in the ranks of mid-level and top-level management. Whether succession involves hiring new executives, promoting individuals from within, or transferring management to other units within a hospital or multi-institutional system, such changes may bring with them considerable change in the power structure of an organization. A new manager often brings a new set of alliances or values that can upset existing alliances and working relationships, as well as previous agreements among organizational personnel. From another perspective, managerial hiring or promotion can be used as a strategy to enhance one's political position if the new manager has allegiances or values consistent with those of particular coalitions in the organization (Pfeffer, 1981, 1992). Politically based promotions are often apparent when "unobvious" choices are picked for advancement. This means that the candidate may be chosen for promotion not based on her skills, expertise, or experience but on her loyalty or similarity to the dominant political coalition in the organization.

On the surface, resource allocation should be made on the basis of rational considerations such as allocating funds to those activities or units most central to the achievement of key organizational or strategic goals. However, the value of resources within organizations is so high that survival of various individuals and departments often depends on obtaining adequate resources. Resource allocation and budgeting become, in effect, the battlegrounds over which organizational priorities are debated (Davis, Dempster, & Wildavsky, 1966). The allocation of resources, the budgeting process, and political influence in setting the organization's agendas are inextricably interrelated. Such political action becomes particularly important in periods of resource decline. If resources are plentiful, all departments potentially receive an allocation that permits them to pursue their own goals and interests. However, as the pie gets smaller, a zero-sum game mentality sets in such that resources allocated to one department are viewed as resources denied another. As illustrated below, this sets the stage for considerable political activity within organizations (Hills & Mahoney, 1978).

CONSOLIDATION OF POWER

The distribution of power in organizations is not a fixed but a dynamic phenomenon that requires constant monitoring and adaptation on the part of managers and others who would effectively use it. Opportunities to gain power and use influence shift with changes in resource availability, contingencies that must be addressed, and the effects of others to gain control over resources, decision premises, and information. Several strategies are available to consolidate or expand power bases by groups or individuals to ensure that their power is maintained.

- *The use of organizational structure to build one's own power or stall the acquisition of power on the part of others in the organization.* Plans for organizational differentiation and integration, designs for centralization and decentralization, and the tensions that can arise in matrix organizations often entail hidden agendas related to power, autonomy, or interdependence among departments and individuals. For example, fragmenting opponents' power bases by adopting a functional structure is a common tactic that some-

IN THE REAL WORLD:
COMPETING GOALS AND CONFLICTING CULTURES

As head of this region's largest radiology group, George Watts had worked at Fairhope Medical Center for over 15 years. So when owner Medmark Corp., a large investor-owned system, sent in a new administrator, Mr. Wade Baron, last year, Dr. Watts paid what he expected to be a friendly courtesy call. But as the doctor now recalls it, the visit was neither friendly nor courteous. "You don't want me for an enemy," he says the new hospital chief executive warned him.

The context of the exchange soon became clear. Dr. Watt's group has long provided radiology services to other hospitals in addition to Fairhope, including Medmark's archrival. Without warning, the new chief executive issued an ultimatum: Split away from your group and practice only at Medmark—or leave. While the same mandate was issued for other physicians in other specialties at Fairhope, Dr. Watts emerged as Mr. Baron's chief foe. He and other members of his group continue to practice at the group's outpatient facility, at several other hospitals and, for the moment, at Fairhope.

"I'm offended that a businessman is trying to tell me when or with whom I can be a doctor," Watts states. Mr. Baron counters: "No one likes change and here's a new guy nobody knew wanting to institute change." Each boasts decades of health care experience. Each claims the moral high ground, saying that if his opponent wins, patient care will suffer.

times has no basis in rational organizational design. Viewed from the opposite perspective, the rigidity and inertia of organizational structures sometimes reflect the tendency to preserve existing structures in order to protect the power that individuals or groups derive from them. Resisting revisions in job descriptions or organizational designs or the adoption of certain new technologies or programs are examples of inertial reactions based on preservation of power or authority in the organization (Hannan & Freeman, 1984). An illustration of this tendency is evident in resistance to the implementation of total quality management (TQM) among middle managers who do not have a clear role in quality improvement efforts and who may feel threatened by new relationships that result from program activities.

- *Expansion of organizational boundaries or domains of activity.* An HMO marketing department, for example, may choose to expand its power by taking on the function of strategic planning, which some view as a natural extension of the marketing function. A move into strategic planning would clearly give marketers access to key information and enable them to influence top-level decision makers of the organization, thereby increasing their power. In health services organizations, the dynamics of power, acquisition, development, and use are often expressed in the relations between different occupational groups and their attempt to improve their professional position and status through expanding their domains of activity and responsibility. Nurses, for example, are becoming more highly trained and seek to increase their prestige vis-à-vis physicians. At the same time, nurses must fend off encroachments to their professional domain by medical technicians. Technicians, in turn, seek to establish their power through enhancing their professional legitimacy within the organizational hierarchy, often at the expense of nurses.
- *The principle of* **co-optation.** To diffuse the influence of rivals or to gain support from important groups, managers will often appoint influential members of these groups to special committees or task forces that are controlled by the manager. By giving them legitimate roles in a context supportive of the goals and interests of the organization, members of competing factions are co-opted into accepting these goals

and/or the legitimacy of the current authority structure (Pfeffer, 1992). In health services organizations, some managers maintain that appointing physicians to the board of trustees is a way to co-opt them into accepting official organizational goals as well as to reduce conflict and tension based on disparate interests between medical staff and the organization.

THE STRUCTURE OF POLITICAL ACTIVITY IN ORGANIZATIONS

Power may be converted into political influence within the organization. The exercise of such influence is often described as a set of "games," each with its own structure and rules that are played outside the legitimate system of authority (Allen, Madison, Porter, Renwick, & Mayes, 1979; Maccoby, 1976; Mintzberg, 1983). Mintzberg (1983) has described these games as structured in the sense that they have established positions, paths through which individuals gain access to positions, and rules that could constrict the range of decisions and actions that are acceptable. The most common **political games** and the reasons they are played are listed in Table 9.3.

The insurgency games are usually played to resist authority, or as a means to affect or prevent change in the organization. Frequently they are played at the point where decisions made at the upper levels of the authority hierarchy have to be implemented. They may be played by lower-level participants who attempt to circumvent, sabotage, or manipulate elements of the authority system and are often played by managers who distort or limit the amount of information sent to superiors in the authority structure. They can be played subtly by individuals or small groups or aggressively by a large number of participants willing to take unified visible action.

The insurgency games are sometimes met by attempting to increase authority (that is, by tightening personnel and bureaucratic controls and by administering sanctions). They may also be countered in a retrospective or prospective fashion by the counterinsurgency games. The most frequent are limiting the amount of information available to subordinates, fostering competition among subordinates to maintain control, and various forms of co-optation.

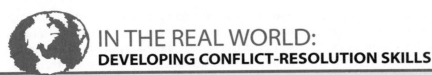

IN THE REAL WORLD:
DEVELOPING CONFLICT-RESOLUTION SKILLS

Like many other U.S. hospitals faced with decreasing occupancy rates and pressures to further reduce health care costs, Northwest Healthcare System and Parkway Memorial hope to establish a formal affiliation. Senior managers and board members believe that such a partnership will increase their bargaining position with managed care companies and other insurers, as well as make possible a number of efficiencies in services delivery.

During the past eight months of frequently heated meetings, it has been difficult trying to overcome the barriers resulting from decades of differing organizational cultures, practice patterns, and decision-making styles. A management consultant has been brought in to help facilitate discussions by clinical chiefs from the two hospitals regarding how to integrate services. But to make matters worse, the

clinical chiefs have found the consultant's "management jargon" exasperating. When counseled at one particularly long meeting to "think out of the box" in efforts to develop a common "mission and vision," the chief of psychiatry shot back: "In my line of work, only schizophrenics have a vision, and we give them medication."

The laughter that followed among the clinical chiefs helped break the tension. But the remark also helps underscore an important lesson: Managers seeking to resolve differences or mediate conflicts can't rely on management terms that seem unfamiliar to the individuals involved. Ideas must be translated by the manager into a vocabulary that is understood and comfortable for the participants—such a process of developing a "common language" almost always precedes finding common ground.

There are a variety of political games played to build power bases. Sponsorship games have simple rules: The individual attaches himself or herself to a rising star—or one already in place—and professes loyalty in return for a piece of the action. The alliance-building game is played by individuals or groups who negotiate with their peers implicit contracts of support for each other. The empire-building game is played by individuals to enlarge their power base by collecting subunits or loyal subordinates. In her study *Men and Women of the Corporation*, Kanter (1977) found that individuals who wanted to have significant influence on the organization had to play at least one of these three games: "people without sponsors, without peer connections, or without promising subordinates remained in the situation of bureaucratic dependency."

Budgeting games are used to acquire more resources for the positions or units the individual already has under his or her control. They are the best known of the political games, probably because they are the most visible and have the most well-defined rules. With respect to operating budgets, a variety of strategies are used to gain the largest possible alloca-

tion (e.g., always requesting more than required in the knowledge that a given percentage will be cut in the final negotiations). In the case of capital budgets, methods are typically found to underestimate costs and overestimate benefits (Table 9.4).

Professionals may play a variety of games in which their expertise is exploited as a political means of influence. These games are played offensively by emphasizing the uniqueness and importance of their skills and knowledge and defensively by both limiting the access of others to their expertise and discouraging attempts on the part of managers and others to rationalize or routinize it (i.e., to disaggregate it into easily learned steps). The lording games involve the utilization of legitimate authority or certified expertise for illegitimate, usually personal reasons.

Games to defeat rivals, such as the line vs. staff or rival camp games, are zero-sum struggles for control over organizational resources, decisions, and/or activities by weakening or sometimes eliminating competitors.

The strategic candidates game is the most common of the games played to effect organizational change.

Table 9.3. Political Games

Games to resist authority	Insurgency games
Games to counter the resistance to authority	Counterinsurgency games
Games to build power bases	Sponsorship games (with superiors)
	Alliance-building games (with peers)
	Empire-building games (with subordinates)
	Budgeting games (with resources)
	Expertise games (with knowledge and skills)
	Lording games (with authority)
Games to defeat rivals	Line vs. staff games
	Rival camps games
Games to effect organizational change	Strategic candidates games
	Whistle-blowing games
	Young Turks games

SOURCE: Adapted from Henry Mintzberg, *Power in and Around Organizations*, copyright © 1983, p. 188. Reprinted by permission of Prentice-Hall, Inc., Englewood Cliffs, New Jersey.

An individual or group seeks a strategic change by promoting through the legitimate systems of influence its own project, proposal, or person as a "strategic candidate." The decision-making process involving strategic decisions often is relatively unstructured, thus encouraging political influence attempts. Furthermore, power within the organization is frequently redistributed during periods of strategic change, usually in favor of those who initially proposed and fought for it. Although strategic candidates in this game are promoted through the legitimate channels of influence, it is important to note that they are supported, at least in part, for nonlegitimate reasons (e.g., in order to defeat rivals or to facilitate empire building).

The whistle-blowing game is usually played by an individual at a relatively low level in the hierarchy of authority who questions the legitimacy of actions by superiors and appeals to powerful individuals outside the organization for support. In the young Turks game, a small group, often with a significant power base, uses political means in attempts to effect fundamental changes in the organization's mission or in the systems of authority, expertise, or ideology. For example, in one religiously sponsored multi-institutional system, a group of newly hired M. B. A. graduates working at the corporate level engaged in a campaign to shift the emphasis of the system toward a bottom-line orientation and away from a traditional, mission-driven orientation.

Most health care organizations must coordinate the activities of a diverse group of highly trained professionals. The traditional system of formal authority tends to be relatively weak in these organizations. Specifically, there is often ambiguity in how to operationalize or prioritize organizational goals, particularly with respect to the curing, caring, and rehabilitation functions of health services organizations. In addition, because of the difficulties involved in measuring outcomes of professional performance, when goals are imposed on professionals by a managerial hierarchy, they are often easy to deflect. Second, among highly trained professionals, identification with a discipline and professional society may well be stronger than with the organization. When many types of professionals are present, intergroup conflict is likely as factions develop along lines of varying professional interests, orientations to patient care, or status distinctions among such groups. Third, highly skilled professionals have a tendency to invert means and ends—to focus on maintenance and further development of their own skills rather than broader organizational objectives. Further, although the skills themselves may be well-defined, the situations to which they may be most appropriately applied often are not. As the opening case illustrates, this situation may lead to territorial disputes over patients, clients, and activities among different disciplines and specialties within health services organizations. Finally, professionals traditionally have been expected to give the highest priority to the needs of their own individual patients or clients—an expectation likely to generate conflicts both with other professionals serving as patient or client advocates and with managers espousing

Table 9.4. Budgeting Games

Strategy	Description
Games to Obtain Funding for New Programs or Equipment	
Foot in the Door	Initially request funding for a modest program. Conceal its actual magnitude until it has gotten underway and built a vocal constituency.
Keeping Up with the Joneses	Base the budget request for new program funding on the rationale that the organization must stay abreast of the competition (whether or not there is a demonstrated need for the new program).
Keeping Up to Date	The rationale is based on the argument that the organization must be a leader and therefore must adopt the latest technology. An actual "Jones" need not be found and cited.
Call It a Rose	Utilize appealing (but misleading) labels. A classic example is the strategy used to obtain additional space by the National Institutes of Health in the early 1960s. During this time period it was impossible to obtain budget approval for new building construction, but it was possible to get funding to build "annexes." It is probably not surprising that at least one "annex" is more than double the size of the original building.
Games to Maintain Programs at Their Current Levels and to Resist Budget Cuts	
Sprinkling	Increase budget estimates by only a few percent, either across-the-board or in areas difficult to detect. Frequently this is done in anticipation that arbitrary cuts will be made. The goal is to attain a final budget allocation that is at the level it would have been without "sprinkling" or arbitrary reductions.
Create a Public Outcry	When budget reductions are ordered, decrease or eliminate a popular program in an effort to elicit client support and divert attention away from less popular program areas where cuts might indeed be feasible. A common example is the reduction of firefighter and police force positions that big city mayors often make when asked to reduce their budgets. The action is often taken in an effort to elicit popular support for budget restorations.
Witches and Goblins	Make the assertion that, if the budget request is not approved, dire consequences will follow. Appeals are based on emotion, not evidence.
We Are the Experts	Assert that the proposed budget must be approved because it reflects expert knowledge that "mere managers" cannot hope to understand. This strategy is frequently used by professionals of all types, including scientists, military officers, professors, and physicians.

SOURCE: Adapted from Robert Anthony and Regina Herzlinger, *Management Control in Nonprofit Organizations* 3rd ed. (Irwin, 1980), pp. 344–353.

organization-wide objectives. This combination of weak formal authority and highly developed systems of expertise creates strong catalysts for the use of politics as a means for achieving organizational goals or implementing major decisions.

The ambiguities and conflicts generated by strong expertise and weak authority systems are most likely to give rise to those political games in which peers compete with each other for the allocation of resources. Alliance and empire building, budgeting, ri-val camps, and strategic candidates games tend to be particularly important. It is also important for managers to note that they can often exercise considerable influence in health services organizations not by relying on the formal system of authority but by their centrality in the organization and a willingness to engage in the political process. When conflict resolution emerges as a critical organizational function, managers may attain influence commensurate with their skills in mediation and negotiation.

POWER STRATEGIES AND TACTICS

The actual use of power to affect organizational decisions or to implement those decisions is, in practice, a subtle, artful process. Power is most effectively used when it is employed as unobtrusively as possible (Pfeffer, 1992). For example, implicit threats by physicians to withdraw their patients or to send them to other institutions are most effective when such threats remain unspoken and not expressed overtly or presented as an ultimatum. A second principle related to the use of power is that attempts to influence are most effective if they are cloaked in an aura of legitimacy and rational purpose. That is, although personal or subunit preferences may drive the exercise of power toward a certain decision, outcome, or implementation process, the outward arguments presented for such outcomes or processes must be based ostensibly on achieving legitimation of actions or decisions. A third type of power strategy involves increasing support from other powerful actors in the organization for a particular decision or action.

The first two strategies, unobtrusive use of power and legitimation of decisions or actions, can be accomplished through a variety of means. One of the most common is to advocate the use of criteria that favor one's own position. This is a particularly common tactic in situations where multiple measures for assessing alternatives are available. Physicians operating in a high-cost, technology-intensive cardiac care facility may advocate the use of quality-related criteria for budget-allocation decisions rather than efficiency-related measures. The key point here is that by politically advocating that a certain set of standards or criteria be applied to a rational process, the use of power becomes legitimated through a standard organizational practice such as budgeting. A related strategy frequently employed in health services organizations is the use of outside experts or consultants. Such consultants can permit power to be used to affect decisions in a less visible way as well as lend to the decision-making process an aura of legitimacy fostered by the expertise of the consultant. At the same time, however, consultants may be carefully chosen to represent certain positions advocated by particular groups or interests within the health care organiza-

tion. For example, a manager interested in adopting a diversification strategy in his hospital may hire consultants known for their expertise in this area.

The third major strategy, coalition building, reflects the processes through which power and support are developed for political contests within organizations. Somewhat ironically, it is the interdependencies that exist within organizations that promote coalition building just as these interdependencies promote the conflict that leads to political action and influence attempts in organizational settings. In health services organizations, the formation of coalitions or alliances between groups and individuals is particularly central to the implementation of organizational decisions because power itself tends to be widely diffused in these types of organizations. The diffusion of power suggests that it is unlikely that any one individual or group will have the requisite degree of power or influence to effectively push the organization toward change or to implement an important strategic decision. For example, to effectively implement a decision to diversify into long-term care, hospital management may be required to build coalitions among key groups of physicians, nurses, and ancillary personnel who share an interest in this arena and who can help to defend this decision and overcome resistance by those groups who are more oriented toward acute inpatient care. The facts that multiple groups are affected by such decisions and that power is diffused so broadly among different subunits and occupational groups within the hospital suggest that coalition building is a necessary strategy for decision implementation, particularly for far-reaching and important decisions.

A frequently overlooked aspect of coalition building in health care organizations is that such coalitions may be externally as well as internally based. Many health care organizations are highly dependent upon important actors and organizations in their environment such as regulatory bodies, major purchasers of health care, key community leaders, and members of the board of directors. Thus, many subgroups in health care organizations often attempt to develop relationships with external stakeholder groups as a way of enhancing their power within the organization and as a means of gaining support for their positions in

MANAGERIAL GUIDELINES

1. *Recognize different sources of power.* In the majority of health care organizations, power is derived from multiple sources—formal authority, control over critical resources, expertise, and to a lesser extent, individual charisma. Effective health care managers must be able to distinguish among different types of power, be sensitive to the source of their own power, and be careful to keep their actions consistent with others' expectations.

2. *Use power selectively.* Effective health care managers must understand the costs, risks, and benefits of using each type of power and must be able to recognize which to draw on in different situations and with different people.

3. *Power and influence are not inexhaustible.* Influence in health services organizations should be considered a finite rather than an unlimited resource. Managers should direct their influence attempts toward those issues of highest priority or where the greatest benefits are likely to result and be willing to defer in other areas.

4. *Position yourself centrally in communications networks.* The highly complex and professional nature of most health services organizations usually results in multiple power centers. Managers can often exercise considerable influence not by relying on the formal system of authority but rather by establishing themselves in a central position vis-à-vis other power holders and being willing to engage in the political process.

5. *Use negotiation and mediation skills to control conflict.* The diffuse power arrangements and multiple goals of health services organizations may lead to recurring conflicts among individuals and groups. When conflict resolution emerges as a critical function, managers who have developed negotiation and mediation skills may attain considerable influence.

6. *Develop power by controlling strategic contingencies and resources.* Be aware of less visible but important power relations that occur outside the formal system of authority in organizations. Increase individual and departmental power by effectively dealing with strategic contingencies that face the organization.

7. *Political behavior and conflict are normal aspects of organizational change.* Regard political behavior and conflict as expected, normal aspects of organizational life. To be an effective agent for change, use power through building coalitions, co-optation of influential members of the organization or external stakeholder groups, and the control of decision-making premises.

8. *Use politics under conditions of ambiguity and uncertainty.* Employ principles of the rational model of organizations when goals are well defined and easily measured, when alternatives are clear, and when the relationship between means and outcomes is unambiguous. When these conditions are not present, consider using the political process to achieve desired ends.

organizational decisions. Medical staff members of a hospital may, for example, attempt to develop friendships with key members of the hospital's governing board in order to exercise influence over the purchase of a new piece of medical technology or, in some cases, express displeasure over the behavior of the hospital CEO. The hospital CEO may attempt to develop a relationship with key local purchasers of health care who would support him in key decisions affecting the strategic direction of the hospital. In developing any external alliance, managers must be prepared to weigh the trade-offs between the utility of these alliances and the potential influence exercised by external actors versus the cost that cultivating external sources of support might be construed as a disloyal act by others in the organization.

POWER, POLITICS, AND ORGANIZATIONAL PERFORMANCE

This chapter began with the claim that many managers view the use of power and politics in their organizations as dysfunctional for the attainment of organizational goals and positive organizational performance. Recent writings, in contrast, have maintained that the use of power and politics in organizational settings can serve to facilitate the implementation of important decisions in these organizations. In all likelihood, the truth probably lies somewhere between these two extremes. There is no doubt that influence attempts can be expensive and time consuming. Engaging in political activity, for example, may dissipate the energies and focus of management in health care organizations, restrict the flow of important information to decision makers, and distort perceptions about the opinions of others in the decision-making process. Indeed, in organizations that appear to be operating effectively and efficiently, the use of politics and informal influence is likely to make the organization more inefficient. Managers of successful health services organizations who desire to reduce inefficiencies stemming from political activity in their organizations might choose several approaches.

- If possible, increase the level of slack resources in their organizations to reduce conflict and to allow subunits to attain their own goals.
- Reduce differentiation and heterogeneity among organizational members and units so as to promote consensus in organizational goals, common views

of means to achieve these goals, and a common culture to bind organizational members together.
- Divide organizational rewards more evenly so that nothing substantial is to be gained from attempts at political influence.

Such strategies for reducing the level of influence and politics in organizations are also appropriate for managers who simply do not feel comfortable or have the skills associated with using power in organizational settings.

However, in the current health care environment, few organizations can be successful without adapting, often in significant ways, to the changing demands imposed by stakeholders, regulators, or competitors. In situations where major changes in strategy, technology, approach to the market, and management of the workforce are required, power and influence processes may be useful and even necessary to achieve such transformations. Over time, power may become institutionalized in health services organizations (that is, imbedded strongly in certain individuals, occupational groups, or departments). This is likely to result in a situation characterized by status quo orientation and inertia. Those in power will strive to keep that power by advocating positions that maintain the structures, strategies, and activities that brought them to power in the first place. As illustrated below, change and adaptation typically come only after great internal political struggle. Thus, to effect change that will ultimately benefit the organization, managers must be prepared to utilize power in a fashion to overcome inertia, resolve turf battles, and channel the diverse interests of organizational members and stakeholders.

DEBATE TIME 9.1: WHAT DO YOU THINK?

Trauma services in Maryland are coordinated by the state's Institute for Emergency Medical Services, a broad network that includes the State Shock-Trauma Center, other trauma centers strategically located in hospitals across the state, and the ambulance and helicopter personnel who

transport patients. Since its founding a quarter of a century ago, the 130-bed shock-trauma facility has been reserved for the most critical trauma patients, many of whom are flown in from all regions of the state with life-threatening injuries due to auto accidents. The Shock-Trauma Center also performs medical triage for the statewide Emergency Medical Services (EMS) system.

For some years the Shock-Trauma Center shared facilities with the state's major University Hospital. Although they were both governed by the same not-for-profit corporation, the Shock-Trauma Center operated with considerable autonomy. In 1984 the state granted approval for a new $35 million separate facility for the Shock-Trauma Center. Part of the agreement included the decision to transfer all trauma care provided in the University Hospital Emergency Department, including patients with knife and gunshot wounds, to the Shock-Trauma Center, which would be located only a few blocks away. The rationale for this decision was to conserve resources by not duplicating trauma care personnel and equipment.

Although the move to the new building was completed in 1989, Shock-Trauma physicians resisted treating a category of patients that they perceived as diluting the center's main mission. In 1992 a new director for the Shock-Trauma Center was hired by the not-for-profit corporation that governed both that facility and the University Hospital. The Shock-Trauma Center was ordered by top managers of the corporation to begin treating all trauma injuries that would in the past have been seen in the University Hospital Emergency Department. Three prominent Shock-Trauma physicians who resisted these changes were fired. At a well-attended news conference defending these changes, the new director, Dr. Bradley, explained that in an era of dwindling resources and soaring health care costs, it was important to end duplication and to move the Shock-Trauma Center into a closer collaboration with the adjacent university medical center.

Since the initial organization of the state's EMS system, the Shock-Trauma Center had assumed responsibility for medical triage, including directing the personnel transporting trauma victims to the most appropriate facility with available resources. The proposal to tighten the relationship between Shock-Trauma and University Hospital generated considerable concerns among other trauma system members regarding whether "patients would continue to be sent to where they could get the best treatment." Separate news conferences were called by a group of physicians representing other hospitals with trauma centers and by the state's volunteer firefighters responsible for the transport of trauma patients. The firefighters complained that they had not been consulted about recent changes in the EMS system. In addition, in separate statements to the press, conflicting positions on these issues were adopted by the governor who supported the new Shock-Trauma director, and several key legislators who sided with the fired surgeons in their belief that broadening the center's focus would dilute its quality.

At this point in the conflict, the state's largest newspaper published an article comparing Dr. Bradley to the original founder of the Shock-Trauma Center, Dr. Gordon, who "was a one-man wrecking crew if someone got in his way." According to the newspaper, Dr. Gordon:

> ... did not suffer fools or foes for very long. As he told colleagues, "Only a dog needs to be loved." The results, not his popularity, were all that mattered.
>
> And he succeeded brilliantly. Over the vehement opposition of other hospitals, jealous physicians, possessive bureaucrats and busy-body legislators, he carved out a new field of medicine— emergency medical services.
>
> Employing innovative techniques, he declared war on behalf of critically injured accident victims. By getting patients into the operating room in that first "golden hour," and by throwing teams of surgeons into the battle, he performed miracles. More often than not, he won the war. Thousands of lives were saved.
>
> Along the way, he collected enemies. It didn't faze him. He was smart enough to win the loyalty of a governor, key legislators, firefighters, and paramedics. Only when he was slowing down, when his own Shock-Trauma doctors turned against him in 1989 for creating "general chaos," did he step down. He died last fall.

Now some of the same doctors are seeking another scalp: Dr. Bradley's. Their complaint is ironic: they don't want Shock-Trauma to change. Yet this is an institution created out of change—a dramatic rethinking of how to treat critically injured accident victims. Dr. Gordon's whole life at the Shock-Trauma Center was about change. He kept the place in constant turmoil.

Time, especially in today's high-tech medical world, does not stand still. This is an era of severe government deficits, a time when the public is demanding accountability. Yet Shock-Trauma had been notorious for its lack of accountability and its free-spending ways. It insisted on total independence. That is now changing. Interdependence is the key word. And there is a strong effort to depoliticize what are essentially medical matters.

Dr. Gordon was superb at getting what he wanted from the politicians and winning public acclaim. At this stage, Dr. Bradley lacks the political skills that served Dr. Gordon so well. The circus at Shock-Trauma is likely to continue. Dr. Bradley's foes will see to that. But, what the heck. As Dr. Gordon used to say, "You can tell the pioneers by the arrows in their backs."

Fortunately, most political conflict in organizations does not reach the level of intensity displayed in this example. It does provide a vivid illustration, however, of the types of conflicts that may be encountered in determining organizational goals, as well as the fragility of the balance of influence in many multi-institutional arrangements.

SOURCE: *Adapted by permission from Barry Rascovar, "Shock and Trauma at the Shock-Trauma Center,"* **The Baltimore Sun** *August 9, 1992.*

Discussion Questions

1. Using concepts from the chapter, can you identify the various political strategies used by Dr. Gordon and Dr. Bradley?
2. As illustrated in Debate Time 9.1, what are some of the functions and some of the possible dysfunctions of using political strategies to effect change in organizations?
3. Do you agree that a strong effort should be made to "depoliticize what are essentially medical matters"?
4. Do you agree with Dr. Gordon's statement, "You can tell the pioneers by the arrows in their backs"? Is this type of outcome inevitable for change agents? (You may want to base your reasoning on concepts from this chapter and Chapter 12.)

References

Alexander, J. A., Morrisey, M. A., & Shortell, S. M. (1986). The effects of competition, regulation and corporatization on hospital-physician relationships. *Journal Health and Social Behavior, 27*, 220–235.

Allen, R. W., Madison, D. L., Porter, L. W., Renwick, P. A., & Mayes, B. T. (1979). Organizational politics: Tactics and characteristics of its actors. *California Management Review, 22*, 66–83.

Anthony, R., and Herzlinger, R. (1980). *Management control in nonprofit organizations,* 3rd ed. Columbus, OH: Irwin Publishers.

Bacharach, S. B. (1980). *Power and politics in organizations.* San Francisco: Jossey-Bass.

Bennis, W., & Nanus, B. (1985). *Leaders: The strategies for taking charge.* New York: Harper and Row.

Blau, P. M. (1964). *Exchange and power in social life.* New York: John Wiley.

Bloom, S. L. (1991, Winter). Hospital turf battles: The manager's role. *Hospital and Health Services Administration, 36*(4), 590–599.

Brass, D. J. (1984). Being in the right place: A structural analysis of individual influence in an organization. *Administrative Science Quarterly, 29,* 518–539.

Buck, V. E. (1966). A model for viewing an organization as a system of constraints. In J. D. Thompson (Ed.), *Approaches to organizational design.* Pittsburgh, PA: University of Pittsburgh Press.

Burns, L. R., Andersen, R. M., & Shortell, S. M. (1989). The impact of corporate structures on physician inclusion and participation. *Medical Care, 27*(10), 967–982.

Cialdini, R. B. (1984). *Influence: Science and practice* (2nd ed.). Glenview, IL: Scott, Foresman.

Crozier, M. (1964). *The bureaucratic phenomenon.* Chicago: University of Chicago Press.

Cyert, R. M., & March, J. G. (1963). *A behavioral theory of the firm.* Englewood Cliffs, NJ: Prentice-Hall.

Davis, O. A., Dempster, M. A. H., & Wildavsky, A. (1966). A theory of the budgeting process. *American Political Science Review, 60,* 529–547.

Edelman, M. (1964). *The symbolic uses of politics.* Urbana, IL: University of Illinois Press.

Eisenhardt, M., & Bourgeois, L. J. (1988). Politics of strategic decision making in high-velocity environments: Toward a midrange theory. *Academy of Management Journal, 31,* 737–770.

Fligstein, N. (1987). The intraorganizational power struggle: Rise of finance personnel to top leadership in large corporations, 1919–1979. *American Sociological Review, 52,* 44–58.

Gamson, W. A. (1961). A theory of coalition formation. *American Sociological Review,* Vol. 26 No. 3, 373–382.

Glandon, G. L., & Morrisey, M. A. (1986). Redefining the hospital-physician relationship under prospective payment. *Inquiry, 23,* 175–186.

Hackman, J. D. (1985). Power and centrality in the allocation of resources in colleges and universities. *Administrative Science Quarterly, 30,* 61–77.

Hannan, M. T., & Freeman, J. (1984). Structural inertia and organizational change. *American Sociological Review, 49,* 149–164.

Heydebrand, W. V. (1973). Autonomy, complexity, and nonbureaucratic coordination in professional organizations. In W. Heydebrand (Ed.), *Comparative organizations* (pp. 158–159). Englewood Cliffs, NJ: Prentice-Hall.

Hickson, D. J., Hinings, C. R., Lee, C. A., Schneck, R. E., & Penning, J. M. (1971). A strategic contingencies theory of intraorganizational power. *Administrative Science Quarterly, 16,* 216–229.

Hills, F. S., & Mahoney, T. A. (1978). University budgets and organizational decision making. *Administrative Science Quarterly, 23,* 454–465.

Hinings, C. R., Hickson, D. J., Pennings, J. M., & Schneck, R. E. (1974). Structural conditions of intraorganizational power. *Administrative Science Quarterly, 19,* 22–44.

Izraeli, D. N. (1975). The middle manager and the tactics of power expansion: A case study. *Sloan Management Review,* 57–70.

Jacobs, D. (1974). Dependency and vulnerability: An exchange approach to the control of organizations. *Administrative Science Quarterly,* Vol. 19, Iss. 1, 45–59.

Kanter, R. M. (1977). *Men and women of the corporation.* New York: Basic Books.

Kanter, R. M. (1979). Power failure in management circuits. *Harvard Business Review, 57*(4), 65–75.

Kotter, J. P. (1977). Power, dependence and effective management. *Harvard Business Review, 55*(4), 135–136.

Kotter, J. P. (1978). Power, success, and organizational effectiveness. *Organizational Dynamics, 6*(3), 27–40.

Kotter, J. P. (1985). *Power and influence: Beyond formal authority.* New York: Free Press.

Kouzes, J. M., & Posner, B. Z. (1988). *The leadership challenge: How to get extraordinary things done in organizations.* San Francisco: Jossey-Bass.

Lourenco, S. V., & Glidewell, J. C. (1975). A dialectical analysis of organizational conflict. *Administrative Science Quarterly,* vol. 20, Iss. 4, 489–508.

Maccoby, M. (1976). *The gamesman*. New York: Simon & Schuster.

MacMillan, I. C. (1978). *Strategy formulation: Political concepts*. St. Paul, MN: West Publishing.

March, J. G., & Olsen, J. P. (1976). *Ambiguity and choice in organizations*. Bergen, Norway: Universitetsforlaget.

McNeil, K. (1978). Understanding organizational power: Building on the Weberian legacy. *Administrative Science Quarterly*, Vol. 23, Iss 1, 65–90.

Mechanic, D. (1962). Sources of power of lower participants in complex organizations. *Administrative Science Quarterly*, 7, 349–364.

Mintzberg, H. (1983). *Power in and around organizations*. Englewood Cliffs, NJ: Prentice-Hall.

Moore, T., & Wood, D. (1979). Power and the hospital executive. *Hospital and Health Services Administration*, 24, 30–41.

Morgan, G. (1986). *Images of organization*. Beverly Hills, CA: Sage.

O'Donnell, C. (1952). The source of managerial authority. *Political Science Quarterly*, 67, 573–588.

Perrow, C. (1961). The analysis of goals in complex organizations. *American Sociological Review*, 854–866.

Perrow, C. (1963). Goals and power structures: A historical case study. In E. Friedson (Ed.), *The hospital in modern society*. New York: Macmillan.

Perrow, C. (1970). Departmental power and perspectives in industrial firms. In M. N. Zald (Ed.), *Power in organizations* (pp. 58–59). Nashville, TN: Vanderbilt University Press.

Pfeffer, J. (1981). *Power in organizations*. Marshfield, MA: Pitman Publishing.

Pfeffer, J. (1992). *Managing with power: Politics and influence in organizations*. Boston: Harvard Business School Press.

Pfeffer, J. (1997). *New directions for organization theory*. New York: Oxford University Press.

Pfeffer, J., & Davis-Blake, A. (1987). Understanding organizational wage structures: A resource dependence approach. *Academy of Management Journal*, 30, 437–455.

Pfeffer, J., & Salancik, G. R. (1974). Organizational decision making as a political process: The case of a university budget. *Administrative Science Quarterly*, 19, 135–151.

Pfeffer, J., & Salancik, G. R. (1978). *The external control of organizations: A resource dependence perspective*. New York: Harper and Row.

Roscovar, B. (1992, August 9). "Shock and trauma at the Shock-trauma center." *The Baltimore Sun*.

Roemer, M. I., & Friedman, J. W. (1971). *Doctors in hospitals*. Baltimore: Johns Hopkins University Press.

Salancik, G. R., & Pfeffer, J. (1974). The bases and use of power in organizational decision making: The case of a university. *Administrative Science Quarterly*, 19, 453–473.

Salancik, G. R., & Pfeffer, J. (1977). Who gets power—and how they hold on to it: A strategic contingency model of power. *Organizational Dynamics*, 3–21.

Scott, W. R. (1982). Managing professional work: Three models of control for health organizations. *Health Services Research*, 17, 213–240.

Shortell, S. M. (1992). *Effective hospital-physician relationships*. Ann Arbor, MI: Health Administration Press.

Tannenbaum, A. S. (1968). *Control in organizations*. Englewood Cliffs, NJ: Prentice-Hall.

Tushman, M. L., Newman, W. H., & Romanelli, E. (1986). Convergence and upheaval: Managing the unsteady pace of organizational evolution. *California Management Review*, 29, 29–44.

Weber, M. (1947). *The theory of social and economic organization*. New York: Free Press.

Young, D. W., & Saltman, R. B. (1985). *The hospital power equilibrium: Physician behavior and cost control*. Baltimore: The Johns Hopkins University Press.

PART

4

Renewing the Organization

THE NATURE OF ORGANIZATIONS: FRAMEWORK FOR THE TEXT

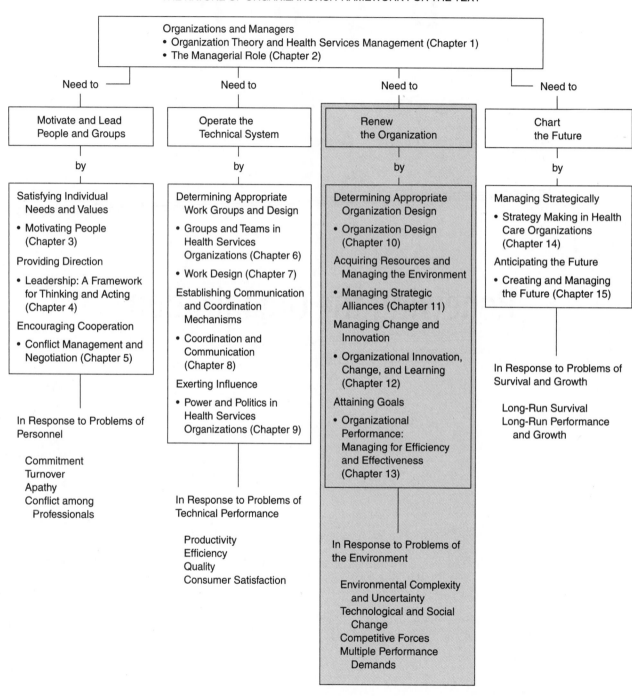

Organizations and Managers
• Organization Theory and Health Services Management (Chapter 1)
• The Managerial Role (Chapter 2)

Need to ———   Need to   Need to   └── Need to

| Motivate and Lead People and Groups | Operate the Technical System | Renew the Organization | Chart the Future |

by   by   by   by

Satisfying Individual Needs and Values
• Motivating People (Chapter 3)

Providing Direction
• Leadership: A Framework for Thinking and Acting (Chapter 4)

Encouraging Cooperation
• Conflict Management and Negotiation (Chapter 5)

In Response to Problems of Personnel

    Commitment
    Turnover
    Apathy
    Conflict among
      Professionals

Determining Appropriate Work Groups and Design
• Groups and Teams in Health Services Organizations (Chapter 6)
• Work Design (Chapter 7)

Establishing Communication and Coordination Mechanisms
• Coordination and Communication (Chapter 8)

Exerting Influence
• Power and Politics in Health Services Organizations (Chapter 9)

In Response to Problems of Technical Performance

    Productivity
    Efficiency
    Quality
    Consumer Satisfaction

Determining Appropriate Organization Design
• Organization Design (Chapter 10)

Acquiring Resources and Managing the Environment
• Managing Strategic Alliances (Chapter 11)

Managing Change and Innovation
• Organizational Innovation, Change, and Learning (Chapter 12)

Attaining Goals
• Organizational Performance: Managing for Efficiency and Effectiveness (Chapter 13)

In Response to Problems of the Environment

    Environmental Complexity and Uncertainty
    Technological and Social Change
    Competitive Forces
    Multiple Performance Demands

Managing Strategically
• Strategy Making in Health Care Organizations (Chapter 14)

Anticipating the Future
• Creating and Managing the Future (Chapter 15)

In Response to Problems of Survival and Growth

    Long-Run Survival
    Long-Run Performance and Growth

Organizations operate within a complex and dynamic environment. Health care executives thus manage the environment as well as the operations within their own organization. The four chapters in this section highlight the nature of the managerial role in terms of understanding and developing strategies for effective intervention.

Chapter 10, "Organization Design," focuses on fundamental principles, evolution, and alternative designs in terms of their strengths and limitations. The chapter addresses the following questions:

- What is organization design? What is the role of management in the design and redesign of organizations?
- What are the components and characteristics of design?
- What designs are available, and what are their strengths and weaknesses relative to different environments?

Chapter 11, "Managing Strategic Alliances," deals with the emergence and operations of such alliances. The chapter focuses on the following questions:

- What are the types and forms of alliance structures?
- What are the processes and dimensions that distinguish these structures?
- What are the stages or processes involved in the development of an alliance?

Chapter 12, "Organizational Innovation, Change, and Learning," presents an analysis of the change process and the various types of changes involved in health services organizations. Among the questions it addresses are the following:

- What are the stages of the change process, and what factors facilitate or inhibit that process?
- What are the different types of changes that may occur, and what strategies are appropriate to ensure successful implementation and institutionalization?

Chapter 13, "Organizational Performance: Managing for Efficiency and Effectiveness," provides an overview of the various dimensions of performance and the issues that face health care managers and their organizations. Among the questions addressed are the following:

- What is organizational performance?
- What criteria are appropriate to differential performance?
- What can managers do to improve quality and increase value?

Upon completing these four chapters, readers should understand the fundamental design of organizations, their relationship to other organizations, and how this relationship affects organizational performance and change.

CHAPTER

10

Organization Design

Peggy Leatt, Ph.D.
Stephen M. Shortell, Ph.D.
John R. Kimberly, Ph.D.

Chapter Outline

- The Meaning of Organization Design
- Levels of Organization Design
- Systematic Assessment before Design
- Designs for a Variety of Health Services Organizations
- Influences on Future Organization Designs

Learning Objectives

After completing this chapter, the reader should be able to:

1. Understand the principles of organization design.
2. Have an awareness of the evolution of organization design.
3. Use a framework for understanding organization design considerations.
4. Analyze common organization designs in terms of their applicability, strengths, and limitations.
5. Consider guidelines for changing organization designs.

Key Terms

Assessment for Design
Bureaucratic Organization
Centralization and Decentralization
Collectivist-Democratic Organization
Cultural Assessment
Design Process
Divisional Design
Environmental Assessment
Functional Design
Human Resources Assessment
Levels of Organization Design
Matrix or Mixed Design
Organization Design
Parallel Design
Political Process Assessment
Product-Line or Program Design

Chapter Purpose

The purpose of this chapter is to explore ways in which organizations, especially health services organizations, make decisions about redesigning organizational structures. Given the complex nature of the external environment in which organizations must operate in order to survive, managers must actively decide who has responsibility for making which decisions at various levels. In other words, who will have power in the organization and for what purposes? The focus of the chapter is on exploring a variety of organization designs that are typical of health services organizations and analyzing where the designs seem to work best. Given the changing environment of health care, designs that will help organizations maintain high performance during times of transition are highlighted. Consider the challenges at Sunnybrook Health Science Centre.

THE MEANING OF ORGANIZATION DESIGN

Design Is Dynamic

Organization design refers to the way in which the building blocks of organization—authority, responsibility, accountability, information, and rewards—are arranged or rearranged to improve effectiveness and adaptive capacity. Organization design and redesign are dynamic, being simultaneously *both outcome* and *process*. As outcome, organization design can be represented by the boxes and lines on an organization chart. These represent how the building blocks are arranged. As many organizations face increasingly uncertain and rapidly changing environments, new ways of representing organization are emerging, replacing boxes and lines. Intersecting circles, inverted triangles, and lattices are alternative ways of describing the outcomes of design and redesign.

Design outcomes, however, are generally transitory. Top management of most organizations is always searching for more effective ways to carry out their mission, and as external circumstances change, redesign may well be indicated. In effect, then, design and redesign constitute a process whereby current arrangements are evaluated and new ones are introduced, in some cases almost continuously.

Although we might like to think of organizational design as a rational, deliberate, and planned series of activities in which men and women of vision create organizational arrangements supportive of mission and strategy and performance-enhancing, in reality—particularly in a sector as volatile as health care—the **design process** reflects the realities of change. Changes in leadership, changes in goals and strategies, and pure accident are all reasons why a change in design may occur on other than a perfectly "rational" basis (Kimberly, 1984).

Management's Role in Organization Design

Management's primary task is to maintain and improve performance. In fact, management texts refer to organization design as one of management's most critical functions (Daft, 1998; Morgan, 1997; Nadler, Gerstein, Shaw, & associates, 1992). Usually, the activities of design are seen as the responsibilities of senior management; however, the most successful designs appear to be those that have been built with input from a broad range of organizational members, including key external and internal stakeholders and persons at all levels within the organization. Outside consultants are

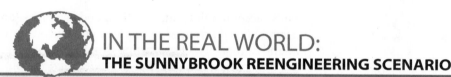

IN THE REAL WORLD:
THE SUNNYBROOK REENGINEERING SCENARIO

Sunnybrook Health Science Centre is a fully accredited academic health science center affiliated with the University of Toronto. Built in 1948 as a veterans' hospital, its ownership was transferred to the University of Toronto in 1966, and it became a fully affiliated teaching hospital. Since 1987, Sunnybrook has developed strategically focused programs in six major areas—cancer, trauma, aging, heart and circulation disorders, mental health, and community services.

Sunnybrook's annual operating budget in 1997 was approximately $265 million, and over $23 million per year was allocated to research. Sunnybrook employed over 4,000 people and had a geographic full-time medical staff of approximately 300. The hospital had approximately 1,000 beds providing a variety of adult services in both acute and long-term care. At that time, Sunnybrook averaged about 360,000 ambulatory visits annually.

In the early 1990s, senior management observed that over the previous four years, the Ministry of Health transfer payment—accounting for approximately 70% of the hospital's revenue—had been reduced by approximately $50 million over what would have been necessary to match cost increases. Management further noted that the government's deficit reduction plans would likely limit funding throughout the 1990s. In addition to this, consumers' overall expectations had been changing rapidly, and they demanded improved quality and service, which was reinforced when patient complaints were analyzed: 75% of the complaints were about system or administrative problems, not quality of care.

To add to this, a restructuring effort in the late 1980s, which decentralized decision making closer to the point of service and created eight clinical units with physician and nursing directors, left Sunnybrook with confusion over roles and budget control. Further, the clinical units created during the restructuring had no real authority over modification of work processes.

Enter Reengineering

As a result of these concerns, Sunnybrook's senior management in February 1992 reviewed the various alternatives to the clinical unit model, involving an extensive benchmarking of different approaches in a variety of jurisdictions. At this time, early results from reengineering attempts at six patient-focused hospitals in the United States were being reported. After lengthy consultation, senior management decided to restructure Sunnybrook so that it would both build on the experience learned through the clinical directorate model and harness the far more radical restructuring and reengineering being attempted in the patient-focused pilot hospitals. The announcement of the restructuring was made in October 1992 and implemented initially in April 1993. Changes have continued at a rapid pace since that initial announcement.

In describing the approach taken to reengineer Sunnybrook, President and CEO Tom Closson said, "You don't cut $22 million without looking at every single thing you're doing and how can you be doing it differently. What we're trying to do is get front-line staff, from nurses . . . to physicians to people who work in accounts, trying to get them involved in a discussion [on] how we can do things differently. When you say patient-focused care at Sunnybrook, what we're really trying to do is find out what the patients want us to be doing for them and then try and design what we do around what they want. . . ."

The result was a five-pronged approach. First, 14 operating units were created that were centered around meeting the needs of specific groups of patients—Sunnybrook's primary mission. Each unit began to think about patients as customers. Each unit grouped similar patients who could be served through an integrated organization, such as cardiology and cardiac surgery patients. The units became decentralized operating units, each with the budgets, the free-

sometimes brought in to provide technical advice on the range of designs that might be considered.

Often organization design has been thought of as a "once and for all event" parallel to an architect or en-

gineer designing and constructing a new building. In our view, when a new organization is formed, a new design will be created; however, the redesign of the organization is an ongoing process in which the de-

dom, and the flexibility to use information and quality improvement tools to better serve their customers.

Second, services were provided as close to the patient as possible; services were brought to the patient rather than taking the patient to the service.

Third, the concept of shared governance was promoted, in support of the intention to devolve authority. Shared governance is a model that places accountability for practice decisions at the level of the practitioner. It is supported by an infrastructure that provides for shared decision making and by an organizational philosophy that values and respects all staff.

Fourth, the roles and scope of practice of staff were expanded. For example, Sunnybrook had five different types of service employees who provided support functions on individual patient units. These included separate housekeeping, foods service, materials management, and nursing aid positions. Each had a different job description and limitations on activities performed and equipment used. Following reengineering, these duties have been consolidated throughout the hospital into one position—a service assistant who provides all these services to a specific set of patients. A similar consolidation took place for the accounting, documentation, admitting, and patient record functions (Trerise and Lemieux-Charles, 1996).

Finally, it was vital to ensure that the reengineered organization would still be true to the strategic direction designed for the hospital and that the inherent clinical programs and client groups were still a priority.

Lessons Learned

1. *Even with good planning, reengineering takes time. The review of the old system was conducted in 1991, and the new arrangements started in 1993 following training and education. In 1997, changes were still being made consistent with the original goals.*
2. *Communication is important, especially in a diverse population. There are no easy solutions to this dilemma, except to communicate in many ways, simultaneously and frequently.*
3. *The transition period is the most difficult time. It is during this destabilized period of moving from one state to the other that the organization is most vulnerable to the "organizational terrorist" who opposes the changes and will challenge and undermine it in the hope that it will lead to failure and abandonment. The only strategy to counteract this is to have clearly defined goals and to move as swiftly as you can through the transition period without losing sight of them.*
4. *Although there was much enthusiasm about giving service employees multiple skills, there was a reluctance to tackle multiskilling clinical staff across traditional professional lines.*
5. *Changing to patient-focused care in academic health science centers is more complicated because schools are organized on traditional professional models.*
6. *Undergoing reengineering did not happen without significant pain and grieving. As Sunnybrook's CEO and COO have said, "We have learned to be humble and recognize that we do not know everything. We were honest at the beginning in explaining that these changes required a leap of faith. . . ."*

Adapted from "Realigning around the Patient: The Application of Restructuring and Process Reengineering at Sunnybrook Health Science Centre," by P. H. Ellis and T. Closson, in Program Management and Beyond: Management Innovations in Ontario Hospitals, edited by P. Leatt, L. Lemieux-Charles, and C. Aird. By permission of publisher.

A version also appeared in Leatt, P., Baker, G. R., Halverson, P. K., and Aird C. "Downsizing, Reengineering and Restructuring: Long term implications for health care organizations." Frontiers of Health Services Management, Vol 13(4), Summer 1997, 2–37.

sign needs will change as the organization's needs change. The idea that designing organizations may be a recurring activity is most important for managers who may not only have responsibility for redesigning their organizations but also for ensuring that the design is implemented.

The design process is not carried out in isolation from other management activities. In fact, ideas about the type of design that might be appropriate should be derived from the organization's mission and strategic planning process (Pearce, 1982). For example, if a pharmaceutical company decides to expand its product lines, it may be necessary to reorganize its research and development division. If the Department of Public Health decides to close down its immunization program, it may be necessary to regroup ongoing services within the organization.

The way in which an organization is designed also has considerable importance for the nature and content of the information system needed by the organization. Since an organization design specifies who has power to make which decisions, it also indicates which positions need what types of information and at what times. Organization design also has implications for how performance will be evaluated and especially for the degree to which the reward system of the organization matches achievement or performance. Finally, the knowledge gathered from performance indicators will be fed back to subsequently influence the organization's mission. The relationships of organization design to these other management activities can be seen in Figure 10.1.

When Should an Organization's Design Be Rethought?

There are a number of circumstances that would suggest a manager should be reconsidering the appropriateness of an organization's design. Some examples of triggers or indicators that the best design may not be in place include:

- *The organization is experiencing severe problems.* Indicators of inadequate performance may be presented to the manager from external reviews such as accreditation processes and customer satisfaction surveys or from internal reviews such as financial statements and clinical audits. These problems may be identified at varying levels within the organization, for example, for a particular position, a work group or team, a department, or a total organization.
- *There is a change in the environment that directly influences internal policies.* In some circumstances, there

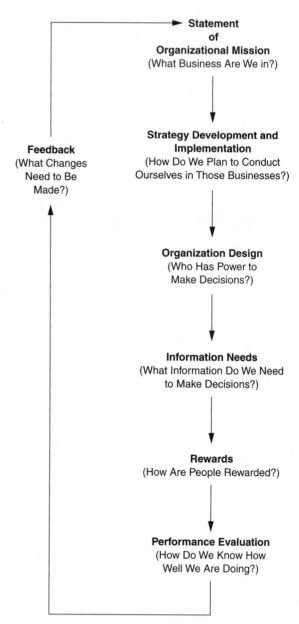

Figure 10.1. Organization Design in Relation to Other Management Activities.

may be major changes in the environment, such as capitation payment for all health services received by a given population or new policies regulating pharmaceuticals. These changes may require a redesign and refocusing of key organizational groups.

- *New programs or product lines are developed.* When an organization recognizes certain markets or product lines as high priority, an organization design change may be necessary to infuse resources into the new areas. Conversely, when old programs are to be dropped, new structural arrangements may be necessary.
- *There is a change in leadership.* New leadership may provide considerable opportunity to rethink the way in which the organization has been designed. New leadership tends to view the organization from a different perspective and may bring innovative ideas to the reorganization.

In summary, health services organizations are being redesigned to adapt to an environment where prevention of disease and promotion of healthy lifestyles are encouraged, incentives exist to redirect patients to utilize more cost-effective ambulatory care services, and there is a market pressure to provide high-quality care at a competitive price while improving patient satisfaction (Gillies, Shortell, & Young, 1997; Shortell, Gillies, Anderson, Mitchell, & Morgan, 1993).

LEVELS OF ORGANIZATION DESIGN

Several aspects of an organization can be redesigned or changed. For example, decisions can be made to change the overall size of the organization, the number and types of units or departments within, and how these units may be grouped. We can also decide to change the span of control of individual managers, reorganize tasks, specify rules and procedures in a formalized or standardized way, reallocate decision-making authority, alter communication channels, change mechanisms of control and reward, and determine how coordination will be achieved.

We typically think of design being achieved for a whole organization, such as a nursing home, a hospital, or a public health unit; however, design may take place for a particular group of departments, for an individual unit or department, or for a specific position (also see Chapter 7). Mintzberg (1983) has pointed out that the design of individual positions forms the basic

building blocks on which the design of a whole organization is developed. On a wider scale than a single organization, we may also create a design for a network of organizations in a given community or for a system of organizations (also see Chapter 11). These interlocking **levels of organization design** are illustrated in Table 10.1.

Designing a Position

In terms of designing individual positions in the organization, there may be hundreds from which to choose, depending upon the organization's size and complexity. For example, a new manager might be hired into a health services organization as an executive assistant to the president. If you were in this position, you would likely be excited about the possibilities and ask the president for a copy of your job description. The president, being amused, might inform you that your first task is to prepare a draft of your own position description for management's approval.

In designing an individual job or position for any level within an organization, it is necessary to identify the breadth and scope of tasks that can be performed and the extent to which the work can be standardized. Both of these factors have implications for the skills and training that will be necessary for the persons filling the job. Some of the basic parameters that should be identified include the major responsibilities and roles inherent in the position, to whom the position is accountable, for whose work the position is accountable, and the relationship of other peer positions to it.

Designing a Work Group

Several authors have noted an increase in the use of teams in health services organizations, which are seen as more responsive than traditional methods in competitive environments (Katzenbach & Smith, 1993; Mohrman, Cohen, & Mohrman, 1995). Quality improvement teams are often cross-functional, which can examine work processes that cut across organizational units (Gaucher & Coffey, 1993; McLaughlin & Kaluzny, 1999; Melum & Sinioris, 1992).

Table 10.1. Levels of Design in Health Services Organizations

Renewing the Organization	
Levels	*Some Illustrations*
Individual positions	Managers
	Staff positions
	Health professionals
	Other workers
Work groups	Task forces and committees
	Teams
	Units and departments
Clusters of work groups	Division of two or more units
	Medical staff organization
Total organizations	Hospitals
	Primary care centers
	Public health units
	Long-term care facilities
	Health maintenance organizations (HMOs)
	Multispecialty group practices
Network of organizations	Strategic alliances between physicians and health systems
	Organizations providing services for oncology patients
	Preferred provider organizations (PPOs)
	Affiliated groups of hospitals
Systems	A group of hospitals under single ownership
	All home health services in a state
	A national system of health services
	An integrated health system

Managers are often placed in the position of creating a task force or team to solve a complex problem in a short time frame. For example, a health services manager may be interested in identifying approaches that could be used to examine work processes that could improve the speed with which the results of blood tests are reported. A quality improvement team could be formed for this task. The manager should clarify the specific purpose of the work group, the time frame for completion of the problem solving, and the boundaries of the group's authority. Depending upon the complexity of the problem at hand, the manager should make decisions about the skills and knowledge necessary to complete the task. For example, to investigate the issue with the results of blood tests, it may be appropriate to use a multidisciplinary approach that includes a nurse, a physician, a laboratory technician, a hematologist, an orderly, or other health workers. A similar design approach may be used for deciding upon more permanent work groups, such as clinical units, strategic business units, departments, or other groups. These issues are further discussed in Chapters 6 and 7.

Designing a Cluster of Work Groups

In some circumstances it may be necessary to redesign a cluster of departments or units within an organization or a system. One of the most important design decisions to be made in clustering work groups involves the most appropriate grouping of units to achieve integration. Grouping of units implies that the units will share a common manager, common resources, and common performance measures. To illustrate the various ways in which units may be grouped, we use the example of the physician-organization arrangements (POAs). POAs are structural mechanisms (joint ventures) to facilitate integration of physicians into a network of integrated health systems (Alexander et al., 1996; Zuckerman et al., 1998). Shortell, Gillies, Anderson, Erickson, and Mitchell (1996) found that greater physician integration was significantly related to higher inpatient productivity and higher levels of integration. POAs may be designed in a number of ways. For example, physician groups may be grouped by knowledge and skill or by specialty and subspecialty (such as all medical specialties and all surgical specialities). Physicians may also be grouped by work process, for instance, by placing the operating rooms, emergency departments, and radiology under the same management, where they have a common patient flow. Ambulatory care clinic physicians may be grouped by time because they tend to hold clinics in the same time frame. Physicians may be grouped by commonality of clients or patients, for example, cardiovascular surgery and cardiology. Finally, physicians may be grouped because they are geographically located in the same hospital or facility. Chapters 6–8 provide further discussion of these issues.

Designing and Redesigning a Total Organization

The parameters of design decisions at this level of analysis have already been mentioned. The challenge at this level is enormous, and the amount of investment necessary to manage the redesign process is extensive. Perhaps most important, the process has to unfold in such a way that behaviors, not just formal structures, change. And, as Paul Allaire, the chief executive officer (CEO) of Xerox and the principal architect of the redesign of that company, said, "If you talk about change but don't change the reward and recognition system, nothing changes" (Howard, 1992).

Designing a Network

A network of organizations comprises those organizations that exist in a particular community or environment, which may be loosely or closely connected to achieve a common purpose or serve a common clientele (Kaluzny, Morissey, & McKinney, 1990). An example is the network of health and social services that may exist in a community to provide services to individuals with dementia and their families. Types of organizations within the network may include an acute hospital, a psychiatric hospital, a nursing home, home health services, day care services, meals on wheels, housing and transport services, social services, and so on. The objective in the design of the network is to ensure coordination of services and smoothness of client flow between organizations to maximize effectiveness. One of the key tasks in designing a network involves the identification of the target population, such as individuals with dementia, to be served by the network. The main demographic and health characteristics of the specific target population must be identified including age, sex, cultural group, language, morbidity and mortality rates by specific diseases, and so on. At the network level, the design process is relatively complex because it involves examining the nature of the relationships among the organizations in the network (Gittell & Weiss, 1997). Design decisions may include analyzing the interorganizational relationships in terms of deciding which organizations should have the most power, which resource transactions may take place, and how innovations will be diffused. These issues are also considered in Chapter 11.

Designing an Organized Delivery System

An organized delivery system (ODS) is a network of organizations that provides or arranges to provide a coordinated continuum of services to a defined population and is willing to be held clinically and fiscally accountable for the outcomes and the health status of a population served (Gillies et al., 1997). At the system level, design decisions are even more complex, depending upon the purpose(s) of the system and the heterogeneity of the programs provided. One of the most important factors to be analyzed at the system level is concerned with the degree of **centralization and decentralization** of decision making. For example, given a system that may include as many as 80 acute health care organizations or groups, it is essential to clarify which decisions will be made at the corporate level and which decisions will be made at the regional or individual organization level. Such decisions can be further categorized as those involving the setting of policy (e.g., wage and salary guidelines), initiating activities (e.g., hiring new staff), and granting final approval (e.g., capital budgets). Where the majority of decisions are centered at the corporate office, the organization is said to be vertically centralized. In high-technology industries such as health care, greater vertical decentralization is expected because of the expertise at lower levels in the organization. As a general rule, decisions should be made at the lowest possible levels, especially when the majority of workers are professionals. Horizontal decentralization refers to the extent to which influence and decision making is shared laterally. In the example of the ODS, an important design factor may be deciding upon the extent to which individual operating units can develop their own strategic plans separately from those developed by the corporate office. A major part of the activities at the decentralized level are concerned with the implementation of policies and ensuring quality.

SYSTEMATIC ASSESSMENT BEFORE DESIGN

Earlier in this chapter, the need to match a design with the organization's mission and strategies as well as obtaining participation from major stakeholders was emphasized. An organizational model or conceptual framework is an essential tool to guide analysis and action. Most people who have been exposed to organizations have an implicit experience-based model; however, organizational theorists and researchers have now developed general models for thinking about organizations as total systems. The major factors

that are essential to consider in an organizational **assessment for design** are shown in Figure 10.2. These factors recognize that organization design decisions should not be made in a vacuum; they need to be made in the context of a broad managerial framework in which several factors are assessed simultaneously. The factors are **environmental assessment,** organizational assessment, **cultural assessment, human resources assessment,** and **political process assessment.**

The Mission

One of the first and most important considerations in beginning an organization design strategy is to identify the mission of the organization. The mission may have been established through a strategic planning process in which a wide range of stakeholders worked together to provide a clear statement of the vision for the organization. Usually a mission statement identifies "what business the organization is in"

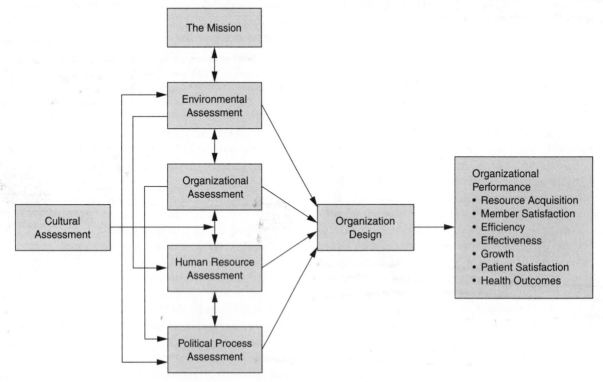

Figure 10.2. Overall Framework for Organization Design Considerations.

and what business it is not in. It may also include statements about the values and ideology of the organization in terms of client services and management. A mission statement usually outlines some more specific formal goals for the organization. Gellerman quotes the American architect Louis Sullivan, writing in 1890, who said, "Form follows function." Gellerman (1990) reaffirms that this principle also applies when designing organizations—they should be designed for a specific purpose or function, hence the importance of the mission statement (1990).

Environmental Assessment

The environment of an organization is considered increasingly important if the organization is to achieve desired levels of effectiveness. Environments are considered complex, which means that both instabilities in the environment and the heterogeneity of components of the environment create uncertainties that result in different organization designs. Environmental uncertainty affects the degree of formality of structure, the nature of interpersonal relationships, and the time orientation (short versus long run of employees). As uncertainty increases—that is, as environmental conditions become less stable—organizations may divide into specialized operating units along functional lines. As a consequence, the units may develop varying priorities and have different time horizons. To ensure expected levels of effectiveness, managers must design a variety of mechanisms to achieve integration across operating units. Absence of such mechanisms may lead to conflict and diminished performance.

What design options are available to the manager faced with the consequences of increasing environmental uncertainty? Lawrence and Lorsch (1967) advocate the creation of lateral relations such as direct managerial contact across functions, interfunctional teams (either permanent or temporary), liaison roles, and integrating departments. Such design strategies have the ultimate effect of decentralizing decision making so that it takes place at the level of the organization where the necessary information exists. As we discuss later in this chapter, Stein and Kanter (1980) have suggested a parallel organizational design as one mechanism for integrating persons from all levels

in the organization in the decision-making process. As Robert Howard's (1992) interview with Paul Allaire, the CEO of Xerox, indicates, increasing environmental volatility calls for an organization design that pushes responsibility, resources, and accountability as close to the market as possible.

It has also been recognized that organization design may be contingent upon the technology of the organization. Rapidly changing treatment and diagnostic therapies as well as changing information technologies in the environment of health services organizations demand more complex, flexible, and nimble designs that can adapt quickly to innovations.

Organizational Assessment

An important stage in preparing to redesign an organization is to identify the strengths and limitations of the organization. Since every organization is different, this assessment can be carried out in a number of ways. A frequently used approach is to conduct focus group discussions of the most important strengths and weaknesses of the organizations. Most organizations will try to build on their strengths. Focus groups for this kind of task are usually multidisciplinary and are made up of key stakeholders of the organization.

Cultural Assessment

Greater attention is being given to the importance of organizational culture to organization success, especially in bringing about organizational change. Culture has been variously defined as the values and beliefs, norms or behaviors that characterize the work of the organization. Culture essentially addresses the question of "what is it like to work here?" Strong cultures may provide greater cohesion for organizational members and allow easier achievement of mission and goals. Different cultures may evolve or exist at different operating units in an organization. Most complete organizations are "multicultural." **Cultural assessment** is a difficult measurement task and may be best achieved through a combination of focus groups for brainstorming, assessment instruments, and observation. Indications of an organization's culture can include employees' favorite stories about heroes of the organization, the celebrations and traditions, language used, and other indications of patterns of behavior that make the organization a good or bad place to work (Siehl & Martin, 1990; Zammutto & Krakower, 1991).

Human Resources Assessment

Organizations are made up of people who give life to the organizations. The availability of individuals with appropriate knowledge and skills to carry out the mission of the organization is critical. It may not be possible, under some circumstances, for an organization to obtain highly specialized expertise at the exact time it needs it. Accordingly, organization designs are influenced by the availability of critical human resources.

Political Process Assessment

All organizations have informal organizations as well as a formal one. It is important that managers understand the nature of the informal organizations that exist, who the key leaders are, and how this network can influence changes in organization design. For example, key leaders can facilitate or create barriers to the implementation of a new organization design; therefore, it is essential for managers to be aware of the informal political processes underpinning the organization's life.

In the framework shown in Figure 10.2, we see the systematic assessment of mission, environment, organization, culture, human resources, and political process being necessary in order to tailor an organization design for the specific needs of the organization. With this systematic approach, it is more likely that the design will facilitate the organization to achieve high levels of performance.

The VNA case provides an example of a health services organization that is facing changing times and is thinking about changing its organization design. How should this organization reconsider its mission in relation to the changing environment? What strengths and weaknesses does the organization have? What is the prevalent culture? How might the work of the nurse-managers be propagated?

IN THE REAL WORLD:
THE VISITING NURSE AGENCY, A CHANGING ENVIRONMENT

The Visiting Nurse Agency (VNA) was founded over 40 years ago by Jennie Johnson. Johnson's mother and grandmother before her had been known in their local community as persons who had always been called by neighbors to help deliver babies or provide support when family members were sick. Johnson saw VNA as an opportunity to carry on the family tradition by providing expert nursing services to those in need of care when sick in their homes.

The VNA was located in a rapidly growing suburb of a large city. During the initial years, VNA concentrated on two goals: first, attracting enough families to provide services to mothers with new babies and elderly persons requiring personal care at home; second, developing a reputation for providing a high-quality, personal, and caring service. All patients and clients appeared content with the

service, and the agency, a private nonprofit organization, was in a financially stable situation.

During the early 1990s, VNA's growth slowed. While VNA was perceived to provide good care in the home, there were a number of new nursing services being provided by private agencies. These agencies were providing more extensive home visits for postnatal care in the evenings and on weekends. Nurses were providing extensive nursing services in conjunction with a local nursing home and a home for the aged on an outreach basis. Their services were available 24 hours a day, seven days a week. The local community general hospital was also experimenting with health promotion clinics where services were being provided at a minimal charge to local residents. The VNA was seen as a very traditional "nursing" agency with rather specialized nursing services in the home and insufficient flexibility to meet the new needs of the community.

The VNA's hours of operation were Monday to Friday, 8:30 A.M. to 4:30 P.M. In 1994, VNA employed 51 registered nurses and five nurse-managers. The agency prided itself on the fact that all the nurses were registered nurses, and about half of them had a university education. Johnson, however, was becoming increasingly concerned by the decreasing demand for their services.

By 1995, Johnson had begun to replace some of her nurse managers, hoping to bring in new energy and fresh ideas. She still believed that the agency was respected because of its high quality of nursing services and the good relationships the agency enjoyed with established families in the community. Johnson called in the nurse-managers and stressed the importance of the quality philosophy to them. She emphasized the need for careful supervision of the nurses. She said all nurses must arrive at their house calls on time; punctuality was very important. She stressed the need for all nursing procedures conducted in the home to adhere to predefined standards. She pointed out the importance of the need for regular performance evaluations for the nurses so that they could be given immediate feedback on areas in which they were not following the exact protocol of the agency.

As new nurse-managers gained experience in VNA, they began to propose changes. One nurse-manager suggested that they establish an advisory board to serve as a liaison between the VNA and the local community. The advisory board would be made up of Jennie Johnson and key people from the local area, such as business people, women, minority group members, and senior citizens group members. The nurse-manager who proposed the idea argued that advisory board members could counsel prospective clients about the nursing services and in general provide a public relations function for VNA.

Another new nurse-manager proposed that the VNA engage in more advertising and marketing strategies. She argued that the agency nurses should become more involved in community groups such as the community center's senior citizen events. She also argued that the VNA should be prepared to respond to proposals for contracts with HMOs.

As Johnson considered these and other proposals, the government announced approval of funding for a major expansion of the Metropolitan Home Care Program. Home care programs had been successful in other metropolitan areas and had been shown in some cases to be an excellent alternative to inhospital care, especially because a range of community support services could be provided. The new funding seemed to favor the provision of a variety of professional services in the home including nursing, medical, rehabilitation, and several homemaker services. The new funding was to be available on a competitive basis to both for-profit and not-for-profit agencies.

Jennie Johnson and the nurse-managers were very concerned about whether they could compete and the impact these developments could have on VNA.

In January 1998, Jennie Johnson felt overwhelmed and wondered whether she was up to managing the VNA. The agency had grown little over the past five years and was receiving fewer and fewer referrals from its long-standing clients. The impact of the expanded Home Care Program was difficult to anticipate, and she was not sure how VNA should respond. Two of the sharpest nurse-managers had been to see her about a change in strategy. They encouraged the creation of several internal committees to study the problems. They also suggested that VNA begin planning the formation of specialized teams, organized around clients' needs and more appropriately able to respond to special interest groups. "The home nursing service industry is becoming more complex and is very competitive," one nurse-manager argued, "and if we don't adapt to it we will be left behind: we need to find partners!" Jennie Johnson thought the best thing might be to retire and get out of the provision of visiting nurse services—so dear to her family tradition.

DESIGNS FOR A VARIETY OF HEALTH SERVICES ORGANIZATIONS

Figure 10.2 provides the overall framework for organizational design considerations. This framework is from contingency theory, which indicates that the design must be tailored to the individual needs of the organization. Two main requirements of contingency theory are that organizations must cope simultaneously with needs to differentiate work and needs to integrate work (Charnes & Smith-Tewksbury, 1993). Differentiation is the requirement to divide work into specialized parts or functions; integration is the requirement to coordinate the work across different operating units or functions. Common forms of organizational designs may be described along a continuum, as shown in Figure 10.3. The designs arranged along the continuum emphasize differentiated designs at one end (the left side of Figure 10.3) and integration at the other end (the right side of Figure 10.3). All of these designs may be found at the different levels of organization design shown in Table 10.1. It is recognized that most organizations' designs are less neat and tidy than these illustrations.

Specific design options available for health services managers depend on environmental demands, the organization's strategies, how activities can be grouped, and how decisions will be made.

Functional Design

A **functional design** exists when labor is divided into departments specialized by functional area. An example is shown in Figure 10.4. This kind of design is typical of a nursing home, chronic-care facility, or small (less than 100 beds) community general hospital. In Figure 10.4 the basic hotel services are separated from the clinical services. The actual number of functional departments (and departmental manager positions) depends upon the size of the organization. The functional design is most useful when the organization has only a few products or goals. From the management's viewpoint, the functional design enables decisions to be made on a centralized, hierarchical basis. Departmental managers are usually promoted from within the organization and have a depth of technical knowledge in the functional area.

The functional design is most appropriate when an organization is in a relatively simple, stable environment in which there are few changes taking place and there are a limited number of other organizations with which the organization has contact. Clearly, a functional design becomes unsuitable when an organization grows and begins to diversify its services because interdepartmental coordination tends to be poor and decisions pile up at the top. If the environment becomes unstable, the functional design cannot cope because it does not have the facility to handle rapid information input or output and the response time is generally too slow. This type of design was most commonly seen in health care organizations 20 years ago. It is uncommon today because of increasing environmental uncertainty.

Divisional Design

The **divisional design** is often found in large academic health science centers (AHSCs) that operate under conditions of high environmental uncertainty exacerbated by relationships with the medical school and high technological complexity because of intensive research activities (Heyssel et al., 1984). It is also

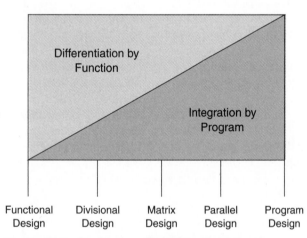

Figure 10.3. Continuum of Organizational Design
SOURCE: Adapted from Charnes and Smith-Tewksbury, *Collaborative Management in Health Care*, San Francisco: Jossey-Bass, 1993, p. 28, Figure 2.1 Continuum of Organizational Configuration.

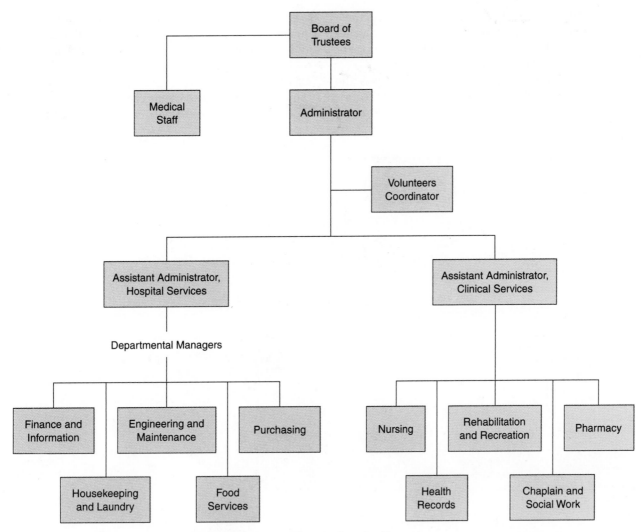

Figure 10.4. A Functional Design: Nursing Home or Chronic-Care Facility.

frequently found in pharmaceutical companies and health supplier organizations where a large variety of products and markets are involved. It is most appropriate for situations where clear divisions can be made within the organization and semiautonomous units can be created. Traditionally, in teaching hospitals the way of grouping units has been relatively clear-cut: Units have been grouped according to the traditional medical specialities, such as medicine, surgery, pediatrics, psychiatry, radiology, and pathology. More recently, AHSCs are beginning to question the appropriateness of these traditional groupings and are moving toward defining product lines that cross traditional boundaries. Examples of "new" product lines are those organized around health promotion; disease prevention programs; or diagnostic, therapeutic, and rehabilitation services; or those grouped around services to specific target groups, such as the elderly or persons with cancer. Similarly, in pharmaceutical companies, divisions are being created among related drugs. Divisionalization decentralizes decision making to the lowest level in the organization where the key expertise is available. Individual divisions have considerable autonomy for the clinical and financial operations. Each division has its own internal management structure, as illustrated in Figure 10.5.

The model illustrated in Figure 10.5 shows the physician in charge of each clinical service as the person with direct authority over all divisional opera-

tions. Each division has a manager of nursing or patient services, a manager of administrative services, and a finance officer. These managers work as a team to direct the division's operations. The managers are also accountable to the vice presidents of their disciplines. In some health science centers, a collaborative model is used to provide leadership of the team at the

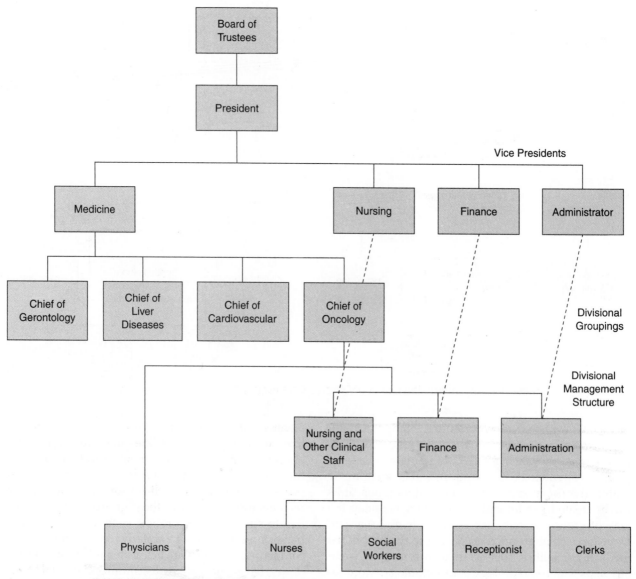

Figure 10.5. A Divisional Design: An Academic Health Science Center.

divisional level—that is, physicians, nurses, and administrators combine their skills to ensure knowledge of both the clinical and financial operations.

This operating unit structure enables the specialized units to handle relevant elements of the environment directly, enhancing the organization's capacity to exchange information with the environment and to develop strategies tailored to the product lines. In many instances the divisions "purchase" central services from within the hospital and are provided incentives to operate their units cost effectively. At the same time, the central service units are driven to operate efficiently; otherwise, the divisions may choose to purchase services outside the hospital at a better rate.

Difficulties with the divisional design tend to occur in times of resource constraints, when priorities must be set at higher organizational levels. For example, an academic health science center may have difficulty arriving at a consensus about which patient programs should be given priority if divisional managers cannot see the perspective of the whole organization. In times of resource constraints, greater sharing of resources between divisions is required, and more effective horizontal integrating mechanisms need to be established (Smith, Leatt, Ellis, & Fried, 1989).

Matrix Design

To overcome some of the problems of the functional and divisional designs, **matrix** or **mixed designs** have evolved to improve mechanisms of lateral coordination and information flow across the organization. An example of a matrix organization for a psychiatric center is provided in Figure 10.6.

The matrix organization, originally developed in the aerospace industry, is characterized by a dual-authority system. There are usually functional and program or product-line managers, both reporting to a common superior and both exercising authority over workers within the matrix. Typically, a matrix organization is particularly useful in highly specialized technological areas that focus on innovation. The matrix design allows program managers to interact directly with the environment vis-à-vis technological developments. Usually each program requires a multidisciplinary team approach; the matrix structure fa-

cilitates the coordination of the team and allows team members to contribute their special expertise.

The matrix design has some disadvantages that stem from the dual-authority lines. Individual workers may find having two bosses to be untenable since it creates conflicting expectations and ambiguity. The matrix design may also be expensive in that both functional and program managers may spend a considerable amount of time in meetings attempting to keep everyone informed of program activities. Additional costs may also be incurred because of the frequent requirement for dual accounting, budget, control, performance evaluation, and reward systems.

The use of the matrix design in health services organizations is becoming more common, particularly in organizations in which multidisciplinary approaches to patient care are being encouraged. To some degree, most health services organizations have many characteristics of a matrix organization, although their design may not be formally named as such. For example, multiple authority over patient care is clearly apparent in most hospitals. Most health professionals—such as nurses, psychologists, physiotherapists, pharmacists, occupational therapists, and social workers—have formal reporting relationships to their functional departments but are also accountable to physicians for the quality of care provided. Multidisciplinary teams, which facilitate lateral communication and coordination of work, are an essential feature of almost all health services organizations, including community health, long-term care, home care, and hospitals. As a result, learning to manage matrix structures is particularly important for health services managers.

Parallel Design

The parallel structure was originally developed as a mechanism for promoting quality of working life in organizations (Stein & Kanter, 1980). The **bureaucratic** or functional **organization** retains responsibility for routine activities in the organization, while the parallel side is responsible for complex problem solving requiring participatory mechanisms. The parallel structure is a means of managing and responding to changing internal and external conditions. It also provides an opportunity for persons occupying positions

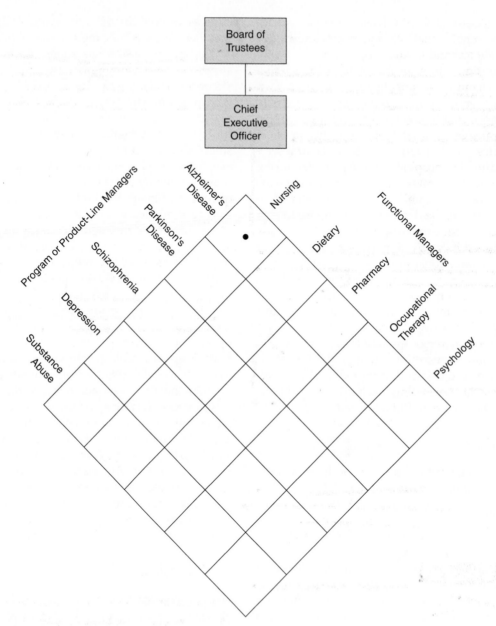

Figure 10.6. A Matrix Design: A Psychiatric Center. An individual worker in this example is part of the Alzheimer program as well as a member of the nursing department.

at various hierarchical levels in the bureaucratic structure and across functional areas to participate in organizational designs.

The **parallel design** is one we commonly see being used by organizations implementing CQI/TQM (continuous quality improvement/total quality management) approaches. CQI/TQM places the clients or patients and their concerns at the center of the organization. The parallel side of the organization is often headed by a quality council made up of members of the bureaucratic side of the organization. The quality council then identifies areas where CQI/TQM teams may be established to investigate work processes where improvements in client services may be made. Representation on the teams is drawn from all levels in the hierarchy and from all departments that are involved in the work process under investigation. An example of a parallel structure for an acute general hospital is shown in Figure 10.7.

Advantages of the parallel structure to individual staff members are perceived to include expansion of their power, opportunities to affect the organization's decisions, the feeling of being involved in organizational issues, and the potential for individual growth through broadening of the range of work activities. Advantages to the organization are potentially those of increased performance and quality. Some possible disadvantages of the parallel structure are (1) organization members may spend too much time in meetings, thus increasing costs of operations; (2) the parallel structure may begin to assume responsibilities for routine decisions, consequently overriding the bureaucratic structure; and (3) conflicts over perceived priorities and resource allocation may occur between the bureaucratic and parallel structures.

Product-Line or Program Design

Product-line management is defined as the placement of a person in charge of all aspects of a given product or group of products. The product line is a revenue and cost center, and the person in charge is responsible for all budgetary and financial responsibilities associated with the product. The person is also responsible for coordinating all the functional resources (e.g., planning, marketing, human resources) re-

quired to successfully manage the product line. Product-line management can provide important advantages by increasing operational efficiencies and enhancing market share. Operational efficiencies can be gained by analyzing cost and revenues across related product lines so that redundancies will be eliminated and synergies captured. Market share can be enhanced by targeting marketing strategies to the group of products and being able to promote these to different segments of the market as appropriate (e.g., the elderly, women, and children).

The major challenges health services organizations face in implementing product-line management include educating the relevant groups to the change, choosing criteria for grouping the products, and selecting and training the product-line managers. These changes require board and top management support and appropriate involvement and support of key leaders throughout the organization. People must see it as a better way to manage resources, maintain or enhance quality, and increase overall value.

While many criteria can be used for grouping products, the most common are similarity of technology, similarity of markets, similarity in the production process, similarity in the distribution process, and similarity in the use of human resources. By grouping products with these kinds of similarities, economies of scale and synergies ($2 + 1 = 5$ solutions) can be generated. Based on these criteria, for example, a hospital can consider the following product-line candidates: women's care, oncology, cardiology, rehabilitation, substance abuse, long-term care, and health promotion.

The selection and training of the product-line managers is particularly important. Individuals must be identified who have good technical knowledge of the product line and good analytical and interpersonal skills. In particular, they must be innovative, feel comfortable with ambiguity and complexity, and be able to work with more than one manager. The latter is reflected in Figure 10.8. This chart shows a matrix-type organization in which the product-line managers work with both the functional department heads and the product-line assistant vice president. Recognizing that many problems and issues cut across the product lines, hospitals may establish a committee to deal

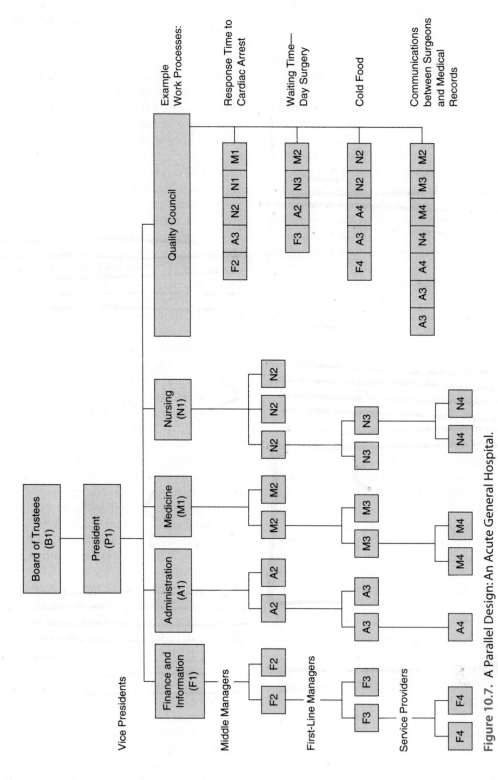

Figure 10.7. A Parallel Design: An Acute General Hospital.

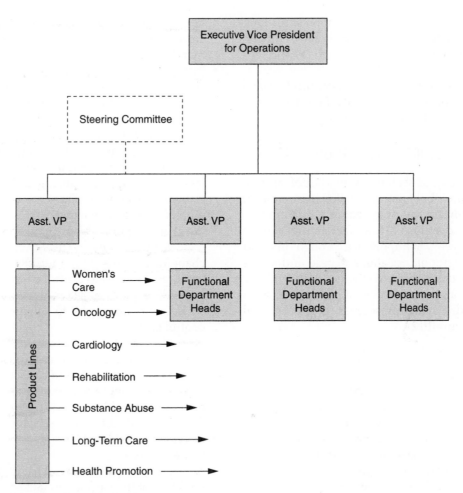

Figure 10.8. Product-Line Manager Design.

with these issues. This committee can be composed of both product-line managers and functional department heads and charged with reviewing the overall performance of the product lines and recommending addition, deletion, or modification of existing product lines.

Key success factors for this **product-line** or **program design** include

- a strong management information system that links clinical, financial, and volume data by product
- a strong budgeting-financial system that can disaggregate costs and revenues so that accountability can be appropriately assigned

- reward systems to encourage innovation and risk taking
- relevant clinical involvement of physicians, nurses, and other health professionals to deal with new technology, diagnosis and treatment patterns, quality, and patient convenience issues
- a strong support staff, particularly in the areas of marketing, finance, and planning
- the need to align authority and responsibility
- the need for integrative mechanisms that cut across product lines; hence, the development of the steering committee
- the need for a concerted management development program that emphasizes the ability to work with

more than one manager, communication skills, conflict-management skills, computer literacy, and creativity (Leatt, Lemieux-Charles, & Aird, 1994).

In addition to their use in hospitals, product-line management designs are frequently found in pharmaceutical and health care supplier organizations.

INFLUENCES ON FUTURE ORGANIZATION DESIGNS

Based on the previous sections, a number of suggestions can be made about particular factors, somewhat unique to health services organizations, that may influence design decisions. These factors are generic and are likely to vary in importance through time and in various geographic locations. These influences may be classified according to whether they originate from the mission, the environment, the organization itself, the culture, human resources, or the political process (see Figure 10.2).

The Mission

The most important factor relating to the mission of health services organizations is concerned with the level of specificity of the mission in determining what will be an appropriate design. As noted previously, health services organizations are beginning to narrow their focus and identify key market-driven areas in which they will operate. The move to identify specific target populations where inputs and health outcomes can be measured is a trend toward increasing the accountability of organizations for a social contract with the community.

The Future Environment

The future environment for most health services organizations is predicted to be both complex and dynamic (see Chapters 1 and 15). A variety of pressures will be exerted externally that will, by necessity, influence design decisions. Some of the most important pressures will be as follows:

- changing demographic characteristics of the population being served with an increase in the proportion of elderly persons needing services

- greater sophistication of the general public and consumers of health services in terms of their demands on the system
- increasing range of services being provided outside of traditional hospitals including ambulatory care programs, home care, long-term care, community health centers, and so on
- growing involvement with the community to address underlying health issues, such as teenage pregnancy, substance abuse, and violence
- increasing competition among health services organizations providing similar services in the same geographic location to maximize their market share
- increasing attempts by governments at all levels to regulate the quantity and quality of services provided
- changing systems of reimbursement to health services organizations to control costs
- expanding private sector involvement in health services organizations to augment services and control costs
- increasing involvement of trustees, physicians, and other health professionals in the strategic planning and management of health services organizations
- increasing attempts by external professional associations and accrediting bodies to set standards for professional conduct in health services organizations
- increasing demand for outcome accountability and greater value
- rapidly developing medical technologies and proliferation of increasing specialized services
- increased information demands, development of real-time information processing systems to relate to the external environment, and growth of artificial intelligence systems

The Organization

Internal to most health services organizations are a series of structural and operating processes that provide opportunities or constraints on design decisions. For example:

- greater emphasis on team work
- greater accountability for the governance of the organization in terms of a social contract
- increasing corporatization of the structure of health services organizations

- demands to continuously improve the quality of care
- demands to control costs, operate efficiently, and increase productivity and overall value
- increasing need for comprehensive and integrated clinical and financial information systems
- constrained financial resources
- changing working relationships to create more situations with two or more supervisor systems
- increasing need to coordinate activities internally and to manage conflict creatively
- increasing needs for integration of functions and for clinical and physician services.

Culture

As radical reform takes place in health services organizations, the culture of organizations will also change. The values that are held in high esteem will be modified. For example:

- increasing emphasis on the "customer" with implementation of processes for patient-focused care
- increasing use of patient/client satisfaction surveys to modify care processes
- greater emphasis on the development of broad sets of indicators (such as the balanced scorecard) to monitor performance
- increasing understanding of the value of community-based care
- increasing use of evidence, such as health outcome measures to modify care processes
- increasing emphasis on challenging traditional ways of doing things and the willingness to experiment
- value of employees who are committed to the organization
- value of employees who are adaptable and able to embrace change
- increasing value will be placed on nonhierarchical leaders who can lead change processes
- increasing emphasis on cultures that facilitate teamwork and collaboration with nontraditional partners
- increasing value of the need to integrate functions and clinical processes
- increasing importance of physicians and other health professions to collaborate in developing trust in health services organizations

Human Resources

The particular characteristics of employees and other service providers available now or in the future may strongly affect the types of design decisions that may be made. For example:

- greater emphasis on cross-skill training versus traditional professional training
- greater emphasis on horizontal teams and collaborative practices
- greater pressure to substitute "cheaper" health care workers for more expensive health professionals
- greater numbers of women in managerial positions requiring flexibility such as accessibility of day care and job sharing
- greater ethnic and cultural diversity of the workforce
- greater need to experiment with new work arrangements such as self-managed work teams and CQI/TQM strategies
- many physicians who historically have had considerable autonomy becoming employees
- shortages of key health services professionals; for example, pharmacists, physical therapists, and occupational therapists
- increasing need for managers with professional training
- increasing unionization of workers in health services organizations
- closer scrutiny by unions as some health services organizations undergo retrenchment
- increasing need to educate all levels in strategic management and in adopting a marketing orientation
- the need for succession planning, career planning, and management development programs linked more closely to the organization's strategic plan
- escalating pressures to provide continuing education programs to health professionals, especially clinical managers

The Political Process

Because of the uncertainty and ambiguities that may exist in health services organizations and the variety of professional groups involved, the informal network within organizations may be particularly active.

Informal leaders may be especially helpful to managers in identifying how a change in organization design might be received. Informal leaders may be useful in communicating ideas about change to the grass-roots level in the organization or in repressing incorrect rumors that could damage the implementation process. Through the informal network, managers can identify which units or departments might be most or least receptive and attempt to involve key players in the redesign process. Additional suggestions are discussed in Chapter 9.

Although these factors are perhaps not comprehensive of all situations or applicable in all circumstances, they are potentially important when considering a new organization design. Most importantly, they emphasize the need for designs that are flexible and that can breathe and grow with the organization.

Organizations in Transition

Life/Cycles

Until now our discussion has focused on the importance of designing organizations in keeping with their mission, environment, information needs, culture, human resources, and politics; however, these factors all change. To a certain extent, organizations go through relatively predictable cycles that have different design implications. For example, Starkweather and Kisch (1971) suggested four phases through which health services organizations pass. The first is the search phase, which is characterized by newness, innovation, and a sense of ascendency as the organization procures resources and seeks to establish its identity. The organization design of an organization in this phase is typically open and informal. The success phase is characterized by achievement in procuring patients, staff, and financial resources. The design of the organization during this phase becomes somewhat more formalized to manage the usually larger scale of operation. The bureaucratic phase is characterized by a relatively rigid conformity to rules and procedures; the organization is isolated from its clients in that it receives little feedback from them. During this phase the organization may begin to decline because of its inability to respond to changes in

the environment or to alter the environment to fit its needs. The succession phase is characterized by the development of new ways of providing services, often through the development of new units within the organization.

Kimberly and Miles (1980) raise important questions about organization design issues associated with such stages of the life cycle. Given that managers wish to design organizations for optimal performance, it makes sense that different designs are more appropriate at different stages of an organization's development. For example, a functional structure might be appropriate for a new organization during its search phase. As the organization grows, achieves success, and perhaps diversifies, a different design such as a product line or program design may be appropriate. During periods of temporary or permanent decline, the organization may need to consider the appropriateness of a parallel design to help generate new ideas and maintain quality of services. These issues are critically important for organizational viability.

Downsizing, Reengineering, Restructuring

Given the highly competitive environment of health services organizations in the United States, Canada, and worldwide, organizations are striving to contain costs and retain market share, as well as quality of care. Future health services organizations must be designed to be lean and yet responsive to changing circumstances. This means that health services organizations are experimenting with transitions beyond the "normal" life cycle of events. Many health services organizations are experiencing "transitions" through downsizing, reengineering work processes, and/or restructuring. The term *downsizing* includes strategies such as across-the-board cuts, early retirements, outsourcing, use of temporary employees, and delayering and organizational redesign. Reengineering involves process redesign and quality improvement techniques. It often necessitates the redesign of individual roles and teams. Restructuring in its broadest sense includes rethinking strategies, which may involve developing new programs and dropping old ones. Table 10.2 shows the main differences between downsizing, reengineering, and restructuring.

Table 10.2. Comparisons among Downsizing, Reengineering, and Restructuring

	Downsizing	Reengineering	Restructuring
Focus of change	Cost reduction	Radical process redesign	Focus on core competencies
Key assumption	Too many people	Ineffective and inefficient processes	Inappropriate strategic focus
Output/input goal	Same output/fewer resources	More output/fewer resources	Different output/fewer or same resources
Scope of change	Moderate	Broad (cross-function)	Broad (across functions and units)
Primary target	Head count reduction	Process redesign for customer needs	Organizational restructuring
Key enabler	Reduce personnel	Improve information technology	New and reformed strategic business units
Strategy	Reactive	Proactive	Proactive
Implementation time	Short	Medium	Medium to long
Direction	Top-down	Top-down and bottom-up	Top-down
Infrastructure change	Ignore	Critical	Critical
Improvement goal	N/A	50%–100%	30%–50%
Key risks	Employee burnout Loss of employee trust Lower productivity Decreased patient-care quality	Process design failures High costs with little return Loss of employee trust Decreased patient-care quality	Lack of return in new/renewed business Financial investment Loss of employee trust Loss of patient loyalty

SOURCE: Leatt, P., Baker, G. R., Halverson, P. K., and Aird C. Downsizing, Reengineering, and Restructuring: Long term Implications for Health Care Organizations, *Frontiers in Health Service Management*, Vol 13(4), Summer 1997, 2–37.

These transitions, often at a rapid pace, have implications for the types of organizational design, which will evolve and for the processes by which they will be developed. Vertically integrated delivery systems (as discussed in Chapter 11) will become the norm as integration becomes a key factor in health services. These systems will require the design of network models that will be developed on the basis of core building blocks of redefined roles and teams/work groups. While traditionally the responsibility for organizational design has been with the CEO and the senior management in a "top-down" process, it is likely that the process of organizational design for the future will place greater emphasis on a "bottom-up" process. In reality, the process will necessitate the involvement of front-line staff in designing their own roles and teams so that larger structures for whole organizations and systems can build upon these.

The following "In The Real World" provides a case study of centralization and decentralization issues facing a vertically integrated health system. The case highlights the importance of fluid organization designs that can adapt to changing circumstances. Such designs must address the organizations' needs for both differentiation and integration. The case underscores the contingent nature of organization design.

IN THE REAL WORLD:
CENTRALIZATION AND DECENTRALIZATION IN A VERTICALLY INTEGRATED SYSTEM: THE XYZ HOSPITAL CORPORATION

- At a recent administrative board meeting, it was realized that two system hospitals within the same city were each planning to develop a separate air transport service.
- The medical staff of a large system hospital unanimously passed a no-confidence vote in the administration of that hospital.
- An administrator with 17 years of service in a rural system hospital was asked to resign.
- System hospitals and long-term care facilities located in different states are required to conform to individual state statutes and market conditions. Increasingly, the compliance is inconsistent, if not in direct conflict, with overall corporate policy.
- While the corporation historically enjoyed a AAA bond rating by Standard and Poor's, there was some concern that the rating might be downgraded to AA.

The system was obviously facing design problems, and it was becoming painfully clear that

- problems were not being recognized in a timely fashion,
- the president of the corporation and his corporate colleagues were being involved and often consumed with specific institutional issues,
- a variety of strategic issues and opportunities were not getting the attention they deserved,
- there appeared to be a great deal of conflict among administrators and corporate-level personnel, and
- corporate policy was unable to reconcile conflicting statutes and guidelines affecting member institutions operating in different states.

The System

The XYZ Hospital Corporation is a religious multi-institutional network in which 24 health care institutions are owned and operated; one is managed, and one is leased. Sixteen of these institutions are hospitals, and eight are long-term care facilities. The system has 4,470 licensed acute and long-term care beds and employs 12,931 full-time equivalent (FTE) employees. The facilities are located in four coastal states with all facilities near major population centers. Of the sixteen hospitals, three have more than 400 beds, five have fewer than 100 beds, and the remainder average about 230 beds per hospital. Of the eight long-term care facilities, three have more than 150 beds, and the remainder have less than 50 beds.

In addition to operating these facilities, the system in 1985 joined with three other health care systems to create a health maintenance organization (HMO) called the Wellness Health Network. The provider group of the network comprises hospitals owned by the sponsoring health systems as well as several community hospitals. The network has developed managed care programs, or outreach health plans, in two of the regions served by the system. One program currently enrolls more than 25,000 people and has 900 participating physicians providing care, and the other involves more than 600 primary care physicians and dentists with services offered to 98 employer groups, enrolling approximately 20,000 people.

The corporation has a history of providing care to the poor and underserved in the community. While many hospitals have done well financially, other hospitals have reported substantial losses in providing such care, given the economic conditions in many communities. Despite their losses, the corporation has chosen to subsidize the institutions by reallocating profits rather than closing or selling such facilities.

Under the current corporate structure, the executive vice president is the chief operating officer (COO) for the corporation, and theoretically, all institutional administrators are accountable to the corporation through this position. In reality, however, the COO position has never been fully accepted by both corporate and institutional personnel, and many administrators relate to both the president and executive vice president, depending on the issue. In fact, some of the administrators from the larger institutions relate solely to the president, thus bypassing the executive vice president.

How to Proceed?

The CEO had recently proposed a regional structure, and the corporation's board had voted not to implement such an effort at that time. Under this proposal, the four states were defined as regions since each geographic area presented a unique set of problems and opportunities. These problems continue. The group reviewed the options and decided that although the board had already voted against a regional structure, perhaps this was the time to review the options and revisit the decision. It was decided that a special meeting should be called, not to arrive at a decision but to review the options.

The agenda for the day was to:

- Develop a perspective on organization design. What is it, and why is it important?
- Clearly identify problems that result from an inappropriate structure.
- Review structural design options against specific criteria.

A perspective on design

Organizational design was designed as

the arrangement and the process of arranging activities, roles, or positions in the organization to coordinate effectively the interdependencies that exist and to improve the effectiveness of the organization.

This definition of design stresses both the arrangement (i.e., the particular configuration) of the organization as well as the process of arriving at that configuration. The process is particularly critical since a design is never finished. Rather, it represents the balancing of the organization's differentiation and coordination needs over time.

These design features are extremely important factors that affect the basic performance of the organization. In fact, in one review of the literature that looked at a number of factors affecting quality, it was concluded that

Changing the process of care at the individual level is not the only nor necessarily the best means of improving quality of care. To the extent that structural characteristics [design] determine the quality of care, efforts to improve care in the long-term through changing the structure of care [design] may prove to be most cost effective than short-run, quality assurance programs. (Palmer and Reilly, 1979)

Design is important in that it provides a map reflecting the past power struggles within the organization and perhaps holds the clue to future events within the organization. At the risk of being somewhat presumptuous, one could hypothesize that some of the problems that the system is currently facing could have been predicted given the existing structure of the system.

Finally, design is important since it provides the basis for setting realistic limits within which managers function. Structure sets the tone within which basic ongoing processes and culture emerge. Moreover, managers operate on the margin and as the environment changes, structure or restructuring efforts represent the paradigm [or the paradigm shift] within which management operates to adjust to environmental changes. If this structure is inappropriate to the environment, the structure greatly limits the ability of management to be effective, given the challenges that the organization is facing.

While structure is important, the understanding of its role vis-à-vis operations as well as overall performance is embryonic. This understanding is greatly complicated by the fact that there is little agreement on what constitutes effectiveness since different constituent groups within the organization apply different criteria to effectiveness. Moreover, the systematic study of structure vis-à-vis criteria is relatively new, and finally, one cannot overestimate the level of complexity. The notion of design encompasses technical, sociological, political, and psychological factors, and few have the level of sophistication in all these relevant disciplines, thus making this a very slow and difficult area in which to work.

The appropriate structure is largely contingent on the character of the environment within which the organization functions and the nature of the organization's goals (Duncan, 1979). For example, when the nature of goals and environment is simple and fairly static, a more functional type of organization characterized by high levels of centralization is appropriate. On the contrary, when the environment is complex but in fact can be segmented into more homogeneous components, a more decentralized configuration would be most appropriate. When the design does not fit the environment, organizations tend to experience a number of problems, such as an inability to anticipate problems, an inability to get information to the *right people at the right time, or an inability to take corrective action quickly.*

The following issues and subsequent problems were identified.

- *There is too much distance between administrators or operating institutions and the governing board: administrators do not have access to the board of directors; response time between the corporate and the hospital levels is too lengthy; those at the corporate level cannot measure the institutional climate and culture or initiate appropriate preventive actions; and the corporate structure does not allow for meaningful input of the board of directors of physicians from the various institutions in administration or of administrators on the governing board.*

- *There is an ambiguity of roles and difference in perspectives: corporate personnel see the system as highly decentralized while personnel at the institutions see it as highly centralized; there is a lack of common criteria for important policy decisions about resources; there is a lack of consistent criteria for evaluating administrative personnel; the CEO and the board of directors have become too involved with operational activities that do not require their attention. This crowds out other activities and puts their credibility at risk; the CEO and the board of directors have failed to address important policy issues like a strategy for managed care and for long-term care and a cohesive approach to legislative affairs; and the roles of vice presidents involved with planning, operations, mission effectiveness, and public affairs at the corporate level are ambiguous. There is less ambiguity surrounding financial and legal activities.*

Structural options

Any decision on structure must be judged against a set of criteria. The board developed the following criteria, which were originally developed as part of the initial discussions on regionalization.

- *Strengthen the collective effectiveness and market position of the XYZ System institutions in each area by unifying strategic planning, financial planning,*

program development, marketing, and the coordination of services.

- *Take full advantage of collective resources in seeking out and responding to mission opportunities and market pressures.*

- *Enhance the effectiveness of the XYZ Corporation institutions by providing greater management oversight and staff support.*

- *Unify and strengthen the XYZ Corporation voice in state and local public policy affairs and advocacy on behalf of the poor.*

- *Enhance the effective utilization of management resources.*

- *Recognize and retain senior executives who are at the top of their organization, thereby providing promotion opportunities for senior associate administrators.*

Each of these criteria were discussed and used as a background against which structural options were reviewed.

Discussions, Issues, and Questions

Given the problems facing the XYZ Corporation and the above criteria:

- *What structures would be most appropriate?*
- *What are the advantages and disadvantages of each structure vis-à-vis the criteria?*
- *Speculate on the advantages and disadvantages of selecting one of the existing administrators within the region and having him or her fulfill the vice presidential responsibilities along with his or her ongoing administrative functions within an existing institution. Given the obvious disadvantages, how could these difficulties be minimized, and what structural mechanisms (i.e., committees, review processes) could be developed to resolve problems that you have identified?*

Kaluzny, A. D. Centralization and Decentralization in a Vertically Integrated System: The XYZ Hospital Corporation. In Strategic Alignment: Managing Integrated Health Systems (Eds. D. A. Conrad and G. A. Hoare). Ann Arbor: AUPHA Press/Health Administration Press, 1994, 125–131.

DEBATE TIME 10.1: WHAT DO YOU THINK?

The Oriole Women's Shelter is a not-for-profit corporation and registered charity that began its operation in 1984 as a crisis-care facility for physically and emotionally abused women and their children. The staff is organized as a feminist collective and works in conjunction with a volunteer board of directors. The collective was founded by a group of women and front-line social agency workers concerned about this unmet need within their community. Some had themselves been victims of domestic violence; others came to the group because of feminist social philosophy and commitment to effect change at a grass-roots level. The total annual budget for the facility is approximately $1.4 million. The mission statement of the shelter states:

> The Oriole Women's Shelter is committed to reducing the incidence of violence and oppression against women and children. It is an emergency crisis facility for abused women and their children, which provides safety, counselling, information, advocacy, and other assistance in a supportive environment, in times of personal or family crisis.

Community outreach and political action are significant components of the collective's work.

The population served by the shelter is extremely diverse ethnically, and a significant proportion are refugees and new immigrants to the country. Issues that have arisen include the need for increased funding for translation services, ethnic foods, and more staff to accompany residents to legal, immigration, and other interviews. Residents and staff have had to address serious issues surrounding racism in addition to the emotional, mental, and physical stresses of working with clients who have been victims of abuse.

The problem of physical and emotional abuse of women and children by men has become more widely publicized in the years that the shelter has been in operation. This publicity has led to increased success with in-house fund-raising, as well as greater ease in obtaining government funding for the work

of the shelter. Nevertheless, the slumping economy of the past year has taken a toll on all publicly funded programs, with the shelter being no exception.

From its inception, the shelter has rejected the concept of a traditional hierarchical structure, which is believed by the founders and staff to reflect a male-dominated social structure that has contributed to power imbalances in society. These imbalances are felt to allow segments of the population to be oppressed and abused. Instead, the staff is structured as a collective, with decisions made on the basis of consensus. The key characteristics of a **collectivist-democratic organization** are described in Table 10.3 (Rothchild and Allen, 1989). All staff (11 full-time equivalents) receive the same salary, regardless of prior education, experience, or seniority within the organization. There is no identified manager, no model of supervision; performance reviews are controversial and conducted by the collective in the context of staff meetings. Weekly staff meetings are facilitated (led) in turn by collective members. The meetings tend to be long, emotionally charged, and perceived by some to be inefficient in conducting the business of the collective. Decision making is laborious and in many cases inconsequential.

Staff interactions have become exhausting and time-consuming. Staff meetings therefore evoke negative emotional reactions from the collective members. Fears of isolation or appearing to be out of tune with the culture of the organization are regularly expressed, and there is a tendency to see fault as lying elsewhere.

Anyone who assumes a leadership role, proffers skills or competence in certain areas, or expresses a political viewpoint that counters the prevailing attitude is seen as attempting to take control. Having power is seen as negative and abusive and a source of anxiety or fear on the part of those who perceive themselves as not having power. Although there is a strong commitment in principle to the collective process, many staff members believe that an informal hierarchy does exist. This has its basis along

Table 10.3 Comparisons of Two Ideal Types of Organization

Dimension	Bureaucratic Organization	Collectivist-Democratic Organization
1. Authority	1. Authority resides in individuals by virtue of incumbency in office or expertise; hierarchical organization of offices. Compliance is to universal fixed rules as these are implemented by office incumbents.	1. Authority resides in the collectivity as a whole; delegated, if at all, only temporarily and subject to recall. Compliance is to the consensus of the collective, which is always fluid and open to negotiation.
2. Rules	2. Formalization of fixed and universalistic rules; calculability and appeal of decisions on the basis of correspondence to the formal, written law.	2. Minimal stipulated rules; primacy of ad hoc, individuated decisions; some calculability possible on the basis of knowing the substantive ethics involved in the situation.
3. Social control	3. Organizational behavior is subject to social control, primarily through direct supervision or standardized rules and sanctions, tertiarily through the selection of homogeneous personnel, especially at top levels.	3. Social controls are primarily based on personalistic or moralistic appeals and the selection of homogeneous personnel.
4. Social relations	4. Ideal of impersonality, relations are to be role-based, segmental, and instrumental.	4. Ideal of community; relations are to be wholistic, personal, of value in themselves.
5. Recruitment and advancement	5a. Employment based on specialized training and formal certification.	5a. Employment based on friends, social-political values, personality attributes, and informally assessed knowledge and skills.
	5b. Employment constitutes a career, advancement based on seniority or achievement.	5b. Concept of career advancement not meaningful; no hierarchy of positions.
6. Incentive structure	6. Remunerative incentives are primary.	6. Normative and solidarity incentives are primary; material incentives are secondary.
7. Social stratification	7. Isomorphic distribution of prestige, privilege, and power (i.e., differential rewards by office); hierarchy justifies inequality.	7. Egalitarian; reward differentials, if any, are strictly limited by the collectivity.
8. Differentiation	8a. Maximal division of labor: dichotomy between intellectual work and manual work and between administrative tasks and performance tasks.	8a. Minimal division of labor; administration combined with performance tasks; division between intellectual and manual work reduced.
	8b. Maximal specialization of jobs and functions; segmental roles. Technical expertise is exclusively held; ideal of the specialist-expert.	8b. Generalization of jobs and functions; wholistic roles. Demystification of expertise: ideal of the amateur generalist.

SOURCE: (67) Rothchild, Joyce and Whit J. Allen. *The Co-operative Workplace. Potentials and dilemmas of organizational democracy and participation.* Cambridge University Press, 1989. Reprinted with permission of Cambridge University Press.

lines of seniority, race, personal characteristics, and depth of commitment to the political beliefs of feminism and collectivism.

The board consists of eight professional and business women who could be described as successful in their respective professions. (Men are not accepted as board or staff, and a release regarding this policy has been obtained from the Human Rights Commission.) The personal and corporate culture of members of the board is typically hierarchical, and they are often in conflict with the organizational culture of the shelter. All agree with and support the concepts of feminism and collectivism but have difficulty reconciling the legal and practical requirements for structure with the collective's wish for its values to be supported and honored. Lack of accountability, responsibility, and commitment to task completion are problems identified by the board, which relate to the collective structure as it now stands.

During the past three years, there have been increasing difficulties with intrastaff and staff-board communication, perceived staff stress, and anger in the workplace. Serious problems have arisen in the areas of administrative activity and accountability. No single individual willingly accepts responsibility for specific tasks or assignments. Although attempts have been made to address individual issues, no long-term or comprehensive solutions have been achieved.

1. What is the nature of decision making in this organization? What are its strengths and weaknesses?
2. Is designated leadership essential to the operation of an organization? Can power and accountability be shared?
3. What might be the impact of a formal organization design on this organization?
4. What mechanisms might preserve the values or culture of the organization while facilitating decision making?

Leatt et al. op. cit

 # MANAGERIAL GUIDELINES

Design Preparation

1. The organization must have a clear understanding of its mission (i.e., it should be clear to everyone what business the organization is in and what it is not).
2. The external environment of the organization must be assessed in terms of its uncertainty. The social, technological, political, economic, legal, cultural, and ecological characteristics of the environment could have important consequences for the choice of organization design.
3. It is important to understand the strengths and weaknesses of the organization so that the design strategy leverages the organization's competitive advantages.
4. It is essential that managers understand the culture(s) of the organization and have a vision for creating a culture for the future that will facilitate organizational change.
5. Assessment of the human resources available in the organization is essential to the task of organization design. There must be systematic understanding of the human resource capability, especially at the senior management level. It may be necessary to consider both short- and long-term succession planning as part of the preparation for redesign.

(continued)

MANAGERIAL GUIDELINES

6. The informal network inside the organization should be assessed so that key informal leaders can participate in the design process and, therefore, contribute to its success.

Design Process

1. Key organizational leaders must anticipate that the process of organization design may take several weeks or months depending upon the individual circumstances of the organization.
2. Some organizations may find it useful to establish a task force or a team to consider alternative organization designs. Key members of senior management and major stakeholders may be members of this team, recognizing that the task force is advisory to the CEO. It is often helpful to expand the membership of the task force to selected individuals at other levels of the organization. For example, it may be useful to have representation from middle managers, unions, and client groups.
3. An external consultant can also be useful in outlining the design options for the organization. Ultimately the decision on the actual acceptability of the design for the organization rests with the organization.
4. It is important to recognize that the building blocks for future organizational designs will likely evolve from the "bottom-up" with individuals designing roles and work groups designing teams.
5. During the design process, it is important to identify the ramifications of any new design. Who will stand to gain or lose from the changes being made?

Design Outcome

1. Once an appropriate organization design has been agreed upon, it is important that a plan be developed for the communication of the design, its implementation, and evaluation.
2. The new design must be communicated to everyone inside and outside the organization who is likely to be affected by the changes. Many organizations develop elaborate, staged plans to communicate the changes so that the individuals most affected by the design hear first.
3. Implementation of the new design will vary depending upon how different the new design is from the old one. Implementation may evolve quickly or may be staged during three to five years in large complex organizations when the new design is radically different and when there is a need for extensive education of individuals to fill new roles. All the principles of implementing change, outlined in Chapter 12, are applicable to implementing new designs.
4. Although not often carried out in the past, it is important to formally monitor the implementation of the design and assess the effect of the design on organizational performance. Recognizing that organization designs exist to help work get done and to achieve the mission of the organization, it is essential that an evaluation process be defined in order to assess the effects on clients, employees, and other relevant stakeholders.

Discussion Questions

1. You have been hired as an assistant to a new CEO of an academic medical center. You have been asked to recommend a variety of organization designs for the 300-bed inpatient facility. The academic medical center is fully affiliated with the medical school, which is internationally renowned for its work in cardiovascular diseases, neurosciences, and transplant programs. The CEO's main objectives in the reorganization are to decentralize decision making to physicians and other clinicians, to pave the way for more effective information systems for monitoring quality and cost, and to break down traditional

barriers between professional hierarchies and groups. What are your recommendations?

2. As administrator of a home care program in a city of 500,000 persons, you are planning to expand your services. Your program has been in operation for about five years, and until now you have focused on clients with relatively short-term needs. Clients' average length of time in the program is 25 days. The expansion will consist of providing comprehensive services to persons who are chronically ill and who consequently require long-term home care. On the basis of a preliminary survey, you estimate that the size of your program will triple within a year. The chronic-care clients will most likely have problems of the circulatory system, neoplasms, or diseases of the musculoskeletal system. Most clients will need long-term nursing services, physiotherapy, occupational therapy, homemaking services, and a variety of supplies and equipment. Your organization is currently structured according to function (nursing, physiotherapy, homemaking, administration, finance). You have a staff of over 200, but with the new program you will probably need to double your staff. You are wondering about changing your organization design in preparation for the expansion. What would be the advantages and disadvantages of a program design for the home care program? On what basis might you group activities and personnel (e.g., by type of clients, by geographic area of the city, or by services)?

3. Pharmaceutical companies globally are faced by a set of similar strategic and organizational challenges: the cost of the research and development required to develop a new product, the amount of time it takes to get a new product to market, differential regulatory hurdles in different markets, changes in who the purchasers of their products are, and variably complex distribution arrangements from one country to the next. Pick any one of the above challenges and discuss how organization design principles might be used to meet it effectively.

4. You have just taken over the management of a rehabilitation center where the main clientele are those persons requiring rehabilitation services for posthip and knee replacement surgery, postcardiac surgery, trauma accidents, and head and back injuries. These patients require a range of multidisciplinary services including medical, physical therapy, nursing, occupational therapy, psychology, and social work. How would you go about designing the teams to provide the necessary services?

5. Consider an organization you are familiar with (preferably one you have worked in). Reflecting on your experience in this organization, define at least one problem in its design. What were the symptoms of the problem? What might be (or should have been) done to solve the problem? Why do you think that nothing was done?

References

Alexander, J. A., Vaughn, T., Burns, L. R., Zuckerman, H. S., Anderson, R. M., Torrens, P., & Hilberman, D. W. (1996, March). Organizational approaches to integrated health care delivery: A taxonomic analysis of physician-organization arrangements. Medical Care Research and Review, 53(1), 71–93.

Charnes, M., & Smith-Tewksbury, L. J. (1993). *Collaborative management in health care.* San Francisco: Jossey-Bass.

Daft, R. L. (1998). Organization theory and design (6th ed.). St. Paul: West Pub. Co.

Duncan, R. (1978, Winter). "What is the right organization structure? Decision tree analysis provides the answer" *Organizational Dynamics, 7*(4), 59–80.

Ellis, P., & Closson, T. (1994). "Realigning around the patient: The application of restructuring and process re-engineering at Sunnybrook Health Science Centre" In Program Management and Beyond: Management Innovations in Ontario Hospitals. P. Leatt, L. Lemieux-Charles, & C. Aird (Eds.). Ottawa: Canadian College of Health Service Executives.

Gaucher, E. J., & Coffey, R. (1993). Total quality in health care. San Francisco: Jossey-Bass.

Gellerman, S. W. (1990). In organizations, as in architecture, form follows function. Organizational Dynamics, 18(3), 57–68.

Gillies, R. R., Shortell, S. M., & Young, G. L. (1997, Fall). Best practices in managing organized delivery systems. *Hospitals and Health Services Administration, 42*(3), 299–321.

Gittell, J. H., & Weiss, L. (1997, November). How organization design shapes informal networks: The case of patient care coordination. Working paper.

Heyssel, R. M., Gaintner, J. R., Kues, I. W., Jones, A. A., & Lipstein, S. H. (1984). Decentralized management in a teaching hospital. New England Journal of Medicine, 310(22), 1477–1480.

Howard, R. (1992, September-October). The CEO as organizational architect: An interview with Paul Allaire. Harvard Business Review, 107–121.

Kaluzny, A. D. (1994). Centralization and decentralization in a vertically integrated system: The XYZ hospital corporation. In D. A. Conrad and G. A. Hoare (Eds.), Strategic alignment: Managing integrated health systems (pp. 125–131). Ann Arbor: AUPHA Press/Health Administration Press.

Kaluzny, A., Morrissey, J., & McKinney, M. (1990). "Emerging organizational networks: The case of the Community Clinical Oncology Program," in S. S. Mick and associates (Eds.). Innovations in the Organization of Healthcare: New Insights into Organiza-tional Theory. San Francisco, CA: Jossey-Bass.

Katzenbach, J. R., & Smith, D. K. (1993). *The wisdom of teams*. Boston: Harvard Business School Press.

Kimberly, J. R. (1984). The anatomy of organizational design. *Journal of Management, 10*(1), 109–126.

Kimberly, J. R., & Miles, R. H. (1980). *The organization life cycle: Issues in the creation transformation and decline of organizations*. San Francisco: Jossey-Bass.

Lawrence, P., & Lorsch, J. (1967). *The organization and its environment*. Cambridge, MA: Harvard University Press.

Leatt, P., Baker, G. R., Halverson, P. K., & Aird, C. (1997, Summer). Downsizing, reengineering, and restructuring: Long term implications for health care organizations. Frontiers in Health Service Management, 13(4), 2–37.

Leatt, P., Lemieux-Charles, L., & Aird, C. (1994). *Program management and beyond: Management innovations in Ontario hospitals*. Ottawa, Canada: CCHSE.

McLaughlin, C. P., & Kaluzny, A. D. (1999). *Continuous quality improvement in health care: Theory, implications and applications*. Gaithersburg, MD: Aspen Publishers.

Melum, M. M., & Sinioris, M. K. (1992). *Total quality management: The health care pioneers*. Chicago: American Hospital Publishing.

Mintzberg, H. (1983). *Structuring in fives: Designing effective organizations*. Englewood Cliffs, NJ: Prentice-Hall.

Mohrman, S. A., Cohen, S. G., & Mohrman, A. M., Jr. (1995). *Designing team based organizations: New form of knowledge work*. San Francisco: Jossey-Bass.

Morgan, G. (1997). *Images of organization*. Thousand Oaks, CA: Sage Publications.

Nadler, D. A., Gerstein, M. S., Shaw, R. B., & associates. (1992). *Organizational architecture: Designs for changing organizations*. San Francisco: Jossey-Bass.

Palmer, R. H., & Reilly, M. C. (1979). Individual and institutional variables which may serve as indicators of quality of medical care. *Medical Care, 17*, 693–717.

Pearce, J. A. (1982, Spring). The company mission as a strategic tool. *Sloan Management Review, 23*(3), 15–24.

Rothchild, J., & Allen, W. A. (1989). *The cooperative workplace: Potentials and dilemmas of organizational democracy and participation*. Cambridge: Cambridge University Press.

Shortell, S. M., Gillies, R. R., Anderson, D., Erickson, K. M., & Mitchell, J. B. (1996). *Remaking health care in America: Building organized delivery systems*. San Francisco: Jossey-Bass.

Shortell, S. M., Gillies, R. R., Anderson, D., Mitchell, J., & Morgan, K. (1993). Creating organized delivery systems. The barriers and facilitators. *Hospital and Health Services Administration, 38*(4), 447–466.

Siehl, L., & Martin, J. (1990). Organizational culture: A key to financial performance? In B. Schneider (Ed.), *Organizational climate and culture*. San Francisco: Jossey-Bass.

Smith, T., Leatt, P., Ellis, P., & Fried, B. (1989). Decentralized hospital management: Rationale, potential and two case examples. *Health Matrix, 7*(1), 11–17.

Starkweather, D., & Kisch, A. (1971). A model of the life cycle dynamics of health service organizations. In M. F. Arnold, L. V. Blankenship, & J. M. Hess, (Eds.), *Administering health systems*. New York: Aldine Atherton Press.

Stein, B. A., & Kanter, R. M. (1980). Building the parallel organization: Creating mechanisms for permanent quality of work life. *Journal of Applied Behavioural Science, 16*, 371–386.

Trerise, B., & Lemieux-Charles, L. (1996). An assessment of the introduction of a multiskilled worker into an acute care setting, Health Care Management Forum, 9(3), 43–48.

Zammutto, R. F., & Krakower, J. Y. (1991). *Quantitative and qualitative studies of organizational culture. Research in organizational change and development*. Greenwich, CT: JAI Press, 83–114.

Zuckerman, H. S., Hilberman, D. W., Andersen, R. M., Burns, L. R., Alexander, J. A., & Torrens, P. (1998, Spring). Physicians and organizations: Strange bedfellows or a marriage made in heaven? *Frontiers of Health Services Management, 14*(3), 3–34.

CHAPTER

11

Managing Strategic Alliances

Edward J. Zajac, Ph.D.
Thomas A. D'Aunno, Ph.D.
Lawton R. Burns, Ph.D.

Chapter Outline

Learning Objectives

After completing this chapter, the reader should be able to:

1. Better understand why strategic alliances are increasing in use, particularly among health care organizations.
2. Distinguish between different types or forms of strategic alliances, using a number of dimensions.
3. Classify an alliance both in terms of what it looks like and what it is meant to do.
4. Understand how alliance motivation is often related to alliance structure and outcomes.
5. Identify whether your motivations for a strategic alliance are compatible with those of your alliance partner.
6. Think about strategic alliances in terms of the likely stages of development that alliances often experience and the critical issues that you may face at each stage.
7. Distinguish between an alliance problem and an alliance symptom and recognize the different implications for managerial intervention.
8. Understand both the pros and cons of alliances.

Key Terms

Alliance Problems versus Symptoms
Cost Reduction versus Revenue Enhancement
Ownership versus Control
Partner Orientation
Pooling versus Trading Alliances
Strategic Alliance
Symbiotic versus Competitive Interdependence
Turbulent Environment
Uncertainty Reduction

Chapter Purpose

There is no doubt that the U.S. health care environment is undergoing major changes that could be characterized as turbulent. The word *turbulence* was originally used to depict highly complex and rapidly changing environments; and it has been somewhat vaguely used to describe many industry contexts (Emery & Trist, 1965). However, a closer inspection of the Emery and Trist definition reveals that the term applies when two general conditions are met: (1) organizations are highly interconnected with one another, and (2) organizations are highly interdependent with the society in which organizations find themselves.

This emphasis on connectedness and interdependence is an important basis for viewing a specific organization's environment not as some amorphous external force but rather as the set of other organizations that are interconnected or interdependent with it. This organization, in turn, is part of the environment for the other organizations. In other words, when an organization looks out with concern or anticipation at its **turbulent environment**, what it sees is other organizations looking out at that organization (Shortell & Zajac, 1990)!

This conceptualization of organizational environments suggests the need to focus more attention on how specific organizations interact with one another. This chapter emphasizes one such type of interaction—cooperative interorganizational relations. Longest (1990), in discussing what he terms "interorganizational linkages in health care," distinguishes between market transactions, voluntary relationships, and involuntary relationships. We focus most of our attention on those interorganizational relations that are noncoercive and entered into primarily for strategic purposes, that is, that are important to an organization's mission and expected to enhance organizational performance. We term such relationships **strategic alliances,** which are defined as any formal arrangements between two or more organizations for purposes of ongoing cooperation and mutual gain.

ALLIANCES IN HEALTH CARE

Alliances are often viewed as facing high failure rates; some claim 50% to 80%. For example, some have argued that strategic alliances, by their very nature, are risky endeavors (Harrigan, 1985). The cooperative linkages between two or more organizations are viewed as somewhat fragile, exposing each party to the risk that the other party or parties may not continue to cooperate as expected. The business press has also had a penchant for describing, in detail, particular joint ventures or other alliances that failed. (For example, one of the authors was approached several years ago by a reporter who wanted to do a story on the five biggest joint venture failures.) The failure of a cooperative alliance between two organizations often involves considerable drama, as interorganizational cooperation turns to conflict.

Although it is important to recognize the pros and cons of alliances (see Debate Time 11.1), we believe that the usual fixation on the likely failure and inherent riskiness of alliances may be misguided. Specifically, we contend that any assessment of the *risk of strategic alliances* should be balanced with an assessment of the expected return or benefit of the alliance in terms of improved financial performance, innovation, and organizational learning, and the opportunity cost of not engaging in a strategic alliance. Regarding the first point, while financial performance is an obvious outcome to consider when analyzing the success or failure of a strategic alliance, it is not clear that it should be

IN THE REAL WORLD:
THE YANKEE ALLIANCE: DEALING WITH ADVERSITY AND CREATING GROWTH

The Yankee Alliance began in 1983 with a few community hospitals in New England. By 1998, Yankee had grown to include 23 member and affiliate hospitals, along with many other nonacute care (nonhospital) health care providers. Among these are 43 long-term care facilities, 11 community health centers, and hundreds of physician offices. This alliance now represents $2.4 billion in members' operating revenues.

It would be easy—and wrong—to think that Yankee's growth and success provide a simple blueprint for others to follow. Rather, Yankee's 15-year history reveals a great deal of complexity that has challenged its members and the management staff that has guided the Alliance from its inception. Indeed, the issues that Yankee has faced illustrate several key concepts and themes in this chapter.

To begin, though the Alliance had added several hospital members in the years after its founding, by 1995 growth in membership had not only stopped, but the size of the alliance actually decreased. One hospital left the Alliance when it joined a for-profit health system. Some members left due to mergers, and still others decided to join a competing national alliance (Voluntary Hospitals of America [VHA]). Further, some CEOs of member hospitals left their positions, and their replacements were not familiar with the Alliance. As Paul O'Neill, president of Yankee since its founding, put it: "One of the greatest challenges we faced was the changes within our own ranks."

At the same time, changes continued to occur in the environment of the Alliance and its members. Two of these changes figure prominently in Yankees' history. One is that hospital alliances, just like their member hospitals, merged to increase their size and market power. Specifically, in early 1996 there was a merger of three large, mainly hospital-based alliances: Premier, American Healthcare Systems (AmHS), and the Sun Health Alliance. This new national alliance is called Premier and includes about one-third of all community hospitals in the nation (1,700 hospitals with 315,000 licensed beds), with $70 billion in annual revenues.

Yankee Alliance had been a member of AmHS for ten years. As a result, the merger that created Premier also created new opportunities—but also threats. One clear opportunity for Yankee was to take advantage of the size and market power of the new national alliance. To do this, however, Yankee members had to sign formal letters of commitment that obligated them to comply with contracts that Premier signs with various suppliers of goods and services. To benefit from the market power (lower costs) that comes from shared purchasing of materials, individual organizations must yield some autonomy. Otherwise, alliance size means relatively little.

The threat to Yankee stemmed from the fact that Premier's founding forced individual hospitals and health care systems to consider if they wanted to join Premier or its major competitor, VHA. Thus far, Premier and Yankee have fared well in this competition.

Premier's founding typifies the complexity of alliances in today's health care industry. Local hospitals and health care providers are members of regional alliances (such as the Yankee Alliance), which, in turn, are nested within larger national alliances (such as Premier).

A second major change that affects Yankee continues to unfold: Hospitals face increased pressure to reduce their costs. Many hospitals have responded by attempting to build integrated health service systems that hold the potential to provide more comprehensive and efficient care. Similarly, most of Yankee's growth in recent years has focused on nonacute care services. This growth in long-term and ambulatory care means that Yankee is much more than what we term a "pooling alliance" in this chapter; these alliances consist of members who are primarily in the same business (such as community hospitals). Rather, Yankee now is also a "trading alliance" that consists of organizations that have different resources to contribute. This change shows that alliances can, and often should, adapt to meet their members' needs as these needs vary over time.

DEBATE TIME 11.1: WHAT DO YOU THINK?

There are a few facts and many more unknowns about strategic alliances. One fact is that we are witnessing a substantial increase in strategic alliances in health care. An unknown, however, is whether this fact reflects a positive or negative development. An interesting recent example of a debate on this issue is found in Duncan, Ginter, and Swayne (1992). In this section, we consider some of the arguments swirling around the use of strategic alliances. Kaluzny and Zuckerman (1992) argue on the positive side for alliances, while Begun offers counterarguments on the negative side. The following list of issues summarizes their points of disagreement.

POSITIVE

1. Alliances reflect a fundamental shift in how health service organizations do business; namely, a change from thinking in terms of control to thinking in terms of commitment, trust, shared risk, and common purpose.
2. Alliances provide organizations with a way to manage growing complexity and interdependence while maintaining a fair amount of individual organizational autonomy.
3. Alliances enable organizations to transcend the existing organizational inertia that is often created by complexity and vested interests seeking to maintain the status quo.
4. Alliances have been found to be effective in other sectors of our society, and failure to apply these concepts to health services would be a missed opportunity for meeting the challenges in the future.

NEGATIVE

1. Alliances distract organizations from their basic goal, which is to clobber your competitors or at least behave as if you have that need. Managers like the thrill of the competitive chase, and competition creates loyalty and team spirit in an organization.
2. Alliances are essentially a fad whose benefits have been exaggerated, similar to Theory Z, the pursuit of excellence, product-line management, and total quality management.
3. Alliances can lead to collusion between otherwise competing organizations, can lead to legal problems relating to antitrust challenges, and are attractive only to lazy organizations that are not interested in competition.
4. The process hassles of initiating and managing alliances are tremendous and costly, and these arrangements are quite fragile.
5. Governing an alliance means governing by committee, which we know to be an ineffective way to run a business. In particular, this problem reduces the speed and flexibility of an organization.
6. Cooperative strategy makes sense for large, multinational firms seeking to enter new and unknown markets or share expensive research and development projects, but not for health care organizations that face well-known local markets and do not need to finance much research and development.

Which of the above perspectives do you favor? How would you justify your position?

---

considered the most important, direct outcome. For example, innovation may be a driving force behind strategic alliances, and more generally, alliances may be viewed as a desirable way for organizations to learn about new markets, services, and ways of doing business (Zajac, Golden, & Shortell, 1991). These may actually be negatively correlated with financial performance, at least in the short run (Shortell & Zajac, 1988). This issue is discussed in greater detail in the section on how strategic intentions drive alliance activity.

In terms of opportunity cost, the relevant question is not, Is it risky?, but rather, Which is riskier: going it alone, doing nothing, or engaging in an alliance? Riskiness is not necessarily a problem. For example, the virtues of entrepreneurship are often extolled, despite the high risk and high failure rates involved. Strategic alliances may appear risky when the baseline comparison is not made explicit, but when compared with attempting a *de novo* entry into a new market or ignoring the market altogether, the alliance may actually seem like a relatively low risk proposition (Shortell & Zajac, 1988). In fact, as subsequently discussed, the creation of a strategic alliance is often motivated by an organization's desire to reduce uncertainty.

The issues raised above are particularly relevant for health care organizations, which have seen an explosion of alliance building in the last decade (Zuckerman & D'Aunno, 1990). Alliance building is not limited to hospitals (Alter & Hage, 1993; Zuckerman & Kaluzny, 1991). There are alliances between hospitals and physician groups, between hospitals and health maintenance organizations (HMOs), and between hospitals, physicians, and agencies of the federal government (Shortell, 1988; Kaluzny, Morrissey, & McKinney, 1990). Nor are alliances limited to providers of care. Alliances known as business coalitions have emerged among buyers of care, that is, employers who band together to increase their effectiveness as purchasers of care for their employees. The variety of possible alliance partners is quite high, given the myriad of interdependencies between organizations in the health sector (see Table 11.1).

The causes for this outburst of activity are not difficult to identify. Perhaps the most important and obvious factor is that health care organizations are experiencing what Meyer (1982) has referred to as a series of "environmental jolts." These are relatively abrupt, major, and often qualitative changes in an environment that threaten organizational survival. The introduction of the Medicare Prospective Payment System, for example, qualifies as an environmental jolt and has led to massive changes in the strategies of hospitals in recent years (Shortell, Morrison, & Friedman, 1990; Zajac & Shortell, 1989). Further, a growing

Table 11.1. Interdependencies between Organizations in the Health Sector

In the health sector, focal organizations have potential interdependencies with organizations such as:

Accrediting agencies
Affiliated organizations
Alternative health systems
Competitors
Confederated organizations
Consortia members
Consumer representatives (public and private)
Employee representatives (unions)
Fiscal intermediaries
Financial organizations (bond rating)
Foundations
Government (all levels)
Health maintenance organizations (HMOs)
Independent practice associations (IPAs)
Insurance companies
Joint venture partners
Media
Physician-hospital organizations (PHOs)
Multi-institutional systems
Other partners
Owners
Political groups
Preferred provider organizations (PPOs)
Suppliers (including capital, consumables, equipment, and human resources)
Third-party association (TPAs)
Trade associations
Utilization management companies

SOURCE: Adapted from Longest B. Interorganizational linkages in the Health Sector. In *Health Care Management Review*, 1990; 15:17–28, with permission of Aspen Publishers, Inc., © 1990.

number of hospitals have closed. Other jolts include increased competition, a surplus of hospital beds, concern with cost containment, an increase in the number of uninsured patients, an aging population, and the AIDS epidemic.

These jolts create great uncertainty for health care managers. Alliances may reflect the reality that it is sometimes better to face life's uncertainties with partners than to go it alone (Kaluzny, Zuckerman, &

Ricketts, 1995; Zuckerman, Kaluzny, & Ricketts, 1995). Of course, alliances are but one response to the environmental changes described above. There has also been a marked increase in other types of multiorganizational arrangements, particularly multihospital systems (Shortell, 1988). Further, other strategic adaptive responses to environmental change have emerged, including vertical integration and diversification (Clement, 1987). In short, as Starr (1982) argued over a decade ago, the landscape of the health care field is itself changing: Where there were once many small and independent organizations there are now clusters of organizations, including alliances and other types of multiorganizational arrangements.

TYPES AND FORMS OF ALLIANCES

While the incidence of strategic alliances has increased dramatically in recent years, it would be an exaggeration to say that they are a new phenomenon. Strategic alliances in a wide range of shapes and sizes have been historically observed in many industries, particularly in health care. Given the variety in types of alliances, it is therefore not surprising that early research on alliances devoted considerable initial attention to the categorization of interorganizational relations (often called multi-institutional arrangements) found in the health care industry, much in the way that a botanist might develop an organizing schema for classifying plants. The earliest approaches toward understanding these arrangements were usually interested in establishing a continuum upon which the arrangements could be located for purposes of comparison and contrast (Brown & Lewis, 1976; DeVries, 1978; Starkweather, 1971). DeVries (1978), for example, arrays multi-institutional systems on a continuum of "less commitment, more institutional autonomy" to "more commitment, more system control," in the following order

- formal affiliation
- shared or cooperative services
- consortia for planning or education
- contract management
- lease

- corporate ownership but separate management
- complete ownership

Ownership versus Control

DeVries (1978) and others have arrayed multi-institutional systems on a continuum of more autonomy to more **control.** However, these rankings often really reflect the degree of **ownership,** with complete ownership being equated with the highest form of control. While it seems reasonable to view ownership as related to control, we argue that this can sometimes be misleading.

For example, it is well known that McDonald's Corp. is very interested in maintaining control over its raw materials to ensure that quality is highly consistent. In dealing with its exchange partners who supply these raw materials, one might therefore expect that McDonald's would prefer an interorganizational arrangement that would involve substantial ownership interest in suppliers in order to have greater control. This is not the case, however. Even with no ownership interests, McDonald's simply communicates its quality requirements to the supplier organizations, and the organizations are typically quick to oblige.

How can this be? Two factors seem to be relevant. The first is obvious. McDonald's, by virtue of its size, enjoys substantial relative power in its relationship with suppliers; McDonald's represents a very large portion of a food supplier's business. This obviates, at least in large part, the need for McDonald's to also own some or all of the suppliers' assets. Ownership and control are essentially separated in this case. The second reason has much less to do with the relative power of the organizations involved and more to do with the establishment of a tradition of mutual gain and cooperation. Specifically, McDonald's has made it a policy to be loyal to high-quality suppliers and to use its size to protect the supplier from dramatic swings in sales revenue. In this way, both parties have incentives to ensure a long-term cooperative relationship—with no ownership interests.

This simplified example is not intended to show that ownership and control are usually unrelated, of course. Rather, the example demonstrates that tight control can exist even in cases where there is no ownership interest. The lesson here is twofold: There are many dimensions upon which one can categorize strategic alliances, and one must exercise caution in interpreting what the dimension really represents. The discussion to follow addresses several additional dimensions upon which one can distinguish one type or form of strategic alliance from another.

Number of Members

Alliances vary greatly in size. They can consist of two organizations, but they often consist of many more. For example, Voluntary Hospitals of America (VHA) is a national hospital alliance that has 100 original members. Size makes a substantial difference in several ways. Larger alliances are more difficult to govern because it is more difficult to represent all members on a single board of directors. Larger size may also entail greater diversity among members, which in turn may make it more difficult to find common ground on important issues ranging from alliance strategy (i.e., what are the overall purpose and goals of the alliance) to the management of alliance programs. Further, even when agreements are reached on alliance strategy and operations, larger size makes it difficult to coordinate members' efforts.

On the other hand, size has virtues. It creates power, as noted earlier. Larger alliances typically have more purchasing power because they can buy in larger volume (assuming, of course, that all members can agree on a particular vendor, which is often difficult). Similarly, larger alliances have more clout in lobbying at various levels of government. Further, larger alliances can generate capital easier simply from having a larger number of members' fees to collect.

Nonetheless, the costs and benefits of alliance size are difficult to assess in the abstract. What often matters most in determining an effective size for an alliance is its strategic purpose and particular situation. For example, a local or regional hospital network will have a relatively small number of members compared to other hospital alliances (e.g., VHA). Yet, it may have exactly the number of members it needs for its purpose, which is to provide the local area with a comprehensive service system.

Governance Structure

In the case of an alliance with two members, it is often not necessary to be concerned about establishing a way to govern alliance activities so as to give them direction. But beyond the simple case of a two-party alliance, governance issues can be considerably complex.

The governing bodies of many alliances, especially hospital alliances, tend to include at least one member from each participating organization, often the director or CEO of the member organization. This practice stems largely from important distinguishing features of alliances; that is, that they are a form of organization in which the members are equal and have a great deal of autonomy.

Further, the boards of health care organizations traditionally have been based on what Fennell and Alexander (1989) term a philanthropic model, which assumes that "bigger is better." In other words, boards were viewed as a key link to the local community and its resources; having more individuals on a board provided a hospital, for example, with greater community support and access to donors. Similarly, we have observed that alliance boards often are large so as to represent various interest groups.

Indeed, as Carman (1992) reports, alliance boards often have physician representatives, board members from participating organizations, and community members as well. Moreover, Carman argues persuasively that alliance boards should not consist entirely of CEOs. He points out that there is enough turnover among CEOs so as to create instability for an alliance if its governance rests only with them (Alexander, Fennell, & Halpern 1993). In contrast, organizational commitment to the alliance is enhanced if it is represented in alliance governance by leaders other than CEOs.

As just noted, however, this means that larger alliances can have boards with dozens of members that in turn, can make it difficult to achieve consensus and can slow decision making. Of course, large alliance boards can, and sometimes do, have executive committees that consist of a smaller subset of elected members who have the authority to make key decisions. Thus, an important choice for larger alliances is whether to represent all or some members on the alliance board and to determine what kinds of individuals (CEOs, physicians, trustees) should be alliance board members.

Mandated vs. Voluntary Participation

Another important dimension on which alliances vary is whether they are voluntary or mandated by an external group with legal or legitimate authority (Provan, 1983). Most health care alliances are voluntary. These alliances reflect the efforts of individual organizations to strategically adapt to external changes by choosing to band together. But, it is important to recognize that even voluntary alliances may emerge in large part as a result of external pressure from powerful actors.

A central issue to note in comparing mandated and voluntary alliances is the extent to which the former are characterized more by style than substance and by instability than longevity. Scott (1987) argues that mandated forms of organization tend to be adopted only superficially and, as a result, also tend to be short-lived. Many international alliances (including the League of Nations and the United Nations) come to mind in this regard. Superficial compliance with a mandate to form an alliance is especially likely to occur when the participating organizations lack other motives for forming a relationship (Oliver, 1990). In general, managers and other organization members chafe under external constraints and regulation, even when such rules have some merit.

Discussion

Existing typologies have been useful in documenting and describing the common and different features of a wide range of interorganizational arrangements in health care. However, it is also important to ask what difference an organization should expect to see if it were to choose one form versus another.

This seemingly simple question is actually quite difficult to answer. More specifically, we believe that gaining an understanding of the various forms of alliances is only part of understanding the fuller picture of strategic alliances. An additional piece of this puzzle lies in asking not only, What do they look like?, but also, What are they meant to accomplish?

In other words, an exclusive focus on the different types or forms of health care strategic alliances implicitly assumed that certain forms imply certain functions, and even outcomes. Otherwise, if a single form could actually serve multiple functions, there would not be such an interest in discussing the differences among forms. Zajac (1986), in an analysis of contract-management arrangements, argues that organizations choosing to engage in a similar type of strategic alliance may have widely varying strategic intentions and that expected performance will vary correspondingly. This suggests that it may not be reasonable to expect a particular form of interorganizational arrangement to translate into a particular performance result.

The form of alliance used may be much less important in suggesting particular performance outcomes than the strategic intentions, as articulated by key decision makers, that motivate that choice of alliance. In other words, the form of the alliance is not necessarily a good predictor of what the alliance can achieve.

WHAT ARE ALLIANCES MEANT TO DO?

Pooling versus Trading Alliances

Most broadly, one can distinguish between **pooling alliances** that bring together organizations seeking to contribute similar resources and **trading alliances** that bring together organizations seeking to contribute different resources (Nielsen, 1986). This distinction is more precise than the often-made statement that organizations generally seek " complementarities" in alliances. The term *complementarity* suggests differences, but it is important to remember that similarities can often drive alliance activity as well. An example of a pooling or similarity-driven strategic intent for an alliance is one that seeks to gain purchasing power over a supplier or group of suppliers. Such alliances are often seen in health care, in the form of business coalitions (against hospitals) or hospital alliances (against health care supply organizations).

Examples of a trading or difference-driven alliance are a physician group–hospital joint venture, where each party contributes something distinct to the alliance, and a joint venture between two health care supply firms, such as Johnson & Johnson and Merck, where the former is known for its marketing expertise, the latter for its product development skills. These examples also highlight how strategic intent can often drive the form of a strategic alliance. Pooling strategies tend to involve more organizations and take the form of federations, consortia, or coalitions; and trading strategies tend to involve fewer (often only two) organizations and take the form of joint ventures, licensing agreements, and related arrangements.

Cost Reduction versus Revenue Enhancement

The strategic intent of alliances can also be examined in terms of their expected outcomes. An emphasis on expected alliance outcomes is relevant for several reasons: The success of an alliance will generally be defined by the degree to which the desired outcomes are achieved; some performance outcomes may be largely incompatible with others; and one alliance partner's perception of the expected outcome may not be shared by that of other partners.

The first and most basic expected outcome refers to financial performance and addresses the issue of whether the alliance is primarily conceived for **cost reduction** or **revenue enhancement.** While this is not to say that the two outcomes are mutually exclusive, there are differences in the challenges for success for alliances, in how one gauges success, and in how cost-reducing versus revenue-enhancing alliances might be organized.

For example, consider a local alliance of four hospitals with historically complementary specialties (or distinctive competencies) that is seeking to increase the volume of patients to be treated in these specialties. Compare this alliance with a similarly sized and similarly located hospital alliance seeking to share the costs of providing indigent care to the local community. One would not measure success the same way, nor would the interaction between partners be the same in the two alliances. One might expect that the alliance motivated by the desire to increase patient volume would require substantial coordination, given that there is a reciprocal interdependence between the partners. In the case of the cost-sharing alliance, one would likely observe a combining of sim-

ilar resources requiring relatively less active coordination, given that there is a pooled interdependence among the partners (Thompson, 1967).

Quality, Innovation, and Learning

Another way of classifying the intent of an alliance is the degree to which the alliance seeks to enhance outcomes such as innovation, organizational learning, and quality (Prahalad & Hamel, 1990; Zajac et al., 1991). These outcomes are distinct from those discussed above in that, while they may lead to revenue enhancement or cost reduction, their relationship to such financial performance measures may be difficult to discern, or in a more extreme case, may be negatively related to financially oriented targets (Shortell & Zajac, 1990).

For example, Zuckerman and D'Aunno (1990) noted that hospitals can increase their reputation for quality by joining a strategic alliance that involves other prestigious organizations. Membership in such an alliance may require only a minor contribution of time, effort, or capital. An interesting feature of such an alliance is that one partner's actions can damage the reputation of another by not delivering the expected level of quality. This suggests the need for appropriate screening of partners in terms of their commitment to quality.

There may also be regional differences in the degree to which membership is prestige-enhancing. One of the authors was involved in a research project on multihospital systems in which a voluntary membership affiliation with a large national, for-profit hospital system was viewed by the local community as an asset to the hospital. The name of the hospital system was proudly displayed at the hospital entrance and on hospital stationery. However, another hospital affiliated with that same system—but located in a different part of the country—made every attempt to downplay that affiliation. No signs were posted with the system name, and no trace of the system could be found on hospital stationery. The reason for this very different treatment? In the first example, the region had many for-profit affiliations, and several of the major hospital chains had their headquarters in that region of the country. In the second example, for-profit hospitals were much less common in the region and were viewed somewhat suspiciously by many in that environment. The point to be made is that, before seeking membership in an alliance for purposes of increasing actual or perceived quality, an organization must be aware of the limits of that benefit.

Other motives driving alliance activity, such as innovation and learning, are also conceptually distinct from other more straightforward motives. The payoffs from alliances that are driven by innovation and learning motives are often slow to emerge. This requires a particularly high level of partner commitment and patience. An additional factor to consider is that many organizations underestimate the involvement necessary to realize benefits such as innovation and learning. In these alliances, a more substantial personnel flow between partners can often accelerate the learning and innovation process.

Power Enhancement, Uncertainty Reduction, and Risk-Sharing

Power enhancement and **uncertainty reduction** are grouped together because one often has implications for the other. Specifically, alliances can be motivated by an organization's desire to gain influence over (or reduce dependence on) an aspect of the organization's environment. This reduction in dependence may also represent a reduction in uncertainty, although the two are conceptually distinct. An organization might be dependent on another organization, but if the more powerful organization is reliable, then the dependent organization may face little uncertainty.

This perspective can be seen in much of the early literature on interorganizational relations in health care. Longest (1990), for example, views the growth of multi-institutional systems as the result of an "external dependency relationship" between the hospital and its environment. In doing so, Longest is applying the resource dependence perspective to the health care industry (Pfeffer & Salancik, 1978). Longest (1990) uses the term *stabilization strategy* to characterize multihospital arrangements, which he explains are "formulated by people for a hospital that exists in relation to an external environment upon which the hospital is highly dependent."

Uncertainty reduction as an alliance motive can also be compared with a similar, yet distinct, motive: risk-sharing. The difference between the two motives is that the former highlights one organization's attempts to reduce its own uncertainty, whereas the latter emphasizes the joint reduction of uncertainty for both (or more) partners. Not surprisingly, the former is equated more with gaining influence of an exchange partner, while the latter is used more in terms of pooling resources to reduce common risk.

Summary

It is important to note that the above-mentioned strategic intentions that can drive alliance activity are not mutually exclusive. For example, a business coalition may be formed because it wants to gain influence over local area hospitals, but it also has as its major objective a reduction in the cost of health care that the coalition members have had to pay. Thus, power and cost-reduction motives are both driving alliance formation. Similarly, a joint venture between a hospital and a multispecialty physician group may have as its objective the creation of new innovative services, yet also have the intent of increasing revenues (Longest, 1990).

Understanding the strategic intent of an alliance can be a critical success factor for the alliance. The understanding has several components, including understanding your own motivation for considering an alliance, expressing this understanding to your alliance partner, eliciting and then listening carefully to your partners' expression of their strategic intentions, and examining the compatibility (which could be compatibly similar or compatibly different) of your intentions and those of your partners. The lack of an articulated mission statement is often cited as the root of many failures in organizational strategy. The same is equally if not more true for strategic alliances, particularly given the potential for incompatible intentions across partners.

Physician-Hospital Trading Alliances

Physician-hospital alliances have spread across the health care system in response to several environmental jolts. The Medicare Prospective Payment System (PPS) altered the financial incentives of hospitals by using fixed, per-case payments but left physician incentives untouched. Because physicians control (directly or indirectly) up to 80% of hospital expenditures, hospitals began to develop relationships with their physicians in order to influence their thinking and practice behavior. The rapid increase in managed care (e.g., penetration by HMOs) in the late 1980s and early 1990s provided an additional spur to alliance formation. As HMOs sought to reduce their inpatient costs (e.g., through lower payments), hospitals looked for ways to cut costs through partnerships with their physicians. Moreover, some HMOs looked to pass on to providers the financial risks for their enrollees. Physicians and hospitals sought to develop alliances to accept and manage this risk. Finally, by the mid-1990s, HMO consolidations served to increase managed care's bargaining power over providers in local markets. Providers have responded to this threat by forming vertical alliances to pose a countervailing force (Burns, Bazzoli, Dynan, & Wholey, 1998).

Physician-hospital alliances take many forms, which contribute to the growing list of acronyms managers must now understand. Physician-hospital organizations (PHOs) constitute joint ventures designed to develop new services (e.g., ambulatory care clinic) or, more commonly, attract managed care contracts. Management services organizations (MSOs) constitute vehicles for the transfer of managerial expertise and administrative systems to physicians in small practices, and sometimes capital for expansion. Integrated salary models (ISMs) constitute vertically integrated arrangements in which the hospital purchases the physician's practice, establishes an employment contract with the physician for a defined period, and negotiates a guaranteed base salary with a variable component based on office productivity, with some expectation (or anticipation) that the physician will refer or admit patients to the hospital.

These alliances serve many purposes. They are generally designed to reduce uncertainty for both parties in dealing with an increasingly competitive and threatening environment. One major, specific objective is revenue enhancement: to increase the trading partners' success in obtaining managed care contracts and capitated revenues. Providers have anticipated the widespread use of capitation by HMOs, which has yet to materialize, and have therefore sought to develop a continuum of services that payers and their enrollees will require. At a minimum, this continuum includes inpatient hospital care and ambulatory physician care. A second specific objective is to provide a platform for future physician-hospital collaboration in such areas as quality improvement and cost containment. Alliances are thus a vehicle for physicians and hospitals to begin working together in a risk-based environment. Because every physician is different, hospitals typically offer physicians a menu of alliances from which to choose (Dynan, Bazzoli, & Burns, 1997).

How well have these alliances performed? If success is gauged by provider interest, alliances are doing quite well. Recent evidence highlights the diffusion of alliances across U.S. hospitals, with continued high growth particularly among MSOs (American Hospital Association, 1998; Burns, Bazzoli, Dynan, & Wholey, 1997; Morrisey, Alexander, Burns, & Johnson, 1996). Other evidence, however, suggests that alliances have failed to achieve their specific objectives. With regard to managed care contracting, for example, barely half of all PHOs have risk-based contracts with HMOs, and most of the PHOs' "covered lives" are in PPO contracts that entail no capitation and little or no financial risk (Ernst & Young, 1995). PHOs and MSOs alike typically have fewer than 12,000 at-risk lives under contract. With regard to collaboration, hospitals have succeeded in enlisting their physicians to join these vehicles. PHOs, for example, typically include 80% to 90% of the medical staff. Such wide-open participation is actually detrimental to the PHO's purposes, however, since the hospital is seeking physician partners who can practice more cost-effective medicine than the medical staff as a whole. Additional evidence suggests that PHO participation does not significantly increase the physician's perceived alignment and identification with the hospital (Burns et al., 1996).

Why are the results so disappointing, especially given the prevalence of alliances and the attention received in the trade literature? One reason is the structural form used to implement the alliance. These alliances are typically organized, financed, and controlled by the hospital with little physician participation. Not surprisingly, physicians balk at partnerships' in which they have not participated. Another reason (stated above) is the sheer size of the physician panel. Alliances that fail to carefully screen their members resemble the medical staff at large and thus represent "business as usual." A third explanation is the lack of infrastructure found in many alliances. Too often hospitals will develop the alliances as external contracting vehicles to approach the managed care market, but fail to develop the internal mechanisms that will help the alliance partners to manage risk. Such mechanisms include physician compensation and productivity systems, quality monitoring and measurement, and physician selection (Burns & Thorpe, 1997). These findings suggest that implementation of the alliance is critical for the success of any alliance that physicians and hospitals form.

THE ALLIANCE PROCESS: A MULTISTAGE ANALYSIS

Previous studies of alliances have focused primarily on why they emerge, how they are structured, and what they do. Less attention has been given to how alliances evolve and behave over time (D'Aunno & Zuckerman, 1987a; Luke, Begun, & Pointer, 1989; Provan, 1984; Sofaer & Myrtle, 1991; Zajac & Olsen, 1993). Thus, we develop models that managers can use to understand how alliances develop as they do and what can be done to improve their chances for success.

Alliances can be considered within the context of a life cycle model (Table 11.2). This model suggests that organizations often move through predictable stages of growth, with one or more factors triggering such movement. Further, each stage brings distinctive tasks that alliance leaders and members need to address.

Emergence: Finding Partners

In the first stage, environmental threats, opportunities, and uncertainty lead organizations with similar ideologies and dependencies to seek out each other. Further, this dance often begins when the potential partners relate to each other **symbiotically** as well as **competitively** (Hawley, 1950; Pfeffer & Salancik, 1978). In other words, alliances may be more likely to emerge when one organization uses some services or

Table 11.2. A Life Cycle Model of Organizational Alliances in Health Care

Stages			
Emergence	*Transition*	*Maturity*	*Critical Crossroads*
Key factors in development at each stage			
Environment poses threat to and uncertainty about valued resources	Motivation to achieve purposes of the alliance	Willingness to put alliance interests first	Increased centralization and dependence on alliance motivates members to seek hierarchy or withdraw from alliance
Organizations share ideologies and similar dependencies	Increased dependence on alliance for valued resources	Members receive benefits from previous investments	
Examples of tasks at each stage			
Define purposes of the alliance	Hire or form a management group	Attain stated objectives	Manage decisions about future of the alliance
Develop membership criteria	Establish mechanisms for coordination and control	Sustain member commitment	

products of the other as opposed to the case when two organizations are vying for the same resources. A common example of symbiosis is a rural community hospital that refers cases for tertiary care to an urban teaching hospital.

Interorganizational exchange processes involve distinct stages (Zajac & Olsen, 1993). For example, in the early stage each organization engages in the process of projecting exchange into the future and constructing net present valuations of alternative exchange relationships on a continuum ranging from markets (i.e., arms-length transactions with another independent organization), through strategic alliances (i.e., a formal cooperative arrangement between organizations, preserving the independent identity of each partner), and finally to hierarchies (i.e., the merging of two or more organizations into one organization) (Macneil, 1983). Perceptions of what each exchange partner seeks also emerge more clearly, enabling the more precise identification of similarities and differences that can form the basis for mutually beneficial exchange.

Thus, in the early stage there is preliminary communication and negotiation concerning mutual and individual organizational interests. An organization's behavior in this stage can set a precedent for future exchange and provide information through which a firm can learn about the expected behavior of its partner. During this phase, initial relational exchange norms are being forged and commitments tested in small but important ways to determine credibility (Macneil, 1983). To summarize, in this initial stage, the purposes and expectations of the partners are stated, membership criteria are established, and group norms begin to evolve.

Though it is important for expectations to be realistic, it turns out that many young alliances have broadly stated goals that do not necessarily coincide with their activities. This is because goal statements reflect compromises made among members who are, as of yet, not willing to subordinate their interests to those of the group as a whole. Further, broad goal statements may attract other partners, and early members want to have the advantages that popularity typically affords.

Thus, in many cases, the criteria for alliance membership are selective and designed to ensure homogeneity among members. This reduces some of the governance and management problems discussed above. Further, many alliances seek to limit overlap in market areas so as to minimize competition among members and avoid antitrust issues.

At this initial stage, most alliances are not likely to form or hire a management group to direct their activities (D'Aunno & Zuckerman, 1987a), because organizations must initially identify and agree on a set of purposes. Organizations are also reluctant to yield authority and commit resources to a management group. Nonetheless, this is typically what happens in the second stage of alliance development.

Transition

In this stage the alliance establishes mechanisms for coordination, control, and decision making. This often entails forming or hiring a management group, moving the alliance to a form that Provan (1983) and D'Aunno and Zuckerman (1987b) term a "federation." The transition may be rocky because, as just noted, organizations are reluctant to grant authority to others or to sacrifice their own autonomy. It is thus critical that alliance managers ensure that their efforts and programs are responsive to members' needs. During this stage the governance structure also takes shape. This may also be threatening to members, especially if they are not directly represented on the governing board.

Alliances vary in the extent to which their members are willing to commit resources to initiate and sustain programs and activities. An important weakness of many alliances is their inability to gain adequate commitment of members' resources. For example, there may be free-rider problems in that some members make little commitment but yet can benefit from the investments of others. It is likely that such problems are directly proportional to the value that members perceive in committing resources to the alliance. The more value that members perceive from active participation, the more resources (including autonomy) they are willing to commit to the alliance.

Of course, this leads to a challenging "chicken and egg" dilemma. On the one hand, members increase their commitment in proportion to threats from their environment and the alliance's ability to reduce threats and uncertainty. On the other hand, for the alliance to be effective in meeting members' needs, it may require the investment of valued resources from members as well as their willingness to coordinate efforts with each other. At some point, alliances require an investment of resources that are risked by members who have no certainty of return equal to their investment. At this point, trust becomes particularly important.

Maturity

The third stage of an alliance's life cycle is that of maturity and growth. In this stage it is critical that the alliance begin to achieve its objectives and aid members in coping with external threats. Such success enables an alliance to continue and to grow. It is also central that members be willing to put the interests of the alliance, at least sometimes, ahead of their own interests. This is necessary because alliances cannot meet the needs of all of their members, at least not simultaneously. Members must recognize that they will not necessarily benefit equally from alliance activities; it is essential, however, that they benefit as equitably as possible.

As alliances seek to attain objectives and sustain member commitment, several issues may arise. For example, alliances that add many members may find it impossible to avoid having members with overlapping market areas. If such overlap does occur, what role, if any, should the alliance play in mediating disputes that may arise among members?

Relationships between the members and alliance managers (if there are any) also become more complex. For example, are new programs initiated through the alliance manager's office, individual members, or both? If through the alliance office, what happens to similar programs already developed by individual members? For instance, suppose that a hospital alliance wishes to develop an alliance-wide HMO, but some members already have HMOs. Further, are there or should there be incentives for members to produce innovative programs that can be shared by all alliance members? In the absence of such incentives, how will the alliance develop innovations in management or services?

Zajac and Olsen (1993), in their discussion of the development of interorganizational relationships, note that alliances in this stage of development face some particularly sensitive issues because value is not only created but also claimed and distributed. Surrounding the issue of claiming and distributing value is the question of interorganizational conflict. Explicit or implicit norms for managing the divergence of interest will often arise (Zajac & Olsen, 1993). To the extent that these norms—defined as "shared and reasoned expectations that may arise from agreement or past acts"—emphasize the importance of joint value maximization, this should lead to searches for mutually satisfactory resolutions of conflict situations (Kaufmann, 1987). On the other hand, if these evolving norms do not develop in this way, the pursuit of individual firm interests would lead to an escalation of conflict that could ultimately be destructive to the strategic alliance. As noted in Chapter 5, the accepted use of conflict-resolution systems can limit the potential damage of interorganizational conflict (Ury, Brett, & Goldberg, 1988).

The continued development of trust is a key issue in this stage of interorganizational exchange. Trust stems from a growing confidence in a firm's expectations of the future (Luhmann, 1979). Schelling (1960) also notes that "trust is often achieved simply by the continuity of the relation between parties and the recognition by each that what he might gain by cheating in a given instance is outweighed by the value of the tradition of trust that makes possible a long sequence of future agreement."

Trust and conflict-management systems are subsets of other relational norms underlying the process exchange over time. These norms include shared expectations of reciprocity between alliance partners and a growing sense of the value of preserving the relationship (Macneil, 1983, 1986). These norms set the tone for the continued execution of contracts.

Critical Crossroads

As they evolve into the fourth stage of development, alliances move to what may be a critical crossroads. Up to this point, members became increasingly dependent on each other for needed resources, and there was growing pressure for greater member commitment to the alliance and more centralized decision making. In many ways, however, these developments run counter to the reasons why many organizations join an alliance. That is, alliances are attractive because they provide a relatively low-cost vehicle to reduce resource dependence while maintaining organizational autonomy. Thus, this stage may be a critical crossroads at which some members conclude that the price of belonging to an alliance is too high and withdraw. Indeed, it appears that at least one hospital alliance collapsed precisely on this point (Ury et al., 1988). In contrast, others may decide that it is necessary to move toward more hierarchical arrangements to gain the full benefits of collective action.

The underlying issue is whether there is sufficient commitment or "glue" to hold alliances together over time (Zuckerman & Kaluzny, 1991). Though there may be common goals, ideologies, values, and inducements that keep members together, alliances typically remain loose arrangements. Can the degree of commitment required of members be secured in the long run? Will members be willing to sacrifice autonomy to allow for greater discipline in decision making? What coordination mechanisms are most appropriate and under what circumstances (Alter & Hage, 1993; Kaluzny & Zuckerman, 1992)? To survive, alliances must balance the need for and benefits of collective action with the need for individual members to retain adequate autonomy.

This critical crossroads represents a reconfiguring stage in the developmental process of a strategic alliance (Zajac & Olsen, 1993). It is usually triggered by reaching the end of the expected duration of the relationship or by changes in the partners' perceived level of the relationship's value. Reconfiguring may imply that an exchange partner will choose to leave, or it may mean that partners will join more tightly together by widening the scope of interorganizational exchange processes. For example, a group of hospitals may move from a shared purchasing arrangement to developing a joint preferred provider network.

With respect to perceived changes in the value of the strategic alliance, such changes may emerge from a new and changing environment or a historical comparison of actual to expected value creation. While this performance gap can lead to a reevaluation (positive or negative) of the interorganizational relationship itself, it may simply lead to a reassessment of the developmental processes. In other words, the reconfiguring stage may not involve a change in the type of strategic alliance *per se* but only a change in the process of interaction within the existing strategic alliance. These change options suggest that this stage may loop back to either the emergence stage, where value forecasts are respecified and strategic motivations are clarified for a new forecast period, or the transition stage, where the forms of exchange are revised and updated based on the continued experiences of the partners. Thus, the process model of strategic alliance development outlined here does not propose a one-way, deterministic path for alliances; instead, it highlights a sequence of likely phases that many alliances may experience and emphasizes a set of critical issues that health care organizations may face at the various stages of alliance development.

FRAMEWORKS FOR ANALYZING ALLIANCE PROBLEMS

A major difficulty that organizations face in addressing alliance problems is actually their inability to identify the problem correctly! By that we mean that individuals within an organization often don't know or disagree strongly on what the problem is, and this is compounded by differences of opinion between partners in alliance problem identification and diagnosis. These disagreements, we contend, can often lead to false diagnoses and the treatment of **alliance symptoms** rather than the root **alliance problems** facing the alliance. These incorrect interventions subsequently lead to greater friction, gridlock, and ultimately an increased likelihood of alliance failure. The three simple frameworks offered below are intended to lessen the likelihood of such failure.

Locating the Problem

If one were to ask several involved individuals why a particular alliance was in trouble, it is possible that one would get a uniform response. In such cases, locating the problem is simple. We argue, however, that

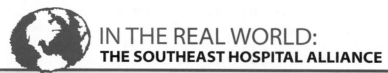

IN THE REAL WORLD:
THE SOUTHEAST HOSPITAL ALLIANCE

The Southeast Hospital Alliance (SHA) was formed by a dozen relatively large teaching hospitals about 10 years ago. It began as an alliance founded by the hospital CEOs, and it did not have a management group. Further, members were geographically distant from each other, enough so that their market areas did not overlap. The original members perceived common threats to teaching hospitals, especially from increased competition from community hospitals that were growing in sophistication and tertiary services.

After a few years, it became clear to the founding members that they needed a management group to help them move beyond discussion to develop useful programs. Further, there were several other hospitals that wanted to join the alliance. A well-regarded management consulting firm, led by a very capable individual, was hired to provide leadership and technical expertise to the alliance.

The new management group suggested adding new members, and the alliance tripled in size. SHA, under the direction of its management group, began to realize large savings from group purchasing of various supplies. The management group, flush with its initial success, continued to develop new programs. However, subtle but increasing discontent began to develop among many of the CEOs. Further, beyond the initial programs, it was not clear what overall direction SHA should take. The SHA manager contacted an external consultant to develop a strategic plan for SHA.

The consultants soon discovered some of the causes for the CEO's discontent. The SHA management group, through its original and main line of business—management consulting—was leasing mobile MRI and CT scan equipment to rural hospitals. The leased equipment effectively helped the rural hospitals to compete with SHA members. Moreover, in an effort to increase its size to support its group purchasing program, SHA had admitted several members whose market areas overlapped with each other.

such agreement is the exception rather than the norm. Typically there are a host of possible reasons why an alliance might be facing difficulties. Without some way of organizing these reasons, there may be little hope of remedying the situation. We propose that alliance problems can be viewed as generally falling into the following categories (Johnson, 1986):

- environmental problems
- strategy problems
- structure problems
- behavior problems

These categories follow a macro to micro continuum, but more important for purposes of this chapter, they also tend to follow an uncontrollable to controllable continuum. For example, SHA faced controllable problems. The problems first appeared to stem from competitors in the environment. But, closer

analysis showed that the SHA management group was fueling the competition for its own members; thus, a change in management's behavior was needed. Further, SHA had a structural problem: members with overlapping market areas. This problem was also under SHA control.

Consider also the problems in health care alliances that require collaboration among professional groups with different training, time horizons, and economic incentives. For example, trading alliances between physicians and hospitals are particularly vulnerable to these difficulties. A recent analysis of six integrated systems in Illinois suggests that physician-hospital alliances have polarities to be resolved rather than problems to be solved (Burns, 1999). These polarities consist of nine areas in which the integrated system must seek to manage in two directions simultaneously (i.e., pursue the physicians' interests simultaneously with the hospital's interests). For example, the hospital system seeks to expose its physicians to practicing in a risk-based environment; at the same time, it is purchasing primary care physicians who are then given guaranteed salaries for several years—in effect, exempting them from all risk. As another example, the hospital system wishes to become "an organization of physicians," and yet the system is developed and controlled almost exclusively by hospital executives and serves primarily hospital purposes in the short term. For such alliances to be credible to physicians and work effectively, they need to satisfy the interests of both parties simultaneously. In terms of our framework, the problems lie not in uncontrollable environmental issues, or in the basic strategy of deepening physician/hospital relationships, but in the fundamental structural decisions made and the behavioral problems created or exacerbated by those structural decisions.

The framework can be particularly valuable in highlighting disagreement as to what fundamental problems are facing a strategic alliance. We use an interesting nonhealth care example of an alliance failure to further illustrate this point.

In 1990, a consortium called U.S. Memories was conceived to provide a secure supply of chips for U.S. computer makers who were unhappy with the occasional shortages and price fluctuations brought on by Japanese chip makers, who controlled almost 90% of the DRAM market. This alliance, made up of U.S. chip buyers and a few U.S. chip makers, never got off the ground, as initial players backed out and new players refused to commit resources. Analysts offered several reasons as to why the alliance failed. Some attributed the failure to the fact that, once the temporary chip shortage was over, the alliance had no purpose. Others said it was ill-conceived and that the United States could never have competed with the more efficient Japanese chip makers. Some said that not enough players were involved; some said *too many* players were involved; and others said that the deal was not well structured. Finally, some blamed the leader of the consortium, saying that he was not well suited for such a position.

What do we make out of this mess? Could this alliance have been salvaged? Basically, we can start by using the framework above to categorize the myriad of alliance problems into environmental ("the market changed"), strategic ("it was a bad idea from the beginning"), structural ("it wasn't organized correctly"), and behavioral ("we had the wrong person at the top") problems. The point here is that, from a managerial perspective, a person responsible for gathering information about the alliance, processing that information, and making a decision on whether or how to intervene, can begin to piece together problems into useful clusters or categories.

Secondly, the categories themselves are useful in assessing the degree to which intervention can be effective. For example, after analyzing the categorized reasons, a manager may believe that the primary problem is environmental—that is, the market conditions no longer support the alliance. This is largely an uncontrollable factor and, therefore, suggests that the alliance is not likely to succeed. On the other hand, the manager may believe the primary problem is structural—that the number or composition of the alliance is not right (as in the SHA example) or that the incentives for participation are inadequate. This is more of a controllable factor and suggests that the alliance can be modified and thus face improved odds for success. In this way, the Environment→Strategy→Structure→Behavior framework can be a useful tool in identifying and diagnosing alliance problems.

Separating the Root from the Symptom

If you had a rash and were to go to a physician, what would be the first thing the physician would do? Treat the rash or first ask a set of questions to discern why you have the rash? Hopefully, the latter approach is the more common. Unfortunately, many organizations involved in strategic alliances take the former approach. There's a problem; let's fix it. This "can do" attitude is laudable in one sense, but potentially reckless (even rash?) in another sense. Specifically, when one observes friction in strategic alliances, we argue that the most important response is to first delve more deeply to understand the source of that friction before attempting to treat the problem.

This advice regarding diagnosis before treatment may seem obvious, but it often is not done in alliances. The reason it is often not done stems from alliance partners' unwillingness or inability to put themselves in their partners' shoes. In the SHA example, it was the

MANAGERIAL GUIDELINES

1. In assessing the risk of forming or entering an alliance, managers should compare the potential costs and benefits of alliances to doing nothing or to alternative strategies that involve going it alone; alliances may well be less risky than other strategies.

2. The form or structure of alliance should follow from its function—that is, what it is intended to do.

3. Managers should consider their options with respect to several important aspects of alliance structure, including ownership and control, number of members, governance structure, and mandated versus voluntary participation.

4. Many of the benefits of control in interorganizational relationships can be achieved without ownership; trust, commitment, and even power may be important substitutes for control based on ownership.

5. Increased size brings greater complexity and often more difficulty in coordinating efforts, but larger alliances tend to be more powerful for certain purposes (e.g., lobbying, purchasing in volume).

6. Large alliances often need more complex governance structures, and a key issue is who will be represented on an alliance board. It may be a mistake to have only CEOs or executive directors on alliance boards because the interests of other groups may be neglected; further, turnover among top

managers is common and may disrupt the alliance if the board has no other types of members.

7. Mandated participation in an alliance is often less preferable to voluntary participation. Alliances are not likely to succeed if members' only or most important motive for participation is to comply with external demands.

8. Recognize that alliances can be created to achieve one or more of the following objectives: to pool similar resources (e.g., as in joint purchasing arrangements); to trade dissimilar resources (e.g., as in a symbiotic relationship between a hospital and physician group); to reduce costs; to enhance revenues; to promote innovation, learning, or quality of services; or to enhance power, reduce uncertainty, or share risks among members.

9. From the above list, it is important to understand your own motives for seeking an alliance and to express these motives to potential or current partners.

10. Similarly, managers need to listen carefully to the intentions of potential or current partners in order to assess compatibility; failure to articulate a shared mission is an important reason for alliance failure.

11. Two kinds of problems are typical when it comes to alliance objectives. First, even though alliance objectives may be shared by members, the objectives

(continued)

management group that was not putting itself in members' shoes. By this we mean that signs of noncooperative behavior from a partner are often viewed with hostility on the part of other partners. The other partners then devise their own response strategy before an analysis or diagnosis is done as to why the partner may appear to be acting noncooperatively. Quite simply, we are stating that the noncooperative behavior is only a symptom of a deeper problem.

The obvious questions then become, What could the deeper problems be, and how do we treat them? We propose that there are at least four categories of problems:

- parochial self-interest
- misunderstanding and a lack of trust
- different assessments
- low tolerance for ambiguity

These categories, interestingly, match discussions of problems that exist in managing change (Kotter & Schlesinger, 1979). While the categories are not mutually exclusive, they are quite distinct from one another. For example, the first category represents rational, calculative, noncooperative behavior in which one partner knowingly acts in his own interest to the

MANAGERIAL GUIDELINES

may conflict with each other, especially over time. Second, there may be lack of consensus among members concerning alliance objectives. Both problems highlight the need for effective communication.

12. Recognize that alliances often develop in several stages that each bring distinctive threats and opportunities.

13. In the first stage (emergence), it is important to define the purposes of the alliance and select partners accordingly. Clear communication and acknowledgment of interests are critical.

14. After forming an alliance, managers must find ways to coordinate and control activities; this may entail hiring or forming a management group to focus specifically on alliance concerns.

15. As alliances mature, managers are likely to face complex issues about how much individual members must conform to and, indeed, place alliance interests ahead of their own. Further, there may be conflict about how to distribute the benefits (resources) that alliances have generated. Thus, managers need to focus on ways to sustain member commitment through trust, goal attainment, and the use of appropriate mechanisms to resolve conflict.

16. Mature alliances face the task of measuring up to members' original and changing expectations. Such alliances need to rethink their structure and objectives to make sure that they keep pace with members' needs.

17. More specifically, managers can diagnose alliance problems according to whether they are primarily environmental (i.e., stemming from external sources such as shift in market demands); strategic (i.e., concerning the overall purpose and direction of the alliance); structural (i.e., alliance form fits poorly with its purposes); or behavioral (i.e., skills are not adequate for carrying out alliance activities).

18. It is important to match alliance problems with appropriate means to deal with them, ranging from educating members to negotiating with them to coercing them.

19. Alliances can be just a management fad—be careful that you are forming one for the right reasons.

20. Recognize that alliances have their costs for managers in terms of time spent in understanding and negotiating with potential and current partners. In fact, alliances can slow decision making and make organizations less flexible—precisely what they are designed to avoid.

21. Select partners and develop ways of relating to them so as to avoid charges of collusion and antitrust problems.

22. Don't let alliance arrangements make your organization lazy and lose its interest in continuous improvement.

detriment of the other partner. The second type of problem is based less on selfishness than on the absence of accepted and well-developed norms; that is, a trusting relationship between partners has yet to emerge. The third category differs from the first in that, while the first category (i.e., selfish, noncooperative behavior) reflects disagreement on ends and means, the third category reflects agreement on ends but not means. In other words, partners may share the same goal but diverge in their views on how to achieve that goal. Lastly, some alliance partners simply feel uncomfortable with the ambiguity and fluidity of alliances. The absence of full control, as is typical in strategic alliances, may not agree with some reluctant partners.

Identifying different categories of problems is in and of itself useful as a way to move beyond the symptom and toward the problem. Treating the problem is the next step, and we propose a simple principle: The treatment should match the problem. Again, while this seems obvious, we find that all too often in alliances the treatment is either insufficient or too harsh.

Both of these situations are unfavorable. There are at least six ways of dealing with alliance problems:

- education
- participation
- facilitation
- negotiation
- co-optation
- coercion

Matching this set of treatments with the set of problems identified earlier represents a step toward effective alliance management (Kotter & Schlesinger, 1979). Consider the case where a partner faces a particularly calculative, self-interested partner. That partner is not lacking information; she knows what the situation is but does not want what her partner wants. In this case, an approach that emphasizes negotiation or co-optation is likely to be more effective than one that emphasizes participation or education. Contrast such a case with a partner whose actions are based on a misunderstanding. Here, negotiation as a response does not address the root problem; education and participation are more appropriate. We invite the reader to draw further matches between problem and treatment.

Know Thy Partner

A third framework that can be useful in addressing potential and ongoing alliance problems focuses more directly at understanding your partner's "type." Specifically, we suggest that it is a mistake to assume that your partner thinks about your alliance the same way that you do. Ideally, you will know what type of alliance partner you are dealing with at the earliest stages of the alliance. Unfortunately, it is our experience that many times a partner fails to take into adequate account the variety of partner types or **partner orientations** that exist. In our experience, there are five types of partners, ranging from the most desirable to the least desirable; each is discussed briefly below.

The Cooperative Partner

This partner is primarily interested in maximizing the joint gains in the alliance relationship, and recognizes that such maximization requires attention to what you need to achieve in the alliance. Thus, this partner will work with you in helping you achieve your goals, as well as his own. This is what you hope you have in an alliance partner, but it may be more rare than one thinks. This partner sees the alliance as win/win, and is interested in seeing that both sides win.

The Quasi-Cooperative Partner

This partner is interested in making sure that you receive just enough value from the alliance so that you will not exit. By providing you with the minimally acceptable amount of value, you still prefer the alliance above other alternatives, but not by much. This relationship is unbalanced in terms of power and dependence, but can be stable, albeit not as rewarding for the weaker party. This partner sees the alliance in terms of keeping you interested, but barely.

The Indifferent Partner

This partner—for better or worse—is not particularly interested in your strategic aspirations at all. The partner sees the alliance primarily as a vehicle for the achievement of his/her strategic goals, and you are simply along for the ride. The partner has no objections to your expending effort for your purposes, as long as (1) he/she does not need to help you do this, and (2) the attainment of his/her objectives are not impeded as a result. This partner sees the alliance in terms of "I'll get mine, you find yours."

The Competitive Partner

This partner is worse than indifferent, insofar as he/she perceives your gains as implying a loss for him/her, even when really there is no such trade-off. This person is oblivious to the positive-sum possibilities of the alliance, and very sensitive to the zero-sum aspects. This partner cannot abide any asymmetry in alliance success that might favor you, even if such variation is a natural or short-term occurrence. This partner is so fixated on the relative comparison aspects of the relationship that he/she sees the alliance in terms of "your gain must mean my loss."

The Vengeful Partner

This partner is even worse than a win/lose partner, because he/she is primarily focused on ensuring that you lose, even if he/she loses, as well. You might not think that such partners exist, and it is unlikely that you would knowingly ally with such a partner, but a partner can develop this orientation when problems in the alliance become personalized and negative emotion plays a larger role. Note that we readily accept the notion of positive emotion in alliances when we claim that trust between partners is a beneficial aspect of an alliance relationship. However, we suggest that when one partner feels that the other has somehow violated that trust, a sense of betrayal emerges that can lead a partner to act irrationally. This partner sees the alliance in terms of "I may lose, but you'll lose more."

As you can see, there are multiple partner types, and most of them are not particularly attractive! So, how can you "know thy partner" in advance? First and foremost, you must pay careful attention during the alliance emergence process for cues from your alliance partner that suggest one type versus another. For example, we have observed in working with health care organizations that some alliance partners have little idea what their partners' strategic goals are. A cooperative partner would know this, and a lack of interest in the partner's goals is an early indication that your partner is indifferent, or worse. Similarly, explore with your partner alternative scenarios for the alliance, including some in which you do better initially, and gauge your partner's reaction. If your partner objects to the slightest asymmetries in alliance outcomes, this suggests a problem that will likely emerge again and again.

Finally, assuming you are comfortable with your partner's orientation at the inception of the alliance, you must still be vigilant to changes in that orientation that may arise due to changes in the context of the alliance, whether it be changes in environmental conditions or in personnel. Ideally, this type of "early warning system" will serve you well as the alliance relationship evolves. However, we also encourage you to utilize another valuable feature of strategic alliances: Be sure to have a clear written statement of exit provisions, by which you and your partner can extricate yourselves from an alliance that may no longer be serving its intended valued purpose.

Discussion Questions

1. Under what circumstances would you agree with someone who said that alliances are very risky?
2. What dimensions would you use to classify the various types of strategic alliances? Why those dimensions?
3. Which alliance motivations do you think are the most compatible with each other?
4. What do you consider to be the likely stages of strategic alliance development? Does every alliance have to go through each stage?
5. What is the difference between an alliance problem and an alliance symptom, and what does this difference mean in terms of managerial intervention?
6. When can you tell if your partner is not likely to have a cooperative orientation?

References

Alexander, T. A., Fennell, M. L., & Halpern, M. T. (1993, March). Leadership instability in hospitals: The influence of board-CEO relations and organizational growth and decline. *Administrative Science Quarterly,* 74–99.

Alter, C., & Hage, J. (1993). *Organizations working together.* Beverly Hills, CA: Sage.

American Hospital Association. (1998). *Hospital statistics.* Chicago: American Hospital Association Publishing.

Brown, M., & Lewis, H. L. (1976). *Hospital management systems: Multi-unit organization and delivery of health care.* Germantown, MD: Aspen Systems Corporation.

Burns, L. R. (1999). Polarity management: The key challenge for integrated delivery systems. *Journal of Healthcare Management,* 44(1), 14–33.

Burns, L. R., Alexander, J. A., Zuckerman, H. S., Andersen, R. A., Torrens, P., & Hilberman, D. (1996, June). *The impact of economic integration on physician-organization alignment.* Paper presented at annual meeting of Association of Health Services Research, Chicago, IL.

Burns, L. R., Bazzoli, G. J., Dynan, L., & Wholey, D. R. (1997). Managed care, market stages, and integrated delivery systems: Is there a relationship? *Health Affairs, 16,* 204–218.

Burns, L. R., Bazzoli, G. J., Dynan, L., & Wholey, D. R. (1998, June). *HMO impact on integrated provider networks.* Paper presented at annual meeting of Association of Health Services Research, Washington, D.C.

Burns, L. R., & Thorpe, D. P. (1997). Physician-hospital organizations: Strategy, structure, and conduct. In R. Conners (Ed.), *Integrating the practice of medicine* (pp. 351–371). Chicago: American Hospital Association Publishing.

Carman, J. M. (1992). *Strategic alliances among rural hospitals.* Berkeley, CA: Institute of Business and Economic Research, University of California, pp. 92–103.

Clement, J. P. (1987). Does hospital diversification improve financial outcomes? *Medical Care, 25,* 988–1001.

D'Aunno, T. A., & Zuckerman, H. S. (1987a). The emergence of hospital federations: An integration of perspectives from organizational theory. *Medical Care Review, 44*(2), 323–343.

D'Aunno, T. A., & Zuckerman, H. S. (1987b). A life cycle model of organizational federations: The case of hospitals. *Academy of Management Review, 12,* 534–545.

DeVries, R. A. (1978). Strength in numbers. *Hospitals: Journal of the American Hospital Association, 55,* 81–84.

Duncan, W. J., Ginter, P. M., & Swayne, L. E. (1992). *Strategic issues in health care management: Point and counterpoint.* Boston: Kent Publishers.

Dynan, L., Bazzoli, G. J., & Burns, L. R. (1997). Assessing the extent of integration achieved through physician-hospital arrangements. *Journal of Healthcare Management, 43,* 242–262.

Emery, F., & Trist, E. (1965). The casual texture of organizational environments. *Human Relations, 18,* 21–32.

Ernst and Young. (1995). *Physician-hospital organizations: Profile 1995.* Washington, DC: Author.

Fennell, M. L., & Alexander, T. A. (1989). Hospital governance and profound organizational change. *Medical Care Review, 46*(2), 157–187.

Harrigan, K. R. (1985). *Managing for joint venture success.* Lexington, MA: Lexington Books.

Hawley, A. H. (1950). *Human ecology: A theory of community structure.* New York: Ronald Press.

Johnson, D. E. L. (1986). American healthcare systems. *Modern Healthcare, 16,* 78–82.

Kaluzny, A., Morrissey, J., & McKinney, M. (1990). Emerging organizational networks: The case of the community clinical oncology program. In S. Mick & associates (Eds.), *Innovation in health care delivery.* San Francisco, CA: Jossey-Bass.

Kaluzny, A., & Zuckerman, H. (1992, Winter). Strategic alliances: Two perspectives for understanding their effects on health services. *Hospital and Health Services Management, 37,* 477–490.

Kaluzny, A. D., Zuckerman, H. S., & Ricketts, T. C. (1995). *Partners for the dance: Forming strategic alliances in health care.* Ann Arbor, MI: Health Administration Press.

Kaufmann, P. J. (1987). Commercial exchange relationships and the "negotiator's dilemma." *Negotiation Journal, 3,* 73–80.

Kotter, J. P., & Schlesinger, L. A. (1979). Choosing strategies for change. *Harvard Business Review, 57,* 106–114.

Longest, B. B. (1990). Interorganizational linkages in the health sector. *Health Care Management Review, 15,* 17–28.

Luhmann, N. (1979). *Trust and power.* New York: John Wiley and Sons.

Luke, R. D., Begun, J. W., & Pointer, D. D. (1989). Quasi firms: Strategic interorganizational forms in the health care industry. *Academy of Management Review, 14*(9), 19.

Macneil, I. R. (1983). Values in contract: Internal and external. *Northwestern University Law Review, 78,* 340–418.

Macneil, I. R. (1986). Exchange revisited: Individual utility and social solidarity. *Ethics, 96,* 567–593.

Meyer, A. (1982). Adapting to environmental jolts. *Administrative Science Quarterly, 27,* 515–537.

Morrisey, M. A., Alexander, J. A., Burns, L. R., & Johnson, V. (1996). Managed care and physician-hospital integration. *Health Affairs, 15,* 62–73.

Nielsen, R. P. (1986). Cooperative strategies. *Planning Review, 14,* 16–20.

Oliver, C. (1990). Determinants of interorganizational relationships: Integration and future directions. *Academy of Management Review, 15*(2), 241–265.

Pfeffer, J., & Salancik, G. R. (1978). *The external control of organizations: A resource dependence perspective.* New York: Harper & Row.

Prahalad, C. K., & Hamel, G. (1990, May–June). The core competence of the corporation. *Harvard Business Review, 68*(3), 79–82.

Provan, K. G. (1983). The federation as an interorganizational linkage network. *Academy of Management Review, 8*(1), 79–89.

Provan, K. G. (1984). Interorganizational cooperation and decision making autonomy in a consortium multihospital system. *Academy of Management Review, 9,* 494–504.

Schelling, T. C. (1960). *The strategy of conflict.* Cambridge, MA: Harvard University.

Scott, W. R. (1987). The adolescence of institutional theory. *Administrative Science Quarterly, 32,* 493–511.

Shortell, S. M. (1988). The evolution of hospital systems: Unfulfilled promises and self-fulfilling prophecies. *Medical Care Review, 45*(2), 177–214.

Shortell, S. M., Morrison, E. M., & Friedman, B. (1990). *Strategic choices for America's hospitals: Managing change in turbulent times.* San Francisco: Jossey-Bass.

Shortell, S. M., & Zajac, E. J. (1988). Internal corporate joint ventures: Development processes and performance outcomes. *Strategic Management Journal, 9,* 527–542.

Shortell, S. M., & Zajac, E. J. (1990). Health care organizations and the development of the strategic management perspective. S. Mick & associates (Eds). *Innovations in health care delivery: New insights into organization theory* (pp. 141–180). San Francisco: Jossey-Bass.

Sofaer, S., & Myrtle, R. C. (1991). Interorganizational theory and research: Implications for health care management, policy, and research. *Medical Care Review, 48,* 371–409.

Starkweather, D. B. (1971). Health facility mergers: Some conceptualizations. *Medical Care, 9,* 468–478.

Starr, P. (1982). *The social transformation of American medicine.* New York: Basic Books.

Thompson, J. T. (1967). *Organizations in action.* New York: McGraw Hill.

Ury, W. L., Brett, J. M., & Goldberg, S. B. (1988). *Getting disputes resolved.* San Francisco: Jossey-Bass.

Zajac, E. J. (1986). *Organizations, environments, and performance: A study of contract management in hospitals.* Unpublished dissertation, University of Philadelphia, Pennsylvania.

Zajac, E. J., Golden, B. R., & Shortell, S. M. (1991). New organizational forms for enhancing innovation: The case of internal corporate joint ventures. *Management Science, 37,* 70–184.

Zajac, E. J., & Olsen, C. P. (1993). From transaction costs to transactional value analysis: Implications for the study of interorganizational strategies. *Journal of Management Studies, 30,* 131–146.

Zajac, E. J., & Shortell, S. M. (1989). Changing generic strategies: Likelihood, direction, and performance implications. *Strategic Management Journal, 10,* 413–430.

Zuckerman, H. S., & D'Aunno, T. A. (1990). Hospital alliances: Cooperative strategy in a competitive environment. *Health Care Management Review, 15*(2), 21–30.

Zuckerman, H. S., & Kaluzny, A. (1991, Spring). The management of strategic alliances in health services. *Frontiers of Health Services Management, 7*(5), 3–23.

Zuckerman, H. S., Kaluzny, A. D., & Ricketts, T. C. (1995). Alliances in health care: What we know, what we think we know, and what we should know. *Health Care Management Review, 20*(1), 54–64.

CHAPTER

12

Organizational Innovation, Change, and Learning

S. Robert Hernandez, Dr. PH.
Arnold D. Kaluzny, Ph.D.
Cynthia Carter Haddock, Ph.D.

Chapter Outline

Learning Objectives

After completing this chapter, the reader should be able to:

1. Describe the nature of organizational change, innovation, and learning within health care organizations.

2. Identify and understand various types of change.

3. Describe the nature of the change process and the factors that are involved in that process.

4. Identify and describe the tools and strategies that help organizations develop the capacity to innovate, change, and learn within a complex and uncertain environment.

Key Terms

Structural Change Strategies
Awareness
Confrontation Meeting
Continuing Education
Continuous Quality Improvement (CQI)
Diversity Training
Human Resources Change Strategies
Identification
Implementation
Institutionalization
Performance Gap
Process Consultation
Responsibility Charting
Stages of Change or Innovation
Stakeholder Mapping
Survey Feedback
Task Analysis
Team Development
Total Quality Management (TQM)
Learning Organization

Chapter Purpose

Health care organizations face constant change and unrelenting challenges. As illustrated by Ms. Connie Livingston (see In the Real World, p. 332), organizational success or failure depends upon how effective health service executives are at creating and managing an organization that allows it to adapt and respond to changing conditions. Understanding of change and the ability to manage the change process depends upon the perceptions managers have of the problems their organizations are facing and their understanding of the best methods for dealing with change in an uncertain and complex environment. As described by Stephen Covey (1990), "What managers see as the problem is the problem."

The objective of this chapter is to provide an understanding of the change process from the perspective of the **learning organization**. Using this perspective, change is not a rational process under the sole control of management, but a complex and uncertain phenomena involving a range of events, activities, and processes that involve all personnel

within the organization. The chapter will differentiate different types of change, provide an understanding of the change process and its distinguishing characteristics, and present a set of tools and strategies for building an organization that can better accommodate the type and level of change occurring within health care organizations. The chapter concludes with a series of managerial guidelines for improving the ability of the organization to meet the challenges of the millennium.

CHANGE IN AN UNPREDICTABLE, UNKNOWABLE WORLD

Health services organizations are facing continuous and fundamental change. An expanding technology, changing consumer expectations, limited resources, and an unrelenting need for adaptability challenges our prevailing assumptions of rationality and predictability in the provision of health services.

McDaniel (1997, p. 23), for example, asserted that "traditional paradigms on management have relied on Newton and Locke's vision of an orderly and predictable world governed by natural laws." In this classical view of the world, organizational change and innovation should be an orderly process under the control of management. An alternative view suggests that ideas from quantum theory and chaos theory may be more appropriate for our understanding of organizations in the twenty-first century.

Quantum theory tells us that the world is not only unpredictable but that it is also fundamentally unknowable. It also tells us that any measurement of a phenomenon affects the phenomenon itself and that relationships between the elements of a system are more critical to understanding the system than are the elements themselves. Chaos theory assumes that we cannot predict or know how the world will unfold over time. It also tells us that small differences in initial conditions can quickly lead to large differences in the future state of a system.

What does this mean for management in health services organizations as they are increasingly forced to deal with an unpredictable and unknowable world? From quantum and chaos theories, we can gain several new perspectives.

IN THE REAL WORLD:
MEETING UNEXPECTED CHALLENGES

Ms. Connie Livingston is a 31-year-old woman living with breast cancer. Her cancer was diagnosed several years ago, and, following a lumpectomy and adjuvant therapy, she was doing quite well. . . . Well enough to plan a future involving marriage.

The wedding was planned, and the date was set. A license was obtained, guests were invited, and the endless details usually associated with such events were slowly coming into place. Unfortunately, shortly before the wedding, Ms. Livingston developed a pulmonary embolism and was rushed to a university hospital located in an adjacent state. After being admitted to the emergency room, the attending oncologist was called, and arrangements were made to transfer her to the oncology unit. Her condition was critical and was deteriorating rapidly. Fearing the worst, Connie and her fiancée, Jim Smith, requested that the marriage be conducted in the university hospital chapel. They insisted that this be a "legal marriage," not just a ceremony.

The legal marriage required a marriage license (issued in the county where the marriage took place) and new blood tests and certification. It also required the scheduling and coordinating of a group of people, both within and outside the hospital, who just minutes earlier had no idea who Connie Livingston and Jim Smith were—and time was running out. The administrator-in-charge contacted the county registrar to obtain a marriage license and the state laboratory for certification of the required blood test. What typically is done in weeks was now occurring in minutes. Physicians, nurses, and hospital managers also played key roles in coordinating and expediting the wedding. Timing was critical, and any one of these individuals could have created a delay ending the effort. Instead, "things did happen." The wedding occurred . . . a wish fulfilled . . . and three hours later, Mrs. Livingston-Smith died.

Graber, D., and Kaluzny, A., Developing a High Involvement Organization for the Future: Integrating Theory and Practice. In Kilpatrick, A. and Johnson, J. (Eds.), Handbook of Health Administration, New York. Marcel Dekker, 1999.

- Knowing the present situation about an organization and its environment tells us nothing about the future. The problem is not that we do not know enough about the present or past to predict the future, but rather that no matter how much information we have about the present or past, we cannot predict the future. As a result, leaders of health services organizations cannot expect to be in complete control of change processes and various organizational outcomes.
- In addition, the more we try to know more about a situation by measuring various aspects of it, the more we sacrifice our ability to know about other aspects of the situation. Health services executives must be very cautious about drawing conclusions based on organizational measurements to be sure they know what is truly important in a situation.
- We cannot understand an organization and environment better by understanding the individual elements of each better. Understanding relationships and connections among the elements is the reality we need to address to understand the system as a whole. This is particularly true in health services organizations, where the elements of patient care are so highly interdependent.
- Because small changes in initial conditions can produce such large changes in the future state of a system, it is unlikely that a health services organization can follow another's example and achieve the same results.

So, where does this leave health services executives in thinking about organizational change? It tells us that models and strategies for organizational change based on a rational view of organizations may give us some helpful ideas, but in the end they will present an incomplete picture for managing and leading in the twenty-first century. What is required is the creation of learning organizations as a more appropriate model for organizational change and innovation (McDaniel, 1997) and the recognition that "learning is at the heart of a company's ability to adapt to a rapidly changing environment" (Prokech, 1997, p. 148). In a learning organization, change and innovation are seen as part of the normal way of doing business; it is an input that leads to greater learning (McGill & Slocum, 1993).

The Learning Organization

Although organizational learning has been discussed by various scholars and theorists for some time (Fiol & Lyles, 1985; Hedberg, 1981; Jelinek, 1979; Stata, 1989), it was Peter Senge (1990a, p. 1) who popularized the term *learning organization*. In his book, *The Fifth Discipline*, he described learning organizations as places where "people continually expand their capacity to create the results they truly desire, where new and expansive patterns of thinking are nurtured, where collective aspiration is set free, and where people are continually learning to learn together." In reducing this rather utopian vision to its basic meaning, Senge said that a learning organization was "an organization that is continually expanding its capacity to create its future." Garvin (1993, p. 80) further clarified this definition by defining a learning organization as "an organization skilled at creating, acquiring, and transferring knowledge, and at modifying its behavior to reflect new knowledge and insights."

Multiple definitions of learning organization have been given by various writers, and several perspectives to learning organization have evolved. Three perspectives are most relevant (DiBella & Nevis, 1998).

- The *normative perspective* views the learning organization as a particular type of organization characterized by a certain specific set of internal conditions. This perspective assumes that executives intentionally design and build learning organizations and that the learning organization is a form to which organizations should strive if they want to improve their chances for success.
- The *developmental perspective* is related to the normative perspective and places the learning organization within the context of an organization's his-

tory. The learning organization is a later phase of development as an organization moves toward an optimal stage of self-renewal.
- The *capability perspective* assumes that all organizations are learning organizations. This perspective views the question to be what learning style or pattern is most appropriate for a specific organization (Ulrich, Jick, & Von Glinow, 1993) and is therefore much less prescriptive than the other two.

While each of these perspectives takes a bit of a different approach to the concept of a learning organization, there are basic insights for health services executives that are common across the three perspectives (DiBella & Nevis, 1998). These include the need to enhance factors that promote learning in organizations, the need to provide a mechanism for change and innovation, the development of learning styles and capabilities, and the need to depict in a descriptive way how learning takes place.

It is important to understand what makes organizational learning truly organizational and differentiates it from individual learning (DiBella & Nevis, 1998). First, in organizational learning, new skills, attitudes, and behaviors are created or acquired over time. These new ways of thinking are created from the organization's own experiences and the experiences of others. Since organizations lack the consciousness of individuals, awareness of organizational learning may come after the fact. Second, what is learned becomes the property of the collective unit. And, third, what is learned remains within the organization or group even if individuals leave. Organizational learning is about collectively working together to gain experience, build competence, and avoid the repetition of mistakes and errors.

Types of Organizational Learning

Two types of learning have been identified: adaptive, or single-loop, learning, and generative, or double-loop, learning (Senge, 1990b). Adaptive learning focuses on solving problems in the present without examining the appropriateness of current learning behaviors. Adaptive learning is very much a stimulus-response pattern of behavior. For example, a problem in the organization's operations is encountered, and a solution is crafted and implemented to address the problem. Adaptive learning typically has as its outcomes incremental improvements to an organization's existing products, markets, services, or technologies, in line with the organization's previous history and past successes. This sort of learning is the type used by most organizations.

Generative learning emphasizes continuous experimentation and feedback in an ongoing examination of the way organizations define and solve problems. Generative learning involves transformation and expands an organization's capability to learn. Adaptive learning is about coping with a problem or issue the organization currently faces by building on the past, while generative learning is about creating new ideas and new solutions as well as greater capability for learning in the future (Senge, 1990b). It is about something we already know, but generative learning leads to something new. In a learning organization, adaptive learning must be joined by generative learning, with each used appropriately for various organizational circumstances.

The Disciplines of Learning Organizations

What are the components of the learning organization? In *The Fifth Discipline,* Senge (1990a) proposed five disciplines or "component technologies" that are needed. These five are systems thinking, personal mastery, mental models, shared vision, and team learning.

- Systems thinking is a discipline for seeing wholes, interrelationships rather than individual elements of systems, patterns of change rather than time-isolated snapshots.
- Personal mastery is a discipline that connects personal, individual learning with organizational learning. It involves each individual organizational member's continual clarification of personal vision, focusing of energy, developing patience, and seeing reality objectively.
- Mental models are the assumptions and theories that individuals, teams, and groups in organizations hold. In a learning organization, the discipline of understanding these ingrained mental models and changing them when necessary must be practiced.

- Shared vision binds people together around a common identity and sense of direction for the future. This kind of shared vision motivates organizational members to do things because they want to do them rather than because they are forced to do them.
- Team learning refers to the organizational group or team working together to become smarter and more intelligent than any single individual in it. In learning organizations, groups or teams are the fundamental learning units. If members of groups or teams cannot work collectively to learn together, then organizational learning cannot take place.

Managers in the Learning Organizations

What is the role of the management in a learning organization? The traditional, rational view of the manager is the person in control, the one who sets direction, makes decisions, and motivates others in the organization. This view does not fit the world of organizations as described by quantum and chaos theories or the learning organization, with its focus on systems, team learning, and shared vision. In a learning organization, the critical roles for the manager are designer, teacher, and steward (Senge, 1990b).

The manager as designer is first responsible for building a foundation of purpose, vision, and core values. It has been asserted that this is the most important element of building an effective learning organization. The second design task involves crafting policies, strategies, and structures that will move the foundational ideas into action. The third design task involves creating effective learning processes that engage all organizational members in the first two design tasks and in their continual improvement. In a learning organization, the goal is for everyone to contribute (Gozdz, 1998).

The role of manager as teacher does not imply that the manager in a learning organization is the authority or expert telling others what to do or think. Rather, the manager as teacher helps organizational members gain a better view of reality and assists individuals in surfacing their own mental models and testing them against a reality to determine their appropriateness. The manager in a learning organization is a facilitator, coach, and guide, rather than a controlling expert. Cohen and Tichy (1998) have suggested that teaching is at the very heart of effective management.

The manager as steward is a servant leader (Green-leaf, 1996). In a learning organization, the manager has a sense of stewardship for the people he or she leads and for the mission of the organization. Because of the commitment members of a learning organization feel for a shared vision, the manager needs a special sense of responsibility for them. Stewardship for the organization's mission comes from the manager's own personal mastery and commitment to the shared vision.

TYPES OF CHANGE

While organizations are involved with unprecedented change requiring organizational learning, all change is not the same, and different types of change present different challenges to those involved in the change process (see Debate Time 12.1). To classify an almost endless array of activities, consider the means-ends classification scheme in Table 12.1. *Technical change*

refers to the internal modifications of ongoing structure and process in order to enhance organizational operations and performance. *Transition* refers to the modification of goals and/or products of the organization, with minimal or no modification in ongoing functional form and or fundamental technology of the organization. Finally, *transformation* refers to the modification of the internal structure and processes as well as change in organizational mission, goals, and service/product mix. The three types of change have different characteristics and make different demands on managers and the various providers who lead and manage the change and learning process.

Below, we examine each type of change in greater detail and then go on to consider some of the strategies and tools that help build the learning organization to meet the challenges of change and innovation.

Technical Change

Organizations are constantly involved or at least challenged by some modification in the means by which

---

DEBATE TIME 12.1: WHAT DO YOU THINK?

Change and innovation are not one-dimensional or simple linear processes over time. Consider just a few of the changes occurring in various health services organizations.

- Unrelenting flow of technology such as the availability of the gamaknife (GK) radiosurgery, photodynamic therapy, interstitial laser photo coagulation, and endoscopic ultrasonography, to name a few
- Greater attention to health promotion and early detection activities such as genetic screening and counseling, sigmoidoscopy screening, and measuring and maintaining quality of life throughout all health care encounters.
- Evolving administrative and managerial arrangements including greater use of outsourcing, joint equity ventures, on-line

prescribing, tele-medicine, and computerized "paperless" medical records.
- Downsizing and cross-training among existing personnel at the same time that new roles are being created.

Is there a sequence to the types of changes that occur? Are some changes or innovations prerequisites for other types of changes? What factors affect each type of change? Is it likely that factors that facilitate problem recognition and thus lead to the identification of one type of change may limit implementation or institutionalization? Given the types of change and innovation, are some types more likely to occur easily in some organizations or in some units within organizations yet present major difficulties in other organizations or units?

Table 12.1. Types of Change

	Means	Ends
Technical	Change	No change
Transition	No change	Change
Transformation	Change	Change

SOURCE: Adapted from Kaluzny and Vency. (1977).

the normal and usual activities of the organization are carried out. These changes represent challenges to the "technical core," which is concerned with doing the primary work of the organization (Thompson, 1967). Changes may vary in focus, cost, and potential impact and include a range of task and structural alterations such as the implementation of a satellite clinic anticoagulation protocols, an interdisciplinary chronic illness management team, or a computerized patient record—all of which affect operations but remain consistent with the overall mission and goals of the organization. While each of these changes is directed at improving operations, the organization itself attempts to protect its routine activities and reduce uncertainty by sealing off the core from its environment. The technical core standardizes work flow and processes, stockpiling resources so that its operations will not be disrupted. Individuals involved prefer reutilization of activities so that they can do repetitive tasks well.

Health care organizations like Intermountain Health Care Inc. (see In the Real World, p. 337) are constantly involved in trying to improve operations. The challenge for management is to introduce new methods that will improve the internal efficiency of their organization without unintentionally creating difficulties or disrupting the work patterns, norms, and values of professionals within the technical core. Identifying solutions for technical performance problems, identified from either internal or external sources, requires guidance and direction from those intimately involved in providing care and an organization committed to the learning process.

Transitions

A second type of change focuses on a change in organizational mission and goals, but not in the essential means or work processes of the organization. Increasingly, health service organizations are being challenged to reaffirm their fundamental mission to meet changing expectations and the intense competition for patients and physicians in the community. In these situations, the fundamental technology and basic structure (the organizational means) are already in place within the institution, and while there may be some modification, the major focus is to change the mission of the organization. These changes occur less frequently; however, when they occur they are associated with increased stress and trauma (relative to technical change) since organizational mission, and goals are usually identified with some powerful groups within the organization.

Redefining Mission and Goals

The reliance on values as the core of a health services organization's philosophy is a major strategy for achieving successful transitional change in today's environment. Values contribute to the successful change by providing a sense of common direction for employees and serving as a guide for day-to-day activities. Adaptation to a new mission and goals appears to be enhanced because employees can identify with, embrace, and act on the new values of the organization.

Organizations must communicate their goals and values to employees and must implement mechanisms to encourage a sense of membership in the organization. Attention to these issues is especially important in today's health services environment, which has seen increased emphasis on cost containment, competition for market share, downsizings, consolidation, ethical issues in health care operations, and other activities that were foreign to health services 10 to 15 years ago. A reemphasis and strengthening of the culture and values of the organization help employees to gain a sense of stability in a changing and uncertain environment. More importantly, they also help organizations undergoing a mission and vision change to communicate a new mission, vision, and values to employees.

Health services organizations that use strong values programs to communicate mission and direction changes have an explicit philosophy statement or set of values, devote considerable time and energy to

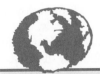

IN THE REAL WORLD:
CLINICAL INTEGRATION AT INTERMOUNTAIN HEALTH CARE, INC.

Intermountain Health Care (IHC) is a nonprofit integrated delivery system based in Salt Lake City, Utah. The system was turned over to the community in the early 1970s by the LDS Church and has maintained a strong presence in three western states despite the entry and growth of major competitors. This fully integrated delivery system is divided into four regions—Urban North, Urban Central, Urban South, and Rural. IHC provides a full continuum of health care services across an extremely diverse rural-urban continuum in Utah, Wyoming, and Idaho. The realities of this highly competitive health care environment for a health care system struggling to profitably maintain its community health mission led visionaries at IHC to move forward with the clinical integration initiative.

Leaders at IHC strategically chose to define their core business in terms of clinical medicine rather than facility management whereby they are primarily managing the processes of care. This process orientation reduces select treatment pathways to a series of interlocked processes. Creating a transparent linkage (to the patient) of interrelated clinical processes in the eight service areas that account for the bulk of care delivery at IHC is intended to improve quality of care, enhance patient satisfaction, and establish competitive distinction in the region.

The key tasks for clinical integration include: (1) arriving at best care; (2) building a network for clinical integration (i.e., programs and structure); and (3) achieving cost effectiveness through quality care. The complete value equation proffered by key champions at IHC is:

Best outcome + Best service + Low cost = Best care

The clinical integration framework rests on a strong primary care foundation. Development of the primary care model has been led by a carefully selected physician leader, who has worked closely with a series of committees with representatives from all IHC regions. Building upon this foundation, the system has sought to define the best care for an array of related services called clinical programs. Corporate leaders have carefully identified physician leaders to serve as champions, spokespersons, educators, and developers in designing the care process models for each clinical program. These physician leaders are selected based on their leadership abilities and professional reputation in the select clinical service area. These leaders are teamed with a high-level nurse administrator, who works closely with the physician in developing and disseminating the evidence-based care process models. Physician and staff participation are sought at every step in the development process, and IHC is currently struggling with the dissemination phase of the initiative. Two care process models—women's and newborns and heart services—are currently being phased in and monitored closely.

Information management is a critical component of this initiative. As one physician said, "You can't manage what you can't measure," and for this reason, IHC is investing resources in developing the information systems necessary to provide feedback in the form of key measures. Preliminary feedback data have indicated rapid and demonstrable progress in quality improvement and cost savings in each of the first two care process models that have been rolled out thus far. Clinical integration champions at IHC are encouraged and have plans to proceed in light of the fact that each care process model is developed, disseminated, adopted, and adhered to more readily than the previous one as the system continues to learn and innovate.

Savitz, L., and Kaluzny, A. (1999). Dissemination and Utilization of Clinical Process Innovations. Working Paper, School of Public Health. University of North Carolina, Chapel Hill.

shaping the values, and exhibit evidence that these values are known to employees. Four or five key statements of values are usually identified by the organization as reflecting the essence of their new core philosophy. The statements are developed to illustrate some of the unique characteristics of their health services organizations.

What makes statements more than slogans is the degree to which these phrases capture something in which health services workers can believe deeply. Within organizations with strong values programs, these words take on rich and concrete meaning. These phrases are core values because they become the essence of the organization's philosophy. These values and beliefs are closely linked to the basic concept

of the business and provide guidelines for employees to follow in their work.

Typically, a health services organization's mission statement and/or values are distributed, discussed, and interpreted during new employee orientation. They are also published on different documents, employee handbooks, policies, and procedures manuals. This process is adequate for introducing new employees to an existing mission; however, significant more energy must be expended to communicate modifications in a mission to employees. In addition, attention must be devoted to reinforcing this mission throughout the organization. An example of this process is illustrated by the Baptist Medical Centers–Birmingham presented below.

IN THE REAL WORLD:
REEXAMINING VALUES AND MISSION

Baptist Medical Centers–Birmingham believes that its Christian values and mission have been important since the system's founding. Senior leadership within the organization felt that the organization was shaping itself too much in the image of others and that it was time to revisit the mission. A strategic long-range planning retreat was held, and a new mission statement was developed. This statement, rewritten in consultation with senior management, was then approved by the board. The new mission statement as described by one member of the board is "simple and straightforward." You be the judge. . . .

As a subsidiary of the Baptist Health System, and as a witness to the love of God, revealed through Jesus Christ, Baptist Health Centers, Inc., (BHC) is committed to promoting these values as they relate to quality care, individual dignity, cost efficiency and community support. It is the purpose of Baptist Health Centers through striving for the goals set forth below, to be recognized as the premiere physician practice management organization in our region:

- *Quality Care—To partner with physicians in striving for the highest standards in the delivery of healthcare while utilizing state-of-the-art resources and techniques.*
- *Individual Dignity—To serve all patients and employees of BHC with respect and dignity.*

- *Cost Efficiency—To provide the most cost-efficient healthcare available through an innovative and performance-based work ethic.*
- *Community Support—To enhance the lives of those living in the communities served by BHC through the provision of compassionate and high-quality healthcare.*

The mission was communicated and reinforced to employees in a number of ways. Every employee received a copy of the mission statement from his/her department head and saw a videotape in which the chief executive officer discussed the mission statement. A series of promotional tactics were used to reinforce the new mission. First, employees who signed a statement saying they had read the mission statement received a mug (90% response rate). Second, employees responding to examples of administrative decisions with ties made to the mission statement received a candy dish. Third, employees who identified ways that they could support the mission received a box of candy (75% response rate). Finally, employees were asked to nominate a fellow employee who "lived the mission." Winners and those who nominated them, in each division, were awarded savings bonds.

Transformation

The most dramatic form of change is transformation. Change occurs in the ongoing structure and processes the organization uses to fulfill its mission, and also in the mission and objectives themselves. For example, long-term care facilities have augmented traditional custodial/skilled nursing services with a greater attention to the continuum of care at varying levels of need that a population may require. The development of retirement centers, assisted living centers, adult daycare centers, and outreach programs for the community have greatly expanded the scope of services available to the community. These organizations are no longer focusing solely on the needs of the vertical patient, but on the broader needs of an aging population. These changes represent both a different mission and a change in structure and process to achieve that mission.

In a similar manner, hospitals have been implored to "reinvent" themselves as health care systems rather than to continue to operate as inpatient acute care facilities (Shortell, Gilles, & Devers, 1995) and many health care organizations have changed or modified their traditional not-for-profit status. These changes will likely require new governance and management structures, including population-based needs-assessment methodologies, new relations with physicians, the reengineering of clinical processes, use of continuous quality improvement (CQI)/total quality management (TQM), a shift of focus to health outcomes, and development of management information systems. While transformational changes occur less frequently than other forms of change, when they do occur they involve a fundamental modification in both the overall direction of the organizational and its structure and processes and is usually accompanied by different perspectives and considerable controversy (see Debate Time 12.2).

THE CHANGE PROCESS

Health care executives, clinical providers, and support personnel are involved in various types of changes and innovations, ranging from the introduction of new pieces of equipment or programs to redefinition of the goals of the organizations. Change is different from innovation. Change is a generic concept that deals with any modification in operations, structure, or ends of the organization. Innovation is more restricted and is defined as any idea, practice, or material artifact perceived to be new to a relevant unit of adoption-organization, work group (Rogers, 1995). Not all change is innovation, but all innovation represents some form of change, and both innovation and change involve organizational learning.

Whether change or innovation, the organization or relevant unit within the organization is involved with a learning and change process. The process involves a number of distinct **stages of change or innovation** (Smith & Kaluzny, 1986).

- **Awareness** is the initial stage of the process in which individuals recognize that there is a discrepancy or gap between what the organization or work unit is currently doing and what it should or could be doing. This awareness may be sparked internally by the expectations of participants or externally by community or regulatory pressures affecting the performance of the organization.
- **Identification,** the second stage of the process, involves an attempt to address the discrepancies or **performance gap** identified in the prior stage. This may occur at various points within the organization, and the critical challenge is to ensure that identified solutions are quickly moved to implementation.
- **Implementation** involves the very presence or operations of the change within the organization or the relevant work unit within the organization.
- **Institutionalization** refers to the integration of the change into ongoing activities of the organization. Many changes are implemented but fail to truly be internalized within the organization.

Figure 12.1 indicates a sequence of stages and the factors that influence each stage. Three points are critical. First, the stages involve a sequential process in which any change or innovation is at risk of not proceeding to the next stage of the process. There is considerable loss throughout the process in that many more problems are recognized than ideas, practices, or material artifacts *identified* to address these problems; many more ideas, practices, or material artifacts identified than actually *implemented*; and finally, many more

DEBATE TIME 12.2: WHAT DO YOU THINK?

Investor-owned hospitals have set a new competitive standard (The Advisory Board Company, 1996), and perhaps this is most vividly presented by Columbia-HCA Healthcare Corp. Unrelenting emphasis on patient volume, financial results, and growth represent a profound change in how health care is provided. Below are two perspectives on that change. What is your perspective?

"Humana on Steroids." That's how Marc Gardner described Columbia HCA's spectacular rise in the world of health care.

Who is Marc Gardner? Mr. Gardner is a 33-year-old former Columbia HCA executive who says that he is willing to testify under oath that Columbia HCA violated numerous laws as it assembled a vast chain of hospitals and piled up unprecedented earning as competitors strained under price cuts and consolidation. Mr. Gardner says of his own behavior, "I committed felonies every day," and alleges:

• Despite federal laws against self-referral, Columbia allowed doctors to buy shares in a group of hospitals and clinics where they worked, shares that would rise in value if earnings did.
• The Columbia "scorecard" ranked and rated each hospital each month on nearly a dozen measures, from cost of supplies to number of surgeries, but not on quality of care.
• A big Columbia hospital limited treatment of uninsured patients, discouraging expensive tests and unpaid drug prescriptions.

Marc Gardner received his degree in hospital administration from Cincinnati's Xavier University, began his career working in a Catholic hospital, and moved on from there to a for-profit hospital owned by Humana, which subsequently was purchased by Columbia HCA. Mr. Gardner had a brief and spectacular career with Columbia HCA. He was a manager at three Columbia hospitals over three years—clearly an individual who was able to meet the challenge. After his first year, his job evaluations gave him "outstanding" ratings in eight of the 11 categories, and his supervisors praised him as an extremely resourceful and an extremely supportive individual.

By early 1996, Mr. Gardner reports that he took a buyout in a consolidation and quit in March; however, Columbia offered him an opportunity to be an aide to David Vandewater, the president of Columbia HCA. He was interviewed; however, the job remained unfilled, and Mr. Gardner went on to assume a position as a chief operating officer of North Lake Regional Hospital in Atlanta. Just a month into his new job at his third Columbia hospital, Mr. Gardner quit again and started writing a tell-all book entitled, *The Columbia Malignancy.*

(Adapted from Lagnado, 1997).

A contrasting view is presented by Keith Sandlin (1997), the chief executive officer of Columbia Cartersville Medical Center in Cartersville, Georgia. He writes, "As a Columbia CEO for four years and having worked in hospital administration for 20 years, I can't imagine a more rewarding profession. Certainly, I am held accountable for generating a fair return to the hospital owners, but I am held accountable by the citizens in my community to see that my hospital provides compassionate, high-quality, cost-effective care." He goes on to say, "Health care is a rapidly changing, tough, competitive business, and you had better have well-honed skills or you will not survive. Just as important is that you have a passion and respect for the business you are in. Columbia is initiating many changes in the industry and is reared and respected by many. This is an industry that most people would agree needs to be changed and as a trailblazer, Columbia is a threat to an over-regulated, inefficient, bureaucratic health care system and the people, agencies and facilities that have benefited for years from this system."

Mr. Sandlin concludes by saying, "For the record, I have never been encouraged to compromise patient care, put earning before quality care or to break any law on behalf of Columbia."

ideas, practices, or material artifacts implemented than *institutionalized*. Moreover, while the process is theoretically interactive—such that institutionalization is contingent on implementation, implementation is contingent on identification, and identification is contingent on awareness—there is always the reality that implementation occurs, bypassing awareness and identification. Organizations have implemented many changes and innovations that have failed to be institutionalized—in part because the implementation has not been linked to the recognition of a problem and the identification of the change to the resolution of that problem.

Second, the process is affected by a complex set of interacting factors. The prevailing structure and processes, such as degree of complexity and formalization, as well as levels of communication, coordination, and availability of resources, all influence whether a change or innovation moves through the sequential stages of the process. These interactions may be paradoxical. For example, organizational complexity provides the diversity within the organization by which personnel are likely to be aware of any discrepancy between what the organization is doing versus what it could or should be doing along with the ability to identify solutions. However, this very same complexity may inhibit the actual implementation and institutionalization of the required change. The diversity of resources within the organization may create conflicting expectations and priorities limiting the amount of change that actually occurs (Scott, 1990). Moreover, change is not an undifferentiated phenomena. Certain types of innovation and change, and the attributes of that change or innovation, may be more consistent with a particular structure and set of process and thus

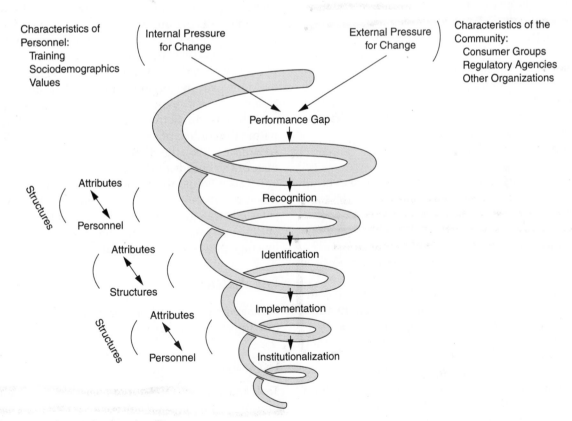

Figure 12.1. Change/Innovation Process.
SOURCE: Adapted from Kaluzny and Hernandez, 1988.

move through the various stages in a much easier manner. For example, change that is compatible with the existing activities of the organization—and perceived as having a relative advantage to the idea, practice, or material artifact that it replaces—are more likely to be implemented and institutionalized.

Finally, change is a continual process. Given the dynamic environment within which the organization functions, changes are institutionalized and require continual assessment and learning, resulting in subsequent awareness of any discrepancy between what the organization is currently doing and what it should be doing, thus reinitiating the process.

BUILDING BLOCKS OF LEARNING ORGANIZATIONS

What are the activities that can help build learning organizations to better prepare for the various types of change and the change process? Consider the following five main activities of learning organizations (Garvin, 1993).

- Systematic problem solving
- Learning from their own experience and past history
- Learning from the experiences and practices of others
- Transferring knowledge quickly and efficiently throughout the organization
- Experimenting with new approaches

While most organizations engage in one or even all of these activities, a manager in a learning organization must consciously create a learning process that incorporates all of these activities into its daily operation—up, down, and across the organization. The learning organization must also provide support for these activities by ensuring that the members of the organization have training in the knowledge, insights, habits, and skills that will be needed. In addition, it is important to provide support for the emotional side of learning and the anxiety that may accompany it (Schein, 1993).

Another activity that can help build a learning organization is learning from others. For example, John Browne, the chief executive officer of British Petroleum, suggested that it is crucial for a learning organization to learn from all possible sources: an organization's own experience, contractors, suppliers, partners, customers, and companies outside the organization's line of business (Prokech, 1997). Creating learning histories can also be an important tool for collective learning from experience (Kleiner & Roth, 1997, p. 173). A learning history is a "written narrative of an organization's recent set of critical episodes: a corporate change event, a new initiative, a widespread innovation, a successful product launch, or even a traumatic event such as a major reduction in the workforce."

Communities of practice (Senge & Kim, 1997; Wenger, 1996, 1998) provide an approach to collective learning by bringing together groups within and across organizations so that there is a social context for informal dissemination of information. Cross-training and rotating clinical and administrative personnel can expedite knowledge transfer in health services organizations (Barnsley, Lemieux-Charles, & McKinney, 1998). Not all organizations will employ the same tools in building a learning organization but instead will use those that most appropriately fit the organization (Wishart, Elam, & Robey, 1996).

Finally, a variety of tools and strategies exist for building learning organizations and facilitating the change process. Experimentation with different approaches is an activity that differentiates change within the context of the learning organization. David Lawrence (1998), the chief executive officer and chairman of the boards of Kaiser Foundation Health Plan and Kaiser Foundation Hospitals, has even suggested that it is sometimes better to experiment than to plan. Selected strategies and tools are presented below, focusing on task, structural, and human resources as leverage points within the organization.

Task Strategies

Management has a number of tools available for improving systematic problem solving.

Task Analysis

Task analysis focuses on the redesign of tasks within the organization to facilitate change and improve performance. Division of work into simple, specialized jobs was first suggested by the scientific management school to increase internal efficiency. This specialization allowed tasks to be differentiated, resulting in greater organizational control over individual behavior, selection of less skilled workers, and routinization of work flow to improve coordination.

However, routine jobs that require few skills and provide no challenge because of extreme specialization can lead to dissatisfaction, turnover and absenteeism, reduced motivation, and low-quality performance. Jobs may be redesigned by job enlargement (adding more activities) or job enrichment (adding more responsibility to the job). Perhaps this is best illustrated in nursing where job redesign and enlargement both within and outside the hospital setting have had significant implications. A recent study by VHA Inc. and the American Organization of Nursing Executives (Gelinas & Manthey, 1996) found that nurse executives are "at the heart" of organizational redesign. Of the 2,000 nursing executives surveyed, 80% reported an expansion of activities and responsibilities, 60% made redesign decisions jointly with the CEO, and 30% assumed responsibilities for respiratory therapy and social and pharmacy services. These and related issues of work design are discussed further in Chapter 7.

Academic Detailing

Academic detailing is a constellation of principles and techniques that focus on physician behavior change, including the use of market research to develop an understanding of motivational patterns of physicians' use, the sociometric identification of the key decision maker, and the use of basic learning reinforcement techniques (Soumerai & Avorn, 1990). While the approach has important implications for fundamental behavioral change (see "Human Resources Strategies," p. 349), it has received considerable attention as a method to disseminate guidelines and change practice patterns. Emphasis is given to staged intervention, in which the first phase is devoted to the identification of opinion leaders within the particular organization, the promotion of a consensus and commitment to voluntary practice changes among these leaders, and the identification of barriers and approaches to surmounting them. The second stage involves the opinion leaders meeting with nurses and physicians throughout the organization,

usually in small groups. These meetings provide an opportunity to provide performance feedback, identify system barriers attributed to deficits in practice, and, through that process, revise protocols, clinical pathways, and, where appropriate, standing orders. The approach has had a significant effect on accelerating the adoption of some beneficial therapies in the treatment of acute myocardial infarction (Soumerai et al., 1998).

Total Quality Management

Total quality management (TQM) or **continuous quality improvement (CQI),** as it is sometimes called, is another approach to facilitate change. It requires a systematic examination of the internal operations of the organization and focuses on identifying and implementing improvement in performance. It is a participative, systematic approach to planning and implementing a continuous organizational improvement process (Deming, 1986; McLaughlin & Kaluzny, 1999).

The approach is focused on satisfying customers' expectations, identifying problems, building commitment, and promoting open decision making among workers. CQI uses a structured process often known as FOCUS to identify, analyze, and design process improvements; it also uses another known as PCDA to implement and institutionalize improvements. Both FOCUS and PCDA are cyclical processes and provide a simple yet effective shorthand for problem solving and planning based on a systematic and rigorous approach. FOCUS specifies the steps to use in identifying and solving problems:

- find a process to improve.
- organize the team.
- collect information.
- understand variation in the process.
- select improvements.

PCDA reminds team members to:

- plan and try out the change.
- check the results.
- do what it takes to implement the change.
- act to secure the change and to identify new problems.

The analytical tools used in FOCUS-PCDA include Ishikawa (fish bone) diagrams, flowcharts, check sheets, Pareto charts, and run and control charts. The process is also carefully designed to include decision and communication tools such as brainstorming, nominal group process, and consensus formation to institute quality measures and storyboards to communicate the result to others. An example of using CQI to change the way in which a hospital laboratory provides serum potassium results to the emergency room (ER) is shown in Figure 12.2.

Structural Strategies

Task strategies rely heavily upon professional staff for expertise. In contrast, **structural change strategy** is concerned with the fundamental design and structure of health services organizations. This change involves areas such as designation of departmental reporting relationships and authority; the clinical and managerial information systems of the organization: the management control systems used; and the goals, policies, and strategic direction for the organization.

Structural strategies are initiated by senior management in collaboration with key professional and clinical personnel and are characterized as a top-down flow of influence. Top management decides that a change will be initiated and then designates the exact nature of the change to be undertaken. Thus, structural strategies are facilitated by the use of more bureaucratic mechanisms such as centralized decision making and formalization.

Senior management may become aware of the need for change because of internal operating problems. For example, the CEO of a health maintenance organization (HMO) may feel that the decision-making process for the organization operates in a very slow, awkward manner. Further assessment reveals that this is placing the organization at a competitive disadvantage, given other HMOs in the area.

An examination of these issues may suggest several reasons for the inadequate decision-making

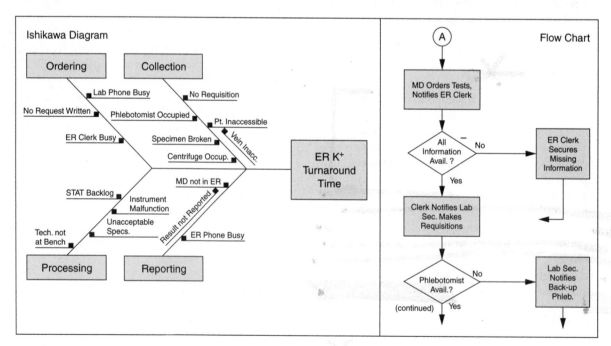

Figure 12.2. Analytical Tools Used in FOCUS-PCDA.
SOURCE: Adapted from Simpson, Kaluzny, and McLaughlin, 1994.

Check Sheet
Delays in production of Se K⁺ results from 1/1/91 to 1/7/91

	Code/Delay Type	Mon	Tue	Wed	Thur	Fri	Sat	Sun	Total
A	Request not Written by Physician	I	I				I		3
B	Lab Phone Busy > 2 minutes	I		I		II		I	5
C	Phlebotomists Unavailable	III	II	III	III	II	IIII	III	20
D	Requisition not Ready	II	I	I	I	I	III	II	11
E	Patient Inaccessible	I	I	II	I		II	I	8
F	Vein Inaccessible	I		II		I	II		6
G	Centrifuge Busy	II		I		I			4
H	Specimen Broken	II		I				I	4
I	STAT Backlog	III			I		II	I	7
J	Tech. not at Bench	II		II		I	II	I	8
K	Unacceptable Specimen	I	I		II		I	II	7
L	Lab. Sec. Unavailable to Report	III		I		I	I		6
M	ER Phone not Answered			I			II		3
N	MD not in ER	II		I		II		I	6
O	MD not Answer Page	I	I	II		II		II	8
P	Results not Reported by ER Sec.	II	I	II	I	III	II	II	13

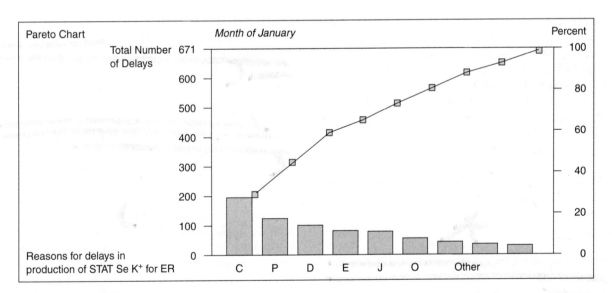

Figure 12.2. *(continued)*

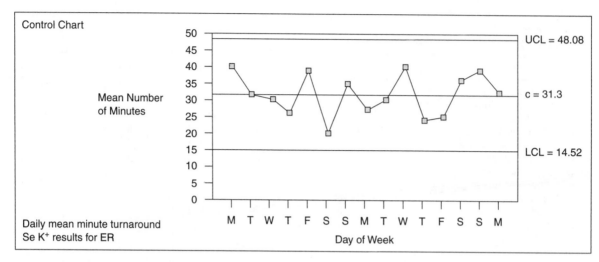

Figure 12.2. *(continued)*

process, as well as potential solutions. The management information system may not be providing managers with timely, useful information with which to make decisions. Thus, management may decide that a new information system is needed, identify the requirements for an improved system (with input from users throughout the organization), and then design the new system to better fit the organization.

The lack of a timely decision-making process may also result from the HMO having too many hierarchical levels or from involving too many groups in the decision-making process. Examination of the administrative ratio for the HMO and the decision-making process may require that the number of hierarchical levels be reduced.

Management has a number of structural strategies for facilitating the change process.

Stakeholder Mapping

Stakeholder mapping attempts to provide a systematic assessment of the variance among personnel as stakeholders. The process involves three key steps (Gilmore, 1991):

1. identifying relevant stakeholders (i.e., personnel who are affected or would be affected by the change)

2. ranking each stakeholder based on attitudes toward the change (i.e., favorable or opposed)

3. assessing each stakeholder's power within the organization to shape and affect its ultimate utilization

Based on this information, relevant personnel are identified and strategies are developed appropriate to each one. Individuals who are found to be in favor and clearly in a strong position within the organization should be mobilized to ensure support of this endeavor. It is critical that they be kept continuously informed of developments and planned activities in order to facilitate support of the activity.

Those individuals found to favor the approach but who are in a weak position within the power structure can be empowered, thereby giving them an opportunity to influence events. For example, to facilitate the implementation of CQI, physicians favoring the change, but marginal to decision making, could be appointed to various ad hoc and/or standing committees in the organization.

Individuals who oppose the idea but are weak may be co-opted into a larger ongoing effort. More difficult, however, are those stakeholders who oppose and are in a strong position within the organization. Gilmore suggests "reframing" or redefining the issue so that they may see it in a different light. For example, if someone in a large teaching hospital is opposed to a management information system, one might frame the change not as an administration control mechanism but as a mechanism to better assist the fundamental research mission of the organization.

Responsibility Charting

Responsibility charting identifies decision-making patterns among a set of actors—individuals, units, departments, or divisions within the organization. Attention is given to identifying areas, actors, and the type of participation in the decision area (Gilmore,

1988; McCann & Gilmore, 1983). The approach provides an opportunity to compare responses of a specific participant about that person's own role with the response of one or more participants about the same participant's role, compare responses across all actors on a specific decision, examine responses of each actor across a set of decisions, and compare actual decision patterns with desired activity.

An example of the use of responsibility charting is illustrated in Table 12.2. A broad range of decisions that are potentially made within Smith Medical Clinic is listed in the left-hand column of the chart. Major offices or groups involved in the decision process are

Table 12.2. Smith Clinic Decision-Making Responsibilities

	Physicians	President	Board of Directors	Department Chairpersons	Executive Committee	Planning Committee	Personnel Committee	Recruiting Committee	Administration	Chief of Staff Med Executive	Hospital Board
Long-range strategy development	A	I	A	DMIS		I			C		
Operational planning development				DMIS			R		C		
Analyze opportunities	I										
Develop business	I		A			R					
Analyze financial data		DMIS	IR		R						
Compile performance data				DMIS			D		IC		
Plan vs. actual reports analysis											
Billing	D			R			I		IC		
Fees policy		R	A		R						
Financial policy and programs		DR	RA		R				C		
Organizational policy and programs			RA	R'DMIS	R	R	R				
Compensation policy			A		R				I		
Board elections	A		R								
Officer elections		IA									
Project management	DMIA		A	DMIS					DMIA		A
Continuity policy	A	I	DR		D	D	D		C		
Malpractice insurance and risk Management					R						
Work loading medical	IR			DMIA			I				A
Work loading nonmedical	S						S				
Manage retirement funds				DA							

Legend: D-Direct; M-Manage; S-Supervise; A-Approve; I-Implement; R-Recommend; C-Coordinate
NOTE: Any physician has the right to make any recommendations to the person who can do something about it.

shown on the top. The roles that might be played in the decision-making process, which are also listed in the legend, follow:

- C = Coordinate: link together various parts of the organization
- D = Direct: set policy and allocate resources
- M = Manage: establish procedures
- S = Supervise: oversee operations
- A = Approve: authority to authorize action
- I = Implement: responsible for performing actions
- R = Recommend: review and recommend a decision

Within the squares of the table are the role(s) that each group play(s) in each decision. As illustrated, some groups or individuals play multiple roles in a decision, while other groups play no role. Examining the patterns of decisions allows the organization to determine if one or two groups have too much power and control within the organization. It also allows the organization to see if the pattern of decisions is rational and fits the culture of the organization.

Responsibility charting is best used in combination with process-type change strategies often associated with human resources change, which is discussed in the next section. It is one thing to identify needed changes and quite another to be able to recognize how decisions are made.

Assessing Organizational Readiness

Organizations are likely to be at different stages of the change process; thus, it is critical to assess the readiness for any restructuring effort (Rummler & Brache, 1995). Since structural strategies will be managed at various levels of the organization including the organization, work processes, and specific job-level activities (Christianson et al., 1997), it is important to assess the readiness for change at each level. As described by Christianson, Taylor, and Knutson (1998) and their restructuring of treatment process for chronic illness, "By answering specific sub-questions, decision makers can assess the readiness of their particular organization to restructure treatment processes . . . and identify areas where changes are possible that would enhance organizational readiness."

Below is a series of questions to help managers assess the readiness of their organization to restructure a particular (X) disease-management process

Organizational Level

- Is the effective management of care for patients with X disease an important part of the overall mission of the organization?
- Are organizational goals and objectives defined over sufficiently long enough time periods to permit new management processes for disease X and demonstrate their effectiveness?
- Are the goals of functional areas within the organization, and the strategies being used to achieve these goals, supportive of the restructuring of care processes for individuals with X illness?
- Are purchasers willing to pay for restructured care processes for X illness? Is reimbursement for the restructured care process possible under existing payment procedures?
- Is the culture of the organization supportive of coordinated team approaches to patient care?

Process Level

- Can the existing process of care for persons with X illness be clearly described and its shortcoming identified? Is the need for restructuring clear in light of these shortcomings?
- Can clear goals be stated for the restructured X illness care process that are reasonable in light of the perceived shortcomings of the existing care process?
- Is there a "process owner" for the restructuring of the X illness treatment process?
- Is their appreciation among all relevant individuals within the organization of the need to devote resources and time to a carefully staged implementation process? Are there likely to be sufficient time and resources available for implementation?
- Is there commitment to the meaningful involvement of patients in the treatment of the X illness? Is there a history of seeking patient input in organizational decisions regarding care delivery? Is there a mechanism in place for facilitating patient involvement?

Job/Performance Level

- Assuming that new positions can be created as part of the restructured treatment process, can measurable goals for the new positions be established? Do the compensation policies of the health care organization allow the linking of compensation to achievement of these goals?
- Are there barriers or constraints that could inhibit the ability of the organization to select individuals with appropriate skill and training to full newly created positions?
- Is the organization ready to commit the resources to training and education that are necessary for restructured care process to function effectively?
- Are there features in the design of existing compensation systems that would discourage clinicians from participating in disease X treatment teams? Can systems be designed and implemented that reward clinician and patients for effective participation on these teams?
- Are changes needed in the responsibilities and incentives of individuals with the health care organization, but not directly part of the care team, in order for the restructured care process to be effective? Can these changes be implemented?

Human Resources Strategies

Human resources change strategies focus on changing the attitudes, values, skills, and behaviors of employees within the organization. Health services organizations strive to create a work environment that is conducive to the delivery of the highest quality service in an efficient manner. A work environment that is supportive, open, and responsive to organizational members provides such a setting. Management should monitor the climate within their organizations and initiate interventions to improve conditions that they perceive as harmful.

Recognition of the need to initiate a human resources change strategy can result from management's perception that the internal climate of the organization is not conducive to effective performance. Alternatively, management may believe that other changes being instituted by the organization such as downsizing, new service additions, or structural change may have

a negative influence on employees and professional staff. Thus, a human resources change strategy may be viewed as critical for the success of other changes being initiated by the organization.

A number of methods might be used by the organization to improve the attitudes, values, or behaviors of employees. Which method is chosen depends upon the problem that perceived by management.

Organizational Assessment and Feedback

Assessment and feedback are mechanisms for systematically gathering data on the ongoing social-psychological conditions of the organization and confronting work groups with the findings. Data usually deal with intergroup relations, communication, supervision, employee satisfaction, employee attitudes, and with more recent efforts, organizational culture (Kraut, 1996). This information is usually gathered using questionnaire surveys of employees, but interview data can also be used. Results are fed back to individual work groups, starting at the top and moving down through the organization. Each group discusses survey results by analyzing potential problems, identifying possible causes, and agreeing upon solutions. The very process of data collection and feedback facilitates the change process (Nadler, 1996). Data collection generates the energy around activities that are being measured, and feedback provides the basis for disconfirming previous-held ideas and prompting people to search for solutions and new ideas.

For effective results, however, three conditions must be met (Katz & Kahn, 1978). First, discussion of findings must occur in a factual, task-oriented atmosphere. Second, each group must have the freedom to consider implications of findings at its own level. Upper-level management should handle general problems, while problems affecting the work group should be handled at the source of the problem. Finally, reports of outcomes must be sent up the organizational hierarchy.

The assumption underlying these conditions is that management cannot directly influence the processes that exist within the organization (Bowers & Franklin, 1977). Individuals and groups must be given the opportunity to see how their units compare with other units of the organization or how their current operations compare with desired expectations, thus understanding their own problems and initiating corrective action themselves.

360-Degree Feedback

Another application of feedback focuses on assessing and changing individual executive behavior. This process involves having peers/colleagues within the focal person's organization evaluate the individual on a number of relevant dimensions such as relationship building, judgment, problem solving, ability to delegate, financial skills, and related management areas. Peers who work with the individual, subordinates reporting to the focal person, and the immediate supervisor all complete surveys describing the individual's behavior. These results are compared with norms for the type of position held and returned to the focal person. Areas needing attention and improvement can be highlighted using this approach (Edwards, 1996; Lepsinger & Lucia, 1998).

Team Development

Because health care requires coordination of many disciplines and complex tasks, conflict can arise within groups involved with the provision of services. **Team development** strategies attempt to remove barriers to group effectiveness, develop self-sufficiency in managing group process, and facilitate the change process (Hambrick, Nadler, & Tushman, 1998). These interventions differ from **survey feedback** techniques in that team development places greater emphasis upon the changing and refreezing stages of the change process and the importance of external consultation.

External consultants are usually involved in all stages of this intervention strategy. Interventions begin with data gathering on leadership behavior, interpersonal processes, roles, trust, communication, decision making, task problems, and barriers to effective group functioning. After data are gathered, meetings are held during which problems are categorized and prioritized, selected problem areas are discussed, and action plans for change are developed.

The assumption underlying team development is that if appropriate attention is given to the process of a group's work, a group can solve their own problems and make a significant contribution to overall performance. Development activities require group participation, staging of the group, self-examination, problem confrontation, and goal setting (LaPenta & Jacobs, 1996).

Continuing Education

Health services are experiencing rapid technological change in the provision of care. Changes require that personnel involved in service delivery stay abreast of innovations so that their organizations can provide state-of-the-art care. **Continuing education** programs will provide health services personnel with the knowledge required to keep themselves and their organizations aware of new technology and service-delivery programs. Change is assumed to be caused by the increased knowledge, awareness, and subsequent perception of a performance gap that results from continuing education activities.

Continuing education programs for physicians, however, have demonstrated no consistent association with quality of performance unless the program directly involved clinical leaders and face-to-face contact on data feedback based on individual physician performance (Lomas & Hayes, 1988). A lack of association between continuing education programs and performance may occur for several reasons. First, participation in continuing education is mandatory in many states for most licensed health professionals. Professionals may attend continuing education programs without expecting substantive new knowledge to be gained from participation. Second, information acquired through these programs may not pertain to what the individual or organization is doing. Therefore, a stimulus for problem identification and corrective action does not exist.

Negotiation and Conflict Resolution

The process of change involves interactions that arouse fear and conflict requiring a set of negotiating skills (see Chapter 5). One particular approach relevant to the change process is the **confrontation meeting,** which brings together a large segment of the organization for immediate problem identification and action planning

(Beckard, 1967). Up to 60 people may be involved. The large group is then divided into small groups, each of which includes individuals from different organizational units. Supervisors are not placed in the same group with their own subordinates. Each group lists organizational problems that require attention. These problem lists are reported to the larger group of participants, which combines the problems into categories with help from an external consultant. Next, new groups are formed along expert and functional lines in accordance with problem categories. The new groups select items to discuss and identify action steps to be initiated. Results are reported to the larger group.

Confrontation meetings provide rapid diagnosis, increase influence and commitment of lower-level personnel in problem identification and problem solving, reduce bureaucratic barriers in decision making, and improve decisions by having those with information solve problems. These meetings require a climate of openness for problems to be confronted by the organization.

Diversity Training

Diversity training is another human resources change strategy that is used to modify attitudes or opinions of personnel within health services organizations. This change activity focuses on those human qualities that are different from those possessed by the focal individual or group, including gender, ethnicity, race, or sexual/affectional orientation (Fottler, Hernandez, & Joiner, 1994). With an increasingly diverse workforce containing greater numbers of women, minorities, and immigrant workers involved in management or delivery of health services, the need for removal of potential stereotypes and biases is significant. This approach seeks to disconfirm old belief structures and replace them with fairer judgments.

Process Consultation

Process consultation involves an outside consultant helping a clinician to perceive, understand, and act upon process events that are occurring (Reddy, 1995). Solutions can be developed to enhance the performance of the organization and can facilitate the over-all change process. This technique focuses on communications, role and function of group members, group norms, and the use of leadership and authority. The strategy, however, has limited effectiveness where individuals and/or groups with high levels of conflict involving disputes over major unresolved issues are involved (Lewicki & Litterer, 1991). For a further discussion of these issues, see Chapter 5.

EVALUATING ORGANIZATIONAL LEARNING: GUIDING THE CHANGE PROCESS

Using the various tools and strategies, managers and health care providers in organizations learn from their own and others' experiences rather than being bound by the past.

So, what difference do the concepts of the learning organization and the use of various tools and strategies make to our understanding of organizational change and innovation? The key objective of the learning organization is to improve organizational performance within the context of an uncertain and complex environment. In considering whether this objective has been met, several issues must be addressed (DiBella & Nevis, 1998).

- Is behavior or cognitive change desired? Or both?
- Are we interested in long-term or short-term outcomes?
- How is "performance" defined? Financial performance? Quality of work life for employees? Quality of patient care? Health status of the community?

Perhaps most important is that learning may become transparent over time, and we may fail to recognize organizational learning. Because organizations do not have a consciousness of learning something new, as do individuals, organizational learning can only be seen from its outcomes. Yet it may be difficult to connect organizational learning directly to its outcomes, given other intervening factors.

If one important outcome of learning is a better learning process, then a longitudinal analysis of learning histories may be one effective way to evaluate whether organizational learning has occurred,

MANAGERIAL GUIDELINES

1. Be clear about the type of change involved. Change is not an undifferentiated phenomenon. Each type of change has a specific set of attributes that need explicit attention from the health services manager. Moreover, these attributes interact with organizational characteristics to confound the change process. Thus, what may intuitively appear obvious, or at least similar to previous situations, may in reality be quite different and require caution because unanticipated consequences may develop.

2. Be conscious of the latent consequences of each type of change and its impact on organizational learning. Consider these latent consequences not as problems but as opportunities. While managers need to be specific about the particular type of change involved, they must also recognize that one type of change may lead to other types having their own anticipated and unanticipated consequences.

3. Do not assume that the environment is a constant, and not to be considered subject to intervention. Managers traditionally have taken a fairly parochial view of the change process. As a result, organizations are often considered the sole focus of change. Attempting to manage the interdependencies within the environment to enhance the operations of the organization may be a more viable strategy. Attention needs to be given to the context within which organizations operate. Enacting environments more compatible with existing organizational operations thus requires less change in the organization to enhance its overall performance. For example, efforts to increase or change the manner in which states reimburse health services organizations for indigent care is an effort on behalf of the providers to create a more friendly environment.

4. Consider intraorganizational change as a process involving a number of different stages. Organizational change is a process involving a set of distinct stages. Managerial attention needs to be given to clearly identifying the stage at which a particular type of change is currently located and to designing interventions that will facilitate or limit the process, depending on the objectives of management vis-à-vis that particular change activity.

5. Recognize that the change process and organizational learning involves several levels of analysis. Organizational change, innovation, and learning occur at different levels within the organization. While we usually consider change innovation and learning as involving the entire organization, they, in fact, take place at various levels, such as work groups, departments, or within individual roles. Attention should be given to clearly designating the level of the organization involved and to not confusing individual change with modifications in organizational variables.

6. Be aware that organizations are sometimes subject to large changes in the environment, which managerial action can do little to affect. Managers need to be cognizant of their own limitations. Not all problems are tractable, and managers have only a limited amount of personal and organizational resources at their disposal. Attention should be given to those situations that are tractable rather than taking the position that resources are infinite and that all are applicable to facilitating or impeding the change process. Failure to make this distinction results at best in an inefficient use of limited resources and, more tragically, the burnout of managerial personnel.

7. Be conscious of time dimensions involved in change and learning. Time, a difficult concept to understand, is particularly deceptive in an organizational setting. Shifting personnel and priorities contribute to the tendency to underestimate the amount of time involved in any change process. For example, what may be expected to take six months may take 12 to 18 months, or may never be completed. The pace of change must be managed—sometimes increased and sometimes decreased. The challenge for health services executives is the management of this process.

and the organization is better able to accommodate the various types of change. Learning audits that include evaluation of cognitive and behavioral changes, as well as performance improvements, can also be done (Garvin, 1993). Learning audits can use surveys, questionnaires, interviews, direct observation, and organizational performance measures.

The future is unpredictable and unknowable; knowledge about the past and present tells us little about the future, and the successes of the past will not ensure success in the future. Health service managers and leaders of the future must be able to suspend their need of control, to see connections between issues and events, to be creative, to be active problem solvers, and to exhibit empathy. Most of all, managers and the various clinical providers must be the creators of learning organizations—organizations that combine adaptive and generative learning to create, acquire, and transfer knowledge—and then modify their behavior to reflect new knowledge and insights to better manage the change process.

Discussion Questions

1. Three types of change have been identified in this chapter. Compare and contrast these types. Which of the three would you consider to be most critical for organizational success? What are their implications for organizational learning?
2. Select a change or innovation in health care delivery with which you are familiar and analyze it as either a technical, transitional, or transformational change. Describe the stages that the change would go through as it proceeds from concept to institutionalization.
3. What arguments can be made to support or refute the statement that "the worst feature of the American health care system is its resistance to change"?
4. As the chief operating officer for a large multispecialty group practice, you have been given the responsibility for selecting and managing the implementation of a new physician compensation program. What strategies might you consider to ensure the successful awareness, identification, implementation, and institutionalization of a program?
5. A critical challenge facing many health service organizations is the integration of functional departments in order to take advantage of the resource expertise in the organization and better realize the expectations of patients and providers both within and external to the organization. What are the inhibiting and facilitating factors involved in achieving integration, and what set of strategies are most appropriate and under what conditions?

References

The Advisory Board Company. (1996). *The rising tide.* Washington, DC:

Barnsley, J., Lemieux-Charles, L., & McKinney, M. (1998). Integrating learning into integrated delivery systems. *Health Care Management Review, 23*(1), 18–28.

Beckard, R. (1967). The confrontation meeting. *Harvard Business Review,* 45:1, 149–155.

Bowers, D. G., & Franklin, J. L. (1977). *Survey-guided development I: Data-based organizational change.* La Jolla, CA: University Associates.

Christianson, J., Pietz, L., Taylor, R., Woolley, A., & Knutson, D. J. (1997). Implementing programs for chronic illness management: The case of hypertension services. *Journal on Quality Improvement, 23*(11), 593–601.

Christianson, J. B., Taylor, R., & Knutson, D. J. (1998). *Restructuring: Chronic illness management, best practices and innovations in team-based treatment.* San Francisco: Jossey-Bass.

Cohen, E., & Tichy, N. (1998). Teaching: The heart of leadership. *Healthcare Forum Journal, 41*(2), 21–25, 75.

Covey, S. (1990). *The 7 habits of highly effective people: Powerful lessons in personal change.* New York: Fireside.

Deming, W. E. (1986). *Out of the crisis.* Cambridge, MA: Massachusetts Institute of Technology.

DiBella, A. J., & Nevis, E. C. (1998). *How organizations learn: An integrated strategy for building learning capability.* San Francisco: Jossey-Bass.

Edwards, M. (1996). *360 degree feedback: The powerful new model for employee assessment and performance improvement.* Washington, DC: AMACOM.

Fiol, C. M., & Lyles, M. A. (1985). Organizational learning. *Academy of Management Review, 10*(4), 803–813.

Fottler, M., Hernandez, S. R., & Joiner, C. (1994). *The strategic management of human resources in health services organizations.* Albany, NY: Delmar, pp. 208–223.

Garvin, D. A. (1993). Building a learning organization. *Harvard Business Review, 71*(4), 78–91.

Gelinas, L. S., & Manthey, M. (1996). *The impact of organizational redesign on nurse executive leadership, Part II.* Irving, TX: VHA.

Gilmore, T. N. (1988). *Managing a leadership change: How organizations and leaders can handle leadership change successfully.* San Francisco: Jossey-Bass.

Gilmore, T. N. (1991). Building and maintaining effective working alliances. In R. Sheldon, & L. Ginsburg (Eds.), *Managing hospitals: Lessons from Johnson & Johnson—Wharton Fellows Program in management for nurses* (pp. 201–231). San Francisco: Jossey-Bass.

Gozdz, K. (1998). Leadership for a learning community. *Healthcare Forum Journal, 41*(2), 30–34.

Graber, D., & Kaluzny, A. (1999). Developing a high involvement organization for the future: Integrating theory and practice. In A. Kilpatrick, & J. Johnson (Eds.), *Handbook of health administration.* New York: Marcel Dekker.

Greenleaf, R. K. (1996). *On becoming a servant-leader.* San Francisco: Jossey-Bass.

Hambrick, D. C., Nadler, D. A., & Tushman, M. (1998). *Navigating change: How CEOs, top teams, and boards steer transformation.* Boston: Harvard Business School Press.

Hedberg, B. (1981). How organizations learn and unlearn. In P. C. Nystom, & W. H. Starbuck (Eds.), *Handbook of organizational design* (pp. 8–27). London: Oxford University Press.

Jelinek, M. (1979). *Institutionalizing innovations: A study of organizational learning systems.* New York: Praeger.

Katz, D., & Kahn, R. L. (1978). *The social psychology of organizations* (2nd ed.). New York: John Wiley.

Kaluzny, A., & Hernandez S. (1988). "Organizational Change and Innovation" in S. Shortell & A. Kalvzny, Health Care Mangement: A Tact in Organization Theory and Behavior. New York: John Wiley & Sons.

Kaluzny, A., & Vency J., (1977, January). "Types of change and hopistal planning strategies," *American Journal of Health Planning* 1:3, 13–19.

Kleiner, A., & Roth, G. (1997). How to make experience your company's best teacher. *Harvard Business Review, 75*(5), 172–177.

Kraut, A. (Ed.). (1996). *Organizational surveys: Tool for assessment and change.* San Francisco: Jossey-Bass.

Lagnado, L. (1977, May 30). Intensive care: Ex-manager describes the profit-driven life inside Columbia HCA: Finding patients and firing nurses, Marc Gardner, finally tired of it all: Death on the hospital lawn. *The Wall Street Journal*, p. 1.

LaPenta, C., & Jacobs, G. (1996, Fall). Application of group process model to performance appraisal development. *Health Care Management Review, 21*(4), 45–60.

Lawrence, D. M. (1998). Leading discontinuous change: Ten sessions from the battlefront. In D. C. Hambrick, D. A. Nadler, & M. L. Tushman (Eds.), *Navigating change: How CEOs, top teams, and boards steer transformation* (pp. 291–308). Boston: Harvard Business School Press.

Lepsinger, R., & Lucia, A. (1998). *The art and science of 360 feedback.* San Francisco: Jossey-Bass.

Lewicki, R. J., & Litterer, J. A. (1991). *Negotiation.* New York: West.

Lomas, J., & Hayes R. B. (1988). A taxonomy and critical review of tested strategies for the application of clinical practice recommendations: From official to individual clinical policy. In R. Battista, & R. Lawrence (Eds.), Implementing preventive services. *American Journal of Preventive Medicine,* 77–94.

McCann, J., & Gilmore, T. (1983). Diagnosing organizations decision making through responsibility charting. *Sloan Management Review, 24*(2), 3–15.

McDaniel, R. J. (1997). Strategic leadership: A view from quantum and chaos theories. *Health Care Management Review, 22*(1), 21–37.

McGill, M. E., & Slocum, J. W. (1993). Unlearning the organization. *Organizational Dynamics, 22,* 67–78.

McLaughlin C., & Kaluzny, A. (Eds.). (1999–2nd ed.). *Continuous quality improvement in health care; Theory, implementation and applications.* Gaithersburg, MD: Aspen Publications.

Nadler, D. (1996). Setting expectations and reporting results: Conversations with top management. In A. Kraut (Ed.), *Organizational surveys: Tool for assessment and change.* San Francisco: Jossey-Bass.

Prokech, S. E. (1997). Unleashing the power of learning: An interview with British Petroleum's John Browne. *Harvard Business Review, 75*(5), 146–168.

Reddy, B. W. (1995). *Intervention skills: Process consultation for small groups and teams.* San Diego: Pfeiffer & Company.

Rogers, E. M. (1995). *Diffusion of innovations.* New York: Free Press.

Rummler, G. A., & Brache, A. P. (1995). *Improving performance: How to manage the white space on the organization chart.* San Francisco: Jossey-Bass.

Sandlin, K. (1997, July 24). As health-care CEO, I'm held accountable (Letter to the editor). *Wall Street Journal,* section A, p. 19.

Savitz, L., and Kaluzny, A. Dissemination and utilization of clinical process innovations. Working paper, School of Public Health. University of North Carolina, Chapel Hill, 1999.

Schein, E. H. (1993). How can organizations learn faster? The challenge of entering the green room. *Sloan Management Review, 35*(2), 17–24.

Scott, W. R. (1990, Summer). Innovation in medical care organizations: A synthetic review. *Medical Care Review, 47*(2), 165–192.

Senge, P. M. (1990a). *The fifth discipline: The art and practice of the learning organization.* New York: Doubleday.

Senge, P. M. (1990b). The leaders new work: Building learning organizations. *Sloan Management Review, 32*(1), 7–23.

Senge, P. M., & Kim, D. H. (1997). From fragmentation to integration: Building learning communities. *The Systems Thinker, 8*(4), 1–5.

Shortell, S., Gilles, R., & Devers, K. (1995). Reinventing the American hospital. *The Milbank Quarterly, 73*(2), 131–160.

Simpson, K., Kaluzny A., & McLaughlin C. (1999). "Total quality and the manage of laboratories" in C. McLaughlin, & A. Kaluzny (Eds.). *Continuous quality improvement in health care: Theroy, implimention & applications.* Gaithersberg, MD: Aspen Publishers, Inc.

Smith, D., & Kaluzny A. (1986). *The white labyrinth.* Ann Arbor, MI: Health Administration Press.

Soumerai, S. B., & Avorn, J. (1990, January). Principles of educational outreach "academic detailing" to improve clinical decision making. *Journal of the American Medical Association, 263*(4), 549–556.

Soumerai, S. B., McLaughlin, T. J., Gurwitz, J. H., Guadagnoli, E., Hauptman, P. J., Borbas, C., Morris, M., McLaughlin, B., Gao, X., Willison, D. J., Asinger, R. (1998, May). Effect of local medical opinion leaders on quality of care for acute myocardial infarction: A randomized controlled trial. *Journal of the American Medical Association, 279*(17), 1358–1363.

Stata, R. (1989). Organizational learning: A key to management innovation. *Sloan Management Review, 30,* 63–74.

Thompson J. (1967). *Organizations in action.* New York: McGraw-Hill.

Ulrich, D., Jick, T., & Von Glinow, M. A. (1993). High impact learning: Building and diffusing learning capability. *Organizational Dynamics, 22,* 52–66.

Wenger, E. (1996). Communities of practice: The social fabric of a learning organization. *Healthcare Forum Journal, 39*(4), 20–26.

Wenger, E. (1998). Communities of practice: Learning as a social system. *The Systems Thinker, 9*(5), 1–5.

Wishart, N. A., Elam, J. J., & Robey, D. (1996). Redrawing the portrait of a learning organization: Inside Knight-Ridder, Inc. *Academy of Management Executive, 10*(1), 7–20.

CHAPTER

13

Organizational Performance: Managing for Efficiency and Effectiveness

Ann B. Flood, Ph.D.
Jacqueline S. Zinn, Ph.D.
Stephen M. Shortell, Ph.D.
W. Richard Scott, Ph.D.

Learning Objectives

After completing this chapter, the reader should be able to:

1. Understand the importance of assessing organizational performance.
2. Define performance measures for organizations.
3. Understand the important issues in defining, measuring, and using performance measures.
4. Evaluate professional work.
5. Compare management models based on quality assurance and quality improvement.
6. Manage for quality improvement in health care.
7. Understand management roles to create high-performance organizations.

Key Terms

Appropriateness
Benchmarking
Cost Effectiveness
Effectiveness
Efficacy
Efficiency
Organizational Effectiveness
Outcome Measures of Quality
Process Measures of Quality
Productivity
Quality Assurance (QA)
Quality Improvement (QI)
Resource Acquisition
Structural Measures of Quality

Chapter Purpose

The demands for high performance in health care are increasing. This is reflected in the increasing demands from insurers—including public insurance programs like Medicare and self-insuring businesses—seeking discounted prices or other forms of cost containment in return for their business. At the same time, decreases in utilization such as dramatically shortened average lengths of stay, alternative sites for care such as same-day surgery and home care programs, and growth in provider availability have led to increased competition among providers. While these trends have stimulated health services managers to focus on the business of health services—that is, on market share, pricing policies, marginal costs, and productivity—a backlash in the form of reduced public confidence and threats to remove the tax-exempt status of hospitals have caused a renewed interest in serving the community—that is, in fulfilling a larger social function.

Ultimately, if health care providers do not hold themselves accountable for performance, performance standards may be imposed on them (Their & Gelijns, 1998). For example, long-standing concerns about the quality of nursing home care prompted sweeping legislative changes, increasing the regulatory burden on facilities. Similarly, managed care organizations (MCOs) face an increasingly hostile public and regulatory environment prompting numerous bills and legislation at both the state and federal level, which are designed to protect patients' rights and constrain MCOs from attempts to implement cost-efficient strategies (Goldberg, 1998; Mechanic, 1998; Shortell, Waters, Clarke, & Budetti, 1998). The objective of this chapter is to review the major issues related to assessing organizational performance, compare and contrast the approaches of quality assurance and quality improvement, and describe the strategies to achieve an effective health care organization.

THE CHALLENGE OF PERFORMANCE

Clearly, a major challenge to the health care executive is to put together an organization that maximizes productivity, quality, and market share while not losing sight of the organization's mission to serve the health needs of the community. Because they operate in an environment of constrained resources, balancing these pressures has meant having to trade off some programs, services, and markets for others. For example, nursing homes struggle to maintain a single standard of care for all residents in the face of inadequate Medicaid reimbursement. A hospital may agree to give up its maternity services in order to expand its medical-surgical services or may share high-technology resources with another hospital in order to concentrate more effort in expanding its ambulatory care programs. Alternatively, a hospital may agree to introduce a service critically needed in the community despite its being a net drain on its resources. Such trade-offs have meant that chief executive officers (CEOs) of today's health care organizations have to manage their organizations in relation to other organizations and the community's needs in addition to considering the performance of individual subunits.

Another set of internal pressures comes from the concerns of committed health professionals—managers, nurses, physicians, and others—to improve professional practice by using their knowledge, skills, and technology to the best of their abilities and to the improved capabilities permitted by advances in medicine. This force is often neglected when considering the other, perhaps more visible, concerns.

IN THE REAL WORLD:
GOOD PRACTICE AND MALPRACTICE: SMITH VS. ACE MANAGEMENT COMPANY

On May 19, 1992, at 9:30 P.M. at Jackson Memorial Hospital (JMH), Jay Smith was born severely mentally and physically handicapped. His 30-year-old mother, Mary Smith, had been admitted to the labor and delivery unit of the hospital at 11:00 P.M. on May 18, 1992; she was 17 days past her due date. At 10:30 A.M. on May 19, Mrs. Smith was examined by Dr. Wood, her personal obstetrician and chief of obstetrics at JMH, who ordered the administration by intravenous infusion of 10 milliunits per minute of Pitocin (oxytocin), a drug that stimulates uterine contractions. The normal dosage Dr. Wood usually gave was 1.0 milliunit—the dosage recommended by the drug manufacturer in the Physicians' Desk Reference. No one either preparing or administering the drug questioned the accuracy or appropriateness of the dosage for Mrs. Smith. Four hours before Jay was born, Dr. Wood attempted to further stimulate contractions by artificially rupturing Mrs. Smith's membrane, at which point meconium-stained amniotic fluid was identified, suggesting that the fetus may have suffered some distress.

The hospital's policy was to require electronic fetal monitoring only for high-risk pregnancies; however, the criteria for judging who was at "high risk" were left largely to the physician. Following a recent uproar in the community about "excessive" use of fetal monitoring at area hospitals, a committee (including Dr. Wood as chair of the department) had reviewed the hospital's policy to be sure that it complied with accreditation standards. So, when Dr. Wood chose not to monitor Mrs. Smith's labor either before or after rupturing her membrane, no one in the labor room questioned the decision.

At delivery Jay was flaccid and could not breathe on his own. He was transferred to Delta Medical Center, a major medical center with extensive perinatal facilities, where he remained for one month. Jay's problems were severe and irreversible. Now seven years old, Jay has undergone extensive medical care throughout his young life and continues to exhibit signs of spasticity, cerebral palsy, mental retardation, blindness, deafness, and a variety of related conditions.

On October 14, 1993, the Smiths filed a $30 million suit against Dr. Wood, JMH, and ACE Management Company, Inc., the group from which JMH contracted for management services to run the hospital. In including the management company in the suit, the Smiths alleged that ACE was negligent in its management of the hospital—specifically, that the company failed to monitor and oversee the treatment and care provided by physicians and employees of the hospital, to enforce the standards of the Joint Commission on Accreditation of Healthcare Organizations, and to monitor, on an ongoing basis, the physicians of its medical staff.

How could this tragedy to Jay have happened? What roles should management have played in this situation to prevent it, to uncover the problem, and to take corrective actions to change the behavior of the providers and the system?

Given the complex nature of hospitals, staff errors with potentially tragic consequences such as those for Jay Smith are not surprising. Patient care in hospitals is characterized by highly subdivided tasks performed by numerous types of professionals and a culture that preserves the autonomy of physician decision making—factors that contribute to ambiguity and apathy about personal accountability and decision making in hospitals. Putting JMH in the hands of a management company responsible for all hospital operations gave a false sense of control but contributed little toward fostering a culture and a team approach, which might have served to prevent the inappropriate orders or at least intervene before damage had occurred.

The fundamental nature of hospitals and the legal bases governing professional behavior make it impossible for management alone to implement a quality assurance (QA) program, which can effectively prevent mistakes by identifying and disciplining providers—particularly physicians—not complying with good practice. Nevertheless, management has an important role in preventing such problems.

The classic definition of management's role in ensuring quality is to design an organization such that professionals are able to control their own performance. With this model, management focuses on the activities of the small groups operating within the hospital. This approach is important, but it is not enough by itself. Clearly this was inadequate to prevent the problems for Jay.

Several groups are promoting a different paradigm: Quality must be viewed as a process, one that requires continuous improvement. That is, management throughout the organization must continuously endeavor to learn about all aspects of a process and use that knowledge to change the process, thereby improving service. What is required is a major shift in how organizations think of quality and how they define the roles of those participating in the processes.

A part of the redefinition needed involves recognizing the role of middle management. Middle managers traditionally have been neglected in favor of executives. For example, although much attention was given at JMH to reviewing the quality assurance standards, less attention was given to the day-to-day activities of the obstetrics and gynecology supervisor and to working relationships among nurses, administrators, and the physicians in the department of obstetrics. A relationship characterized by information sharing and efforts at continuing improvement would have identified opportunities for improvement and initiated corrective action, which could have prevented the medication error and identified Mrs. Smith as benefiting from monitoring.

Managers at JMH basically viewed quality problems as needing "control." Instead, greater emphasis was needed on day-to-day management involving: fostering and learning from individual initiatives, interdisciplinary

skills, information sharing, and thoughtful participation within the larger organization. These types of middle-management activities require the acquisition of new skills in the areas of group process, negotiation, and conflict resolution. Finally, middle management should understand that hospitals are behavioral systems that involve all the complexities of entangled interest groups and coalitions. One technique is for the administration to meet often with physicians, nurses, and other hospital staff to assess the dynamics of the hospital. However, a more formal level of assessment, involving multiple measurements over time and the comparisons of data from similar organizations, can assist hospital managers in the systematic diagnosis of problems and provide perspectives on an organization's performance.

In summary, the probability of the Smith case occurring could have been reduced if the hospital had

- emphasized practices designed to continuously improve quality rather than to satisfy accreditation standards
- recognized the important roles of middle management and other providers as well as physicians
- learned from systematic organizational assessment

Adapted from Kaluzny, A.D. The role of management in quality assurance: The case of Smith vs. ACE Management Company. Quality Review Bulletin. April 1990:134–137. Copyright 1990 by the Joint Commission on Accreditation of Healthcare Organizations, Oakbrook Terrace, Ill. Reprinted from the April 1990 Quality Review Bulletin with permission.

Finally, in addition to these reasons for managers to attend to performance issues, outcomes research and clinical guidelines have gained a new prominence as the federal government also seeks to evaluate health care in an effort to minimize use of ineffective services, contain costs, and yet hold providers accountable for fairly distributed and well-performed services.

More than anyone else, the manager is responsible for the performance of the organization. In a real sense, all of the preceding chapters are building

blocks for assisting the manager to improve organizational performance. As outlined in Chapters 1 and 2, the manager's role includes attending to the performance of the internal environment (i.e., the various departments and activities within the organization that serve each other) as well as attending to external customers. The successful manager needs to guide and oversee all of the subsystems of the organization, not just the maintenance or managerial subsystems, which have been traditionally emphasized in health administration. Thus, the manager can improve performance not only through attending to productivity and maintenance of the human and capital infrastructure but also to boundary spanning activities, adapting the organization to its ever-changing environment and advances in medicine, and governing, or holding the organization accountable for its actions. The performance of health care organizations in the future may increasingly depend on the ability of health care managers to truly lead, not just steer, through obstacles—that is, to mold and innovate within their environment rather than passively react to external changes (Shortell et al., 1996).

All these factors have helped spawn a variety of terms to describe performance in the delivery of health services: efficacy, effectiveness, appropriateness, productivity, and efficiency. Because these terms are often ill-defined, sometimes used interchangeably, and occasionally inappropriate for evaluating organizational performance, it is important to define them for present purposes. Their variety and occasionally contradictory results serve to illustrate why there cannot be a single criterion for organizational success. For example, a productive or efficient organization is not necessarily effective, and an organization that is efficient in some activities is not necessarily efficient at all.

Three terms are widely used to describe the potential health benefits of a given service. *Efficacy* refers to the capability of a health service, under ideal conditions and applied to the right problem, to produce the desired effect. *Appropriateness* focuses on whether an efficacious treatment was applied to the right patient at the right time. **Effectiveness** in this context involves ascertaining the quality with which a service is carried out, assuming that the service was both efficacious and appropriate. Note that these terms, as defined, refer to the evaluation of a particular treatment or set of services or to a provider's ability to carry them out. They do not describe organizational performance.

Organizational performance is generally depicted using four interrelated concepts. The first two terms center on evaluating an organization in terms of the goods or services it produces for external consumption. Both terms characterize the inputs needed, either using dollars or units of resources expended, to produce these goods or services. Note that these in-

puts can depict labor or capital or both components. **Productivity** is defined as the ratio of outputs to inputs. An example of hospital labor productivity is the total number of admissions divided by the total number of nursing staff hours. A comparable productivity measure in the home health setting is the number of registered nurse visits per day. **Efficiency** is defined as the cost per unit of output. An example is the average total labor costs per admission.

There are important and complex issues associated with assessing inputs. For example, should an efficiency measure include the costs of staff not directly involved in treating patients? Or, should productivity include physician hours when they are not paid by the hospital? In the nursing home, ancillary services are frequently provided by outside contractors. Should these services be included in assessing nursing home efficiency? Despite the difficulty of addressing these issues, the biggest challenge is the problem of measuring outputs. For example, consider the output: hospital stays. Since most of the variation in resources or dollars used during specific hospital stays depends on the reasons for hospitalizing the patients and whether they received surgery, two measures of efficiency—one based on 100 normal births and the other on 100 patients with coronary artery bypass surgeries—are clearly not directly comparable. Even within discharge categories, differences in case mix intensity, such as the proportion of high-risk births, make direct comparison of outcomes problematic. The challenge is to create measures of efficiency or productivity that take into account such differences between patient stays that are due to patient-specific needs for care during an admission.

Given cost-containment pressures, all health care organizations face the challenge of becoming more productive and efficient. Existing studies suggest that the factors associated with increased productivity and efficiency include use of

- high standards and goals (Nauert, 1996; Shortell, 1985)
- information and feedback (Nelson, Mohr, Batalden, & Plume, 1996; Wasson, 1998)
- interdepartmental coordination and resource sharing (Shortell, Becker, & Neuhauser, 1976)

- compensation systems oriented toward rewarding productivity or efficiency (Flood et al., 1998; Hornbrook & Berki, 1985; Sloan & Becker, 1981)
- physician involvement in decision making and governance (Shortell, 1983)
- concentration of staff work and activity (Alexander & Rundall, 1985)
- active governing boards that deal with environmental pressures (Choi, Allison, & Munson, 1986)
- type of ownership (Aaronson, Zinn, & Rosko, 1994; Coyne, 1982; Institute of Medicine, 1986; Pauly, Hillman, & Kerstein, 1990; Rosko, Chilingerian, Zinn, & Aaronson, 1995)
- chain ownership and contract management (Connor, Feldman, Dowd, & Radcliff, 1997; Menke, 1997; Miller & Luft, 1994; Zinn, 1994)

Setting high standards for cost containment motivates organizational members, particularly when the compensation systems reinforce attainment of the productivity and efficiency standards. Productivity-based compensation incentives include sharing cost savings resulting from employee suggestions as well as year-end bonuses based on staying within budget or generating net profits beyond expectations. There is a downside to compensation packages, of course, when they inadvertently reward one behavior while hoping to encourage another (Kerr, 1975). While eliminating all financial conflicts of interest from compensation arrangements is not possible, attention to managing the magnitude of the effects from such conflicts is important (Ohsfeldt, 1993).

The second set of terms to evaluate organizational performance is consistent with a broader, open-system perspective of what the organization is trying to accomplish. **Organizational effectiveness** means the degree to which organizational goals and objectives are successfully met. An organization goal to be achieved could be a subobjective (e.g., recruiting a coordinator for the organization's quality assurance–improvement program), an intermediate level objective (e.g., reducing nursing staff turnover on the units), or an ultimate objective (e.g., reduction in risk-adjusted mortality for acute myocardial infarction cases). **Cost effectiveness** is a composite measure that takes into account both cost and the degree of goal attainment. These measures can be sensitive to consumers' goals as well as organizational considerations (e.g., by incorporating quality-of-life outcomes or consumer satisfaction or by weighting the various outcomes by patients' preferences for them).

Assessing effectiveness is complicated because of the problems associated with defining and measuring organizational goals. As Scott (1977) notes, assessing organizational effectiveness largely depends on the kinds of goals organizations adopt and their reasons for doing so. Goals serve many purposes. They may

- motivate organization members to higher performance;
- act as criteria for evaluating performance;
- legitimize organizational activities; and
- indicate to external agencies what the organization is about.

So how should success in reaching a goal be measured? Different goals may be developed to serve these different purposes; alternatively, the same stated goals may be used differently in different situations to serve any or all of the above functions—with varying degrees of success.

The following section examines the major approaches to assessing organizational performance, particularly in regard to effectiveness. It is organized to highlight three types of problems and issues in evaluating performance: definitional (what is measured), technical (how to measure), and managerial (why it is being measured). These sections include a review of the factors that affect performance, focusing particularly on studies of quality in health care organizations. The managerial issues focus on internal strategies aimed to assure quality and to improve it. The chapter concludes with a discussion of high-performing health care organizations and associated managerial guidelines.

ISSUES IN ASSESSING EFFECTIVE PERFORMANCE

Evaluation systems are the principal devices managers have for attempting to influence and improve the performance of their organizations. It is important for managers to become aware of the limitations of any particular system. As Haberstroh (1965) noted,

"First, performance reporting is omnipresent and necessarily so. Second, almost every instance of performance reporting has something wrong with it." These problems can be broadly classified into definitional, technical, and managerial issues of performance evaluation, although as Kanter (1981) remarks, "The most interesting questions in this area are not technical, they are conceptual: not *how* to measure effectiveness or productivity, but *what* to measure" [italics added].

Definitional Issues in Assessment

Fundamental Perspectives about Organizations

The most important definitional issue in measuring organizational performance is related to one's view of the fundamental purpose and nature of organizations because these views affect the most critical assessment questions: *what* will be measured and *why* it is being evaluated? If organizations are conceived primarily as rationally designed instruments for the production of goods and services for external consumption, emphasis is placed on measures of productivity and efficiency. Alternatively, if organizations are viewed as collectivities capable of pursuing specific goals but primarily oriented toward their own survival—toward system maintenance—attention is diverted from output to support goals, such as members' satisfaction or morale or, more generally, the survival of the organization. If organizations are envisioned to be open systems that are highly interdependent with their environments, the key strategies leading to an effective organization involve acquisition of scarce resources (e.g., through the fund-raising activities of volunteers and the choice of well-connected persons to serve on boards of trustees) and the capacity to adapt to a changing environment (e.g., through the creation of slack, or uncommitted resources). This view, by recognizing both an external and internal reality for organizations, underscores the importance of knowing why an evaluation is being performed: for internal consumption (e.g., to take corrective action to solve a quality problem) or external (e.g., to demonstrate to an external group that accreditation standards were met).

Juxtaposing these different views of organizations not only exposes multiple ways to conceptualize effectiveness but also highlights the potentially conflicting features of performance in an organizational system. Two issues leading to discrepancies help illustrate this point.

First, the measures may not be mutually compatible. For example, efficiency in the attainment of specific goals may not be consistent with maximizing participants' satisfaction. More specifically, a teaching hospital, organized to maximize opportunities to train and take advantage of the availability of residents, can lead to greater dissatisfaction of patients as they experience a depersonalized and discontinuous array of providers and of nurses as they relinquish some valued aspects of their roles to inexperienced residents (Fleming, 1981). Similarly, while injuries may be reduced by the use of physical restraints in nursing homes as a safety measure, they may also negatively impact the quality of residential life and morale.

Second, different time frames for evaluating effectiveness can lead to discrepant evaluations. Particularly in a time of rapid environmental change, the organization that is well suited to deal with today's demands may by that very fact be ill-equipped to handle tomorrow's challenges. Weick (1977) notes that organizational features that preserve adaptability "look ugly and wasteful" in the present context but can prove invaluable when conditions change. Finally, the organization itself is seen as having a life cycle and all of its subunits are subject to changes that develop over time (Kimberly & Miles, 1980). Cameron and Whetten (1981) proposed that effectiveness varies according to the stage of organizational development. Effectiveness in earlier stages depends primarily on creativity and mobilizing resources; later stages emphasize commitment and cohesion among members; still later, formal processes of control and efficiency come to the fore; and finally, structural elaboration, decentralization, and flexibility receive emphasis.

Domain of Activity

Once a general framework or model has been selected to guide the investigation, it is necessary to determine which particular functions or activities will be evaluated. Most complex organizations serve a variety of aims and objectives. Modern hospitals, for example, not only provide a variety of types of patient care, including broad categories of services such as outpatient, inpatient, and emergency care, but many also pursue educational goals (e.g., residency training), research goals, and preventive and community service goals. Departmental and work group subdivisions often reflect—and protect—these differentiated purposes, with different subgroups and types of personnel performing quite divergent tasks and pursuing quite distinct objectives.

In some cases, these goals and the activities of the various groups are highly interdependent—in either negative or positive ways. Training objectives sometimes conflict with patient care as noted above, but they can also support and complement good care by making available advanced technology or encouraging providers to investigate unexpected results. In other cases, the goals and activities may be quite independent, the policies and practices of a labor and delivery center may be largely unaffected by those of the hospice program. In either situation—even if the same concept of effectiveness is being applied—the same organization may perform extremely well in one domain of activities but relatively poorly in another. For example, while long-term care settings provide both medical and social services for their residents, they may not provide both with equal effectiveness. The diversity of products in modern managed care organizations and integrated systems likewise exponentially increases the challenge to do all things well. Simply put, no organization can be equally effective with respect to all the objectives it pursues. Two implications are that there is no simple measure of overall effectiveness for a health care organization, but there is always room to continuously improve at least some aspect of performance.

Different Levels of Analysis

A third critical factor influencing conceptions of organizational performance is the level of analysis selected to guide the assessment. An important insight gained from open systems theory is that all complex systems tend to be nested units, systems within systems. Thus a hospital is composed of departments, and the departments are composed of work units, and the hospital as a whole is part of one or more larger systems, such as a multiunit hospital or regional health system. The boundaries that separate these levels are seldom clear and are often rather arbitrary. Further, many of these boundaries are not organized in neat concentric circles but frequently overlap and cross-cut one another. Individuals in modern societies are not completely contained within any single organization but instead are partially involved in several, and professional occupations and union organizations cross organizational boundaries in complex and unexpected ways.

Although there are obviously various possibilities, it is conventional to identify at least three system levels

- the organization itself, such as a health maintenance organization (HMO)
- a larger socially defined unit that contains the organization, such as a community, a health services region, or a system of hospitals
- subunits contained within the organization, such as individual departments or practitioners.

Nerenz and Zajac (1991) propose yet another unit of analysis to assess performance in a variety of vertically-integrated health systems. They propose that the basic unit of data collection should not be a service or a patient but an episode of care that embraces services provided across multiple sites and involving numerous actors. They challenge traditional measures of performance as containing inappropriate assumptions for today's complex systems, such as the presumed association between utilization and revenue or the assumption that the system's effectiveness can be maximized by maximizing the effectiveness of each component organization. They propose new ways to collect information that can aid future attempts to understand the relationship between system performance and system characteristics. An excellent example of the implementation of these concepts is the Self-Assessment for Systems Integration Tool developed by the National Chronic Care Consortium.

The unit of analysis selected can have a profound effect on the assessment of performance. For example, a strategy to measure efficiency of emergency services at the community level may differ considerably from an assessment focused on one hospital's emergency room. Most analyses of organizational performance focus on one or more of these three levels. The critical point, however, is that one should be as clear as possible about what level of analysis is selected.

It is also important to recognize that system performance at any given level may not be analyzable as a simple aggregation of system performance at lower levels. This is one of the principal features of any system: Its performance is determined as much, if not more, by the arrangements of its parts—their relations and interactions—as by the performance of the individual components. A number of highly qualified physicians do not necessarily add up to a high-quality medical staff. Rather, how the staff members are deployed by level of privileges and types of service, how their work is monitored and information fed back to allow improvement, the arrangements for continuing education, and other similar factors may be more decisive for many aspects of medical effectiveness.

One must be careful not to confuse level of analysis with the issue of whose interests are reflected in the determination of assessment criteria. For example, it is possible to focus on the performance of the hospital as a complex system but to assess this performance from the standpoint of the interest of the larger community. Whose interests are served in assessing effectiveness is best treated as a separate topic, a fourth factor that affects one's view of organizational performance.

Stakeholders

Early performance measures, based on small entrepreneurial organizations, focused primarily on profit for the owners or their agents (managers). For publicly traded health care organizations, like many nursing home, assisted living, and home health care providers, stockholder benefit remains a key measure of performance. It was not long before analysts noted that the interests of owners and their agents were far from being perfectly aligned and that other groups—such as professional workers, the public, and external clients—had interests in the organization's performance (Berle & Means, 1932; Burnham, 1941). Cyert and March (1966) described organizations in terms of shifting coalitions of interest groups—some internal, others external to the organization—that are constantly engaged in negotiating and renegotiating the conditions of their participation and thereby affecting the performance of organizations.

In any organization, both internal and external interested parties—stakeholders—have different desires and needs to be met by the organization. They want the organization to score points on different things. They have varying expectations and criteria for effectiveness. For example, internal stakeholders in hospitals include employees, physicians, and boards of directors. Most employees want meaningful work, opportunity for growth, and a reasonable degree of job security. Physicians want up-to-date technology, support services, and an environment in which they are free to practice medicine as they were trained. Physicians, while viewed primarily as internal stakeholders, can also be considered as external stakeholders, depending on the degree to which particular physicians identify with a given health care organization. Health care organizations can also be external stakeholders for other health care organizations. For example, hospitals are a major source of referrals for home health agencies.

Other external stakeholders include suppliers, regulatory groups, competitors, third-party payers, and community groups. Third-party payers expect care to be provided in the most cost-effective manner possible. Patients have varying expectations depending on the severity of their illness, their education, and their financial resources. Regulators will be concerned with the organization's ability to maintain standards and contain costs. Suppliers of capital focus on the institution's bottom line. Given this disparate set of demands and expectations, it is not possible for a given organization to be seen as equally effective by all of its stakeholders or constituent groups at a given point in time.

Recently, researchers have examined performance issues that involve multiple interested parties and coalition formation in health care organizations. Fennell and Alexander (1989) note that a board of trustees is supposed to represent the external stakeholders' interests and monitor and contain any self-interested actions on the part of hospital management and internal stakeholders. However, the stakeholders and customers in hospitals are often difficult to identify and sometimes hard to tell apart, resulting in continuous coalition formation among the interest groups.

This lack of clear-cut boundaries among the interests of various actors is further illustrated by proponents of quality improvement who argue that production of any service or product within the organization—such as filling a prescription or preparing a report for the government—involves a seemingly endless chain of suppliers, processors, and customers (Berwick, Godfrey, & Roessner, 1991). Rather than restrict the term *customers* to end users of an organization's product, this perspective emphasizes the complex web of parties with a stake in performance. This perspective is particularly useful in evaluating integrated delivery systems where complex supplier-customer relationships among system components abound.

Of course, not all interests are equally powerful. In most organizations, one can detect the presence of a dominant coalition whose interests carry more weight than others. But it is still important to note that in most organizations power is more widely dispersed today than in the past, and more diverse constituencies are perceived to be legitimate stakeholders in the enterprise.

One response to the disparate needs of multiple competing interests has been the development of a "community orientation" by health care organizations. Spurred by a variety of factors, there is a growing consensus among third-party payers, employers, community organizations, local governments, and other stakeholders that health services organizations like hospitals must reach beyond a narrow definition of their patients to enhance the health status of the entire population they serve (i.e., of their community). In this context, community includes all persons and organizations within a circumscribed geographical area in which there is a sense of interdependence and belonging. The degree of community orientation can be defined by the extent to which these organizations

generate community intelligence, disseminate it internally and externally, and use it to develop community health interventions.

To summarize, a number of factors have been identified that have clear relevance to the evaluation of organizational performance. Views of the nature of organizations and the impact of time frames, the domains of the activities being evaluated, the level of analysis, and the perspective of interested parties are sufficiently complex that one may expect to find little consensus in the selection of criteria employed to evaluate organizational effectiveness (Campbell, 1977; Flood, 1994; Flood & Fennell, 1995; Steers, 1975).

Technical Issues in Assessment

Having described key definitional issues related to what should be measured, we now turn to problems of how to measure performance. The focus is on the generic problems and concerns that arise during the process of evaluating work performance.

Classes of Measures

Performance assessment requires that evidence be collected upon which evaluations can be based. More than 30 years ago, Donabedian (1966) noted that evaluators of the quality of health care answered the "how to" question by using one of three basic classes of measures: structural, process, and outcome measures. Although he was referring to the evaluation of technical and psychosocial aspects of clinical care, these same categories are useful for evaluating nonclinical performance as well. Table 13.1 provides examples of each class of indicators applied to financial management, clinical care, and human resources management.

Structural Measures

Structural indicators are based on assessments of organizational features or participants' characteristics that are presumed to have an impact on organizational performance. As such, they can be thought of as input measures of an organization's capacity to permit or promote effective work. For example, in the opening scenario of Jackson Memorial Hospital,

Table 13.1. Examples of Performance Measures by Category

	Domain of Activity		
	Clinical Care	*Financial Management*	*Human Resources Management*
Structure	*Effectiveness* • Percent of active physicians who are board certified • JCAHO accreditation • Number of residencies and filled positions • Presence of council for quality improvement planning	*Effectiveness* • Qualifications of administrators in finance department • Use of preadmission criteria • Presence of an integrated financial and clinical information system	*Effectiveness* • Ability to attract desired registered nurses and other health professionals • Size (or growth) of active physician staff • Salary and benefits compared with competitors • Quality of inhouse staff education
Process	*Effectiveness* • Rate of medication error • Rate of nosocomial infection • Rate of postsurgical wound infection • Rate of normal tissue removed	*Effectiveness* • Days in accounts receivable • Use of generic drugs and drug formulary • Market share • Size (or growth) of shared service arrangements	*Effectiveness* • Grievances • Promotions • Organizational climate
	Productivity • Ratio of total patient days to total full-time equivalent (FTE) nurses • Ratio of total admissions to total FTE staff • Ratio of physician visits to total FTE physicians	*Productivity* • Ratio of collection to FTE financial staff • Ratio of total admissions to FTE in finance department • Ratio of new capital to fund-raising staff	*Productivity* • Ratio of line staff to managers
	Efficiency • Average cost per patient • Average cost per admission	*Efficiency* • Cost per collection • Debt/equity ratio	*Efficiency* • Cost of recruiting
Outcome	*Effectiveness* • Case-severity-adjusted mortality • Patient satisfaction • Patient functional health status	*Effectiveness* • Return on assets • Operating margins • Size (or growth) of federal, state, or local grants for teaching and research • Bond rating	*Effectiveness* • Turnover rate • Absenteeism • Staff satisfaction

structural measures of quality would portray the quality and number of staff in the labor and delivery room and the forms of coordination to carry out doctor's orders. Other indicators include the number and types of specialized equipment, such as fetal monitoring; the presence of an active peer review program; and the proportion of the medical staff that is board certified. Until recently, accreditation and certification reviews relied almost exclusively on either structural or process measures of performance; note too that accreditation itself can be used as a structural indicator of performance. For example, many managed care organizations require provider organizations to have accreditation by the Joint Commission on the Accreditation of Healthcare Organizations (JCAHO) as a prerequisite for contract participation.

Process Measures

Process measures of quality are based on evidence relating to the performer's activities in carrying out work. Examples include quality assurance activities such as reviews of physician decision making and orders provided to all patients dying in-hospital or reviewing nurse and physician conformance with standards for cleanliness on units with outbreaks of nosocomial infections. The proportion of residents physically restrained or catheterized are process "checkpoints" that may trigger more rigorous quality review in the federal nursing home certification process. Process measures can be directed at an organization or system of care as well—a review of the system for conducting and reporting the results of urgently requested laboratory tests. Process measures can also be used to assess the nonclinical aspects of performance. Examples in the financial area include liquidity ratios, such as the ratio of current assets to current liability, and activity ratios, such as the ratio of total operating revenue to total assets (Cleverly, 1981).

Outcome Measures

Outcome measures of quality are based on evidence gathered from the objects upon which the work is performed. Since assessments are made to determine whether changes have occurred in their characteristics that can be attributed to the work performed upon them, these can be thought of as measures of the output of work processes. Thus, for clinical care, changes in the patient's health status (to measure technical aspects of care) or satisfaction (to assess the interpersonal care) are assessed; for training institutions, changes in the student's knowledge, skills, or attitudes may be examined. In the financial area, outcome might be measured by the operating margin (ratio of operating income to operating revenue) or the return on assets (Cleverly, 1981).

These three classes of measures are not independent measures of performance, but linked in an underlying model. Structural measures of quality are valid to the extent that they motivate and encourage providers to choose efficacious, appropriate, or cost-effective actions. Process measures in turn are valid if they lead to improved products or better outcomes. This model overstates the simplicity of these relationships, which are loosely coupled at best and certainly should not be mistaken as substitutes for each other. It is important to recognize that each of these types of indicators is imperfect—subject to bias and misinterpretation. Process measures focus on energy and effort expended but neglect effects achieved. Moreover, measures based on process alone can only compare performance values with some specified standard; they cannot themselves assess the appropriateness of the standards employed. If process measures are once removed from effects, then structural indicators are twice removed, since they do not assess work performed or effort expended but only the organization's capacity for work. Presumed competencies may in practice turn out to be ineffectual, and existing capacities may on specific occasions be unemployed or underemployed. Outcome measures have the advantage of focusing attention on changes produced and results achieved. Their drawback is that they do not in themselves provide evidence that can connect observed outcomes to the effects of performance. Particularly in arenas such as medical care, it is common for poor outcomes to occur in spite of superior performance, and vice versa. Causal factors that are beyond the control of the caregiver are at work. And at a more general organizational level, a high proportion of good outcomes—patient recoveries, student achievements, profitability—may be more a function of selection procedures—admitting only the easiest patients or brightest students—than what the organization does. Finally, because full recovery is not the goal for much of health care, such as for chronic or mental illness and for care of the dying patient, a comparison of actual versus expected decline or comfort for such patients may be the most appropriate measure of outcome performance.

It is also important to distinguish objective measures of quality from people's perceptions. For example, a given home health agency may have the highest possible accreditation rating and best patient functional health status outcomes (objective measures) but be perceived by the community as having relatively low quality, perhaps owing to problems of convenience and access to services or an occasional war story of poor care. In the same vein, it is important to recognize that the public's perception of quality may differ from those of physicians and caregivers. For example, the public may give greater weight to access, convenience, comfort, and interpersonal relationships while the professional caregiver places greater emphasis on technical skill. In part, this is due to the public's relative inability to evaluate technical expertise. As a result, they use other criteria as proxy measures or assume technical quality as a given and then make choices based on the nontechnical criteria discussed above. Again, this points out the importance of deciding which stakeholder perspective(s) will be used to assess performance.

Preferences for Classes of Performance Measures

Associations are likely to exist between these classes of indicators and broadly defined categories of constituencies in organizations (Scott, 1977). Executives and managers typically prefer to employ structural measures of effectiveness since these are the types of indicators over which they have most control. Similarly, caregivers are likely to emphasize process measures because these activities are more under their control. By contrast, clients and representatives of the various external publics may prefer to focus attention on outcomes; never mind capacity or effort, what results were actually achieved? Patients, for example, are much more likely to be concerned about remission of symptoms and restoration of function than about the technical correctness of the procedures employed or the formal qualifications of personnel. Despite this preference, patients seldom can obtain good information about the average patient's experience with outcomes and must rely on the physician's judgment or structural indicators such as accreditation. Indeed, for these reasons, executives need to be attentive to such visible indicators of quality—whether they reflect true differences in patient care—since these indicators may be used by prospective customers to choose where they go for care. More broadly, licensing, ac-

creditation, tort law, and regulations associated with quality control abound in health care. Even when they use standards based on widely held beliefs rather than on evidence of their import for quality, they have an ability to influence organizational performance regardless of the validity of the claim.

Factors Associated with Effective Performance

Despite the difficulties involved, studies have identified a number of factors generally associated with higher quality of care (Aiken, Sochalski, & Lake, 1997; Flood, 1994; Flood & Fennell, 1995; Flood & Scott, 1987; Miller & Luft, 1994):

- quality of professional staff
- high standards
- experience with other cases of the same type
- more formally organized professional staffs with well-defined coordination and conflict management processes
- participative organization cultures emphasizing team approaches
- timely and accurate performance feedback
- active management of environmental forces
- type of ownership, competition, staffing continuity, and compensation

Evidence related to peer review through quality assurance and continuous quality improvement is discussed in the following section.

In nursing homes, higher levels of staffing by registered nurses is associated with improved physical functioning, lower mortality, a greater likelihood of being discharged to home, and less unnecessary hospitalizations. In home health care services, it is also associated with greater patient satisfaction. In regard to the quality of professional staff, key factors are recruitment, retention, and having people work within their professional abilities. This involves concentrating the work of professionals in such a fashion that greater experience produces better patient-care outcomes over time. As noted, several studies have found higher volume of patients treated by both institutions and individual physicians to be associated with more positive patient-care outcomes (Flood,

Scott, & Ewy, 1984; Luft, Granick, Mark, & McPhee, 1990).

Setting high standards is compatible with professional values. A key factor involves strict admission requirements and exerting strong control in enforcing standards. More tightly organized professional staffs assist in this process by providing regular forums for problem management and conflict resolution (Shortell & LoGerfo, 1981). In nursing homes, greater control over medical staff admitting privileges is associated with less inappropriate drug prescribing; staffing continuity and compensation are associated with greater resident satisfaction and better physical functioning. Coordination also plays an important role in overall effectiveness.

A participative organizational culture emphasizing team approaches is particularly important when the environment is changing rapidly. An ongoing team approach allows ideas to be communicated and discussed quickly by the professionals that will be most affected by the changes involved. A participative culture helps to develop good work habits on the part of all involved and reinforces appropriate peer group pressure. Further, teams generally do a better job of solving complex problems than individuals. For example, work focused on hospital intensive care units found that efficiency of utilization and perceptions of higher quality of care were related to good conflict management—including communication, problem solving, and leadership—combined with a patient orientation (Shortell et al., 1990). Many studies suggest that structures allowing for greater coordination and communication across disciplines that participate in the care of the elderly contribute to better outcomes. For example, the use of multidisciplinary teams bears favorably on both physical and psychosocial outcomes in nursing homes and patient satisfaction with home health care services.

Timely and accurate feedback raises the visibility of behavior in the organization such that accountability requirements are met, and deviation from performance standards is assessed. Nursing homes and home health agencies are beginning to tie together financial and clinical data in negotiating rates for various levels of services with managed care organizations. A good clinical-financial management information system enables corrective action to be taken more quickly. Finally, more active management of the external environment enables the organization to educate external groups (e.g., licensing and accreditation bodies, regulatory groups, third-party payers) about quality objectives and practices and the associated challenges involved. For example, university teaching hospitals, which have established their own hospital-specific governing boards separate from the university governing boards, have been better able to negotiate with relevant external groups and more clearly communicate their mission and objectives.

As the incentives to form more integrated delivery systems grow, there is great need to assess the performance of such systems from both an efficiency and effectiveness perspective. The existing evidence is largely mixed while the issue of quality of care provided by such systems is largely unexplored (Friedman & Shortell, 1988; Shortell, Morrison, & Friedman, 1990; Zuckerman, 1979).

In sum, managers must recognize the limitations of each class of performance indicator as well as understand the interests of the various constituency groups—including their own—that have a stake in the functioning of their organization. Only such awareness will enable them to correct for these biases and balance the often conflicting interests of the several parties involved.

Managerial Issues in Assessing Performance

The need for managing quality is central to any organization. Health care organizations, coming under increasing pressure to be cost-effective, have been turning away from old models of assuring quality to a new model of quality improvement, which has been effective in helping industries worldwide to improve their products or services. The old model in health care relegated quality to the quality assurance (QA) department; the new model emphasizes quality improvement (QI) teams, which cut horizontally across functions and reach vertically across hierarchical lines to involve the entire management and staff. The old model solved problems and held individuals culpable for mistakes; the new one prevents problems by continuously improving the true source of defects—

the process. The old model was based on peer review and focused on upholding minimally acceptable standards of care; the new borrows from principles applicable to any industry and encourages striving for excellence. The form and function of the old model was required by external accreditors and third-party payers for quality of care; the new permeates all processes and requires a strong internal culture to support it. The differences are profound enough to require a major paradigm shift—not necessarily to displace all of the activities of QA but to restructure most of the way quality is managed. In this section, both models are presented and their strengths and weaknesses contrasted. To set the stage, general issues in evaluating

professionals and other staff and unintended responses to evaluation are presented.

Evaluating Professional Performance: The Professional Model

In the classic professional model, the foremost means to ensure that professionals produce high-quality work is to give them the skills, training, and values needed to produce life-long devotion to excellence. However, to weed out any "bad apples" and to inspire them to continue learning, professional workers can be held accountable by making their work visible to others whose opinion counts. In professional work, peer review is

IN THE REAL WORLD:
STAKEHOLDERS VS. STOCKHOLDERS: VENCOR, INC. "SLAMS THE DOOR" ON MEDICAID PATIENTS

On April 7, 1998, The Wall Street Journal *reported that Vencor, Inc., a publicly traded health care corporation operating 62 hospitals and 310 nursing home facilities, was evicting all residents whose care was paid for through the Medicaid program in 13 nursing homes in nine states. The $3 billion company stated that it needed the beds to attract wealthier patients who can afford the higher level of medical care it plans to provide.*

From its base as an operator of specialty long-term-care hospitals, Vencor expanded rapidly between 1985 and 1995. After an initial public offering in 1989, its stock shot up severalfold in a little more than two years. But regulatory and competitive pressures hurt: Selling at $37 per share in 1995, Vencor sold at $29.50 per share just prior to the eviction notice. The company hoped that higher fees from private-pay patients would help it make a comeback.

However, the evictions created hard feelings in affected communities. In many instances, little assistance or planning preceded the 24-hour eviction notices to residents. Even staff and resident families were not informed prior to resident notification. Residents had to find new places to live on their own, and assumed all expenses associated with relocation. As one family member wrote:

"This matter was handled in a most cold, calculated, and callous way." A Vencor spokesman commenting on the handling of the eviction stated: "My philosophy is that if you have to do something you're better off to face up to it and do it. . . . This is like having to go through an amputation. If you have to cut your hand off, do you do it one finger at a time or just cut your hand off and go on?"

Vencor's tactics drew swift responses from a number of circles. The following is a representative sample:

- *Edie Ousley, spokeswoman for the Florida Agency for Health Care Administration: "This is not about bottom-line profits. It's about resident health and safety. It was made very clear to Vencor that the State of Florida was offended by their corporate philosophy and would not put up with it."*
- *U.S. Senator Bob Graham, D–Fla: "For these people to be told they are going to be dumped is totally unacceptable."*
- *U.S Representative Jim Davis, D–Tampa: "I think there was an enormous temptation on the part of this particular nursing home to put their profits ahead of their patients."*

- *Nursing home resident Betty Nelson: "You're kicking us out because we don't have enough money."*
- *Family member Anna Anello: "I know the almighty dollar is important, but I don't think it should be at the expense of these people."*

These responses prompted a number of state investigations resulting in sanctions and penalties. The State of Georgia recommended that Vencor be fined $533,000 and be barred from Medicare participation by the federal government. Florida fined the company $260,000 and recommended that the federal government fine Vencor an additional $100,000. The Florida congressman quoted above filed federal legislation that would ban the dumping of Medicaid-covered residents and require facilities that participate in the Medicare program to participate in the Medicaid program as well. Kentucky and California also began investigations of the company's discharge practices.

After the public outcry, Vencor made an abrupt reversal. It sent letters to all residents apologizing for the evictions and inviting them to return to the facilities. It also promised that there would be no more evictions. The company agreed to reimburse residents for their relocation expenses. In the words of Bruce Lunsford, Vencor's chairman and chief executive officer: "I'm embarrassed. Our company is embarrassed. We regret what happened."

Vencor still plans to withdraw from the Medicaid program, but will do it gradually through attrition and selective admission policies as opposed to forced eviction.

Why did Vencor decide to take such misguided action initially? Vencor was focused on the needs of one group, its stockholders, to the exclusion of others. However, while stockholders are important stakeholders, not all stakeholders are stockholders. It may be that Vencor assumed that the stakeholder group most affected, the evicted residents, were not powerful enough to retaliate. However, residents and their families were able to form a powerful coalition with legislators and regulators that immediately retaliated against Vencor and set in motion a series of investigations that could impact on the company for a long time to come.

Could they have achieved their objective without incurring the resulting damage? Had they conducted a thorough stakeholder analysis, they may have foreseen the potential reaction, leading them to an alternative approach to withdrawal from the Medicaid program.

Moss M, Adams C. For Medicaid patients, doors slam closed; Langreth R. After seeing profits from the poor, some HMOs abandon them. Wall Street Journal (Eastern Edition) (Apr. 7, 1998) p. B1.

needed because only peers can truly judge the quality of one's work. These notions, for physicians in particular and nurses to a more limited extent, are backed up by a potential for malpractice litigation against substandard care and by financial fines or professional reprimands for poor performance (Hall, 1988).

Health care organizations have always operated by using both professional and bureaucratic forms of control. Some have argued that there are two independent lines of authority, one for physicians and the other for everyone else. In their exposition of work in hospitals, Geogopoulos and Mann (1962) implied that these two lines of authority acted more like a lobotomized brain rather than an integrated right and left brain in coordinating activities. But others, like Scott (1982), describe three alternative models that can be used to embed professionals effectively into an organization: autonomous, in which professionals retain independent authority to control and evaluate themselves as a group; heteronomous, in which professionals are subject to more line-authority control; and conjoint, in which professionals and administrators coexist in a mutually interdependent setting in which each group is roughly equal in power and in the importance of their functions. The hospital that Geogopoulos and Mann were describing fit the autonomous model; but the modern health care organization is moving toward the third model, in which mutual understanding and cooperation play key roles for organizational effectiveness.

In health care organizations, because of the high percentage of professionals involved and their diversity, health care executives need to understand and accommodate the varying professional requirements of each group. Physicians, in particular, have high need for achievement and autonomy in clinical decision making. Other groups have less highly developed claims to autonomy but desire organizational settings in which they can practice their full range of professional skills. Job autonomy, for example, is associated with less conflict, increased job satisfaction, and greater client satisfaction (Weisman & Nathanson, 1985).

Almost all professionals have high standards of excellence, and therefore organizations and managers that emphasize high-performance expectations and provide the necessary support for obtaining excellence are likely to be more effective. Achieving such standards is a function of both specification of rules and procedures as well as informal communication and use of ad hoc task forces that involve relevant groups. Rules and procedures help to define and handle many problems, but because of the complexity and uncertainty of much professional work, informal and ad hoc mechanisms must also be used to deal with nonroutine problems. Examples include emergency cases; patients with multiple diagnoses; elderly patients with chronic care needs that cut across many specialties and even organizations; and patients with illnesses involving complicated moral, legal, economic, or ethical issues.

Involving professionals in the development of standards, norms, rules, policies, and practices is essential. Studies indicate that such involvement is associated with greater professional satisfaction and can play an important role in staff retention. Increasingly, professionals want to be involved not only in deciding what will have an immediate impact on their work but also in some of the larger organizational issues that may affect their future practice. Examples include the organization's relationship with third-party payers, regulators, and competitors. Thus there exists growing physician involvement in management and governance issues and new forms of joint venture relationships (also see Chapters 9 and 11) (Alexander, Morrisey, & Shortell, 1986; Barr & Steinberg, 1983; Shortell, Morrisey, & Conrad, 1985).

In sum, existing studies suggest that evaluating and coordinating professional work is facilitated by high standards and clear expectations, specified rules and procedures combined with job autonomy, flexibility in coordinating work, and a high degree of professional involvement in decision making. These practices place a premium on the manager's conflict management (see Chapter 5), communication and coordination (see Chapter 8), and organization design skills (see Chapters 6, 7, 9, and 10).

Evaluating Nonprofessional Work: The Bureaucratic Model

Comparing observed performance values with established standards is also seldom a simple mechanical process but one requiring experience and judgment. It is to accommodate these skills that the appraisal function is typically assigned to a supervisor—a person selected on the basis of seniority or merit and located close to the work site. Experience and proximity allow these individuals to detect nuances in performers' activities and to take into account special circumstances that affect performance values and their associated outcomes. Many of the complaints and problems associated with supervisor-worker relations may be attributed to disagreements over performance appraisal and may signify both the complexities and the sensitivities associated with this process. In nursing homes, research shows that who does performance evaluation can make a difference. Nurse aide turnover is higher in nursing homes in which the director of nursing, as opposed to the floor charge nurse, writes performance evaluations.

In the modern health care organization, these tasks of evaluating performance—particularly in the context of maximizing organizational performance—are made more difficult by the complexity of occupations and people involved in providing care. More and more, in recognition of the different skills and perspectives necessary to perform such tasks, interdisciplinary teams rather than individuals become the basic accountability unit within the organization, necessitating new means for evaluating work and improving the process.

The Impact of Evaluation on All Types of Performers

All attempts to evaluate a performance may be expected to have effects on that performance. The setting of standards, the selection of indicators, the sampling of performance, and the comparison of performances with standards all affect the performance itself (Dornbusch & Scott, 1975). The primary purpose of any evaluation system is to exert influence on the performance of participants—if not the performance immediately under review, then subsequent ones. But equally important and less obvious are the unintended effects of performance evaluation. People basically prefer to receive a good evaluation; therefore, workers will seek to improve their evaluation irrespective of whether that change actually improves the quality of their performance. Ideally, of course, the evaluations made are accurate and appropriate; but if not, *reactivity* to the performance criteria can result in an appearance of improvement in performance rather than motivating the worker to seek true changes in quality. Or, as W. Richard Scott once paraphrased an old song, "When you're not near the goal that you love, you love the goal that you're near."

These biasing or diverting effects occur because it is often difficult or overly costly to devise evaluation systems and indicators that accurately reflect the complexity of desired outcomes to which the performance is addressed. Thus, although examinations are developed to test learning, their repeated use is likely to influence what is taught or, more importantly, what is learned. And if diagnostic thoroughness is signified by the number of laboratory tests ordered, then the number of tests ordered may far exceed the number required by the patient's medical condition. In particular, hard measures—measures that are specific, capable of being quantified, and easy to observe—tend to drive out soft measures.

Nonetheless, there is some evidence that physicians will respond to evaluations by peers for its own sake. For example, physicians have responded to internally imposed peer review (Wennberg, Blowers, Parker, & Gittelsohn, 1977). Dyck and his colleagues (1977) found that rates of healthy tissue removal associated with appendectomy dropped significantly when criteria about "acceptable" rates were made explicit, absent any need to reprimand physicians. However, physicians knew that peers were going to monitor their rates in the future with undetermined consequences. Physicians have also responded by

dropping the rate of prescribing drugs when a computerized system with the capability to monitor prescriptions was introduced, even though the system was intended for another purpose (Cohen, Flood, Himmelberger, Mangini, & Moore, 1980).

Finally, the work by the Maine Medical Foundation (MMF) and the Minnesota Clinical Comparison and Assessment Project provides many examples of how a study group of physicians, when given feedback on utilization with evidence that some physicians were unusually high, can result in a reduction of the outlier rates over time (Borbas et al., 1990; Keeler, Chapin, & Soule, 1990; Keeler, Soule, Wennberg, & Hanley, 1990). However, there is some recent evidence that suggests that physician profiles showing the relative use rates of services, when divorced of any apparent consequences, appear to have no effect on behavior (Wones, 1987).

Two Models for Changing Performance

Quality Assurance

Quality assurance (QA) refers to "the formal and systematic exercise of identifying problems in medical care delivery, designing activities to overcome these problems, and carrying out follow-up steps to ensure that no new problems have been introduced and that corrective actions have been effective (Brook & Lohr, 1985). In reviewing 25 years of QA activities, Williamson (1988) noted agreement on five principles for assuring quality.

- Successful QA requires individual and organizational commitment to develop the values and incentives of excellence.
- Responsibility for excellence must be decentralized so that the professionals and staff responsible for the care have the power to review and implement necessary changes.
- At the same time, QA requires an approach that is comprehensive of all the groups in the hospital that can affect quality, including education, administration, and support services.
- At the same time, QA is best targeted toward prioritized, specific needs rather than being based on a shotgun approach to identifying problems.

- QA itself should be continuously monitored for its effectiveness and adaptiveness to current organizational needs to ensure that its contributions outweigh its costs.

The evidence that QA has been successful in changing physician's behavior is scant (Jessee, 1984; Luke, Krueger, & Modrow, 1983; Mittman & Siv, 1992). As Luke, Krueger, and Modrow (1983) remarked, "It is clear that quality assurance has until now been both expensive and, in general, marginally effective." The general conclusion is that the primary problem has been a failure to focus on the means to secure changes in organizations or physicians rather than on the techniques to assess quality (Fifer, 1983; Jessee, 1984; Shanahan, 1983; Wyszewianski, 1988). In reviewing the evidence on changing physician's behavior and assuring quality, Eisenberg (1986) discusses the importance of an environment conducive to high quality, including strong professional leadership and diffusion of up-to-date innovations in medicine as well as face-to-face interactions with colleagues—not necessarily found in most QA activities. These arguments have been supported by work based on QA in a primary care setting (Kind, Fowles, & McCoy, 1987; McCoy, Kind, Fowles, & Schned, 1987).

Many are calling for greater integration and coordination of QA activities as well. For example, a study by the U.S. General Accounting Office found several reasons for concern about the systems for monitoring quality in Medicare. There is little evidence of the effectiveness of the review methods being used; there is poor coordination across groups reviewing quality with little or no sharing of information; the data used are of questionable accuracy and generalizability; and there are inadequate strategies for developing the methods and knowledge needed to correct the situation and inadequate resources being allocated to redress these concerns ("Medicare," 1988).

While most have called for increased coordination and integration of these activities as well as standardization of the procedures, others have warned of information overload, which overwhelms the system and stymies action and largely symbolic evaluations—going through the motions of QA—which can attend too centralized and extensive of reviews (Fifer,

1983; Heatherington, 1982; Rosen & Feigin, 1982; Shanahan, 1983; Vuori, 1980). To solve these problems, many propose to increase coordination and integration of these activities as well as standardize the procedures. Others caution against too much information gathering, which can overload the system and stymy action or create largely symbolic evaluations—going through the motions without impacting the substance.

Quality Improvement

Quality improvement is the promise put forward to address the problems—real and imagined—in quality assurance in American health care delivery. **Quality improvement (QI)** is a management philosophy to improve the level of performance of key processes in the organization. It was developed originally by several industrial quality experts and applied successfully in a variety of industries worldwide (Crosby, 1979; Deming, 1986; Juran, 1988). The principles espoused by these experts differ little but have helped spawn several terms used interchangeably with QI: *total quality management (TQM), industrial quality control,* and *continuous quality improvement (CQI).* Key philosophical concepts include:

- Productive work involves processes. Most work implies a chain of processes whereby each worker receives inputs from suppliers (internal or external to the organization), adds value, and then passes it on to the customers, who are defined to include everyone internal or external who receives the product or service of the worker.
- The customer is central to every process. Processes are improved to meet the customer's needs reliably and efficiently.
- There are two ways to improve quality: eliminate defects in the process and add features that meet customers' needs or preferences better.
- The main source of quality defects is problems in the process. Workers basically want to and succeed in carrying out the process correctly. The problems derive from the process being wrong.
- Quality defects are costly in terms of internal losses by lowered productivity and efficiency, increased requirements for inspection and monitoring, and

DEBATE TIME 13.1: WHAT DO YOU THINK?

An article in the *Journal of the American Medical Association (JAMA)* described a study of serious medical "missteps" based on anonymous responses from 114 interns and residents regarding their own most significant errors in the previous year. The main categories of serious missteps and examples of each are indicated below.

It is possible that the problems may *not* have been due to individual error but rather to underlying processes and systems involved in patient diagnosis and treatment. For each category of missteps, develop an argument that the error was due to problems in the underlying process rather than from the individual physician's mistake.

Example	Outcome*
ERRORS IN DIAGNOSIS—38 Cases (33%)	
Failed to diagnose bowel obstruction in patient with fluid buildup in abdomen	Death
Failed to examine and diagnose fracture in crack cocaine user	Delayed treatment
EVALUATION AND TREATMENT—24 cases (21%)	
Treated malignant hypertension on the ward instead of in an intensive care unit	Stroke
Incompletely cleaned a diabetic foot ulcer	Amputation
PRESCRIBING AND DOSING—33 Cases (29%)	
Did not read syringe and gave 50 times the correct dose of a thyroid drug	None apparent
Inadvertently stopped asthma medication at time of hospitalization	Respiratory failure
PROCEDURAL COMPLICATIONS—13 Cases (11%)	
Removed pulmonary artery catheter with the balloon inflated	Small amount of bleeding
Placed intravenous line in main vein without a follow-up X-ray	Fatal lung collapse
FAULTY COMMUNICATIONS—6 Cases (5%)	
Failed to put do-not-resuscitate order in chart and failed to inform spouse	Resuscitation performed against patient's wishes
Failed to obtain consent before placing intravenous line in main vein	Fatal complication after procedure

*Cause and effect cannot be determined.
SOURCE: Adapted from Wu AW, Folkman S, McPhee SJ, Lo B. Do house officers learn from their mistakes? *JAMA*, 265(16):2090. Copyright 1991, American Medical Association.

dissatisfied customers. Preventing defects in the process by careful planning saves resources.

- Focus on the most important processes to improve. Use statistical thinking and tools to identify desired performance levels, measure current performance, interpret it, and take action when necessary.
- Involve every worker in QI. Use new structures such as teams and quality councils to advise and plan QI strategies.

- Set high standards for performance; go for being the best.

Benchmarking is the process of establishing operating targets based on the leading performance standards for the industry or what the Japanese call *dantotsu*, the "best of the best." But it should not simply be a metric—determining a standard against which to measure performance; benchmarking is a philosophy to guide the process of proactive, structured practices needed to achieve excellence. Camp (1989) describes this process in four steps.

1. Know your operation. That is, assess your organizational strengths and weaknesses.
2. Know the industry leaders or your direct competitors.
3. Incorporate the best. Don't hesitate to copy or modify, but be sure you start with the best.
4. Gain superiority.

An example of this philosophy applied to a clinical situation in a hospital is illustrated in the case of Jackson Memorial Hospital.

The philosophical approach of QI in some senses is similar to that of such groups as the MMF (Keeler, Kahn, Draper et al., 1990). Both start with the premise that wide variation in practice indicates that something is amiss—not all rates can be right, even if one doesn't know which rate is right. But the two part company in their philosophical approaches to which rate is right—in the sense of being desirable. The MMF approach targets the outliers (usually high utilization) with the view that outlying providers should alter their performance to look more like the typical performance of their peers. All others are okay as is. The QI approach, in contrast, argues that the outliers on the side of good quality should become the benchmark against which everyone else should strive—to try to be the best, not typical.

The evidence that QI will help improve performance in health care comes mostly from other industries since its application is so new to the health industry. Many groups have turned to QI, and accreditation bodies such as the Joint Commission of Healthcare Organizations has revised its accreditation rules to foster this approach (Roberts, 1992). Berwick, Godfrey, and Roessner (1991) report on demonstrations carrying out QI in 21 health care organizations including hospitals, group practices, and HMOs. While some organizations did not complete their reports and few tackled clinical quality of care issues, most felt that they had made significant progress. The authors (Berwick, Godfrey, & Roessner, 1991, p. 25) conclude:

> The evidence that quality management can help in manufacturing and business processes is overwhelming, and it is a very safe bet that the analogous processes in health care (billing, information transfer, equipment maintenance, and the like) stand to gain as much. . . . The same goes for *service* processes, like making appointments, providing telephone access, and moving patients efficiently from place to place. . . . It requires a little more imagination to see how quality management can help technical medical care . . . yet these areas still await complete exploration.

A study of Pennsylvania nursing homes indicates that quality improvement adopters, when compared with facilities that practice only quality assurance, are more likely to report improvements in the quality of resident care and in employee relationships resulting from their quality monitoring program. In addition, nursing home quality improvement adopters report being more satisfied with their quality control program and are more likely to report reductions in mortality and infection rates, reduction in food delivery times, and reduction in employee absenteeism (Zinn, Aaronson, & Rosko, 1993a, 1993b).

In a study of adoption of quality improvement techniques in hospitals, Westphal, Gulati, and Shortell (1997) found that early adopters reformed programs to suit their own needs, but later adopters took on programs that had become normative. They found that only those who customized programs gained performance efficiencies from their introduction, though later adopters gained legitimacy even if no efficiencies resulted.

In the process of implementing QI, a balance between the basic components—implementing the technique, establishing the culture, and planning appropriate strategy—needs to be maintained to be effective (Berwick, 1991). Sometimes proponents try to implement only one component, such as data gathering and problem solving by the interested parties. But evidence from other industries suggests that the package, to be successful, requires implementation of all features. Based on the experiences with QI at the Henry Ford Health System, Sahney (1992) identified several major barriers to successful implementation and urged preventive or corrective attention be paid by managers.

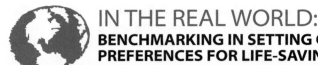

IN THE REAL WORLD:
BENCHMARKING IN SETTING GOALS TO DISCUSS PATIENT PREFERENCES FOR LIFE-SAVING PROCEDURES

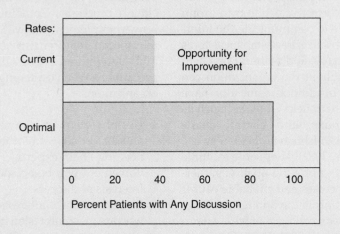

At Jackson Memorial Hospital, all adult patients with serious chronic illnesses and a life expectancy of less than one year or their family members were surveyed to determine how many had had discussions with any provider regarding their preferences about when or whether to use life-sustaining procedures. They found that even among this seriously ill group, only 40 percent had had any such discussions. About 30 percent—some who had had such discussions and some who had not—actually had do-not-resuscitate (DNR) orders placed in their charts during the hospitalization. Arguing that ascertaining preferences for these seriously ill patients was especially important, the QI team set as a benchmark goal for the future that 90 percent of these patients or their surrogates should have had such discussions no later than the first few days of hospitalization.

Adapted from SUPPORT: Study to Understand Prognosis, Preferences for Outcomes, Risks, and Treatment project. Journal of Clinical Epidemiology, 1990, 43 (suppl).

- Middle management is unsure of its role and lets teams tackle insignificant processes or complex problems with insufficient support.
- The pace of improvement is often glacially slow as people brainstorm and flounder on how to proceed. Feedback and rewards for time invested are insufficient.
- Changing the culture is difficult, and members can lose faith in the process.
- Evangelistic devotion to QI can block free discussion and inventive solutions. Likewise, cynical use

of QI can divert resources and energy with no real benefit to the organization as a whole.
- Time availability to carry out QI must be sufficient at all levels, including senior and middle management.
- Results of QI, if not shared broadly internally to the organization, are unknown beyond the few people involved.

A basic premise of QI is that every process has variation in how well it produces a service or product. In order to reduce the variation, the first step involves a careful and information-driven analysis of what can cause a failure of the process, with what frequency such problems occur, and the extent to which problems vary over time. Understanding the process and developing and implementing corrective action by a group process requires being able to communicate the information effectively. Simple and direct statistical tools such as histograms, bar charts, and scattergrams help ensure that anyone throughout the organization can understand and use them. In addition, some tools have been developed specifically to help QI teams, such as flowcharts, Pareto diagrams, and control charts (Batalden & Buchanan, 1989; Ishikawa, 1985; Stewart, 1986; Wheeler & Chambers, 1987). They serve multiple purposes in the process of improving quality: gathering information about processes and probable causes of problems, displaying information and testing theories, and monitoring and controlling a process after a remedy has been applied (Plsek, 1991; Plsek, Onnias, & Early, 1989). One such tool, the cause-and-effect diagram, is used to condense a large array of information about processes in an organized way. The ultimate effect (e.g., an adverse event such as medication errors) is at the end of the arrow. Each major antecedent cause is represented by a branch attached to the arrow. Fig-

ure 13.1 is a cause-and-effect diagram portraying the overall process of producing health services.

Finally, both advocates and critics of QI note the special challenges presented by involving professionals—particularly physicians—in QI systems to evaluate clinical processes. Combining general lessons about how to implement innovations in organizations with the special requirements of professionals, Kaluzny, McLaughlin, and Kibbe (1992) advise taking several precautions when designing QI strategy in health care organizations.

- Use physicians' time wisely. Use them as consultants or on subteams that focus on clinical issues needing their expertise. Recognize that their involvement will be episodic and related to specific interests and topics.
- Peak physicians' interests. Capitalize on physicians who are most interested in QI, nurture their involvement, and focus on issues that make them curious.
- Empower physicians' participation. Involve them early on in the process.
- Respect professional values. Avoid statistics and reviews that threaten physicians' competency. Be flexible. Balance the needs for autonomy with the requirements of QI initiatives.

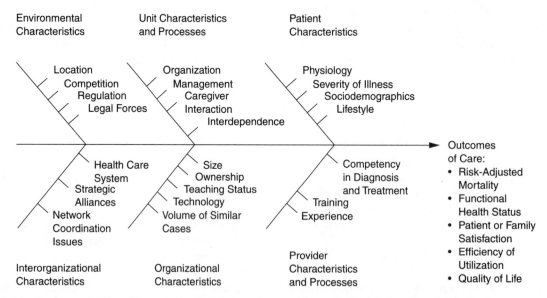

Figure 13.1. Cause-and-Effect Diagram for Continuous Improvement in Health Services Organizations.

DEBATE TIME 13.2: WHAT DO YOU THINK?

Figure 13.1 provides a framework for thinking about quality improvement in health services organizations. Some people believe that the greatest improvement opportunities lie with increasing clinicians' competence and skills. Others believe greater improvement results from changes in the organization and management of patient care units. Still others believe that the quality of care is largely a function of the availability of sophisticated technology or the degree of teaching activity going on. What do you think? Where would you place the most emphasis? What factors, conditions, or variables influence your decision?

• Diagnose and capitalize on which of the four stages of adoption specific units and groups have reached: recognizing a problem in need of a solution, identifying QI as a valued solution, implementing QI strategies related to the problem, or institutionalizing QI thinking and techniques into everyday clinical practice.

THE MANAGER'S ROLE IN CREATING HIGH-PERFORMANCE HEALTH CARE ORGANIZATIONS

The problems in defining and measuring performance, which occur in all organizations, are particularly challenging for health care organizations. This is because, as noted in Chapter 1, the product of health care organizations is frequently difficult to define and measure. In addition, many of the activities that influence the performance of health care organizations are not directly controllable by managers but rather are under the direction of physicians and other health care professionals. Add to this the environmental forces of inflation, regulation, competition, new technology, and changing consumer preferences, and it is no wonder that some have referred to the health care executive's job as attempting to steer a wayward bus down a hill in which physicians control the brakes, and other groups (trustees, third-party payers, etc.) have their foot on the accelerator. Thus it is tempting to wave the white flag and conclude that there is relatively little that managers can do to define, measure, or influence performance. Nothing could be further from the truth.

It is precisely because the task of defining, measuring, and influencing performance is so difficult that

management can play a key role. As discussed in Chapter 4, defining the organization's core values and reasons for being and translating these into operational reality lies at the heart of **transformational leadership.** Transformational leaders think about performance in terms of controllable and noncontrollable factors and constantly work to convert uncontrollable factors into factors that can be controlled. Figure 13.2 provides a continuum of such factors.

As shown, events such as natural disasters, international relations, and national economic policy are relatively uncontrollable by health care executives. In contrast, issues concerning the organization's wage and salary administration, marketing plans, and patient-care policies and practices are, for the most part, directly controllable by executives. In between are factors involving intermediate degrees of control. These include factors largely internal such as the organization's mission and culture, labor mix, and organization design as well as external factors such as system consolidation, growth, and third-party payment trends on the one hand and external regulation, competition, and new technological developments on the other.

A major point of Figure 13.2 is that more effective managers not only focus on variables on the right side of the page that are most directly controllable but also attempt to extend their influence over factors moving to the left, involving health industry trends and external regulatory, competitive, technological, and legal forces. They do this by refusing to accept these forces as givens and viewing them instead as opportunities for expanding their organization's mission and potential effectiveness. For example, many health care companies have

Relatively
Uncontrollable

→

Relatively
Controllable

Natural Disasters	Health Care System	Consolidation	Organizational Mission	Wage and Salary
International Relations	External Regulation	System Growth	and Culture	Administration
National Economic Policy	and Accreditation	Organization Size	Labor Mix	Capital Investment
(e.g., Inflation	New Technological	Ownership Status	Human Resources	Strategy
Unemployment)	Developments	Third-Party Payment	Development	Financial Goals
Population Demographics	Competition	Trends	New Product or New	Marketing Plans
(e.g., Changing Age	Physician Surplus or	Teaching Affiliation	Market Development	Patient Care Policies
Mix of the Population)	Shortage	Medical Staff	Vertical and Horizontal	and Practices
Stock Market	Nurse Surplus or	Organization and	Integration (e.g.,	Problem Identification
Social Problems	Shortage	Characteristics	Acquisitions, Alternative	and Management
(e.g., Riots)	New Legal	Purchaser Demands	Delivery System	Conflict Management
Immigration Patterns	Developments	for Preferential	Development)	Practices
	Societal Preferences	Conditions	Organization Design	QA Practices and
	and Tastes		(e.g., Coordination,	Policies
			Centralization of	
			Decision Making)	

Figure 13.2. Factors Affecting Health Care Organizational Performance Arranged on a Continuum of the Degree to Which Managers Can Exert Control.

developed, on their own or in joint ventures with insurance companies, the ability to provide health insurance services and other third-party financing, which can channel more patients into their delivery system. Many hospitals are changing their size by reducing inpatient bed capacity and converting formerly unused capacity to long-term-care beds or outpatient programs. Nursing homes are rapidly expanding into subacute and rehabilitation services in response to the growth in Medicare managed care.

Other organizations have gained control over new technological developments through linkages with medical schools and research centers and through investment in biomedical and biological product companies. In similar fashion, these organizations are proactive in shaping consumer preferences and tastes through market research and new product-development strategies rather than merely reacting to changes in consumer preferences.

These attempts to broaden the influence base involve macropolitical strategies of networking, coalition building, and joint venturing (see Chapters 9–11 for related discussions). They involve actively managing the environment and not merely managing one's own organization. Priorities must be set, and trade-offs must be made. Nonetheless, all stakehold-

ers would agree that the organization needs to obtain necessary resources (people, money, legitimacy) for its continued existence; to coordinate, manage, and integrate these resources in providing desired services and products; and to achieve a reasonable degree of goal attainment in those areas that are deemed most important. Thus the discussion and guidelines that follow are organized around the issues of acquiring necessary resources, making wise performance trade-offs, and managing a high-performance health care organization for the twenty-first century.

Resource Acquisition

The way in which health care organizations obtain resources has changed radically in the past few years. Philanthropy has declined to the point where it is no longer a major source of support, and much greater emphasis is given to the debt and, for investor-owned organizations, equity markets. At the same time, mergers, consolidations, affiliations, and opportunities to join multihospital systems have enabled many hospitals to obtain resources otherwise not available (Ermann & Gabel, 1984). As a result, it has become increasingly important for health care organizations to have positive operating margins and strong balance sheets regardless of whether they are investor owned or not-for-profit. Overall, **resource acquisition** needs to be more carefully targeted than in the past to conform with the organization's overall strategic plan (see Chapter 14). New areas for strategic growth include same-day surgery, satellite clinics, home health care, diagnostic imaging, ambulatory alcoholism and psychiatric care, health promotion, sports medicine, and related ventures.

The forces listed above have meant a different role in the resource acquisition process for the organization's board of directors. Previously, effective health care organizations selected board members primarily for their ability to provide and maintain rapport with community groups as a linkage to philanthropic sources; today's boards require greater experience and expertise in marketing, finance, risk taking, and entrepreneurship. Taking hospitals as an example, bridges to the community and other links to the external environment are still important, but the linkage requires board members to possess expertise and experience to help hospitals make the transition from acute care inpatient institutions to more diversified health care organizations emphasizing outpatient and primary care. The emphasis shifts from board members being the stewards of the hospital's assets to becoming active builders of a more diversified resource base. This is a particular challenge for rural, inner-city, public, and some university teaching hospitals. These groups face a variety of resource acquisition issues: low occupancy and financial instability (e.g., many rural hospitals), a high percentage of Medicaid and medically indigent patients (e.g., many inner-city and public hospitals), and diminished revenues from state governments coupled with increased competition from surrounding community hospitals (e.g., many teaching hospitals affiliated with state medical schools).

The issues of resource acquisition is particularly important in competitive environments. A study focused on hospitals found that organizations in competitive environments whose boards are entrepreneurial tend to be more successful in obtaining needed resources (money, patients, and staff) than those with boards not so oriented (Barrett & Windham, 1984). This study also suggests that in any environment, whether competitive or noncompetitive, ef-

fectiveness in obtaining resources is increased when there is greater congruence of interests between the CEO and the board chairperson.

Failure of a given organization to attract sufficient resources on its own may result in corporate reorganization, consolidation, merger, affiliation membership, or multihospital system membership. With the exception of internal corporate reorganization, all of these represent to varying degrees a networking strategy designed to attract capital, strengthen political clout, create possible economies of scale, compete for managed care contracts, and perhaps most importantly, achieve integration of clinical services. Failure to successfully negotiate such relationships is likely to result in suboptimal performance and possible closure.

A second important resource acquisition issue involves the ability to recruit and retain physicians, nurses, and related professional staff, which in turn can help attract patients. The existing shortage of primary care physicians represents a major new challenge not only to acquire such staff but potentially to restructure and retrain current staff to meet these needs. To meet this challenge, recruitment efforts need to be carefully targeted. Restructuring efforts may involve nurses playing an even greater role in delivering primary care or some specialists retraining to provide general care. Such restructuring of the professional staff, to be successful, needs to be extra sensitive to issues of control and motivation in professional work (see Chapters 3–5).

Managing Trade-offs

Health care organizations are confronting an increasingly competitive environment in which the public will hold managers accountable not only for the cost of care but for the quality of care provided within their institutions. A natural reaction to this type of demand is to tighten existing controls, define lines of authority, clarify role definitions, and implement a range of performance-evaluation systems. These actions may symbolically fulfill the expectations of those within and outside the organization that somebody is finally taking control. In reality, however, this approach may camouflage serious problems.

What is really needed is a shift in paradigms away from the mechanical model of control based on surveillance, inspection, and discipline to a new model of commitment and a cycle of continuous improvement as previously discussed. Each department in the organization determines who its customers are and what they want. The department then develops systems to meet the needs of its constituent groups and to monitor performance, assuring continuous improvement in the quality of services provided.

Many observers believe that there are inherent trade-offs between efficiency and effectiveness—between containing costs and providing high-quality care. It is felt that attempts to become more efficient and productive will be made at the expense of quality. For example, patients may be discharged too soon, they may receive fewer services, the quality of the services they receive may be reduced, and hospitals may not keep up with the latest technology advances to provide state-of-the-art care. All of these behaviors may indeed erode the quality of care provided as perceived by one group or another.

But a contrasting view may also be taken. Specifically, it is possible that attempts to become more productive and efficient may be associated with improvements in quality. For example, productivity improvements that reduce length of stay may facilitate patient discharge to more appropriate outpatient settings or home environments, which may facilitate the healing process and reduce patients' susceptibility to hospital-acquired infections and illnesses. Fewer tests and procedures reduce the risk of possible side effects and mistakes. It also requires that caregivers be better diagnosticians and provide more focused treatment. Given the lack of evidence supporting strong relationships between process and outcomes of care, it is uncertain how changes in the process of care may affect outcomes, although it is recognized that there are thresholds beyond which outcomes may not improve and may, indeed, even deteriorate. Reductions in the quality of inputs involving patient-care amenities may reduce patient satisfaction but are not likely to affect mortality or functional health status measures. Finally, the fact that not all hospitals will be able to have state-of-the-art technology may actually improve quality by channeling patients to selected high-tech hospitals where more qualified professionals exist to use the technology appropriately and where sufficient volume of cases exist to promote better patient outcomes (Flood et al., 1984; Luft, 1981; Shortell & LoGerfo, 1981).

Which of the scenarios described above is most likely to occur depends on a number of key variables. It would appear that the greatest potential for diminished quality exists in health care organizations that are financially stressed, serve a relatively high percentage of uninsured patients, operate in highly competitive markets, have difficulty recruiting highly qualified staff, and serve a patient population in which there is inadequate home and social support networks.

Existing studies, for the most part, suggest that trade-offs between efficiency and effectiveness need not occur. Some studies find that efficiency is associated with higher quality of care. A common thread underlying these results is effective management. In brief, these organizations have developed many of the management and organization practices discussed in this chapter. For example, several Rochester-area hospitals identified patients who could be tube-fed rather than IV-fed. This resulted in a significant cost reduction while improving patient treatment ("Clinical services improved," 1982). A study of the nursing home industry in New York State revealed that labor-intensive aspects of care involving the quality of nursing and rehabilitation services did not increase costs, perhaps because of careful screening of nurses (which reduces turnover), better staff training, and better coordination (Ullmann, 1985). However, capital-intensive aspects of patient-care quality were associated with higher costs, which is consistent with results from some hospital studies as well.

Existing knowledge regarding the trade-off issue must be viewed with caution. First, it is important to note that almost all of the studies have been done prior to the widespread introduction of Medicare's Prospective Payment System and related incentive-reimbursement arrangements. Thus health organizations were not feeling the pressure to contain cost to the degree they are today. Second, all the studies have been cross-sectional at a single point in time, and thus have not been able to assess the issue of whether a strategy to cut costs at time T1 actually results in a change in quality at time T2. Third, all studies have struggled with the problem of developing valid measures of quality, which adequately take into account the case-mix severity of patients. While great strides have been made, considerable more work needs to be done. Finally, it is important to remember that high cost does not necessarily mean inefficient management but may simply reflect management's desire to provide more amenities to patients and staff, resulting in higher patient and staff satisfaction. More recently, however, the margins for such behavior are being reduced.

It is clear that the trade-off issue will not go away. It places health care managers squarely in the center of the tension between those who view health care primarily as an economic good and those who view it primarily as a social good.

It is also important to recognize that improving the performance of individual health care organizations is not the same as improving an individual's performance or the overall ability of health care systems and communities to deliver cost-effective services. Nonetheless, as the delivery of health care becomes more consolidated both horizontally and vertically, improvements in individual organizational performance are likely to have ripple effects. Conversely, failure to improve performance has pervasive negative effects throughout the system. Thus a major challenge for health care managers in the future lies not only in improving individual organizational performance but in improving the performance of networks, coalitions, affiliations, and systems. In the process, it will be important to remember that there is something wrong with every available measure of performance. Thus effective managers will use many indicators to assess individual, group, organizational, and network performance.

 # MANAGERIAL GUIDELINES

Maintaining and Improving Quality of Care

1. Develop a participative, team-oriented organizational culture that encourages input from professionals and other workers from all levels of the organization.
2. Establish high standards that appeal to professional standards. Link professional values and goals to those of the organization.
3. Develop information systems that provide relevant, timely, and accurate data for purposes of taking corrective action and reaching ever-higher standards. Use statistical thinking and tools to identify desired performance levels, measure current performance, interpret it, and take action when necessary.
4. Look for opportunities to improve quality by detecting and preventing potential problems in the process. Focus on the most important processes to improve.
5. Design work to make the best use of professionals' experience and expertise.

6. Develop reward systems that reinforce participation and high performance. Don't blame individuals for defects in the process.
7. Develop organizational structures that promote communication, coordination, and conflict management.
8. Actively manage the external environment to recruit the best available talent.

Evaluating Professional Work

1. Professionals working in health care organizations are largely self-motivated. Thus setting high standards consistent with professional norms of excellence promotes effectiveness.
2. Any organization requires rules and procedures. In health care organizations, the rules and procedures must be based as much on professional needs, values, and aspirations as on the needs, values, and aspirations of the organization.

(continued)

MANAGERIAL GUIDELINES

3. The professional's need for autonomy must be kept paramount in all organization design decisions.
4. The special needs of professional work demand that flexible mechanisms be used to coordinate such activity.
5. Professionals want to participate in decisions that will affect the professional nature of their work.
6. Increasingly, professionals want to participate in larger issues that will affect the nature of their work in years to come.

Acquiring Resources

1. Boards of directors need to adopt more corporate forms of organization with emphasis given to strategic planning, entrepreneurial, and risk-taking activities.
2. Linkages must be formed with new types of stakeholders, including employers, business coalitions, and special-interest consumer groups.
3. Executives need to make more use of macropolitical strategies involving the negotiation of network relationships, which will form larger resource pools.
4. The effective health care organization needs to become more proactive in managing its environment in order to compete more effectively.
5. The organization needs to become adept at developing specialized market niches and initiating products and services for targeted market segments where sufficient resources exist to gain a distinctive long-run competitive advantage.

6. In order to be effective in the long run, organizations need to learn how to continuously differentiate their product or service relative to competitors.

Improving Productivity and Efficiency

1. Develop accurate, timely, and useful management information systems. Remember that all data are not useful.
2. Concentrate productivity improvement programs in large departments where big payoffs will result.
3. Consider streamlining and consolidating departments and functions.
4. Develop scheduling systems consistent with professional values. Focus on areas where quality can be maintained or even enhanced through better scheduling of staff and support resources.
5. Cross-train staff to gain greater flexibility.
6. Develop productivity-based incentives based on work activities under the control of organizational members.
7. Set high standards by establishing "best practices" in one's own organization as well as using comparisons from competitors and industry leaders.
8. Involve organizational members, particularly professionals, in the development, implementation, and monitoring of productivity and efficiency initiatives.
9. Focus energy on working smarter, not necessarily harder.

Discussion Questions

1. Take the perspective of an HMO executive. Describe three major ways that you could manage the HMO plan to improve the access, quality, and cost containment for your patients. Critique your solutions regarding the extent to which your solutions may cause other problems to surface (what kind?) and the extent to which you as a CEO could (or should) have the power to accomplish these changes.

2. Using a health care organization that you know well, provide three examples each of possible structural, process, and outcome measures of effectiveness. Would you expect these measures to be highly associated? Why or why not?
3. Consider a community hospital, a major teaching hospital, and an HMO. For each, list the major constituency groups (both internal and external). Indicate what kinds of effectiveness criteria each group would be most likely to promote.

4. Hospital A and Hospital B both have as their major goal for this year the implementation of a QI program. Hospital A hired a consultant firm and sent its top managers to a program to learn how to change the corporate culture and to set up quality teams to investigate problems. They formed teams to plan strategies of meaningful QI in two specific areas: billing and use of the emergency room. Hospital B, lacking funds, tried to have study groups and use self-teaching but involved everyone from the CEO to the janitor. Which hospital do you think will succeed in implementing QI? Why?

5. Clinic Q was a large multispecialty group practice with a major emphasis on specialist care. Because they were worried about not having enough referrals for specialist care, their major goal for the year was to set up two new branches of primary care providers. To attract primary care providers, they discovered that they had to offer salaries higher than the average salary of other physicians at the clinic. Start-up costs were also high. Using concepts such as strategic planning, effectiveness, productivity, and efficiency, discuss how to evaluate whether this expansion was a "success" for the organization.

References

Aaronson, W. E., Zinn, J. S., & Rosko, M. D. (1994). Do for-profit and not-for-profit nursing homes behave differently? *Gerontologist, 34,* 775–786.

Aiken, L. H., Sochalski, J., & Lake, E. T. (1997). Studying outcomes of organizational change in health services. *Medicare Care, 35,* NS6–NS18.

Alexander, J. A., Morrisey, M. A., & Shortell, S. M. (1986, September). The effects of competition regulation and corporatization on hospital-physician relationships. *Journal of Health and Social Behavior, 27,* 220–235.

Alexander, J. A., & Rundall, T. G. (1985, March). Public hospitals under contract management: An assessment of operating performance. *Medical Care, 23,* 209–219.

Argyris, C. (1982). *Reasoning, learning, and action.* San Francisco: Jossey-Bass.

Barr, J. K., & Steinberg, M. (1983, Spring). Professional participation in organizational decision making: Physicians in HMOs. *Journal of Community Health, 8*(3), 160–173.

Barrett, D., & Windham, S. R. (1984, Fall). Hospital boards and adaptability to competitive environments. *Health Care Management Review,* 11–20.

Batalden, P. B., & Buchanan, E. D. (1989). Industry models of quality improvement. In N. Goldfield, & D. B. Nash (Eds.), *Providing quality care: The challenge to clinicians.* Philadelphia: American College of Surgeons.

Berle, A. A., & Means, G. C. (1932). *The modern corporation and private property.* New York: Macmillan.

Berwick, D. M. (1991, Summer). Blazing the trail of quality: The HFHS quality management process. *Frontiers of Health Services Management, 7*(4), 47–50.

Berwick, D. M., Godfrey, A. B., & Roessner, J. (1991). *Curing health care: New strategies for quality improvement.* San Francisco: Jossey-Bass.

Borbas, C., Stump, M. A., Dedecker, K. et al. (1990, February). The Minnesota Clinical Comparison and Assessment Project. *Quality Review Bulletin, 16,* 87–92.

Bradford, D. L., & Cohen, A. R. (1984). *Managing for excellence.* New York: John Wiley & Sons.

Brook, R. H., & Lohr, K. N. (1985). Efficacy, effectiveness, variations and quality: Boundary-crossing research. *Medical Care, 23,* 710–722.

Burnham, J. (1941). *The managerial revolution.* New York: John Day.

Burns, J. M. (1978). *Leadership.* New York: Harper & Row.

Cameron, K., & Whetten, D. A. (1981). Perceptions of organizational effectiveness across organizational life cycles. *Administrative Science Quarterly, 26,* 525–544.

Camp, R. C. (1989). *Benchmarking: The search for industry best practices that lead to superior practices.* Milwaukee, WI: American Society for Quality Control, Quality Press.

Campbell, J. P. (1977). On the nature of organizational effectiveness. In P. S. Goodman, & J. M. Pennings (Eds.), *New perspectives on organizational effectiveness.* San Francisco: Jossey-Bass.

Choi, T., Allison, R. F., & Munson, F. (1986). *Governance and management of university hospitals: External forces and internal processes.* Ann Arbor, MI: Health Administration Press.

Cleverly, W. O. (1981). Financial ratios: Summary indicators for management decision making. *Hospital and Health Services Administration, 26*, 26–47.

Clinical services improved. (1982, July/August). *Human-size hospital economics.* Beverly Hills, CA: American Medical International, p. 4.

Cohen, S. N., Flood, A. B., Himmelberger, D. U., Mangini, R. J., & Moore, T. N. (1980). *Development, implementation, and evaluation of the monitoring and evaluation of drug interactions by a pharmacy oriented report system (MEDIPHOR) HS00739.* (Final Report to the National Center for Health Services Research). Springfield, VA: National Technical Information Service.

Connor, R. A., Feldman, R. D., Dowd, B. E., & Radcliff, T. A. (1997). Which types of hospital mergers save consumers money? *Health Affairs, 16*(6), 62–74.

Coyne, J. S. (1982, Winter). Hospital performance in multi-hospital systems: A comparative study of system and independent hospitals. *Health Services Research, 17*, 303–329.

Crosby, P. B. (1979). *Quality is free.* New York: New American Library.

Cyert, R. M., & March, J. G. (1966). *A behavioral theory of the firm.* Englewood Cliffs, NJ: Prentice-Hall.

Deming, W. E. (1986). *Out of the crisis.* Cambridge, MA: Massachusetts Institute of Technology.

Donabedian, A. (1966). Evaluating the quality of medical care. *Milbank Memorial Fund Quarterly, 44*(2), 166–206.

Dornbusch, S. M., Scott, W. R., with Busching, B. C., & Laing, J. D. (1975). *Evaluation and the exercise of authority.* San Francisco: Jossey-Bass.

Dyck, F. J., Murphy, F. A., Murphy, J. K., Road, D. A., Boyd, M. S. et al. (1977). The effect of surveillance on the number of hysterectomies in the province of Saskatchewan. *New England Journal of Medicine, 296*, 1326–1328.

Eisenberg, J. M. (1986). *Doctors' decisions and the cost of medical care: The reasons for doctors' practice and ways to change them.* Ann Arbor, MI: Health Administration Press Perspective.

Ermann, D., & Grabel, J. (1984). "Multihospital systems: Issues and empirical findings: *Health Affairs,* 18:585–596.

Fennell, M. L., & Alexander, J. A. (1989). Governing boards and profound organizational change in hospitals. *Medical Care Review, 46*, 157–187.

Fifer, W. R. (1983). Integrating quality assurance mechanisms. In R. D. Luke, J. C. Krueger, & R. E. Modrow (Eds.), *Organization and change in health care quality assurance.* Rockville, MD: Aspen System Corporation.

Fleming, G. V. (1981). Hospital structure and consumer satisfaction. *Health Services Research, 16*, 43–64.

Flood, A. B. (1994). The impact of organizational and managerial factors on the quality of care in health care organizations. *Medical Care Review, 51*(4), 381–428.

Flood, A. B., & Fennell, M. L. (1995). Through the lenses of organizational sociology: The role of organizational theory and research in conceptualizing and examining our health care system. *Journal of Health and Social Behavior, 36*, 154–169.

Flood, A. B., Fremont, A. M., Jin, K. et al. (1998). How do HMOs achieve their savings? The effectiveness of one organization's strategies. *Health Services Research, 33*(1), 79–99.

Flood, A. B., & Scott, W. R. (1987). *Hospital structure and performance.* Baltimore: Johns Hopkins Press.

Flood, A. B., Scott, W. R., Ewy, W. (1984, February). Does practice make perfect? Part I: The relationship between hospital volume and outcomes for select diagnostic categories. *Medical Care, 22*, 98–114.

Friedman, B., & Shortell, S. M. (1988). The financial performance of selected investor-owned and not-for-profit system hospitals before and after Medicare prospective payment. *Health Services Research, 23*, 237–267.

Georgopoulos, B. S., & Mann, F. C. (1962). *The community general hospital.* New York: Macmillan.

Goldberg, R. K. (1998). Regaining public trust: A health executive's top-ten list of things HMOs must do to regain the public's long-lost trust in health care. *Health Affairs, 17*(6), 138–141.

Haberstroh, C. J. (1965). Organization design and systems analysis. In J. G. March (Ed.), *Handbook of organizations* (p. 1182). Chicago: Rand McNally.

Hall, M. A. (1988). Institutional control of physician behavior: Legal barriers to health care cost containment. *University of Pennsylvania Law Review, 137,* 431–536.

Heatherington, R. W. (1982). Quality assurance and organizational effectiveness in hospitals. *Health Services Research, 17,* 185–201.

Hornbrook, M. C., & Berki, S. E. (1985). Practice mode and payment method: Effects on use, costs, quality and access. *Medical Care, 23*(5), 484–511.

Institute of Medicine. (1986). *For profit enterprise in health care.* Washington, DC: National Academy Press.

Ishikawa, K. (1985). *What is total quality control?* Englewood Cliffs, NJ: Prentice-Hall.

Jessee, W. F. (1984). Quality assurance systems: Why aren't there any? *Quality Review Bulletin, 10,* 408–411.

Juran, J. M. (Ed.). (1988). *Juran's quality control handbook* (4th ed.). New York: McGraw-Hill.

Kaluzny, A. D. (1990, April). The role of management in quality assurance: The case of Smith vs. ACE Management Company. *Quality Review Bulletin,* 134–137.

Kaluzny, A. D., McLaughlin, C. P., & Kibbe, D. C. (1992). Continuous quality improvement in the clinical setting: Enhancing adoption. *Quality Management in Health Care, 1,* 37–44.

Kanter, R. M. (1981). Organizational performance: Recent developments in measurement. *Annual Review of Sociology, 7,* 321.

Keeler, E. B., Kahn, K. L., Draper, D. M. et al. (1990). Changes in sickness at admission following the introduction of the Prospective Payment System. *Journal of American Medical Association, 264,* 1962–1968.

Keeler, R. B., Chapin, A. M., & Soule, D. N. (1990). Informed inquiry into practice variations: The Maine Medical Assessment Foundation. *Quality Assurance in Health Care, 2,* 69–75.

Keeler, R. B., Soule, D. N., Wennberg, J. E., & Hanley, D. F. (1990). Dealing with geographic variations in the use of hospitals: The experience of the Maine Medical Assessment Foundation Orthopedic Study Group. *Journal of Bone and Joint Surgery, 72*(A), 1286–1293.

Kerr, S. (1975). On the folly of rewarding A while hoping for B. *Academy of Management Journal, 18,* 769–783.

Kimberly, J. R., & Miles, R. H. (Eds.). (1980). *The organizational life cycle.* San Francisco: Jossey-Bass.

Kind, E. A., Fowles, J., & McCoy, C. E. (1987, September). *Effectiveness of the primary profile in changing physician practice styles.* Presented at the American Medical Review Research Center Annual Meetings, Washington, DC.

Komaroff, A. L. (1985). Quality assurance in 1984. *Medical Care, 23,* 723–738.

Landau, M. (1973). On the concept of a self-correcting organization. *Public Administration Review, 33,* 533–542.

Luft, H. S. (1981). *Health maintenance organizations: Dimensions of performance.* New York: John Wiley & Sons.

Luft, H. S., Granick, D. W., Mark, D. H., & McPhee, S. J. (Eds.). (1990). *Hospital volume, physician volume and patient outcomes: Assessing the evidence.* Ann Arbor, MI: Health Administration Press.

Luke, R. D., Krueger, J. C., & Modrow, R. E. (1983). *Organization and change in health care quality assurance.* Rockville, MD: Aspen System Corporation.

Managing Hospital Marketing at AMI. (1984, June). Beverly Hills, CA: American Medical International.

McCoy, C. E., Kind, E. A., Fowles, J., & Schned, E. S. (1987). Measuring quality in an HMO: The primary care practice profile. In *Managing quality health care in a dynamic era* (pp. 112–117). Washington, DC: The Group Health Association of America.

Mechanic, D. (1998). The functions and limitations of trust in the provision of medical care. *Journal of Health Politics, Policy and Law, 23*(4), 661–686.

Medicare: Improving quality of care assessment and assurance: Report to the Chairman, Subcommittee on Health, Committee on Ways and Means, House of Representatives. (1988). (GAO/PEMD-88-10). Washington, DC: US General Accounting Office.

Menke, T. J. (1997). The effect of chain membership on hospital costs. *Health Services Research, 32*(2), 177–196.

Miller, R. H., & Luft, H. S. (1994). Managed care plan performance since 1980. *Journal of the American Medical Association, 271*(19), 1512–1519.

Mittman, B. S., & Siv, A. L. (1992). Changing provider behavior: Applying research on outcomes and effectiveness in health care. In S. M. Shortell, & U. E. Reinhardt (Eds.), *Improving health policy and management.* Baxter Health Policy Review, Ann Arbor, MI: Health Administration Press.

Moss, M., & Adams, C. (1998, April 7). For Medicaid patients, doors slam closed; Langreth R. After seeing profits from the poor, some HMOs abadon them. *The Wall Street Journal* (Eastern Edition) p. B1.

Nauert, R. C. (1996). The quest for value in health care. *Journal of Health Care Finance, 22*(3), 52–61.

Nelson, E. C., Mohr, J. J., Batalden, P. B., & Plume, S. K. (1996). Improving health care, Part 1: The clinical value compass. *The Joint Commission Journal on Quality Improvement, 22*(4), 243–258.

Nerenz, D. R., & Zajac, B. M. (1991). *Indicators of performance for vertically integrated health systems: Final report of 1990 Ray Woodham Visiting Fellowship.* Detroit, MI: Center for Health System Studies, Henry Ford Health System.

Ohsfeldt, R. L. (1993). Contractual arrangements, financial incentives, and physician-patient relationships. In J. M. Clair and R. M. Allman (Eds.), *Sociomedical perspectives on patients' care.* Lexington, KY: University of Kentucky Press.

Pauly, M. V., Hillman, A. L., & Kerstein, J. (1990). Managing physician incentives in managed care: The role of for-profit ownership. *Medical Care, 28,* 1013–1024.

Peters, T. K., & Waterman, R. A., Jr. (1982). *In search of excellence.* New York: Harper & Row.

Plsek, P. E. (1991). Resource B: A primer on quality improvement tools. In D.M. Berwick, A.B. Godfrey, & J. Roessner (Eds.), *Curing health care: New strategies for quality improvement.* San Francisco: Jossey-Bass.

Plsek, P. E., Onnias, A., & Early, J. F. (1989). *Quality improvement tools.* Wilton, CN: Juran Institute.

Roberts, J. S. (1992). Peer review and continuous quality improvement. In *Bridging the gap between theory and practice.* Chicago: Hospital Research and Educational Trust.

Rosen, H. M., & Feigin, W. (1982). Medical peer review and information management: The deadend phenomenon. *Health Care Management Review, 7,* 59–66.

Rosko, M. D., Chilingerian, J. A., Zinn, J. S., & Aaronson, W. E. (1995). The effects of ownership, operating environment, and strategic choices on nursing home efficiency. *Medical Care, 33,* 1001–1021.

Sahney, V. K. (1992). Implementation, observed barriers, and management of continuous quality improvement (CQI). In *Bridging the gap between theory and practice: Exploring continuous quality improvement.* Chicago: Hospital Research and Educational Trust.

Scott, W. R. (1977). Effectiveness of organizational effectiveness studies. In P.S. Goodman, & J.M. Pennings (Eds.), *New perspectives on organizational effectiveness.* San Francisco: Jossey-Bass.

Scott, W. R. (1982). Managing professional work: Three models of control for health organizations. *Health Services Research, 17,* 213–240.

Scott, W. R. (1993). The organization of medical care services: Toward an integrated model. *Medical Care Review, 50,* 271–304.

Senge, P. (1990). *The fifth discipline: The art and practice of the learning organization.* New York: Free Press.

Shanahan, M. (1983). The quality assurance standard of the JCAH: A rational approach to patient care evaluation. In R. D. Luke, J. C. Krueger, & R. E. Modrow (Eds.), *Organization and change in health care quality assurance.* Rockville, MD: Aspen Systems Corporation.

Shortell, S. M. (1983). Physician involvement in hospital decision-making. In B. Gray (Ed.), *The new health care for profit: Doctors and hospitals in a competitive environment* (pp. 73–102). Washington, DC: National Academy Press, Institute of Medicine.

Shortell, S. M. (1985, July-August). High performing health care organizations. Guidelines for the pursuit of excellence. *Hospital and Health Services Administration, 30,* 7–35.

Shortell, S. M., Becker, S. W., & Neuhauser, D. (1976). The effects of management practices on hospital efficiency and quality of care. In S. M. Shortell, & M. Brown (Eds.), *Organizational research and hospitals.* Chicago: Blue Cross Association.

Shortell, S. M., Gillies, R. R., Anderson, D. A. et al. (1996). *Remaking health care in America: Building organized delivery systems.* San Francisco: Jossey-Bass.

Shortell, S. M., & LoGerfo, J. P. (1981, October). Hospital medical staff organization and quality of care: Results for myocardial infarction and appendectomy. *Medical Care, 19,* 1041–1055.

Shortell, S. M., Morrisey, M. A., & Conrad, D. (1985, December). Economic regulation and hospital behavior: The effects on medical staff organization and hospital-physician relationships. *Health Services Research, 20,* 597–627.

Shortell, S. M., Morrison, E. M., & Friedman, B. (1990). *Strategic choices for America's hospital: Managing change in turbulent times.* San Francisco: Jossey-Bass.

Shortell, S. M., Waters, J. M., Clarke, K. W. P., & Budetti, P. P. (1998). Physicians as double agents: Maintaining trust in an era of multiple accountabilities. *Journal of the American Medical Association, 280*(12), 1102–1108.

Shortell, S. M., Wickizer, T. M., & Wheeler, J. R. C., Jr. (1984). *Hospital-physician joint ventures: Results and lessons from a national demonstration in primary care.* Ann Arbor, MI: Health Administration Press.

Shortell, S. M., Zimmerman, J. E., Gillies, R. R. et al. (1990, May). Continuously improving patient care: Practical lessons and an assessment tool from the National ICU Study. *Quality Review Bulletin, 5,* 150–155.

Sloan, F., & Becker, E. (1981). Internal organization of hospitals and hospital costs. *Inquiry, 18,* 224–240.

Steers, R. M. (1975). Problems in the measurement of organizational effectiveness. *Administrative Science Quarterly, 20,* 546.

Stewart, W. A. (1986). *Statistical method from the viewpoint of quality control.* New York: Dover Publications.

SUPPORT: Study to Understand Prognosis, Preferences for Outcomes, Risks, and Treatment project. (1990). *Journal of Clinical Epidemiology, 43.*

Their, S. O., & Gelijns, A. C. (1998). Improving health: The reason performance measurement matters. *Health Affairs, 17*(4), 26–28.

Ullmann, S. G. (1985). The impact of quality on cost in the provision of long-term care. *Inquiry, 22*(3), 293–302.

Vuori, H. (1980). Optimal and logical quality: Two neglected aspects of quality of health services. *Medical Care, 18,* 975–985.

Wasson, J. H. (Ed.). (1998). Special issue of *The Journal of Ambulatory Care Management, 21*(3), 1–59.

Weick, K. E. (1977). Re-punctuating the problem. In P. S. Goodman and J.M. Pennings (Eds.), *New perspectives on organizational effectiveness.* San Francisco: Jossey-Bass.

Weisman, C. S., & Nathanson, C. A. (1985, October). Professional satisfaction and client outcomes: A comparative organizational analysis. *Medical Care, 23,* 1179–1192.

Wennberg, J. E., Blowers, L., Parker, P., & Gittelsohn, A. M. (1977). Changes in tonsillectomy rates associated with feedback and review. *Pediatrics, 59,* 821–826.

Westphal, J. D., Gulati, R., & Shortell, S. M. (1997). Customization or conformity? An institutional and network perspective on the content and consequences of TQM adoption. *Administrative Science Quarterly, 42,* 366–394.

Wheeler, D. J., & Chambers, D. S. (1987). *Understanding statistical process control.* Knoxville, TN: Statistical Process Controls.

Williamson, J. M. (1988). Future policy directions for quality assurance: Lessons from the health accounting experience. *Inquiry, 25,* 67–77.

Wones, R. G. (1987). Failure of low-cost audits with feedback to reduce laboratory test utilization. *Medical Care, 25,* 78–82.

Wu, A.W., Folkman, S., McPhee, S. J., & Lo, B. (1991). Do house officers learn from their mistakes? *Journal of American Medical Association; 265*(16), 2090.

Wyszewianski, L. (1988). The emphasis is on measurement in quality assurance: Reasons and implications. *Inquiry, 25,* 424–436.

Zinn, J. S. (1994). Market competition and the quality of nursing home care. *Journal of Health Politics, Policy & Law, 19,* 555–582.

Zinn, J. S., Aaronson, W. E., & Rosko, M. D. (1993a). The use of standardized indicators as quality improvement tools: An application in Pennsylvania nursing homes. *American Journal of Medical Quality, 8,* 72–78.

Zinn, J. S., Aaronson, W. E., & Rosko, M. D. (1993b). Variations in the outcomes of care provided in Pennsylvania nursing homes. Facility and environmental correlates. *Medical Care, 31,* 475–487.

Zuckerman, H. S. (1979). Multi-institutional systems: Their promise and performance. In H. Zuckerman, & L. E. Weeks (Eds.), *Multi-institutional hospital systems.* Chicago: Hospital Research and Educational Trust.

PART

5

Charting the Future

THE NATURE OF ORGANIZATIONS: FRAMEWORK FOR THE TEXT

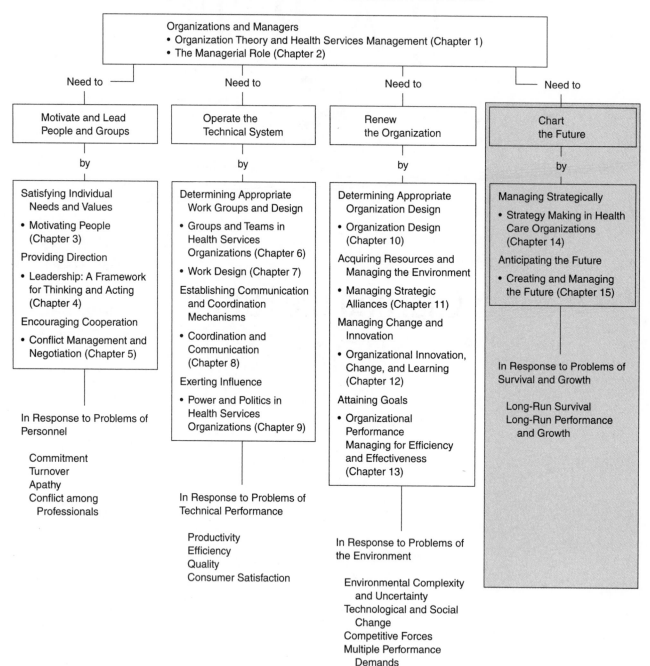

Organizations are components of a larger environment and are influenced by an unfolding series of events over time. Success of an organization depends upon its ability to chart the future given the events of time. The two chapters in this section highlight a number of future trends that will influence health care and various approaches to manage the organization given these trends.

Chapter 14, "Strategy Making in Health Care Organizations," focuses on the idea of strategic management and how the principles of strategic management can increase the effectiveness of the organization in its changing environment. Specifically, the chapter addresses the following questions:

- What is strategic management, and how does it relate to competitive advantage, corporate structure, and market structure?
- What are the major structural features of markets and market structure, and how does this affect the development of a management strategy?
- What strategic models are available, and how might they be used within the health care setting?

The last chapter, "Creating and Managing the Future," identifies the major trends likely to affect the delivery of health care over the next decade. Attention is given to understanding the changing role of health care providers and, specifically, the challenges facing management. Questions include:

- What larger societal forces are shaping the health care system?
- How are the changing roles of physicians, nurses, and other health professionals likely to influence the delivery of health care?
- What are the major future challenges to health care managers?

Upon completing these final two chapters, readers should be able to identify the major trends likely to affect the operations of health services organizations and the strategic approaches required to meet these challenges over the next decade.

CHAPTER

14

Strategy Making in Health Care Organizations

Roice D. Luke, Ph.D.
James W. Begun, Ph.D.
Stephen L. Walston, Ph.D.

Chapter Outline

- Strategic Management
- Strategy
- Market Structure

Learning Objectives

After completing this chapter, the reader should be able to:

1. Define the concepts of strategic management, strategy, competitive advantage, and market structure.

2. Understand the major schools of thought in strategic management and how these address different components of strategic management.

3. Comprehend the effect of environmental turbulence on strategy.

4. Understand the major sources of competitive advantage, including some of the major types of strategy identified with each source.

5. Understand the relationship between strategy and the formation of complex organizations in health care.

6. Understand the major structural features of markets and their relationships to and effects on strategy and be able to apply these to the analysis of strategy.

7. Identify the major sources of threat in the Porter framework and be able to use these in conducting strategy analysis.

8. Gain insight into how strategy and strategy analysis applies to real markets and organizations in the health care industry.

Key Terms

Absolute Power
Acquisition
Buyer Threats
Competitive Advantage
Concentration
Consolidation
Countervailing Power
Declining Market
Emerging Market
Entrant Threats
Entry Barrier
Fragmented Market
Four-Firm Ratio
Growth/share Matrix
Herfindahl-Hirschman Index (HHI)
Horizontal Expansion
Horizontal Integration
Hybrid Organization
Industrial Organization
Market Share
Market Structure
Mature Market
Merger
Monopolistic Market
Niche Strategy
Oligopolistic Market
Pace Strategy
Performance Strategy
Porter Model
Portfolio Strategy
Position Strategy
Potential Strategy
Power Strategy
Relative Power
Rival Threats
Seller Threats
Strategic Alliance
Strategic Management
Strategy
Substitution Threats
Synergies
Vertical Integration

At first glance, the health care and grocery store industries would appear to be very different from one another. However, they do share some common characteristics. For one, both industries engage in retail enterprise and both provide products and services that meet very basic needs of the public. Perhaps more notably, they share a significant strategic reality—in both, small local firms compete successfully against larger, regionally, and nationally distributed rivals. The "In the Real World" illustrates clearly how one local supermarket chain (Ukrops) has dominated its market, even in the face of competition from powerful regional (Food Lion) and national (Safeway) firms. Similarly, we have observed in the decade of the 1990s how locally organized health care providers have competed with considerable success against larger regional and national provider systems and managed care companies. And even the larger systems are now emphasizing local market strategies, thereby gaining many of the same advantages of the locally organized health care systems.

In view of its inherent advantages, the health care industry in the 1990s elevated the strategy of local system building to the level of a major paradigm. There emerged in the industry a near consensus that a powerful new set of rules dictated how health care should be organized, financed, and delivered. It was widely believed that survival would depend heavily on the ability of providers to arrange themselves into comprehensive delivery systems that spanned all geographic sectors of local markets. Also, in some final and ideal stage, hospitals and physicians would join forces and together integrate vertically with payors. Because of its importance, the new paradigm generated an ever-expanding lexicon, which included such terms as integrated delivery systems, seamless delivery, single signature contracting, vertical integration, one-stop shopping, and integrated networks. Significantly, belief in the paradigm spurred widespread market restructuring, as health care providers translated its underlying concepts into specific market strategies.

With the passage of a few years, the paradigm has undergone considerable rethinking. Indeed, the field now appears to recognize a central lesson of strategy

IN THE REAL WORLD:
FROM GROCERIES TO GURNIES—LEARNING FROM THE GROCERY STORE BUSINESS

In 1937, Joe and Ldevia Ukrop opened their first 16-by-32-foot grocery store. Those were difficult times in the general economy, so to survive they gave high priority to customer service. They readily gave credit to shoppers and developed an active delivery service. Having been successful with their special blend of quality products and personal service, the Ukrops enlarged their small store in 1942 to 3,000 square feet, thereby becoming Richmond, Virginia's, first independent, full self-service grocery store. During the ensuing 20 years, they expanded their store still further, added new management staff, and became one of the highest volume supermarkets in the Richmond metropolitan area.

Then came a major change in the Ukrops strategy. In 1963, realizing that they had a winning formula for success, they opened a second store. Within the next 10 years, they added three more stores, one of which was their first move north of the James River (an important geographic barrier that historically has divided the core of Richmond from important suburbs to the south).

The Ukrops company now has 25 food stores, a central bakery, a central kitchen, a downtown café (Ukrop's Fresh Express), a uniform shop (Ukrop's Dress Express), and pharmacies in 15 of their stores. Ukrop's has also added a full-service cleaner to many of its newer locations and is in the process of incorporating full-service banking (First Market Bank) in each of its stores. Importantly, Ukrops recently opened one of its superstores in Fredericksburg, a community located just 60 miles to the north of Richmond. It is also planning stores to the west in Charlottesville and to the east in Williamsburg. These moves outside Richmond represent a major strategic redirection for this local supermarket chain.

The stated vision of Ukrops is ". . . to be a world-class provider of food and services." Its mission is ". . . to serve our customers and community efficiently and effectively while treating our customers, associates, and suppliers as we personally like to be treated. We will achieve profitable growth and long-term financial success while promoting an atmosphere of mutual trust, honesty and integrity." There is every indication that this vision and mission are deeply imbedded within the company's culture, as well as its strategy for gaining competitive advantage.

In the Richmond metropolitan area, Ukrops has established a clear leadership position in the market. As a local chain, it has been able to compete with their larger regional and national competitors (for example, in recent years it has driven Safeways and Farm Fresh out of the market). They have done this by combining a strategy of local market dominance with a strong position for service and quality, excellent internal competencies, efficient and innovative management, and a well-trained and highly loyal staff. Today Ukrops is broadly recognized for its high level of customer service and product quality. In recent surveys of shopper attitudes, Ukrops consistently ranked at the very top on all quality and service-oriented measures (e.g., friendliness of personnel, attractiveness of interiors, quality of meats and produce, cleanliness, convenience, selection, speed of check-out service, value, orderliness of arrangements). Ukrops is also distinguished by its own particular brand of family values—it remains closed on Sundays, does not sell alcohol products or lottery tickets, offers financial incentives in support of local charities, and promotes church attendance.

But the family orientation of this local company does not mean that it has been cautious in its strategic maneuvering. Ukrops has consistently led competitors in the introduction of new product and service innovations, such as scanning, Valued Customer Cards (discount cards), and a wide variety of on-site prepared food and other new product lines. Their in-store food parks (a form of vertical integration) have successfully captured a significant share of the restaurant business in Richmond. With its combination of customer orientation, aggressive innovation, and persistent growth, Ukrops has moved from a market share of 23% 10 years ago to a share of over 30% in the mid-1990s. Clearly, Ukrops has become a dominant player in a single market and is gradually becoming a regional competitor as well.

The achievements of Ukrops have not come easily, nor is a similar pattern of growth guaranteed in the future. One national competitor—Food Lion, a $10-billion company with over 1,000 stores located in 11 states—has staked out a clear low-cost position, causing Ukrops to experiment with both high-quality/service and low-price positions. The key to Food Lion's success has been its ability to establish low-price positions in most of its markets. Through a strategy of rapid growth, it has been able to capture all-important economies of scale. Food Lion claims that when it moves into an area, it causes prices to lower in that area by as much as 15% (via strong price competition thereby stimulated). To do this, Food Lion has aggressively introduced management, production, and delivery strategies including computerized management of energy, labor controls, avoidance of promotional gimmicks, and use of its own fleet of trucks that are designed for fuel efficiency. It has also maintained the practice of expanding only on its geographic margins, emphasizing the need to reduce the costs of transportation and coordination.

A recent competitor (filling the void left by Safeways and Farm Fresh) is Hannaford's, a rapidly growing $3-billion company that has nearly 150 stores located in eight Eastern states. Hannaford is positioned fairly close to Ukrops in terms of quality and service, thus emerging as a strong direct competitor and one that can draw on some significant economies of scale.

In addition to a few grocery store competitors in the area that hold relatively small market shares, Ukrops' leading position in the market is being threatened by big discount stores, especially by the recently entered discount shopping clubs that offer bulk purchases of food products at very low prices.

As Ukrops looks to the future, it will need to assess how, as a relatively small local firm, it can maintain or even expand its current position of dominance. It will also need to consider whether its strong quality and service positions and pattern of aggressively introducing market innovations will hold up under the stress of price competition, the continuing threats of major regional and national companies, and a cloudy economy. And finally, it will need to learn how to compete on a regional basis, an approach to strategy with which it has little experience.

making—that rarely will one grand idea about how to achieve competitive advantage fit all competitors. A great many strategic options are available to health care organizations, ranging from refining internal infrastructures, to building integrated systems, to repositioning in order to attract desired patient populations. And which of these is best will depend on an organization's capabilities and the particulars of its market structure. Also, in a rapidly changing environment—such as currently exists within the health care industry—selecting optimal strategies becomes all the more challenging, uncertain, and unique to individual circumstances.

The purpose of this chapter is not to answer the question of which strategy is best for individual organizations, but to provide the conceptual foundations needed for one to answer that question.

We do this in three steps. First, we discuss strategic management, drawing on Mintzberg's interpretation of the major schools of thought. Second, we introduce the concept of strategy, how it ties to an organization's mission, the marketplace, and internal competencies. We suggest that individual strategies are defined by how competitive advantage is pursued. Third, we explore the dimensions of market structure as well as some of the important interrelationships that exist between strategy and market structure. Along the way, we weigh the various approaches to achieving competitive advantage in light of the dramatic changes taking place in health care markets. It should become clear that individual health care organizations face very distinctive strategic challenges, depending upon the structures and unique conditions of their local markets.

STRATEGIC MANAGEMENT

Strategic management oversees the formulation, implementation, and monitoring of strategy and, as such, involves both internal and external management functions. First, it is intensely internal in its orientation. Effective strategic management requires the extensive participation of an organization's leaders. Top management typically play key roles in conceptualizing and interrelating strategy with organizational goals, missions, and visions, as well as implementing and evaluating strategy. They integrate strategy with internal support functions, the organization's culture, and the motivations of key personnel. And they may even determine that organizational power and interorganizational relationships need to be restructured. We note that many of the underlying concepts of strategic management have been covered in other chapters in this book. For example, Chapter 10 discusses essential concepts of organization design; Chapter 4, the shaping of a supporting culture; and Chapter 11, the design of strategic alliances.

Strategic management is also highly external in its orientation, thereby distinguishing it from most other managerial processes. It focuses on how to survive in market environments, counter threats from rivals, and assure the patronage of valued consumers. It requires organizations to reach well beyond their boundaries, assess competitors, anticipate the future, and predict what market responses will best ensure that they gain competitive advantage in the long term.

Strategic management is unique among managerial processes in that it is at times militant in its orientation. It deals with the tactics of winning territory and defeating enemies. Indeed, its roots can be traced to the maneuvers of war and thus extend as far back as the antiquities (Bracker, 1980; Wing, 1988). Quinn (1988), for example, reached back to 338 B.C. for insights, to the stratagems of Philip and his son Alexander, who attempted to free Macedonia from the influence of the Greeks and themselves to dominate the northern part of Greece. On the other hand, one need not go quite so far back to discover its managerial origins (Montgomery & Porter, 1991). While the rudiments of business strategy appeared very early in the management literature, the fundamentals took root in the mid-1950s through the mid-1960s. Important early works included three books written respectively by Drucker (1954), Chandler (1962), and Ansoff (1965). Despite a clear military pedigree and a growing business literature, strategic management is a very young field, a field that is still in considerable flux and evolution.

While not coined by them, the concept of strategic management received considerable prominence when Shendel and Hofer (1979) proclaimed it the new paradigm for the field of business policy:

> Today, the policy field is in need of a new paradigm that can end the continual and pointless redefinition of concepts used in both practice and teaching. . . . The new paradigm we propose . . . is that of "Strategic Management," and it rests squarely on the concept of strategy.

Strategic management, they explained, involves those entrepreneurial processes that may lead, ultimately, to organizational growth and renewal. They identified six such processes in their groundbreaking work: (1) goal formation, (2) environmental analysis, (3) strategy formulation, (4) strategy evaluation, (5) strategy implementation, and (6) strategic control. In the ensuing years, the number of processes has been expanded and contracted many times. Nevertheless, all formulations link the external analyses of competitors and markets to the internal adjustments organizations must make to implement strategy.

Schools of Thought

In an attempt to synthesize the literature on strategic management, Mintzberg (1990) conceptualized 10 schools of thought. These schools, he suggested, can be grouped into those that are prescriptive, emphasizing how strategies *should* be formulated, and those that are descriptive, characterizing how strategies *actually* are made. Table 14.1 summarizes the 10 schools identified by Mintzberg. Among these, the three prescriptive schools have been more widely developed in the field.

The design school views strategy as the product of the conceptual and analytical efforts of chief executives (Ansoff, 1991; Goold, 1992; Mintzberg, 1991).

Table 14.1. Mintzberg's Ten Schools of Thought in Strategy Formulation

School	Strategy Formulation as a
Prescriptive Schools	
Design	Conceptual process
Planning	Formal process
Positioning	Analytical process
Descriptive Schools	
Entrepreneurial	Visionary process
Cognitive	Mental process
Learning	Emergent process
Political	Power process
Cultural	Ideological process
Environmental	Passive process
Configurational	Episodic process

SOURCE: Table adapted from "Strategy Formulation: Schools of Thought" by Henry Mintzberg from *Perspectives on Strategic Management* by James Fredrickson, Ed. Copyright ©199? HarperBusiness. Reprinted by permission of HarperCollins Publishing, Inc.

Strategy making in this school embodies explicit and simple principles that organizations use to guide them in their organizational structuring and resource-allocation processes. This school especially typifies the approach taken by many management consultants working in the field. The planning school, by contrast, focuses more on the technical processes of strategy analysis. While this perspective recognizes the ultimate role played by chief executive officers in making decisions, it gives considerable weight to the role of planning staffs in developing the plans and supporting rationale for whatever strategies are adopted. Consequently, the executive role is more one of approving than of designing. In this school, strategic planning is both formal and complex. It is a process in which detail and thoroughness become the hallmarks of the successful execution of strategy formulation. The expected end result of the often rational, even machine-like strategic planning process is a detailed blueprint for action, backed by extensive analyses of data (often financial) (Mintzberg, 1994; Steiner, 1979).

In the 1980s, the positioning school became very popular as it brought into the field a whole new set of concepts and frameworks needed for the analysis of competitors, markets, and strategy. Its influence was founded primarily on Porter's (1980) enormously in-

fluential book, *Competitive Strategy*. In another sense, the positioning school is the oldest of them all, as it drew upon the concepts and framework of industrial organization economics (Oster, 1994; Sherer & Ross, 1990). The basic framework of this branch of economics is expressed in Figure 14.1. Based on this framework, firm conduct (which is where organizational strategy is found) is driven by the structures of markets as well as by forces in the environment. Also performance is driven by all of these effects combined. Porter's contribution was to dig more deeply into market conduct and to explore how individual firm strategies are impacted by particular market structures. In so doing, he provided important new insights into how strategy might be conceived and formulated within competitive contexts.

Other significant and more recent schools of thought include the learning, entrepreneurial, and cultural schools (see Table 14.1). The learning school conceptualizes strategy as a product of organizational learning and adaptation. Figure 14.2 presents Mintzberg's (1978; Mintzberg & Waters, 1985) characterization of the processes by which strategies evolve. Realized strategies, he argues, are the combined product of intended, deliberate, and emergent (unintended) strategies. Indeed, the emergent strategies may be the more important among these as they are the products of learning and reality testing, rather than undue

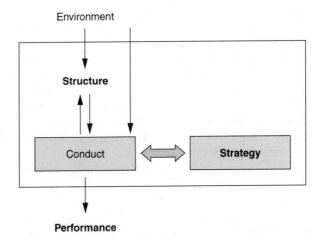

Figure 14.1. Industrial Organization Paradigm: A Framework for Strategy Analysis.

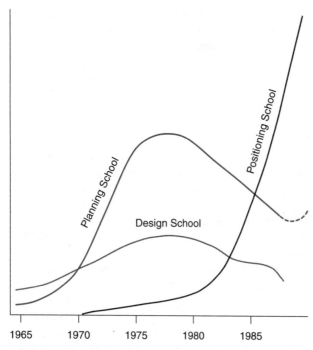

Figure 14.2. Evolution over Time in Prescriptive Schools of Thought in Strategy Formulation.
SOURCE: From "Strategy Formulation Schools of Thought" by Henry Mintzberg from *Perspectives on Strategic Management* by James W. Frederickson. Copyright 1990 by HarperBusiness. Reprinted by permission of HarperCollins Publishers Inc.

"rational deliberateness" (Mintzberg & Waters, 1985). The entrepreneurial school defines *strategy* as a vision of the organization's future, as seen by the organization's leader. From this perspective, strategy is an emergent process, driven by experience and intuition. The cultural school describes how sources of strategic advantage come from a firm's culture. Organizational culture is seen as a key resource, as a core capability that shapes effective strategies.

Since in this chapter we examine strategy primarily from a positioning school perspective, we address some of Mintzberg's criticisms of this school (Mintzberg, Lampel, & Ahlstrand, 1998). He questions, for example, the school's undue reliance on quantification (a tendency to overlook "soft" information) and the frameworks of economics (as against political sci-

ence, sociology, etc.). He also sees biases within the school toward consolidation (overfragmentation), dominance (overniching), and mature markets (overemerging). We suggest, however, that these are not so much limitations of this school of thought, but the biases of scholars and analysts who have preferred to study large organizations and ologopolistic markets.

Two other criticisms, however, deserve attention. The first is a possible overemphasis on external approaches to deriving competitive advantage. At least until recently, the positioning school tended to focus more on approaches to building demand or gaining dominant positions in the markets than on improving internal capabilities, management, and systems. On the other hand, concern with internal processes should not obscure the need to deal with markets and competitors. There is clearly a need to weigh the variety of strategic options in order to determine which are more likely to produce competitive advantage. In this chapter, therefore, we discuss both internal and external approaches to achieving competitive advantage. But it should be noted that this in no way undermines the positioning school approach. Rather, it enhances its applicability to the complexities of strategy analysis.

The second important criticism is a possible overemphasis on analytically derived strategies. The concern is that by taking a more analytical approach, organizations could rigidify commitments to deliberate strategies and create blind spots to new information and emerging strategies. On the other hand, as Mintzberg, Lampel, and Ahlstrand (1998, p. 225) point out, an overemphasis on emerging strategies could lead to a kind of "disjointed incrementalism," a "constant nibbling instead of a good bite" in strategy. They note:

> . . . the task is not to change everything all the time, but to know what to change when. And that means balancing change with continuity. Effective strategy means to sustain learning while pursuing the strategies that work. (p. 227)

Again, there is the need for balance. All organizations need to engage in strategy formulation processes that generate intended strategies. But they also need to take some caution in implementation. They need regularly to reassess, to determine whether their intended strategies fit the changing environment and shifts in their organization's internal capabilities. Given the importance of this point, we develop it further in the context of environmental turbulence.

In sum, all the schools of thought have merit. The challenge to the strategic analyst is to ensure that when attention is given to one aspect of strategy and strategy making, others are not overlooked. Strategy should not be decided and implemented, for example, without taking into consideration possible sources of resistance (the power school), the need for a supporting culture (the culture school), or possible environmental changes (the learning school).

Strategy and Environmental Turbulence

With health care markets currently undergoing major change, it is difficult to predict exactly what kinds of organizations will remain after market restructuring has run its course. Despite this uncertainty, individual organizations must find ways to compete. But what strategies they should pursue will depend on evaluations of their own and competitor strengths and weaknesses. It will also depend on careful assessments of their market environments.

It is common to conceive of two types of external environments—those that are relatively *predictable* and those that are fraught with *turbulence* (Ansoff, 1988; Drucker, 1980). In the more predictable environments, approaches to formulating strategy will tend to be linear. They will likely focus more on the maintenance and fine-tuning of existing, successful strategies, than on the remaking of strategies. In addition, they tend to emphasize the "control" of strategy. Centralized efforts will be made to assure the proper functioning of those organizational subsystems that are involved in the implementation of established strategies (Hayes, Pisano, & Upton, 1996; Lorange, Morton, & Ghoshal, 1986). In predictable environments, the more mechanistic and analytical approaches will tend to be the most applicable. Such was the case during the 1960s, when the health care industry experienced increased funding and growing prosperity. In such environments, it may be sufficient to take a planning approach, combined with the analytics of the positioning school.

By contrast, in turbulent environments—which typify the health care industry since the late 1970s and, especially, the 1990s—competing organizations will often need to rethink and, possibly, redirect their courses of action (D'Aveni, 1994). They will be challenged to find winning strategies in environments in which all competitors are searching aggressively for strategic approaches to assuring their own survival. The simultaneity of search by all will tend to exaggerate the level of unpredictability and threat. In these circumstances, lengthy analytical planning may be the least useful for formulating strategy, and emergent, decentralized strategies may actually be the most effective. There simply will be few readily accessible formulae that will not already have been considered or attempted by an organization's competitors. Strategic planning, as a formal process for decision making, may also be too sluggish for timely responses to rapidly changing environmental conditions.

In turbulent times, the spoils of victory will likely flow to those who have engaged either in careful analysis or, simply, are the beneficiaries of luck—it is said that Napoleon liked generals who were lucky. But because few gamblers win in the long run, thorough analyses, combined with nimbleness, innovativeness, and learning may be required if an organization hopes to outmaneuver tenacious competitors. To do this, the leaders of organizations will need well-honed capacities to analyze the markets in which they operate and to assess the relative advantages and possible actions of major rivals. Here is where the perspectives and tools of the positioning school might need to be combined with those of the learning school. There is always the need to assess markets in such environments, perhaps, even more than at more tranquil times. But there is also the need for some caution, for decisions to be made, reassessed in light of changing circumstances or, if necessary, discontinued.

It is also important to consider how strategy is made in turbulent environments. In such environments, creative processes take precedence, drawing heavily on the gifts of the creative mind (the entrepreneurial school). **Competitive advantage** is temporary, and strategy is constantly changing. Market leaders experiment with new combinations of resources to serve emerging but unstructured markets

(Moore, 1996). To the extent that strategic ideas emanate, perhaps even mystically, from entrepreneurial enterprise, leadership becomes even more important. Efforts will therefore be made to assess the innate skills of leaders, both as visionaries and as analysts. Successful leaders will be seen as those who are best able to generate innovative ideas and well-reasoned solutions that enlighten the road to success or, at least, make better "sense" of the road being traveled (McDaniel, 1998).

While analytical skills can be learned, the skill of visioning is not easily acquired. The trick is for leaders to see beyond the complexities. They need to be capable of grasping the subtle interrelationships that exist between strategy and markets, to be able to assess the distinctive competencies of rivals, and have an awareness of emerging trends in the marketplace. Such skills are essential for good strategists, especially for those who must lead large, complex organizations in highly competitive environments. One very important ingredient of strategic leadership in turbulent times, therefore, is a willingness to change and modify organizational strategies when markets change or in anticipation of their changing (Brown & Eisenhardt, 1998).

In sum, assuming that significant environmental turbulence exists in the health care industry and will continue for the foreseeable future, it follows that the making of strategy in health care will involve more art than science. It should be based more on ideas, conceptualizations, visions, and other nonlinear patterns of strategic thinking (the positioning and learning schools) than on the products of formal analytic processes (the planning school). The formal processes, however, will have their place even under such conditions. In particular, they will be useful for confirming strategic decisions and assisting in the control of strategies once implemented.

STRATEGY

Over the years, the concept of **strategy** has evolved from "policies" to "plans" (Bracker, 1980). In the past decade or so, agreement appears to have been reached that strategy addresses those factors that give organizations competitive advantage over rivals.

Porter's (1980, p. 47) definition of strategy provides a good example of the prevailing viewpoint: "positioning a business to maximize the value of the capabilities that distinguish it from its competitors." This definition draws attention to two important elements of strategy: (1) an organization's distinctive advantages and (2) the strength of those advantages relative to those enjoyed by competitors. Actually, this definition is not too different from one offered by Ulysses S. Grant, who in 1860 is said to have commented that strategy is "the deployment of one's resources in a manner which is most likely to defeat the enemy" (Mintzberg, 1988, p. 17).

Strategy and, correspondingly, competitive advantage has little meaning if it is not juxtaposed against the strategies and capabilities of competitors. This, therefore, leads to our own definition of strategy: *Strategy is an integrating set of ideas and concepts that guide an organization in its attempts to achieve competitive advantage over rivals.*

Consistent with Porter, this definition identifies the object of strategy as achieving competitive advantage relative to rivals (Montgomery & Porter, 1991; Porter, 1985; Powell, 1992, pp. 119–134). All competitors, regardless of ownership type (profit, nonprofit, or public) have rivals. Possible exceptions are those that enjoy monopoly or near-monopoly positions, but even many monopolists must be wary of possible entrants or threats from substitutes or buyers. The above definition also recognizes that strategy is conceptual and not *per se* a plan, a policy, or a specific intended investment. It is an expression of those highly proprietary concepts and ideas that organizations hope will help them achieve advantage.

Strategy—Integrating an Organization's Vision/Mission

Strategy, properly formulated, should provide the central rallying point around which an organization's members can unite to ensure that it survives and thrives over the long term. To achieve its potential as a unifying force, however, any strategy should be consistent with the organization's mission and vision, which themselves embody *an organization's values and aspirations* (Quigley, 1993). The organization's mission and vision frame the strategic options from which one could choose and, presumably, marshal the resources needed for strategic action to be taken.

Once embraced by an organization's members, visions/missions often take on an almost evangelical aura, replete with all the symbolism of inspired thought. In their book on leadership, Kouzes and Posner (1995, pp. 10–11) discuss the visionary role of strategic ideas:

> Every organization . . . begins with a dream. The dream or vision is the force that invents the future.
>
> [Leaders] gaze across the horizon of time, imagining the attractive opportunities that are in store when they and their constituents arrive at a final destination. Leaders have a desire to make something happen, to change the way things are, to create something that no one else has ever created before.

As they also point out, there are many terms—purpose, dream, mission, legacy, calling, personal agenda—that capture the vision or key idea of an organization. But in its essence, the vision should provide the frame for decision making and a basis for inspiring coordinated action.

The integrative link between strategy and mission requires what Ansoff (1965) referred to as the "common thread"—that set of concepts that integrates the activities of a business. The thread, he explained, provides the rationale for many strategic considerations. These include determining in which products and markets a firm should be invested (corporate strategy). More specifically, they include the patterns by which an organization will grow (i.e., into new products, new markets, or sticking to existing strategies), how it will distinguish itself from its competitors, and how multiple business activities might be combined so as to maximize synergies among them. Shendel and Hofer (1979) referred to this integrative thread as the "key idea" or the idea that provides the fundamental rationale for how a firm will develop and, ultimately, survive:

> Any successful business begins with a key idea. . . .
> The "key idea," that product of the entrepreneurial mind, is the central concept. . . .

Without it, there is no business . . . and it is a good strategy that insures the formulation, renewal, and survival of the total enterprise that in turn leads to an integration of the functional areas of the business and not the other way around. . . .

In some organizations, the vision and mission are made explicit and widely shared both internally and externally. But because of their proprietary nature, strategies will often not be shared beyond a select group of an organization's leaders. In fact, Hax (1990, pp. 34–40) has pointed out that even some members of top management and boards of directors may not be privy to the innermost concepts and ideas being considered by the leaders of organizations, and what aspects of strategy are revealed will often vary by the audience. Expressions of strategy by hospital CEOs to boards of directors, for example, may stress financial over tactical issues. Or a CEO concerned with possible reactions of physicians may promote motivational objectives more than share critical market assessments of rivals. Certainly, strategy as expressed in an annual report should correlate with the general sense of where an organization is going. But it will also likely emphasize positive performance expectations and obscure the more proprietary considerations inherent in strategy.

However, if the strategies are to serve as an integrating force for all members of organizations, they must be shared, and in clear and convincing terms. Doing so helps to establish a "strategic intent," as described by Hamel and Prahalad (1989, pp. 63–76), or the mechanisms for establishing "a desired leadership position . . . the criterion the organization will use to chart its progress."

Sources of Competitive Advantage

Brutus: . . . What do you think
        Of marching to Philippi presently?
Cassius: I do not think it good.
Brutus: Your reason?
Cassius: . . . 'Tis better that the enemy seek us:
        So shall he waste his means, weary his soldiers,
        Doing himself offence; whilst we, lying still,
        Are full of rest, defense, and nimbleness.

Brutus: Good reasons must, of force, give place to better.

.

.

.

Our legions are brim-full, our cause is ripe:
The enemy increaseth every day;
We, at the height, are ready to decline.
There is a tide in the affairs of men
Which, taken at the flood, leads on to fortune;
Omitted, all the voyage of their life
Is bound in shallows and in miseries.
On such a full sea are we now afloat;
And we must take the current when it serves
Or lose our ventures.

Cassius: Then, with your will, go on;

In this famous scene from Act IV of Shakespeare's *Julius Caesar*, Brutus and Cassius debate how they should contest the troops of Octavius Caesar and Mark Anthony that are marching upon Philippi. Cassius argued that they should maintain their well-established defensive positions, but he ultimately and mistakenly succumbed to Brutus' arguments that they "take the current when it serves" and attack. Embedded in this fatal exchange between two conspirators in the death of Caesar are several essential elements of strategy. The exchange reveals not only the options of battle, the specific actions to be taken (attack now or hold off on the attack), but also the reasons why those actions might prove victorious ("Tis better that the enemy seek us: So shall he waste his means, weary his soldiers").

Just as Brutus and Cassius did before choosing from among the major options available to them, health care strategists must explore both the available options and their underlying sources of advantage and then choose courses of action they hope will bring success. Here, Brutus' eloquent arguments won the day. They took the offensive, but unfortunately for their side, they lost.

Even though the eloquence or effectiveness of strategic reasoning is no guarantor of success, such reasoning nevertheless is fundamental to the making of strategy. Strategic decisions are highly important (as proved true for Brutus and Cassius) and must not be taken lightly. Any important decision calls for careful analysis and provision of a defensible rationale for action.

The responsibility for articulating the conceptual structures and for choosing from among the alternative courses of action clearly rests with the leaders of organizations. They are the ones who are in the best position to see the "big picture," and they bear the primary responsibility for assuring the long-term survival of their organizations. The cognitive structures that support the formation of strategies thus flow from the insights gained by an organization's leaders as they search for answers as to how best to assure their organization's survival in hostile environments. The soundness of those insights, though, will depend greatly upon the degree to which they understand the bases upon which marketplace advantages can be achieved.

The Five "Ps" of Strategy

Having defined strategy as those ideas and concepts that guide an organization in its attempts to achieve competitive advantage over rivals, we now explore some of the more common sources of competitive advantage. It is useful to distinguish between internal and external sources of competitive advantage, even though they are highly interdependent. Each builds on the other, and both are necessary for success. The importance of both internal and external sources of competitive advantage, for example, is reflected in that well-known strategy acronym, SWOT, where *Strengths* and *Weaknesses*, for the most part, look internally, and *Opportunities* and *Threats* tend toward an external focus (Andrews, 1987; Christiansen, Andrews, Bower, Hamermesh, & Porter, 1987; Stern & Stalk, 1998). Attention to all of these is essential to achieving competitive advantage.

All sources of competitive advantage serve to increase *market power*, which translates directly into a competitor's ability to resist threats from buyers and sellers or to take market actions without fear of reprisal. Positioning, for example, is directly focused on building market power. Firms that are successful in differentiating their products diminish the effect of competitors, thereby increasing their own power in the marketplace.

We therefore discuss strategy in terms of both internal and external sources of competitive advantage. Most of these can be summarized within five major sources. For ease of remembering them, each is labeled with a word beginning with a P:

- *Position*—advantage gained by achieving distinctive value in the minds of consumers
- *Power*—advantage gained through the accumulation and effective consolidation of mass
- *Pace*—advantage gained through managing the timing and intensity of strategic actions
- *Potential*—advantage derived from the accumulation of critical resources and capabilities
- *Performance*—advantage gained through the efficient conduct of operations and the effective implementation of strategy.

Each of these is differentiated by the primary underlying logic required for attaining advantage. As Figure 14.3 shows, power and position are primarily external sources, while potential and performance are primarily internal. Pace applies equally to both.

It should be noted that all organizations draw upon all five sources of advantage, although they may emphasize one or two in their own strategy formulations. For example, an organization might choose to pursue large organizational scale (power) through merger and acquisition, not only to achieve a dominating position in the market, but also to project

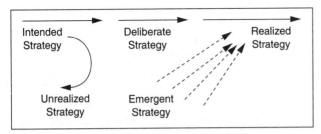

Figure 14.3. Mintzberg's Pattern of Learning in the Formulation of Strategy.
SOURCE: Adapted from Mintzberg H. "Patterns in Strategy Formulation." *Management Science* 1978;24(9):934. Reprinted by permission. The Institute of Management Sciences (currently INFORMS), 901 Elkridge Landing Road, Suite 400, Linthium, Maryland 21090-2109 USA.

a low-cost image in the minds of consumers (position). It may choose to do this rapidly (pace) in order to preempt a rival from taking similar actions, and it may select as acquisition targets rivals that have strong clinical capabilities (potential). Of course, it will need to have a strategy for implementation (performance), recognizing the difficulties of combining organizations that historically were competitors.

Position

Strategies that derive their advantage from the achievement of distinctive value in the marketplace are labeled **position strategies**. According to Porter, distinctive value can be achieved by pursuing one or more of the following three positions—Porter's (1980) "generic" strategies.

- low cost
- high differentiation
- distinctive niche

It has long been recognized that low-cost positions make it possible for competitors to gain **market shares** relative to rivals, to deter potential entrants to their markets, and to achieve other strategic objectives. Less than optimal cost positions can be sustained, but only if positions are protected either by producing goods and services that consumers perceive to have distinctive value or by pursuing protected niches. Organizations achieve low-cost positions in many ways, including by capturing the advantages of scale and/or learning or by introducing tight managerial controls and lean operating systems. In health care, the desire to achieve low-cost positions led many hospitals in the 1970s and 1980s to join multihospital systems (also a power strategy). The evidence is mixed, however, as to whether low-cost positions actually were achieved (Clement et al., 1997; Ginsberg, 1998; Gray, 1986).

Over the years, many health care competitors, especially hospitals and physicians, have tended to avoid low-cost positions, fearing consumers would interpret them as indicating low quality. HMOs have experienced particular difficulties in projecting low-cost position. In that industry, consumers have viewed cost-saving strategies as little more than efforts to constrain utilization, avoid coverage, limit access, or lower the overall quality of care. In recent years, however, changes in reimbursements (for example, DRGs and capitated payments) have motivated many health care organizations to look to low-cost positioning as a key to their strategies.

Positions of high differentiation are achieved by modifying the characteristics (quality, service support, technological sophistication, etc.) of goods and services for the purpose of projecting distinctive value to consumers. Differentiation opportunities can be found not only in product design, but also by making adjustments internally throughout most organizations. The latter is especially true in health care and many other service industries where consumption and production are often performed simultaneously (Carman & Langeard, 1978). Differentiation, therefore, involves far more than modifying product characteristics. It involves structuring all aspects of organizations to achieve differentiated positions. Many health care organizations have in recent years adopted various internal strategies—for example, reengineering, total quality improvement, and system integration—both to increase operating efficiencies and to enhance the quality of care and reinforce positioning. Leaders in health care systems nationwide have been very aware of the simultaneity of production and consumption and the need, therefore, to focus system improvements at many levels within their organizations as part of their positioning strategies.

Ironically, despite the obvious importance of quality for health care providers, few have been able to establish distinctive quality positions. Selected tertiary care providers may be an exception, but because many of these also serve as health care safety nets for the poor and disadvantaged, they have difficulty capitalizing on their ready-made positions of high quality. The expansion of the Minnesota-based Mayo Clinic into Arizona and Florida appears clearly to be based on a strategy grounded on quality positioning. (Because it involves market expansion, it is a power strategy as well.) A high-quality reputation has also been a key factor in the success Houston's Methodist Hospital (and other institutions located on the Texas Medical Center campus) has had in attracting both national and international patients. Although many hospitals are now focusing on improving their quality, it will be interesting to see if they are able to differentiate themselves sufficiently to achieve strong quality positions in their markets.

The forming of integrated systems has also attempted to extend advantages gained from their growing size and complexity to capture positions in the area of quality. In time, this may work, especially if they can effectively market their enlarged local profiles and use improvements from clinical integration to lower costs and enhance their reputations for quality (Shortell, Gillies, Anderson, Mitchell, & Morgan, 1993). Further, if they are successful in capturing the limited number of top-quality clinicians and institutions available in their markets, this strategy could prove very hard to beat. On the other hand, it is possible that these strategies will remain rather transparent, as patients continue to focus on their individual providers and give little weight to broader system interrelationships.

Another positioning strategy being pursued by some integrated systems is the management of community well-being, proclaimed by Conrad and Shortell (1997) to be the emerging issue of the first decade of the twenty-first century for integrated systems. Achieving such a position requires major transformation of information systems, governance, physician participation, and management systems (Griffith, 1997). This strategy may be particularly suited to nonprofit systems in which the community is, at least theoretically, a major stakeholder.

Niching positions are achieved by selecting distinctive segments in the market and orienting one's appeal uniquely to them. That appeal could draw upon one or both of the other two approaches to achieving distinctive positions—low cost and high differentiation. Specialty, public, teaching, suburban, and many other hospitals are good examples of organizations that maintain niched positions. Recently, specialty services such as MedCath in Little Rock, Arkansas, have arisen with claims of lower costs and higher quality. These organizations provide single-specialty, near-exclusive focus on services such as cardiology, rehabilitation, long-term care, neonatal intensive care, cancer, AIDS, and orthopedics. Such strategies promise to provide more thorough and efficient care (Harris, 1998).

Niche strategies have often proved highly successful in health care where a great diversity of products/ services and differentiated client preferences have long existed. Despite the complexity and high levels of specialization required, some niche strategies have come under attack in the restructuring health care markets. Teaching centers, for example, have learned that many of their historically well-defended specialty positions are now subject to assault, especially by the locally forming integrated delivery systems and specialty-oriented PPMCs.

Niching traditionally has been a favored strategy for small competitors (Bowring, 1986). This is true for many small hospitals that compete in markets dominated by large local hospital systems. Lacking the resources needed to compete head to head with larger competitors, they find safe haven focusing on specialized products and services (for example, rehabilitation care), unique locations (such as suburban populations), or a narrow range of consumers (minorities, aged, etc.).

Ultimately, whether the pursuit of quality or any other approach to position strategy will produce competitive advantage will depend on the unique structures of individual markets. Strategies in dominated markets will differ from those in fragmented markets; strategies in markets with high-entry barriers will differ from those with low-entry barriers, and so on. See Debate Time 14.1 to address these interrelationships.

Power

Perhaps the most important source of competitive advantage, and the one that receives the greatest attention in the strategy literature, is the amount of raw power an organization is able to amass in the competitive arena. "Might" has been at the very core of many military and business strategies. General Motors used it to great advantage for years, of course, before the Japanese countered by adopting a superior positioning strategy of building fuel-efficient, high-quality, and reliable automobiles. The battle between IBM and Macintosh similarly has been based largely on might versus positioning (product quality and niching). In this case, might appears, at least so far, to have won. The pursuit of competitive advantage through power is perhaps best represented in the health care field by the steady increases since the 1970s in the numbers of hospitals that have become members of multihospital systems, purchased contracts for management services, joined hospital consortia, formed local systems, and expanded into a great variety of health care and insurance businesses.

Power strategies derive their advantages primarily from one or both of the following: (1) economies of scale and (2) synergies that accrue when different businesses combine. Four strategies are of particular importance here:

- **Horizontal expansion**—expansion in the scale of existing business activities (for example, merger of two hospitals)
- **Horizontal integration**—the pursuit of synergies among different types of businesses that are not vertically related (for example, jointly managing nursing home and hospital businesses)
- **Vertical integration**—the pursuit of synergies among different types of businesses that share input-output relationships (for example, integrating hospital and managed care businesses)
- **Portfolio strategy**—the pursuit of financial synergies among different types of businesses (for example, combining any businesses primarily for financial purposes).

The economies that support vertical and horizontal integration are similar. All draw upon the advantages of larger-scale organizations, but they differ by their primary sources of synergies. Vertical integration derives its advantages by gaining economies of internal control, information, and technological exchange with suppliers or buyers (Walston, Kimberly, & Burns, 1996). Horizontal integration is not restricted to buyer/seller relationships, but it draws heavily upon the synergies of interorganizational coordination. Horizontal expansion (as distinct from horizontal integration) gains its advantages primarily from traditional economies of scale, scope, and learning. In portfolio strategies, any combinations among businesses, whether related or unrelated, take advantage of financial interdependencies (for instance, the spreading of risk across businesses and/or the restructuring of financial flows from established businesses to those that have potential for growth) (Stern & Stalk, 1998).

It is not always easy to determine, simply by observation, which of the four power strategies is being pursued in a given strategy. The joining of nursing home and hospital businesses, for example, could involve horizontal integration, vertical integration, or even portfolio strategies, depending on how the advantages of scale and synergies are pursued among the combined businesses. While it is common in the health care field to characterize such strategies as vertical, in actual practice many involve only limited coordination in production flows (the hallmark of vertical integration) or even the pursuit of synergies across the business units (the essence of horizontal integration). This is because the costs of coordination and compromise (for example, costs of joint decision making, communications, and overcoming interorganizational resistance) can be very significant. As a result, many multibusiness combinations amount to little more than portfolio strategies (Porter, 1985).

Likewise, the expected advantages of horizontal expansion may not be realized, even when the rationale for coordination appears to be significant. Again, this point is reinforced by the evidence that multihospital systems often do not lead to improvements in efficiencies or that the integrated delivery systems are experiencing considerable difficulties in integrating hospital partners, acquired physician practices, and managed care businesses. The transformation of synergies into meaningful strategic advantage represents a major managerial challenge, especially in the health care field where there are so many highly institutionalized autonomies and organizational complexities that act as barriers to interorganizational coordination (see Chapter 11 for further discussion of these complexities).

Absolute versus relative power. It is important to note that power as derived from size can be expressed in either absolute or relative terms. The building of **absolute power** focuses directly on economies of scale, learn-

ing, and scope. Large organizations generally are better able to direct resources to competitive skirmishes than are small organizations. However, if smaller organizations are able to capture high local market shares, then they may be able to override the advantages of large absolute scale. (This was one of the sources of advantage Ukrops was able to use to defeat Safeways and other larger competitors.)

A strategy that leads to the building of large-scale organizations—for example, national strategies pursued by Columbia/HCA or by one of the major physician practice–management companies, Phycor or MedPartners—derives its rationale from the advantages of *absolute* power. On the other hand, one that amasses local market shares without regard to organizational scale is typically the strategy of choice of nonprofit hospital systems. The latter derive their advantages from power *relative* to the competitors in their markets. Importantly, even the large national firms have recognized the advantages of local system formation and sought to build up local market power in many markets across the country (Luke, Ozcan, & Olden, 1995). Also, **relative power** does not appear to be as important in the managed care markets, a lesson being learned by many local hospital systems that have expanded into the managed care area. There, absolute power appears to reign supreme, which may account for the rash of mergers of late among managed care firms.

Pace

Another critical source of advantage is grounded in the timing and intensity of strategic action. The Cassius and Brutus debate demonstrates effectively the validity of that old cliche—"timing is everything." If successful, early movers gain the advantage of working down the learning curve, capturing new demands, gaining customer loyalty, establishing insurmountable positions in the markets, and so on.

Of course, failure to read the markets accurately could prove very costly to early movers. In health care, the evidence is mixed as to whether competitors that made early moves gained the expected advantage. Several leading health care organizations (such as Phycor of Nashville, Intermountain Healthcare in Salt

DEBATE TIME 14.1: WHAT DO YOU THINK?

In the last several years, a considerable interest has been devoted to upgrading quality in organizations at all levels. Variously labeled as total quality management, continuous quality improvement, and reengineering, this new managerial approach to improving the internal workings, quality, and productivity of organizations is also considered by many to be a major approach to strengthening strategic position in markets. Put simply, the view holds that, by imbuing an organization's members with a powerful commitment to improving performance, they will advance the quality of goods and services sold and thereby increase their market shares. A double benefit is this approach will enhance morale among employees, and the consuming public will become more satisfied, thus improving the overall prospects for organizational survival.

Alternatively, there are those who argue that in most markets the issue is not how best to appeal to a wary consuming public; after all, the new consumers are the managed care companies and their customers business, and governmental agencies. Furthermore, the markets are consolidating, and competitors are becoming stronger and stronger. Therefore, they should focus more on how best to defeat a determined competitor bent on gaining market share at their expense. This latter approach argues that organizations should assume an external competitive stance and be ever ready to engage in nihilistic battles against competitors in order to increase the likelihood they will dominate their markets.

Behind such orientations—the internal versus the external strategies—there are a number of issues. One has to do with determining the strategies that might be most effectively applied under various market structural conditions. There is evidence that many health care markets are consolidating, barriers to entry are coming down, product differentiation is becoming more and more difficult to sustain, and substitute products are emerging everywhere. If the structure is changing, strategy should adapt accordingly.

Another issue has to do with values. On the one hand, there is the perspective that health care is not like other industries, that it is imbued with a delicate admixture of *public* and *private interests.* Therefore overt competitive battling could be seen to do harm to the consuming public as well as to those who might engage in such actions. An alternative perspective holds that the only way for a firm to be really strong in the long term is to steel itself in the heat of competitive battle. It also holds that competition is the best way in the long run to improve quality, and that giving excessive attention to quality improvement and cultural enhancements wastes vital organizational energies that might better be spent on winning the competitive war.

Which orientation to strategy—working on the internal capabilities and performance versus expanding market shares through acquisition and merger or repositioning products and services—fits best within the health care field in the first decade of the twenty-first century? Why?

Lake City, and Sentara in Norfolk) appear to have gained considerable advantage by becoming early movers. There are, however, a number of high-profile examples of organizations that have not been so successful: Humana, the hospital company, with entries into formula physician practice and managed care in the 1980s; Columbia/HCA in its attempt to acquire Blue Cross of Ohio, and, overall, develop a national strategy; and Coastal, with its difficulties in combining physician and managed care businesses in Florida.

Differences in orientation with respect to timing and risk-taking behavior were captured in Miles and Snow's (1978) interesting typology of strategy. They identified four strategy types:

- *Prospectors*—organizations that frequently search for new market opportunities and regularly engage in experimentation and innovation
- *Analyzers*—organizations that maintain stable operations in some areas but also search for new

opportunities, often following the lead of prospector organizations

- *Defenders*—organizations that search for additional opportunities for growth and seldom make adjustments to existing, well-established strategies
- *Reactors*—organizations that perceive opportunities and turbulence, but are not able to adapt consistently or effectively.

Strategic orientations such as these are often deeply embedded within an organization's culture and strategic history. As a result, organizations do not easily change their strategic orientations, even when faced with strong environmental pressures (Miles, 1982).

Shortell, Morrison, and Friedman (1990), however, suggested that when organizations do decide to shift from one orientation to another, they are more likely to do so within "strategic comfort zones." In other words, they will shift to that orientation that is least dissimilar from the one they now occupy. This idea is illustrated in Figure 14.4, where the Miles and Snow strategic orientations are arranged to reflect comfort zones. Should defender organizations, for example, decide to become more aggressive in the marketplace, they would be expected to shift to the more proximate

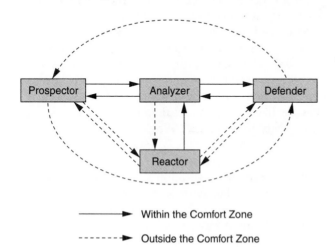

Figure 14.4. Strategic Comfort Zones for Shifting Pace Strategy Orientations.
SOURCE: Adapted from Shortell SM, Morrison EM, Friedman B. *Strategic Choices for America's Hospitals.* San Francisco: Jossey-Bass Publishers, 1990:37.

analyzer than to the more distant prospector orientation. Shortell and colleagues found evidence for the comfort zones in a study of hospital strategic behavior (Shortell, Morrison, & Friedman, 1990; Zajac & Shortell, 1989).

Other useful concepts that fall under the heading of **pace strategy** include the management of surprise, signaling, managing momentum, and timed pacing as well as a variety of strategies associated with deterring entry and initiating counter moves (Amburgey & Miner, 1992; Brown & Eisenhardt, 1998; Day & Reibstein, 1997; Harrigan, 1985). Surprise has often been the key to successful military as well as business strategies. Unexpected attacks catch rivals unprepared, thus producing initial critical advantages for the initiators of surprise. It is vital in managing surprise that competitors have a clear understanding of the landscape of competition. In particular, they need to understand competitor capabilities, difficulties or possibilities of entry, and broad trends in the markets. Vulnerability to surprise is especially acute for competitors engaged in niching and other position strategies. Specialty hospitals, for instance, risk becoming so centered on their specific areas of strength that they fail to recognize moves on the part of general hospitals to offer substitute products or compete directly with them.

There is, of course, a place for announcing strategic actions well in advance. A competitor just beginning to invest heavily in a particular strategic move could chose to make an early announcement of its plans in order to scare away potential rivals. A hospital could announce plans to build a satellite hospital in a suburb, for example, thus signaling to rivals that they should look elsewhere to find opportunities for market expansion. A competitor, however, could also use such announcements to detract attention away from other moves that are being initiated in secret or simply to cause competitors to react unnecessarily to feigned strategic action. Threats of entry must be credible to have market impact. Organizations that announce illogical or empty actions gain no advantage.

Potential

Now we turn to the sources of advantage that are essentially internal to the organization. **Potential strat-**

egy has to do with the distinctive resources and capabilities that might give organizations an advantage as they design and implement their strategies. Some organizations enjoy distinctive strengths in selected clinical areas. Others gain from memberships in multihospital systems, memberships in purchasing alliances, advanced information systems, recognized research capabilities, low debt and high cash reserves, modern and attractive physical facilities, and/or aggressive and effective managerial talent. All of these, and others, can give competitors advantages, depending on the circumstances of their marketplaces. Successful clinical information system development within an integrated system, for example, could create an advantage in the pursuit of low-cost, high-quality provider linkages. Some believe that as a result of the constant change in customer demands and environmental turbulence, organizations have no choice but to look for internal capabilities for competitive advantage (Grant, 1991).

Now all distinctive capabilities, however, can be transformed into long-term competitive advantage. Collis and Montgomery (1995) identified some essential characteristics that may be needed for a resource or capability to become important strategically:

- *Transferability*—it can be transformed into a resource or service that is valued by customers (and thus is similar with positioning)
- *Competitive superiority*—it is truly better than the resources or capabilities of competitors
- *Inimitability*—it cannot be copied easily by competitors
- *Substitutability*—it cannot be replaced through substitution by competitors
- *Durability*—its value does not depreciate quickly.

The resources or capabilities of many competitors may not pass such market tests, or they simply may be unable to provide sustained competitive advantages. Nevertheless, like quality positioning, this is an area that may be inadequately mined by health care strategists. Many health care providers have tangible and intangible assets that go largely undeveloped from a strategic perspective. In fact, viable external strategies may only reach fruition after organizations exploit their internal strengths and shore up their weaknesses. Too often, organizations go through the motions of assessing their strengths and weaknesses without acting sufficiently on their conclusions. Developing internal capabilities almost always takes many years and consistent efforts. Organizations seeking short-term improvements often find external strategies to hold greater appeal.

A new organizational form—the **hybrid organization**—may prove to be an important internal source of advantage (Ashkenas, Ulrich, Jick, & Kerr, 1995; Powell, 1990). Many hospitals, physicians, and other health care organizations and providers, as they have traditionally enjoyed high levels of autonomy, are reluctant to give up prized independence in exchange for gains in strategic power. Because of this, the hybrid or virtual organizational forms have become the method of choice for many of them (Coffey, Fenner, & Stofis, 1997). Providers are able to retain organizational independence, while capturing many of the advantages of larger organizational scale. The precise structures can also be altered to facilitate rapid entry or exit. An additional strategic advantage is that contractual arrangements can be undone as quickly as they are arranged. This is especially valuable in an environment of rapid change, where there is great potential for strategic error to be made. Rapid entry or exit can be facilitated by the relative ease with which organizations can be created by contract.

These structures do have some important drawbacks that could prevent the participants from achieving their strategic objectives (Jarillo, 1988; Luke, Begun, & Pointer, 1989). For one, they often fail to establish a strong strategic head or resolve power differences among the participants. As a result, they are not always able to take timely and significant actions in the marketplace. Relative to more tightly structured organizations, the hybrids can be expected to react slowly to environmental change and competitive threat. They often also lack strong and well-developed interorganizational linkages and systems of management control. Thus they are unable to achieve valued synergies or to realize sufficiently the promise inherent in increased organizational scale. There are exceptions to this, of course. A good example of a hybrid organization that has achieved a good balance between organizational autonomies and the need to centralize power is the Promina Health System in Atlanta. In 1994, Promina was formed when three systems in the Atlanta area (others have joined since) joined into a strategic alliance. They have given considerable power to the system CEO, thereby minimizing the limitations typical of loosely coupled organizational forms. Consequently, Promina has emerged as a powerful competitor in its market.

In general, therefore, an important element on the "potential" side of competitive advantage is the structure of the organization. The way in which organizations are organized can play a major role in either hindering or facilitating strategic response (as observed above for hybrid organizations). Depending on its structure, an organization may or may not be able to move quickly, amass important resources, direct them toward a particular strategic objective, or successfully project a desired position in the market. Organizational structure has become especially important in the health care field where there are numerous determined sources of resistance to the ongoing consolidation of the markets.

Performance

Closely associated with potential as an internal source of competitive advantage is the effectiveness with which strategies are implemented and organizations managed. Chapter 13 deals directly with many dimensions of organizational efficiency and effectiveness, particularly in the realm of health care quality. Implementation and operations are often the keys to the successful execution of strategy. Many great ideas fall far short of their potential, simply because organizations failed to ensure effective implementation of their strategies.

Drawing attention to the importance of the implementation, Porter introduced the concept of value chains. A value chain is a diagrammatic disaggregation of the activities organizations undertake to produce products and services and to carry out their strategies. By carefully assessing their value chains, he suggests, organizations can identify those areas where improvements in performance could lead to more successful execution of strategy. For instance,

carefully managed alliances with suppliers can result in smoother management of pharmaceuticals and other supplies and thus improved efficiencies and quality on the part of physicians, nurses, and other health professionals. This also could lead indirectly to more satisfied patients.

The need to manage and address the implementation of **performance strategy** is especially important for integrated systems. They need to ensure not only that each individual component runs efficiently and effectively, but that each reinforces the others and supports the overall strategic goals of the organization. Fitting the individual parts to the whole is what Porter (1996) referred to as ensuring "organizational fit" within complex organizations. He argued:

> It is harder for a rival to match an array of interlocked activities than it is merely to imitate a particular sales-force approach, match a process technology, or replicate a set of product features. Positions built on systems of activities are far more sustainable than those built on individual activities.

This is the central objective of the integrated system—to generate advantages from the sum of the individual parts. Success may rest as much on implementation as on establishing appropriate organizational structures, incentive systems, or, even, positioning strategies. More particularly, the hard work of integrating physicians into systems, multiple functional units, and clinical care are prerequisites to a successful strategy of vertical integration (Satinsky, 1998; Shortell et al., 1996).

MARKET STRUCTURE

Understanding the external environment is critical in the formulation and management of strategy. The industrial organization framework, as presented in Figure 14.1, offers valuable insight in the analysis of the environment and, more particularly, the markets (Bain, 1956, 1972; Bain & Qualls, 1987; Caves, 1982; Mason, 1939; Sherer & Ross, 1990). We build upon this framework to clarify **market structures,** firm conduct, and their relationship to strategy. As indicated, the performance of firms depends upon: (1) the organization of "economically significant features" of markets—market structure—and (2) the "acts, practices, and politics" firms pursue as they strive for profits—firm conduct. More importantly for purposes of this chapter, the framework recognizes the direct effect of market structure on conduct, which encompasses the strategic behaviors of individual firms.

As shown in Figure 14.1, the conduct or strategy also impacts the market structure itself. The merger, acquisition, and affiliation activities of hospitals, physicians, and managed care organizations perhaps best illustrate this reverse relationship. These actions (conduct/strategy), while driven by existing market structure and environmental forces, alter the market structure by reducing the number of competitors.

The analysis of market structure is properly carried out at the level of individual markets. At the corporate level, analyses are conducted individually for each market in which a company conducts business. However, since many corporations have dominant businesses, they may tend to pay particular attention to their major markets and fail to give sufficient attention to the submarkets in which they are involved. This is increasingly becoming a problem in the health care industry as multibusiness combinations proliferate. For example, a hospital-based integrated system, despite having investments in nursing homes, ambulatory surgery clinics, managed care products, and other health care businesses, may give analytic priority to the study of acute care markets, thereby overlooking the distinctive challenges facing their other businesses. Certainly, strategy needs to be examined at the overall corporate level. However, the markets for each distinct business should be examined and implications for strategy evaluated.

A Typology of Market Structures

Of a number of structural features of markets, three are among the most important:

- *Market concentration*—the degree to which a small number of competitors dominate a market.
- *Entry barriers*—the difficulties encountered by potential new competitors as they consider entering a market.

- *Product differentiation*—the degree to which individual competitors are able to distinguish themselves from one another in ways that are valued by consumers.

In general, the more concentrated the markets, the higher the **entry barriers,** and the greater the product differentiation, the more likely it is that competitors will engage in behaviors that maintain higher prices. This does not mean, of course, that competition goes away—quite the contrary. In markets with high concentration and few competitors (technically known as oligopolistically structured markets), competitors often are highly rivalrous, even if not particularly focused on price competition. Because of small numbers, such competitors tend to be very interdependent—they carefully monitor and react to each other's strategic moves. In health care, managed care and hospital markets tend to be oligopolistic, many having already achieved high levels of concentration. While not there yet, physician markets have the potential of becoming oligopolistic, especially if trends toward consolidation continue.

Each of the above three structural features reflects degrees to which market actors possess and are able to exercise market power. Individual sellers in concentrated markets have greater market power than competitors in less concentrated or atomistic markets. As a result, strategic actions taken by competitors in the more concentrated markets can be expected to have major impacts on their rivals, causing the latter to react and engage in countermaneuvers. By contrast, competitors in less concentrated markets, being more numerous and relatively small in size, will be much less reactive to the actions of competitors. Instead, they will more likely focus their strategies directly on consumers (for example, position strategies). This is a good example of how market structure (in this case, atomistic versus concentrated) determines which source of competitive advantage competitors will emphasize.

The payoff to overcoming fragmentation can be very significant if there exist sufficient economic bases for consolidation (the potential for achieving economies of scale, raising entry barriers, creating strong alliances vertically with buyers, etc.). But where these conditions do not exist, the pursuit of consolidation could prove to be a significant strategic trap. There is already some evidence for this in physician markets, where consolidations of physician practices into integrated systems have not produced the expected economic gains. For example, two of the largest health care systems in Philadelphia reported heavy losses from their physician networks and are beginning to divest many practices (Fernandez, 1998).

Using the above three characteristics, Bain and Qualls (1987) built a useful typology of market structure. As a first step, they divided the first and perhaps most important dimension—the degree of seller concentration—into three subcategories:

1. *Atomistic*—many small sellers (low level of interaction to one another)
2. *Oligopolistic*—few large sellers (high level of interaction to one another
3. *Monopolistic*—single seller.

They then divided the second dimension—the degree of product differentiation in the market—into two categories:

1. *Homogeneous products*—products nearly identical
2. *Differentiated products*—products differentiated by design, quality branding, etc.

The third dimension—ease of market entry—was divided into three categories:

1. *Easy entry*—no barrier to entry
2. *Moderately difficult entry*—barriers appreciably high, but not high enough to permit sellers to act like monopolists
3. *Blockaded entry*—barriers high enough to permit monopoly pricing without attracting additional entry.

Using the degree of seller concentration as the primary organizing characteristic, they combined the above categories, creating nine general market types, as summarized in Table 14.2.

While examples of all nine can be found in the health care field, those involving undifferentiated products are the least likely to be observed. This is be-

cause virtually all health care markets involve considerable degrees of product differentiation. Competitors in hospital markets, for example, differ not only by whether they are members of local and/or multihospital systems, but also by the characteristics of the hospitals themselves. Hospitals vary by their complexity, specialization, ownership (church-sponsored, for-profit, nonprofit, etc.), teaching status, quality reputation, physician affiliations, locations (such as rural, suburban, urban, spatially isolated versus clustered), and even their contractual relationships with managed care companies. Location is perhaps the most important characteristic for differentiating individual hospitals (Luke, 1991). Differences in location are also related to differences in patient populations, physician affiliations, success in contracting, and so on. Nursing home, physician, home health care, and other sectors draw upon similar bases for achieving differentiation. The key point is that higher differentiation increases the overall market power that individual competitors enjoy.

Other characteristics, in addition to the above, play important roles in shaping the strategic behaviors of competitors within the health care industry. Of particular importance is the rate of growth in markets, which is often expressed using the well-known concepts of market stages and/or product life cycle. Because of its importance, we discuss this dimension below. First, however, we examine another well-recognized typology of market structure developed by Porter.

Porter's Five Forces Framework

In his own expression of market structure and its effects on strategy, Porter (1980) focused directly on five key "sources of competitive pressure." As exhibited in Figure 14.5, these include threats from rivals, potential entrants, sellers, substitutes, and buyers. While all five forces are important, their consequences for strategy likely will vary across individual markets.

Rivals

The **Porter model** identified a number of factors that directly impact the intensity of rivalry within markets (including, by the way, all those identified in the Bain

Table 14.2. Major Power Strategy Options

Strategy	Definition	Example
Horizontal expansion	Expansion in the scale of existing business activities	The merger of two or more hospitals
Horizontal integration	The pursuit of synergies among different types of businesses (other than among those that are vertically related); could include business combinations that are either:	
	related (have in common similar technologies, markets, or product functions), or	The combination of hospital and nursing home businesses and centralizing many management functions for both organizations
	unrelated (have in common few or no similarities in technological, market, or product functions)	The combination of hospital and furniture store businesses and sharing marketing and information system capacities
Vertical integration	The pursuit of synergies among different types of businesses that share input-output relationships with each other along the production chain	The combination of hospital and insurance companies to produce HMO products
Portfolio	The pursuit of financial synergies among different types of businesses, regardless of whether related	The combination of hospital and furniture store businesses either to diversify investments or to facilitate excess cash flows to be drawn from one to support growth in the other

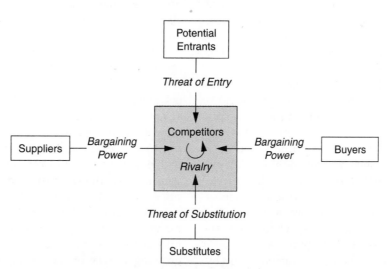

Figure 14.5. Porter's Framework of Five Forces that Affect the Level of Rivalry in a Market.
SOURCE: Reprinted and adapted with the permission of Free Press, a Division of Simon & Schuster, Inc. from *Competitive Strategy: Techniques for Analyzing Industries and Competitors* by Michael E. Porter. Copyright © 1980 by the Free Press.

& Qualls classification scheme). We selectively discuss these in regard to health care markets.

Market concentration. The degree of concentration within a market refers to the proportion of market power held by leading firms. The more concentrated the markets, the more power individual competitors are able to wield against **rival threats,** potential entrants, **buyer threats, substitution threats,** and **seller threats.** Further, as discussed earlier, the more concentrated the markets, the more rivals will react to one another, perhaps paying somewhat less attention to buyers or other strategic concerns.

A number of indicators are available for measuring the degree of concentration in markets (Sherer & Ross, 1990). Two of the most popular are the **four-firm ratio** and the **Herfindahl-Hirschman Index (HHI).** The four-firm ratio is simply the sum of market shares controlled by the top four firms in a market, and the HHI is measured as follows:

$$HHI = \Sigma\, S^2$$

where $\Sigma\, S^2$ is the sum of squared shares of all competitors in a market.

By squaring each competitor's shares (percentages of the market), the shares of the larger firms are more heavily weighted than are those with smaller shares. This has the advantage of emphasizing the strength of the most powerful firms, yielding a good indicator of disproportionate distributions in market power.

Regardless of which measure is used, it is critical that they be applied at the proper geographic level—national, regional, or local. For some industries, especially service and retail markets, concentration is best measured at the local level. This is primarily because transportation costs in such markets limit market exchanges to buyers and sellers located within proximate geographic space. This is also true in much of health care. Possible exceptions are tertiary care, pharmaceuticals, and managed care, where the markets often reach well beyond local boundaries.

We illustrate the measurement of concentration by applying the four-firm ratio (calculated by summing the percentages of hospital patient days controlled by the top four firms per market) to the analysis of hospital markets. Computed at the national level, the top four hospital firms accounted in 1997 for just around 12% of the total acute care, medical/surgical market. (Columbia/HCA had the highest individual share of just under 6%.) As discussed above, measurement at this level could lead to the mistaken conclusion that the hospital market is very fragmented. The more appropriate approach, however, would be to calculate concentration at the local level, which clearly would present a very different picture of concentration.

In examining concentration at the local level, we adopt a broad conceptualization of what constitutes a hospital firm. First, we treat as members of the same firm all hospitals that are either under the same ownership (that is, members of the same multi-hospital system) or are strategically partnered within a market. We call all such combinations strategic hospital alliances (SHAs). Individual firms then constitute either SHAs or free-standing hospitals. Figure 14.6 displays the mean four-firm values averaged across metropolitan statistical areas (MSAs) within geographic regions and categories of population size. As can be seen, the average values are very high. They exceed 96% for MSAs with populations less than 1 million, and the averages across all four regions exceed 90%, with the overall average around 96%.

What does this mean? It means that if hospital concentration is measured at the local level, the level at which patterns of exchange between buyers and sellers generally occur, hospital markets already have achieved very high levels of concentration. When viewed in the context of their other sources of market power—for example, high product differentiation and high entry barriers—hospital markets, while highly rivalrous, lack many of the characteristics needed for price competition to occur. This is one reason why buyers are consolidating and reorganizing (especially, managed care companies and businesses aggregated into coalitions) to countervail the established and growing power of the hospital competitors. It also means that strategy in hospital markets may tend to be directed more at competitors or institutional buyers

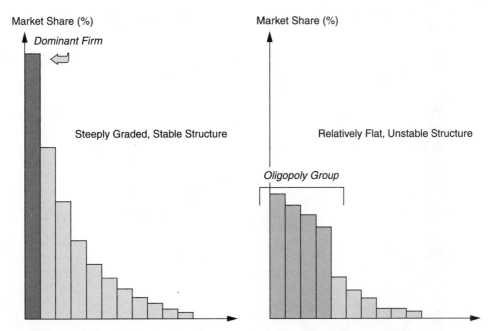

Figure 14.6. Market Structure Patterns Differentiated by Gradients in Market Shares. Shares are calculated as the percent of beds in the market.
SOURCE: William G. Shepherd, *The Economics of Industrial Organization,* © 1979, p. 199. Adapted by permission of Prentice-Hall, Englewood Cliffs, New Jersey.

(for example, power and pace strategies) than at individual consumers (position strategies).

Gradation in market shares. The markets not only differ by level of concentration, but also by the distribution of shares among competitors (Shepherd, 1979). In some markets, the distribution in shares can be very sharply graded, from a dominant player down to very small, relatively weak competitors. In others, the shares may be fairly equal across competitors, resulting in a flat gradation. These two contrasting patterns are illustrated in Figure 14.7.

Ironically, the first of the two patterns (the sharply graded case) may be the more stable of the two, since it has a clearly established pecking order among competitors. Such a clear ordering of market power will tend to reduce the prospects that any one rival will significantly challenge any other. The second or flatter pattern, by contrast, may be less stable. Facing relative equality in power, competitors in this pattern may be tempted to vie with one another for positions

of dominance. Such positions could be achieved in a number of ways, the most dramatic of which would be for one rival to merge with one or two others, thereby adding rapidly to their collective market share. Were this to occur, the structure might evolve toward the first pattern of dominance, reducing competitive tensions and the prospects for overt rivalry.

Strategies in the dominated market structure should also differ from those one would find in the flatter structure. The dominating organizations, for example, could be expected to function as, in effect, "enforcers," pressing for discipline among the other competitors, especially in the volatile area of price competition. Also, the smaller members (with lower market shares) in this model, given their relative inability to exercise power, could be expected strategically to seek safe positions or niches where they hope to be free from the threats of the other, larger rivals. In the flatter structure, rivals could be expected to behave as oligopolists, reacting to one another, even engaging in power strategies.

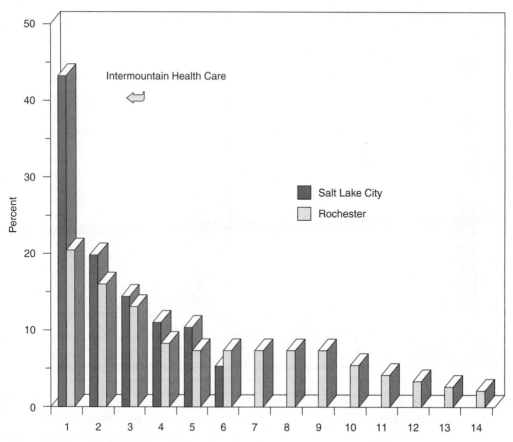

Figure 14.7. Hospital Firm Market Shares of Salt Lake City, Utah, and Rochester, New York. Firms constitute either single hospitals or the combination of those hospitals that are owned, managed, or sponsored by the same multihospital company (e.g., the Intermountain Health Care firm combines a total of five hospitals). Shares are calculated for each as the percent of beds in the market.

Presence of switching costs. Another factor influencing rivalry is the presence of switching costs (the costs incurred when switching from one seller or buyer to another). If there are few switching costs, the likelihood for buyers to shift to one's competition will increase, and this will in turn increase the intensity of rivalry and overall instability of such markets. The costs of switching, on the other hand, can be significant and can stabilize buyer/seller relationships and dampen competitive pressures.

Switching costs are very significant at many points within the health care industry and, therefore, play a major role in diminishing rivalry among competitors.

Some health care firms even attempt to promote switching costs as a centerpiece to their strategies. For example, because referral relationships among physicians or between physicians and hospitals are difficult to create and sustain, many hospital systems have pursued a number of strategies (within legal limits, of course) in order to lock in referral arrangements. Contractual arrangements with physicians often include restrictive agreements that make later separation costly. Likewise, health care providers may enter into contractual and other vertical arrangements with insurance companies to assure directed flows of patients. Once implemented, these arrangements generate administrative mechanisms (information systems and other administrative complexities), the costs of which promote continuity in the relationships. Also, nearly all of the major distribution companies, especially the medical/surgical distributors, seek more involved arrangements with provider systems. They seek not just to sell product, but to offer a wide range of supply-channel management services, including on-site warehousing, product redistribution within systems, just-in-time delivery, and so on. Again, these arrangements introduce administrative costs that, once incurred, make it difficult for providers to switch to other distributors.

Diverse competitors.   Porter (1980) argued that "competitors diverse in strategies, origins, personalities, relationships to their parent companies . . . have a hard time reading each other's intentions accurately and agreeing on a set of 'rules of the game' for the industry." As a result, they may more frequently make wrong strategic choices than might firms located in industries in which there is less diversity. Diversity often generates situations of unpredictability and greater competition.

Within the hospital industry, for example, there is considerable diversity in goals, missions, and other service characteristics among competitors. There are, in particular, substantial differences in ownership, product and service mixes, system arrangements, physician arrangements, and so on. Consistent with Porter's point, such diversity contributes to the unpredictability of market responses and, generally, tends to stimulate rivalry. On the other hand, if diversity leads to differences in, say, market segmentation strategies, this could serve to reduce competitive tensions. For example, teaching hospitals might pursue low-income patients; for profits, middle income suburban populations; and specialty hospitals, other market niches. Nevertheless, it is clear that competitors located in markets composed of diverse rivals are greatly challenged to formulate workable strategies for their organizations.

Exit barriers.   Exit barriers are another important feature of market structure. High exit barriers tend to retain competitors in markets, thus increasing the level of

competition over what might otherwise occur. Exit barriers historically have been very high in many sectors of the health care industry, but there are indications that in certain sectors they may be falling.

Some hospitals have closed over the past 10 to 15 years, though these closures have tended to be in rural markets. It is only in recent years, with all of the **merger, acquisition,** and alliance activities in the hospital industry, that capacity in metropolitan areas appears to be falling. There are numerous anecdotal examples of hospitals, having joined local or national systems, ceasing to provide acute care services and, instead, providing long-term nursing, rehabilitation, or other services. There are also examples of hospitals reducing their capacities, possibly to delay or avoid ultimate closure or conversion. And, of course, some are closed outright.

However, there remain a number of economic, social, emotional, and other reasons why hospitals resist exiting completely from their markets. Some hospitals serve specific population groups (such as inner-city poor, suburban, or ethnic populations) and remain open despite poor economic or quality performance. Others enjoy strong institutional support from sponsors, such as local or county government or church organizations. The resistance to closure for such providers often is very great. By comparison, the barriers to exit are not so high for the nursing home or managed care sectors. In these, the exiting of weaker rivals dampens competitive pressures overall.

It is important for strategists to understand both entry and exit barriers, especially as their organizations enter into new business arenas. One should not assume that one market shares the same entry and exit barriers as another, and it is important to monitor *adjustments* in those barriers. In recent years, the health care industry has undergone significant changes, which in many cases, translate into the restructuring of markets (including altering the height of entry and exit barriers) and the drivers of strategy.

Buyers

The most significant strategic threats facing many health care organizations come from the buyer side. For over a decade, health insurance companies have been intensely engaged in their own strategic maneuvering in response to powerful challenges from their buyers. As is now well known, this has dramatically ratcheted up competitive pressures on providers and, looking further upstream, on health care suppliers as well. Porter has identified a number of mitigating factors that modify the effects of buyers on sellers. We summarize two that are particularly relevant in health care markets.

Seller dependency. Buyers who purchase substantial percentages of the goods and services produced by individual sellers exercise considerable leverage over those sellers. When placed in a local market context, this leads to high seller dependencies. This is a calculation many insurance companies and providers have had to make as they have entered into contracts with one another at the local market level.

Indeed, that such interdependencies might occur was central to the so-called paradigm shift of the 1990s, which included a shift to vertical integration. It was expected by many that buyers and sellers would opt for tightened vertical alignments, producing exclusive flows of patients and services between insurers and providers. To date, however, although some vertically integrated systems have formed, most hospitals and insurers have preferred to enter into contractual arrangements with multiple buyers and sellers, leading to far less seller and buyer vertical dependencies than had been expected. As a result, both provider systems and insurers are freer than expected to maneuver strategically.

On the other hand, there is no guarantee that the expected structuring of vertical relationships will not ultimately begin to develop. The Minneapolis–St. Paul market, where insurers and providers have entered into a high degree of vertical structuring (the Allina Health System and HealthPartners, for instance), remains a striking example of how that paradigm might ultimately shift in other markets. If it does, sellers—and buyers as well—will become far more dependent on one another, significantly restricting their freedom to modify strategies locally.

Market information controlled by buyers. To the degree that buyers have good access to strategically important in-formation about the businesses of their sellers, they will be able to exercise leverage in their negotiations with those sellers. This is a very important consideration in the relationship between health insurance companies and health care providers and, in similar ways, between hospitals and physicians. With the continuing expansion and growing sophistication of managed care systems, information systems, and formal contracting, insurance companies are increasingly able to obtain unusual amounts of information about the demand structures, prices, and production capabilities of their buyers. The same is true for the ability of hospital systems to gain information on physicians.

The free flow of information vertically in the health care industry could have one of two very different consequences. On the one hand, it could facilitate vertical ownership within markets. The free flow of information may bring together compatible parties and facilitate consolidations. Information exchange is essential in any combination of organizations. On the other hand, since information appears so freely available, at least in vertical exchanges, it may be unnecessary for buyers and sellers to integrate formally. Looser, "virtual" relationships may be sufficient to facilitate complex market exchanges and satisfy the requirements of contractual arrangements. Looser arrangements appear to be more common in the current market environment, despite earlier predictions of tighter vertical integration. This, of course, could change in time, as in the Minneapolis–St. Paul case. Strategic analysts must take care to revise regularly their assumptions about existing strategy patterns and market restructuring.

Entrants

New entrants to local markets can rapidly reorder existing market shares and long-held positions in the markets. When entry barriers are low, one can expect to see incumbents and potential entrants engaging in a variety of tactical maneuvers—such as false signaling of strategic moves, use of surprise, predatory pricing, and other hostile behaviors—all designed to alter the likelihood of entry.

As noted by Porter, the most common sources of entry barriers include economies of scale, product differentiation, capital requirements, switching costs, access to distribution channels, and other cost advantages that are independent of scale. In addition, barriers can be created artificially (such as certificate of need laws in health care) or, as suggested above, by strategic maneuvering. These are all important in health care markets, but to varying degrees.

Certainly, the barriers to entering hospital markets historically have been very high; but, as with exit barriers, they appear recently to be declining. There still are substantial barriers to expansion of capacity in most markets; but new entry has occurred as external rivals have acquired local competitors and sought to build systems of delivery at the local market level. On the other hand, Columbia/HCA discovered how high entry barriers (to acquisition) still are in many markets. They experienced little difficulty entering markets in the South and Southwest. But as they attempted to move into other regions, they encountered greater resistance from forces as varied as local clergy, citizen groups, and businesses. This, in effect, severely hindered their progress toward implementing a strategy of becoming a national provider.

By contrast, the barriers limiting entry to physician, dental, and other health professional markets appear relatively low (as are the exit barriers). If local integrated systems succeed in bringing health professionals into institutionally based systems, however, entry barriers for health professional workers could rise precipitously. New entrants might then need to be linked or, at least, closely aligned with such systems in order to secure a patient base. Again, it is essential that strategic analysts keep abreast of changes in the structures and strategic behaviors in their markets.

Substitutes

Substitute products or services are those that, while different in significant ways, serve the same function as existing services or products within an industry. In this rapidly changing health care environment, the threat of substitutes remains very high. For example, substitutes have steadily eroded the traditional acute care business of hospitals. The movement toward unbundling hospital services, including the spinning off of such vital services as ambulatory surgery and high-tech diagnostic procedures, are examples of substitution effects. Interestingly, hospitals, given their considerable financial and manpower capabilities, have to some extent been able to minimize the consequences of substitution by entering themselves into the substitute businesses. Nevertheless, specialized physician practice-management companies and other specialized provider groups still pose significant threats to hospital systems. They threaten to become the providers of choice for lower cost and, possibly, higher quality substitute services.

The threats of substitution are also significant in the insurance industry. Perhaps the most important example of a potential substitute is the provider-sponsored organization (PSO). These entities enable providers to contract directly with buyers, thereby bypassing insurers (at least for the delivery of Medicare, for which legislation has been passed supporting the creation of PSOs). Whether PSOs will reach their full potential, however, is very much in doubt. They effectively pit provider systems against powerful buyers—managed care companies—and stimulate unwanted countermoves on the part of these companies, and providers face high costs when they enter the risky and competitive business of managed care.

The era of substitution in health care is still very much ahead of us. With continuing and, even, heightening pressures to reduce costs and eliminate waste and redundancies, opportunities to offer substitute products and services inevitably will arise. Some, for example, believe that future drug and gene therapies will become direct substitutes for much of current health care and will radically replace many providers. The analysis of substitution then becomes yet another critical area to which strategic analysts need to give attention.

Sellers

Threats from sellers are the inverse of those emanating from buyers, and many of the issues addressed in the discussion of buyers apply here. For most health care providers, the threat of forward integration from suppliers is very remote. Few suppliers (manufacturers, distributors, and others) pose credible threats of forward integration, though they do have significant capacity to negotiate effectively over prices and other product characteristics, given their absolute sizes as companies and the degree to which they enjoy monopoly power for patented drugs, medical equipment, and other items. However, providers over the last decade have increased significantly their purchasing power, having formed integrated delivery systems and joined purchasing alliances.

With regard to providers (as sellers) and managed care companies (as buyers), the balance of power appears to be fairly equal. On the one hand, a number of managed care companies have penetrated markets and engaged in merger activities, becoming very large in absolute terms. They have also captured high market shares in many markets. On the other hand, the providers appear to have countered effectively by forming into systems and capturing considerable relative power at the local market level. As in the grocery store example, presented at the beginning of this chapter, this gives providers a sufficient counterweight, at least to this point, to the power of managed care companies. However, as the markets continue to consolidate, the balance of power could shift. It is improbable in the near term that providers will go much beyond controlling local markets. But managed care companies will likely continue their patterns of national consolidation. Therefore, much will depend on the restructuring of managed care markets.

Stages of Market Growth

In addition to the more traditional structural determinants, a market's growth or decline can alter competitive advantage significantly. Markets are always expanding, declining, or flattening out in their rates of growth. Sometimes this is attributable to short-term or cyclical patterns and at other times, to longer-term causes. It is the latter, of course, that are important from the perspective of assessing markets and strategy. There are a number of reasons why the rates of growth in markets shift over time, including changes in buyer preferences, technology, entry barriers, the viability of substitute products, and the numbers and types of competitors. Changes in any one of these areas can alter demand on near permanent bases, thereby forcing competitors to reconsider and, if necessary, restructure their market strategies.

In one popular classification, markets evolve through three primary stages: emerging, mature, and decline (Porter, 1980). Not all markets flow through each of these stages, and they do not necessarily flow in the prescribed order. It is also important to note that separate business segments may lie in different stages. For example, integrated systems may own emerging stage physician practice-management organizations, mature stage clinics, and selected decline-stage hospital services. Nevertheless, each of these stages presents different forces to which strategic analysts must react in planning strategy.

Emerging markets characteristically experience high rates of growth combined with high levels of uncertainty. The uncertainty stems from many factors, including the presence of new buyers and sellers, new products, high learning costs, and evolving market structures. Ambulatory surgery is an example of a sector within health care that can be said to be in an emerging stage. The performance of physician practice management is still relatively unsettled. As a result, there remains a great deal of uncertainty in this sector. For example, it is not yet known who the major players will be, what clinical areas are best suited for this new model, whether there are economies of scale, how high the entry barriers will be, how rapidly demand will shift toward larger physician clinics, and what counter moves hospitals will take to shore up historic positions in this area.

Because competitors in emerging markets tend to be fairly high up on the learning curve, they face some significant challenges. Market uncertainty means that determining the appropriate pace of strategic development is a critical strategic consideration. In addition to pace, other sources of competitive advantage are important in emerging markets. Having access to the necessary talent, technologies, and resources such as investment capital (potential as a source of advantage) frequently is important to success in these markets. Also, capturing just the right positions in the markets often will be crucial.

Mature markets, by contrast, are characterized by a longer-term slackening in demand, which produces a unique set of challenges for the strategic analyst. Importantly, with limited expansion in demand, competitors discover that growth comes only by drawing market shares away from rivals. This can lead to aggressive patterns of rivalry, especially in early phases of market maturity. Being ill-prepared for the slowing growth, competitors will often make a variety of strategic moves grounded in inaccurate assumptions about market conditions. Having overestimated the growth in demand, for example, many will find themselves with costly excesses in capacity and will overreact to this by vigorously attempting to utilize excess capacities or even investing in more capacity. The management of capacity is a major concern in the early phases of market maturity.

A related and equally common response in the early phases of market maturity is the pursuit of consolidation strategies. Competitors perceive that this will help them not only to eliminate rivals, but also to capture economies of scale and, possibly more importantly, to increase their options for taking capacity out of the markets.

Alternatively, one can expect to find somewhat more predictable, even placid forms of competition within mature markets, especially in their later phases. Often, at some point in the evolution of the markets, rivals will have been driven out (depending, of course, on the height of exit barriers), relative positions of dominance will have been established, and competitors will have exhausted most alternatives to further restructuring shares and power within their markets. With experience, therefore, competitors increasingly will find the costs of direct confrontation far outweigh further gains in shares. Competitors will therefore shift their priorities to performance over growth and their strategic orientations from aggressive to defensive.

Many of the above conditions were observed in hospital markets throughout the 1990s, a period in which the growth in demand for acute care services slowed precipitously. In that period, we observed a rush to consolidation. Slowed growth in demand and increased threats from buyers, intent on winning price concessions, led many hospitals to participate in mergers, acquisitions, vertical integration, portfolio diversification, and hybrid organizations. Many of these power strategies (especially horizontal expansion) have proven to be very effective strategic responses within the maturing hospital industry. However, this is not true for all of the strategies. Some strategies (such as acquisition of physician practices, entering into the managed care businesses, and other integration strategies) appear only to be exacerbating the cost problems of hospitals and hospital systems. Interestingly, there are indications that a heavy emphasis on performance (for example, investing in information systems, clinical management capability, organizational restructuring or reengineering) itself has been more costly than anticipated. It is unclear whether the cost is due to excessive investments in infrastructure and consulting services, complications emanating from unwarranted vertical strategies, and/or failures to resolve internal power conflicts attributable to weak structural arrangements.

Finally, there is the special case of **declining markets.** As with the other market stages, the strategic analyst is mainly interested in changes that are due to long-term and sustained declines in demand. The traditional prescription for decline is a harvest strategy, which refers to "eliminating investment and generating maximum cash flow from a business, followed by eventual divestment (Porter, 1980, p. 254)." But this is not the only option available to competitors under conditions of decline. In part, strategy at this stage depends on the rate at which demand is falling. In most circumstances, decline is a gradual phenomenon, making it difficult to distinguish decline from maturity. For example, some claim that the hospital industry is in decline, pointing to falling admission rates and lengths of stays. Others argue that we are merely observing an adjustment to new patterns of delivery, the entry of selected substitute options (such as ambulatory surgery), and so on. It may be more accurate to say that some elements of the industry are in decline, while others are experiencing temporary shifts in demand and transitions in market restructuring.

Porter identified four strategy options for competitors in markets that are in decline. These are:

- *Leadership*—seek a dominant position in terms of market share
- *Niche*—create or defend a strong position in a particular segment
- *Harvest*—manage a controlled divestment
- *Divest quickly*—liquidate and reinvest elsewhere.

The first, leadership, assumes that competitive advantage can be gained through dominance, a logic similar to that discussed above, whereby a firm might adopt a power strategy to survive at the early stages of market maturity. The second, niche, assumes that there are segments within markets that remain steady or, even, are growing. The harvest strategy refers to gradual withdrawal from a market, primarily by drawing out cash and not reinvesting in a business. This strategy, of course, assumes that such withdrawals would not harm quality or service, which if they did could hasten declines in demand. If there is little reserve for cash withdrawal, then the last strategy, quick divestment, may be all that is left. The motivation for quick divestment is to exit while still financially viable and before the decline progresses too far. This option is likely only available at the earliest stages of decline, which is also when decline is most difficult to predict.

Interdependencies between Market Concentration and Stage of Growth

It is important to recognize that structural factors often combine to affect strategy. To illustrate how this is so, we introduce two of the dimensions of market structure discussed earlier and within each of these, three market models. These two dimensions and their three respective models are (1) degree of concentration (models: atomistic, oligopolistic, and monopolistic) and stage of market growth (models: emerging, mature, and decline). The cross-classification of market concentration and market stage yields nine market types. The types are identified in Table 14.3 along with the sources of competitive advantage

that could be priorities for firms competing within each type.

As can be seen, emerging markets can be atomistic, oligopolistic, or monopolistic, depending on the number of competitors and their relative shares. In emerging/atomistically structured markets, competitors must pay particular attention to the timing of their investments (pace) as well as ensure that they are projecting value to consumers (positioning). They must also be sure that they have assembled the proper capabilities to compete effectively in their new and forming markets (potential). Competitors in emerging/**oligopolistic markets,** where by definition there is only a small number of fairly dominating players, must add power strategies to the strategy mix. Those in **monopolistic markets** need less to worry about immediate rivals, but must ensure that others do not enter. Thus, for them, all of the sources of advantage become important, except, perhaps, power strategies (which, presumably they have already mastered). In general, performance may be less important in

Table 14.3. Bain's Market Typology, Based upon Three Major Dimensions of Market Structure: Seller Concentration, Product Differentiation, and Conditions of Entry.

Market Structure Dimensions	Type
1. Atomistic	
A. Without product differentiation	1-A
B. With product differentiation	1-B
2. Oligopolistic	
A. Without product differentiation	
a. With easy entry	2-A-a
b. With moderately difficult entry	2-A-b
c. With blockaded entry	2-A-c
B. With product differentiation	
a. With easy entry	2-B-a
b. With moderately difficult entry	2-B-b
c. With blockaded entry	2-B-C
3. Monopolized	3

SOURCE: Adapted from Bain JS, Qualls PD. *Industrial Organization: A Treatise, Part A.* Greenwich, CT: JAI Press, 1987;23–24.

emerging markets because of the steady, though uncertain, growth in demand within them.

In mature markets, competitors face a slowing in demand. The primary difference here is that pace ceases to be an important source of competitive advantage (except, perhaps, in the early stages when early recognition of the maturing phase might provide an advantage). A significant difference exists between competitors in atomistic and oligopolistic markets. In the atomistic markets, positioning is critical. While there are many competitors, no one of them is sufficiently large to impact significantly any other. Thus the key to survival is projecting value to consumers. Note, however, that power is a priority source of advantage in atomistic markets. This is because the necessary economic conditions for consolidating atomistic markets (for example, opportunities for economies of scale, high entry barriers, and large and powerful buyers) may be present, and if one or more of the competitors is able to consolidate the markets, they could achieve significant gains in competitive advantage. But, of course, this depends on whether those conditions exist. There is obvious danger in attempting to consolidate a market that does not support consolidation. This could be true, for example, in the physician markets, as a number of the large physician practice-management companies have learned.

By contrast, in mature/oligopolistic markets, competitors are large enough for their strategic actions to affect one another. As a result, they may need to take actions that give them added power to countervail the strength of rivals, and with the slowing in demand, survival for all competitors will depend heavily on their ability to control costs (performance). On the other hand, as has already been discussed, oligopolistically structured markets vary by the steepness of the gradient in market shares (and along other dimensions of structure as well). In the flatter gradient structures, in which there would exist a fairly balanced oligopoly group, the expectations expressed in Figure 14.8 would apply. The leading competitors, perhaps all of them, could be expected to seek ways by which to dominate through the pursuit of power strategies. Alternatively, in situations in which the

gradient is far steeper and one firm occupies an unassailably dominant position (for example, the Mayo Clinic in Rochester, Minnesota), several different strategic responses could be expected. First, the dominant firm, content with its relative market power, could adopt rather passive, shares-maintaining strategies, focusing more on position strategies than power or pace. The smaller or "fringe" firms, accepting the existing division of power, could act in a manner consistent with an atomistically structured market. Perceiving little threat from the passive dominant player, they could, as a result, give somewhat more priority to consumers, especially through product differentiation and niching strategies, rather than attempting to counter directly the dominant competitor.

Again, in monopolistic markets, the objective is to keep entrants out and to keep entry barriers high. As a result, positioning and performance are considered to be key in mature/monopolistic markets. Sole-provider hospitals in rural areas, for example, typically position themselves as being highly responsive to community needs for access to primary and secondary care services, and this becomes all the more important as urban systems reach out to compete for patients in the rural areas. In general, we note that pace, while it could be very important in individual cases, may be less important relative to the other sources of advantage in mature markets.

The Hill Rom corporation headquartered in Evanston, Indiana, offers another example of a firm that enjoys a near monopoly position in a very mature market, but still is very aggressive strategically. Hill Rom dominates the general medical/surgical bed and patient room support-system businesses. Their market shares in these areas are in the 95% range. They do have some important competitors in selected areas, but for the most part they dominate their markets. Hill Rom is very aware that despite their overwhelming market share, they are vulnerable to attack. Technological change in the industry, for example, could alter the formulas currently determining how beds, furniture, and patient support systems are combined in patient rooms. Future advances in computer and other medically related technologies could easily make it possible for new competitors to enter the market, thereby eroding Hill Rom's powerful market positions. The upshot is that Hill Rom, despite enjoying near-monopoly positions, has developed a highly sophisticated capacity to conduct strategy analyses. Hill Rom regularly monitors trends in new technologies and medical applications, assesses consumer attitudes and preferences, and measures the advantages of existing and prospective rivals. The firm illustrates very well the critical interplay between established power and the need to attend to other sources of competitive advantage.

Finally, in markets that are in decline, positioning (particularly, niching) and performance become highly important, regardless of the degree of concentration of the market, because all competitors in these markets must worry about capturing whatever demand remains. But they must take care not to erode quality and service and risk speeding up their own demise. As suggested earlier, a leadership (power) strategy may work under circumstances of decline, because dominant players have the best chance to succeed relative to rivals when markets are weakening.

 MANAGERIAL GUIDELINES

1. Develop a clear understanding of the concepts of and interrelationships among mission/vision, strategy, competitive advantage, and market structure. Strategy is not the mere selection of business opportunities that might have the best financials. Rather, it is a collection of concepts, ideas, and interrelationships that should assist leaders of organizations to better visualize and give meaning to their complex and often very threatening external environments. The vagaries and indirections of market competition can only be understood if interpreted within the context of a valid and workable framework. Such a framework is provided by the positioning school of thought within the strategy formulation field. In the framework, such concepts as strategy, competitive advantage, and market structure can be woven into a powerful set of strategic tools. In particular, Porter's structural framework provides a simple checkoff of major market forces and the interplay among them that should prove useful for those involved in strategy analysis.

2. Develop a clear understanding of the important relationship between organizational structure, implementation capabilities, and strategy. While discussed only briefly in this chapter, a strategic analyst will ultimately be confronted with the challenge of creating an organizational structure and implementation capabilities that will facilitate and sustain the objectives of intended and emergent strategies. This is especially important for complex organizations in which strategy often leads to the combination of multiple business units, and it may be even more important for a health care field that is becoming ever more integrated and elaborate. With the many interorganizational relationships that will need to be managed in the modern health care firm, new structures and approaches to implementation may well become the lynchpin of a successful strategy. It will likely be of little value, for example, to visualize the strategic power of a regionalized health system if there is no way to bring physicians, partnering hospitals, and other health care providers into a unified whole. Structure and implementation skills thus could

(continued)

Clearly, it is important for analysts to be careful not to generalize about strategy based on one dimension of market structure alone. Many dimensions come into play, and the logic for strategy will vary by which dimensions are identified and how they are combined.

CONCLUSIONS

To conclude this discussion of strategy making, we place strategy in a larger context. To do so, we offer three recommendations for managers who bear responsibility for formulating organizational strategies.

These are summarized in the Managerial Guidlines below.

From the Guidelines it should be apparent that neither the prescription of Cassius—" 'Tis better that the enemy seek us: So shall he waste his means, weary his soldiers"—nor that of Brutus—"we must take the current when it serves"—necessarily represent good strategic advice. The diversity of circumstances between competitors and across markets is very great, and the options for response are countless and multidimensional. It is the challenge of the successful strategic analyst to bring coherence and meaning out of the chaos of inexorably changing and often turbulent health care environments.

 # MANAGERIAL GUIDELINES

be the keys to unlocking the full potential of well-conceived strategies in the health care field.

3. Grasp the close linkage between strategic objectives and the public interest in health care. Strategy may well be the equivalent of an ill-shaped suit when fitted onto health care organizations. While health care organizations pursue their individual strategies, they will often be confronted by the question: "Does this strategy serve the community interest?" For example, while power strategies may prove very effective in assuring survival in highly competitive and obligopolistically structured hospital markets, they may not necessarily add to an objective of maximizing competition. A low-cost strategy may not prove to be in the best interest of patients whose lives hang in the balance of critical resource-allocation decisions. Or an aggressive expansion in health care business lines could simply add to the duplication of an already too costly health care system.

Strategy need not, however, be in conflict with the public good. The pursuit of a power strategy in a local market, for instance, could lead to the integration of otherwise fragmented and highly duplicative health care delivery units. Health care providers therefore operate in a unique environment in which there will inevitably exist a tenuous balance between public and private interests. Health care strategists must not carry out their roles with a blind eye to how their decisions will impact the cost, quality, and access of care available to local populations. And for this, collaborative rather than competitive strategies will often offer better prospects for serving local community needs.

As a final precautionary note, we would point out that once commitments are made to particular strategic courses of action, one risks becoming deeply immersed in strategic implementation and control at the expense of engaging in ongoing strategic analyses and reconsiderations of those courses. Strategy analysis should indeed be dynamic. Thinking while doing and doing while thinking should be the hallmark of effective strategy making.

Discussion Questions

1. The Ukrops grocery store company asked you to consult regarding what it should do to maintain and, hopefully, expand its share beyond the Richmond, Virginia, market. Review its current strategy using the concepts developed in this chapter, analyze the strategies of its competitors and possible markets into which it might enter (consider new geographic as well as product options), and recommend what strategic actions it should take to achieve its objectives. Be sure to explain all of the major points in your analysis, especially your recommendations for the future.

2. Select two metropolitan areas in your region, one large (say, exceeding 1,000,000 MSA population) and the other somewhat smaller (say, less than 750,000 population). Then, using the most recent issue of the *AHA Guide to the Health Care Field*, identify the hospitals that reside there, the systems that own them, if any, and their market shares (by hospital and system, using the ratio of their total beds to the total in the market). Be sure to determine what suburban areas and counties are included within those metropolitan areas so that all competing hospitals are identified. Consider also the markets and competitors located in surrounding rural and nearby urban areas, possible regional or national entrants, major managed care players in the market, and major physician groups, if any. Using this information, apply the Porter model in an analysis of the structure of the hospital markets in those areas and predict what strategies might most likely be followed by each hospital/system located in those areas. Defend your analysis.

3. Apply Table 14.3 to health care markets. Identify examples that fit in as many of the cells that you can. Test the predictions as to emphasis on sources of competitive advantage. For each of the examples, identify the leading competitor in that particular market. Also, generally describe the market structures for each using the Porter, Bain and Qualls, and stage of growth structural typologies. Again, defend your analysis.

4. Select a major health care system or hospital in your area and a major merger or acquisition target (hospital or other type of health care organization) in or around the area. Using the insights gained in the preceding chapters, identify three major categories of actors within each organization who might have a strong interest in and could have a powerful effect on the success of the proposed interorganizational combination. Also, assess their likely responses to the proposal and suggest managerial actions that should be taken by the leaders of the system or hospital to initiate the change and to assure the cooperation of each of the identified categories of actors. Also, provide a strategic rationale for the proposed acquisition.

References

Amburgey, T. L., & Miner, A. S. (1992, June). Strategic momentum: The effects of repetitive, positional, and contextual momentum on merger activity. *Strategic Management Journal, 13*, 335–348.

Andrews, K. R. (1987). The concept of corporate strategy (3rd ed.). Homewood, IL: Richard D. Irwin, Inc.

Ansoff, H. I. (1965). *Corporate strategy: An analytic approach to business policy for growth and expansion.* New York: McGraw-Hill.

Ansoff, H. I. (1991). Critique of Henry Mintzberg's "The design school: Reconsidering the basic premises of strategic management." *Strategic Management Journal, 12*(6), 449–461.

Ansoff, H. I. (1998). *The new corporate strategy.* New York: John Wiley & Sons.

Ashkenas, R., Ulrich, D., Jick, T., & Kerr, S. (1995). *The boundaryless organization: Breaking the chains of organizational structure.* San Francisco: Jossey-Bass.

Bain, J. S. (1956). *Barriers to new competition.* Cambridge, MA: Harvard University Press.

Bain, J. S. (1972). *Essays on price theory and industrial organization.* Boston: Little Brown.

Bain, J. S., & Qualls, D. (1987). *Industrial organization: A treatise.* Greenwich, CT: JAI Press.

Bowring, J. (1986). *Competition in a dual economy.* Princeton, NJ: Princeton Press.

Bracker, J. (1980). The historical development of the strategic management concept. *Academy of Management Review, 5*(2), 219–224.

Brown, S. L., & Eisenhardt, K. M. (1998). *Competing on the edge: Strategy as structured chaos.* Boston: Harvard Business School Press.

Carman, J. M., & Langeard, E. (1978, November). *Growth strategies for service firms.* (Working paper). U.C. Berkeley: Institute of Business and Economic Research.

Caves, R. (1982). *American industry: Structures, conduct, and performance* (5th ed.). Englewood Cliffs, NJ: Prentice-Hall.

Chandler, A. D., Jr. (1962). *Strategy and structure: Chapters in the history of the industrial enterprise.* Cambridge, MA: MIT Press.

Christiansen, C. R., Andrews, K. R., Bower, J. L., Hamermesh, R. G., & Porter, M. E. (1987). *Business policy: Text and cases* (6th ed.). Homewood, IL: Richard D. Irwin.

Clement, J. P., McCue, M. J., Luke, R. D., Rossiter, L. F., Ozcan, Y. A., & Bramble, J. D. (1997, December). Strategic hospital alliances: Impact on financial performance. *Health Affairs*, 193–203.

Coffey, R. J., Fenner, K. M., & Stofis, S. L. (1997). *Virtually integrated health systems.* San Francisco: Jossey-Bass.

Collis, D. J., & Montgomery, C. A. (1995, July-August). Competing on resources: Strategy in the 1990s. *Harvard Business Review*, 118–128.

Conrad, D. A., & Shortell, S. M. (1997). Integrated health systems: Promise and performance. In *Integrated delivery systems: Creation, management, and governance* (pp. 3–44). Chicago: Health Administration Press.

D'Aveni, R. A. (1994). *Hypercompetition: Managing the dynamics of strategic maneuvering.* New York: The Free Press.

Day, G. S., & Reibstein, D. J. (1997). *Wharton on dynamic competitive strategy.* New York: John Wiley & Sons.

Drucker, P. F. (1954). *The practice of management.* New York: Harper & Brothers.

Drucker, P. F. (1980). *Managing in turbulent times.* New York: Harper & Row.

Fernandez, B. (1998, August 2). Practices did not make perfect. *Philadelphia Inquirer.*

Ginsberg, E. (1998, September). For-profit medicine: A reassessment. *New England Journal of Medicine, 319*, 757–761.

Goold, M. (1992). Design, learning, and planning: A further observation on the design school debate. *Strategic Management Journal, 13*(2), 169–170.

Grant, R. M. (1991). The resource-based theory of competitive advantage: Implications for strategy formulation. *California Management Review, 33*(3), 114–135.

Gray, B. H. (Ed.). (1986). *For-profit enterprise in health care.* Washington, DC: National Academy Press.

Griffith, J. R. (1997). Managing the transition to integrated health care organizations. In *Integrated delivery systems: Creation, management, and governance* (pp. 91–132). Chicago: Health Administration Press.

Hamel, G., & Prahalad, C. J. (1989, May-June). Strategic intent. *Harvard Business Review*, 63–76.

Harrigan, K. (1985). *Strategic flexibility: A management guide for changing times.* Lexington, MA: Lexington Books.

Harris, M. (1998, April 5). Focused factories: Are you ready for the competition? *Hospitals and Health Networks.*

Hax, A. C. (1990). Redefining the concept of strategy and the strategy formation process. *Planning Review, 18*(3), 34–40.

Hayes, R. H., Pisano, G. P., & Upton, D. M. (1996). *Strategic operations: Competing through capabilities.* New York: The Free Press.

Jarillo, J. C. (1988). On strategic networks. *Strategic Management Journal, 9*, 31–41.

Kouzes, J. M., & Posner, B. Z. (1995). *The leadership challenge: How to keep getting extraordinary things done in organizations.* San Francisco: Jossey-Bass, pp. 10–11.

Lorange, P., Morton, M. F. S., & Ghoshal, S. (1986). *Strategic control.* St. Paul, MN: West Publishing.

Luke, R. D. (1991). Spatial competition and cooperation in local hospital markets. *Medical Care Review, 48*(2), 207–237.

Luke, R. D., Begun, J.W., & Pointer, D. D. (1989). Quasi firms: Strategic interorganizational forms in the health care industry. *Academy of Management Review, 14*, 9–19.

Luke, R. D., Ozcan, Y. A., & Olden, P. C. (1995, October). Local markets and systems: Hospital consolidations in urban areas. *Health Services Research*, 555–575.

Mason, E. S. (1939, March). Price and production policies of large enterprise. *American Economic Review*, 61–74.

McDaniel, R. R., Jr. (1998). Strategic leadership: A view from quantum and chaos theories. In W. J. Duncan, P. M. Ginter, & L. E. Swayne (Eds.), *Handbook of health care management* (pp. 339–367). Malden, MA: Blackwell.

Miles, R. (1982). *Coffin nails and corporate strategies*. Englewood Cliffs, NJ: Prentice-Hall.

Miles, R. E., & Snow, C. C. (1978). *Organizational strategy, structure, and process*. New York: McGraw-Hill.

Mintzberg, H. (1978). Patterns in strategy formation. *Management Science, 24*(9), 934–948.

Mintzberg, H. (1988). Opening up the definition of strategy. In J. B. Quinn, H. Mintzberg, & R. M. James (Eds.), *The strategy process: Concepts, contexts, and cases* (p. 17). Englewood Cliffs, NJ: Prentice-Hall.

Mintzberg, H. (1990). Strategy formation schools of thought. In J. W. Frederickson (Ed.), *Perspectives on strategic management* (pp. 105–236). New York: Harper Business.

Mintzberg, H. (1991). Learning 1, planning 0: Reply to Igor Ansoff. *Strategic Management Journal, 12*(6), 463–466.

Mintzberg, H. (1994). *The rise and fall of strategic management: Reconceiving roles for planning, plans, planners*. New York: The Free Press.

Mintzberg, H., Lampel, J., & Ahlstrand, B. W. (1998). *Strategy safari: A guided tour through the wilds of strategic management*. New York: Simon & Schuster.

Mintzberg, H., & Waters, J. A. (1985). Of strategies, deliberate and emergent. *Strategic Management Journal, 6*, 257–272.

Montgomery, C. A., & Porter, M. E. (1991). *Strategy: Seeking and securing competitive advantage*. Boston: HBS Press.

Moore, J. F. (1996). *The death of competition: Leadership and strategy in the age of business ecosystems*. New York: HarperCollins.

Oster, S. M. (1994). *Modern competitive analysis* (2nd ed.). New York: Oxford University Press.

Porter, M. E. (1980). *Competitive strategy: Techniques for analyzing industries and competitors*. New York: The Free Press.

Porter, M. E. (1985). *Competitive advantage: Creating and sustaining superior performance*. New York: The Free Press.

Porter, M. E. (1996, November-December). What is strategy? *Harvard Business Review*, 61–78.

Powell, T. C. (1992). Organizational alignment as competitive advantage. *Strategic Management Journal, 13*(2), 119–134.

Powell, W. W. (1990). Neither market nor hierarchy: Network forms of organization. In B. M. Straw, & L. L. Cummings (Eds.), *Research in organizational behavior, XII* (pp. 295–336). Greenwich, CN: JAI Press.

Quigley, J. V. (1993). *Vision: How leaders develop it, share it, and sustain it*. New York: McGraw-Hill.

Quinn, J. B. (1988). Strategies for change. In J. B. Quinn, H. Mintzberg, & R. M. James (Eds.), *The strategy process: Concepts, contexts and cases* (pp. 2–9). Englewood Cliffs, NJ: Prentice-Hall.

Satinsky, M. A. (1998). *The foundations of integrated care: Facing the challenges of change*. Chicago: American Hospital Publishing.

Shendel, D., & Hofer, C. (1979). *Strategic management: A new view of business and policy planning*. Boston: Little, Brown, and Co.

Shepherd, W. G. (1979). *The economics of industrial organization*. New York: Prentice-Hall.

Sherer, F. M., & Ross, D. (1990). *Industrial market structure and economic performance* (3rd ed.). Boston: Houghton Mifflin.

Shortell, S. M., Gillies, R. R., Anderson, D., Mitchell, J., & Morgan, K. (1993). Creating organized delivery system: The barriers and facilitators. *Hospital and Health Services Administration, 38*(4), 447–466.

Shortell, S. M., Gillies, R. R., Anderson, D. A., Morgan, K., & Mitchell, J. B. (1996). *Remaking health care in America: Building organized delivery systems*. San Francisco: Jossey-Bass.

Shortell, S. M., Morrison, E. M., & Friedman, B. (1990). *Strategic choices for America's hospitals: Managing change in turbulent times.* San Francisco: Jossey-Bass.

Steiner, G. A. (1979). *Strategic planning: What every manager should know.* New York: Free Press.

Stern, C. W., & Stalk, G., Jr. (1998). *Perspectives on strategy: From the Boston Consulting Group.* New York: John Wiley & Sons.

Walston, S. L., Kimberly, J. R., & Burns, L. R. (1996, Winter). Owned vertical integration and health care: Promise and performance. *Health Care Management Review, 21*(1), 83–92.

Wing, R. L. (1988). *The art of strategy: A new translation of Sun Tzu's classic—The Art of War.* New York: Doubleday.

Zajac, E. J., & Shortell, S. M. (1989). Changing generic strategies: Likelihood, direction and performance implications. *Strategic Management Journal, 10,* 413–430.

CHAPTER

15

Creating and Managing the Future

Arnold D. Kaluzny, Ph.D.
Stephen M. Shortell, Ph.D.

Chapter Outline

- The Organization and the Environment
- Individuals and Groups within the Organization
- The Managerial Role

Learning Objectives

After completing this chapter, the reader should be able to:

1. Identify the major trends likely to affect the delivery of health care.
2. Understand the changing role of physicians, nurses, and other health care professions.
3. Understand the changing role of management and the competencies required to function in the managerial role.

Key Terms

Community Care Networks
Ethnic Composition
Evidence-based Management
Evidence-based Medicine
Future Scenarios
Horizontal Integration
Just-in-time Management (JIT)
Organizational Learning
Organized Delivery Systems
Social Experimentation
Social Norms and Expectations
Strategic Alliances
Technology Assessment
Vertical Integration

Chapter Purpose

Like so many, Mrs. Peterson is a victim of the system (In the Real World, p. 434). How might this have been prevented? Better technology? More caring people? Perhaps, but clearly the structure within which care is provided influences the provision of care; this, in turn, is dependent on larger secular trends. Four future scenarios are presented in Debate Time 15.1 that may influence whether Mrs. Peterson is an isolated event or a constant reminder of a delivery system with fundamental problems (Bezold, 1996). It is likely that elements of each scenario will combine to influence the future provision of health services.

A number of forces will play a key role in the emerging health care system. This chapter begins by considering changes likely to occur in the organization and its environment, discusses the future of individuals and groups within organizations, and ends with consideration of the managerial role. The intent is to be provocative yet realistic, building on issues developed in preceding chapters. A central theme is that health services organizations and their leaders can actively influence their environment and thereby create and actively manage their future, and if past is prologue "nothing is written."

THE ORGANIZATION AND THE ENVIRONMENT

Health services organizations, functioning as corporate actors, are the major repository of power within health services. Health care expenditures represent a significant percentage of the gross national product (GNP), and as federal and state governments and major employers continue to be major purchasers of care, the influence of health services corporate actors will increase. The collective decisions of individual hospitals, multihospital systems, alternative delivery systems, nursing home chains, regulatory groups, suppliers, and other corporate actors within the health services field will significantly affect the basic structure and characteristics of services provided.

Moreover, these organizations will be operating in and affected by an increasingly complex and unpredictable environment, an environment characterized by the difficulty of predicting both the occurrence and content of change. For example, decisions about health care may in fact be made on factors quite independent of the substantive issues involved with health care. Specifically, as health services consume greater portions of the gross national product, their effects on other sectors of the economy are pervasive. Thus, other criteria, such as local employment or employment in a variety of other support ancillary areas, become important criteria affecting decisions within health services.

Along with increasing complexity and unpredictability of the environment will come a demand for greater organizational responsiveness and accountability from different groups. The organization will face the problem of reconciling incompatible objectives. For example, the federal government often defines accountability in terms of cost control, while local consumer groups may see accountability in terms of added facilities and services and greater consumer participation in decision making. In short, the future involves major issues centering on the organization's ability to adapt to divergent demands. This effort will require innovation, the ability to manage external dependencies, and at the same time the ability to learn and restructure relationships. A number of major trends and their implications follow.

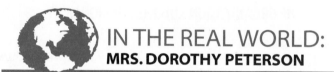

IN THE REAL WORLD:
MRS. DOROTHY PETERSON

Mrs. Dorothy Peterson is a 72-year-old woman living in a retirement community. On February 1, she was found unconscious in her apartment and was taken to the emergency room of the local hospital. While she was a patient at that hospital a few months earlier, hospital personnel were unable to locate her medical record. The ER conducted its first assessment, and within a few hours, she was transferred to the hospital's medical unit.

The medical unit conducted a second assessment, and developed the first nursing plan. Mrs. Peterson progressed nicely, and soon was transferred to the rehabilitation unit where a third assessment was conducted and a second nursing plan developed.

While in the rehabilitation unit, Mrs. Peterson developed a urinary tract infection, and was readmitted to the nursing unit, where still another assessment and nursing plan was developed. Three days later she was discharged to a home care program, where yet another care plan and assessment were conducted.

Two weeks later, she was readmitted to the ER with an elevated temperature and dehydration, where she received her sixth assessment and was admitted to the medical unit. In the medical unit, she was again evaluated, and received yet another nursing plan. Two days later, she was discharged to Beacon Nursing Home and received her eighth assessment and sixth nursing care plan. On the fourth day at the nursing facility, she complained of shortness of breath, and was readmitted to the emergency room, where, despite all efforts, personnel were unable to resuscitate her, and she was pronounced dead.

During these thirty-eight days, Mrs. Peterson experienced a caring staff, state-of-the-art technology, along with eight assessments, six nursing care plans, eight admissions, 14 attending physicians, and 24 separate bills totaling $140,000, of which only $40,000 were reimbursed.

Kaluzny, Zuckerman, & Rabiner. (1998). Interorganizational factors affecting the delivery of primary care to older Americans. Health Services Research, 33 (2), Part II, 381–401.

Changing Social Norms and Expectations

The underlining **social norms and expectations** are important guides to behavior within health services, and changing norms and expectations will serve to shape the fundamental questions and issues that will guide the public policy debate regarding the future character of health services. Questions of access, choice, and accountability will play a central role and be shaped by fundamental norms and expectations. As a society, we have valued equality of access and opportunity as well as placing a great deal of emphasis on individualism. It is unlikely that the future will see a resolution between the underlying values of universal access to health care and individual freedom.

Imposed upon these underlying values is the growing need for accountability and the recognition that accountability must include both clinical and financial criteria. Simply holding down costs without paying attention to the quality of services provided or the impact on patient health status is unacceptable. The new accountability will emphasize value—the relationship between quality and cost or between benefit and cost that meets purchaser and consumer needs and demands. The new accountability, however, will place a significant burden on provider organizations and insurance carriers as they try to track medical treatments and outcomes, presenting a dilemma between accountability and choice. The greater the accountability the more likely the choice of provider will be limited since plans or provider organizations will only reimburse providers meeting accountability criteria (Weinstein, 1998). The level and focus of accountability are not clear. Most likely the country will evolve toward a system of shared accountability involving the private and public sector at multiple levels requiring the active participation of many parties.

DEBATE TIME 15.1: WHAT DO YOU THINK?

SCENARIO 1: BUSINESS AS USUAL

National health care reform was sent back to the states, resulting in great diversity. Expensive advances in technology and therapeutics, including function-enhancing bionics, help health care's share of the GNP grow to 17% by 2005. Health care providers shift to forecasting and then managing illness far earlier and more successfully. Poverty and lack of access to health care persist.

SCENARIO 2: HARD TIMES/ GOVERNMENT LEADERSHIP

Recurrent hard times and a political revolt against health care lead to a frugal Canadian-like health care system. Most states follow Oregon in consciously setting priorities. Heroic measures for terminal patients decline, and more frugal, yet successful, approaches to innovation are adapted. Health care's percentage of the GNP is reduced to 11% by 2001. Thirty percent of Americans "buy up" to affluent, higher-tech care, and two different systems of health care emerge.

SCENARIO 3: BUYER'S MARKET

Many thought the 1980s was the decade of health care's entry into the marketplace and that competition would lead to better, less expensive service. What failed during the 1980s worked very well over the next two decades. Markets, including health care, now do a much better job of giving consumers a range of high-quality services, delivered in convenient ways at relatively low cost over the long term, while maintaining a high degree of innovation. These amazing changes are coupled with better social policies to blunt the inequities and lack of access that accompany the stronger market approach.

SCENARIO 4: HEALTH GAINS AND HEALING

The 15 years before 2010 were a time of vision and design for health care. Health care organizations, their customers, and the communities they served joined to develop and pursue powerful shared visions. These generally lead to health gains, through a variety of paths. This noble activity was reinforced by "smarter markets," which allow consumers and large purchasers to understand the outcomes of health care providers both for individuals and for the communities they serve.

Which of the above scenarios do you believe is most likely to occur? What are the most important implications for health services managers?

The particular configuration is likely to be influenced by two emerging trends:

- *Health care as a political issue*—While the intersection of politics and health is not new, the late 1990s signaled the dramatic shift prompting one observer to comment, "something new is happening in Washington—Congress is practicing medicine." Policy is increasingly being shaped by political personnel and special-interest groups rather than objective scientific inquiry. For example, in 1997, following extensive review by the scientific community, congressional pressure reversed the recommendation of an NIH consensus panel charged to review scientific evidence on mammography screening for premenopausal women (Fletcher, 1997). As health care and medical technology become more important to an aging population, and the population has access to politicians, it is likely that evidence-based decisions are increasingly likely to be influenced by political as well as scientific judgment.

- *Deprofessionalization of the medical care process*—In order to meet the challenges of accountability and competition, health services have increasingly taken on the characteristics of industrial organizations. This is really *part of a larger trend* to redefine health care as a commercial as well as professional activity (Hurley, 1998). Through this redefinition, health care has assumed the characteristics of industrial-type organizations with "product lines," "medical loss ratios," and "finder fees" for terminally ill patients requiring hospice care—to illustrate just a few of the challenges underlying the principles of patient care (Glasser, 1998). It will also require the medical profession to share accountability with numerous other groups including payers, consumers, and the community (Shortell, Waters, Clarke, & Budetti, 1998).

Demographic Composition and Epidemiology

Managing the future requires a thorough understanding of the evolving demographics and epidemiological characteristics of the population. Perhaps most far-reaching is the changing character of the population, and specifically, the increase in the percentage of elderly people in the population. The proportion of the total population composed of those 65 and over is expected to increase in all states. Over a 30-year period, California and Florida would continue to rank first and second respectively in having the largest number of elderly. By 2025, Texas will rank number three, passing New York and Pennsylvania, and Florida is expected to be the "oldest" state with more than 26% of its population age 65 or older. In fact, the number of elderly is projected to double in 20 states between 1995 and 2025 (Campbell, 1997).

Equally important for managing the future is the racial and **ethnic composition** of the population. Two groups of particular importance that will affect our ability to manage the future are African-Americans and Hispanic-Americans. Both groups currently remain outside the mainstream of health services and will greatly challenge the ability of the health system in the future. It is expected that African-Americans will grow as a percentage of the population from 11.8% in 1980 to 14.2% in the year 2025. Although in 1980, the Hispanic-American population was roughly half of the total African-American population, by the year 2025, the two groups will be equal in size and together represent 32% of the U.S. population. Both groups will represent the youngest part of the population requiring services that are fundamentally dif-

ferent from those required by the elderly portion of the population.

The demands of the population will be further reflected in the epidemiological trends of the population. Diseases of aging, lifestyle, and behavior will present major challenges to the delivery system. While heart disease and cancer remain the most common cause of death and will remain a cause of death well into the twenty-first century, age-adjusted reductions in mortality occurred for both heart disease and cancer in 1995–1996. The reduction in heart disease mortality is consistent with a downward trend since 1950; cancer mortality has followed a downward trend only since 1990. It is estimated that in the United States, men have a 1 in 2 lifetime risk of developing cancer, and for women the risk is 1 in 3. Moreover, of the 1,228,600 Americans diagnosed with cancer, 491,400, or 4 of 10 patients, are expected to be alive five years after diagnosis.

Alzheimer's disease (AD) will also present major challenges to the system as the population increases in age. The U.S. Government Accounting Office (1998) estimated that in 1995 at least 1.9 million Americans 65 years or older suffered from some level of AD and projected that by 2015, 2.8 million Americans will have some form of the disease. Total estimated costs are staggering. Using 1991 data, it is estimated (Ernst & Hay, 1984) that direct and total prevalence costs were $20.6 billion and $67.3 billion respectively, and that the long-term dollar losses will exceed $1.75 trillion.

Diseases of lifestyle and behavior will present the most difficult challenges to the health services system. Perhaps most traumatic will be the continued toll taken by acquired immune deficiency syndrome (AIDS). Not even listed as a leading cause of death in 1985, the human immunodeficiency virus (HIV) was the eighth-leading cause of death in 1995. While recent data have highlighted substantial declines in AIDS' incidence and death ("Diagnosis and reporting of HIV," 1998), this decline has not been accompanied by a comparable decline in newly diagnosed HIV cases. The cost in human suffering is immeasurable, and the medical expenses associated with AIDS treatment is estimated to be more than $100,000 per person (Epstein et al., 1995). Current federal spending for

1996 alone exceed $7.3 billion, placing a significant burden on health care providers (National Center for Health Statistics, 1997).

Technology Development, Assessment, and Outcomes

Technology development in both treatment, prevention, and early-detection activities will continue to have a major impact on health services in the future. Such developments will raise questions involving who will have access to new technological developments, to what degree the decision to use new technology will be centralized, what effect new technology will have on provider-patient relationships, and what new ethical considerations must be considered. In addition, more patients and segments of the general population will be using alternative medicine practices such as chiropractic, acupuncture, and homopathy, as well as methods that may be potentially harmful (Cassileth and Chapman, 1996; Cassileth, 1998).

New developments will change our paradigm of disease and health. The paradigm of diagnosis and treatment will be replaced by one of prediction and early-stage management of the illness. Such projects as the Human Genome Project in which geneticists around the world will be conducting a massive cooperative research effort to completely map or at least partially sequence the entire human genome. This process will define the form and function of most of our genes; thus, instead of diagnosing diseases late in the disease process, we will be predicting disease risk based on our genetic inheritance and attempting to manage that risk before symptoms emerge. While the challenges are great, proponents of this project, and particularly those who speculate about its implications for health services, suggest that "within 15 years it will be morally and fiscally untenable to continue to think of disease as an inexorable act of God" (Goldsmith, 1992).

New developments in prevention, early detection, and health-promotion activities will have similarly important implications, particularly as they are implemented in health care delivery systems involving defined populations. Although not as dramatic or as heroic as the basic technological development described above, significant progress is occurring in the control of hypertension, coronary disease, cancer, and certain disabling forms of mental illness. For example, biomarkers and chemoprevention agents—such as the breast cancer prevention agent, tamoxifen, for women at increased risk of developing breast cancer—are important developments having profound implications on the health services system.

Moreover, increasing attention will be given to the role of social factors in determining health. Despite significant improvements in overall health status and an impressive technology, there exists significant—in fact, embarrassing—variation in health status among social groups (Amick, Levine, Tarlov, & Walsh, 1995). Unequal distribution of social resources and well-being are fundamental determinants of health and disease. Emphasizing the role of social determinants of health provides an opportunity to develop and implement more effective social and public health interventions for population-based health improvement. Many of these initiatives will be outside the traditional health community, involving industry, education, and other nonhealth personnel, and have a significant impact on overall health status.

Developments of both conventional and alternative treatments as well as preventive and health-promotion strategies will be accompanied by greater concern for assessment of costs and efficacy. Increasingly, attention will be given to outcomes and the development of evidence-based disease management—that is, an approach to care that emphasizes coordinated, comprehensive care along the continuum of disease and across health care providers in which the approach to practice integrates pathophysiological rational, caregiver experience, and patient preferences with valid and current clinical research evidence (Ellrodt et al., 1997).

Organizational Arrangements

While evolving social norms and expectations, demography, epidemiology, and technologies will affect organizational arrangements, the very nature of the organizations themselves and their interactions will affect the management challenges of the future. New organizational forms will be developed, and existing forms will change, forging new relationships with other organizations in the environment. In the world of health services, a great deal of attention has been given to the configuration of service-delivery organizations transcending existing organizational entities. While both **vertical and horizontal integration** represent interorganizational efforts, to be more responsive to changing environmental conditions, the unrelenting demand of cost containment, improving quality, and assuring technology transfer and accountability, will force managers to increasingly consider other forms of organizational arrangements. These include the development of organized delivery systems (Shortell et al., 1996), community care networks (Weiner & Alexander, 1998) and employer-sponsored delivery systems, or more loosely coupled alliances such as joint ventures, purchasing coalitions (Satinsky, 1997) and alliances to facilitate the transfer of state-of-the-art technology to local communities (Kaluzny & Warnecke, & associates, 1996; Lamb, Greenlick, & McCarty, 1998).

The watchword among many of these configurations has been *integration*. While a growing percentage of health care organizations and providers of various types participated in these arrangements throughout the 1990s, there is as yet little evidence either pro or con of cost savings or improvement in quality or outcomes of care (Health Care Advisory Board, 1997). In fact, a number of specialized disease "carve-out" companies have arisen in areas such as cancer care, heart disease, diabetes, and behavioral medicine. These developments are likely to require a new alignment between organizations and providers designed to achieve some long-term strategic purpose not possible by any single organization (Zuckerman & Kaluzny, 1991).

Particular attention needs to be given to the emerging relationships between "integrated" health systems and single-disease providers in managing the challenges of those with multiple chronic illnesses (see Debate Time 15.2).

While these alliances are not unique to health services, they are clearly different organizational forms from those historically characterizing health services and thus, in profound ways, will change how existing health care organizations operate. Emphasis is given

to the interaction process in which there is a constant exchange of products, information, money, and social symbols with the emphasis being on interaction and interdependency on each other in various ways in an effort to "customize" services to meet the demands and expectations of patients and defined population groups (McLaughlin & Kaluzny, 1997). Clearly these are fragile and emerging relationships with the critical challenge being the way management deals with the issues of commitment, control, performance, communication, information, and participation over time.

While health services organizations—particularly hospitals, integrated health networks/systems, and health departments—have prided themselves on their self-sufficiency, the push for efficiency will force attention to new configurations among providers, suppliers, and vendors (Halverson, Mays, Kaluzny, & Richards, 1997) and further experimentation with subcontracting and outsourcing functions to other organizations in the community. **Just-in-time management (JIT),** in which organizations can benefit from synchronizing inventory with workflow needs, and outsourcing of functions, which has traditionally been part of normal operations, are just a few of the opportunities to realize efficiencies once thought impossible. The managerial challenge will be the development of trust among a variety of participants and particularly involving physicians in positions of leadership at all levels of the organization (Zukerman et al., 1998).

Financing

The changing demographics and epidemiology and new organizational forms will put added stress on the financing of health services and the manner in which providers are reimbursed. Major segments of the population continue to be without health insurance coverage, and health care expenditures consume a significant portion of the gross national product. For example, throughout the entire 1995 calendar year, an estimated 41 million people in the United States (15.4% of the population) were without health insurance—unchanged from the prior year. Moreover, despite the existence of programs such as Medicaid and Medicare, 30.2% of the population (11 million) had no

DEBATE TIME 15.2: WHAT DO YOU THINK?

"The competition of the future isn't between hospitals or big capitated systems," says Bradford Koles, management director of the Advisory Board Co. in Washington. "It's product competition. It's who has the best cancer services. That's what consumers are looking for."

"We're here to serve the whole community and the whole person, not just individual organs that are profitable," snaps Russell Harrington, Jr., president of Baptist Health, the hospital's parent system. Still, he concedes, "it's hard to compete against a provider that focuses on a niche."

He may be right about that: Most of the 63 beds of the Arkansas Heart Hospital have been steadily occupied since the three-story facility opened a year ago, just blocks from Baptist. The heart hospital quickly posted a profit, too. The facility's backbone is the equity partnership between MedCath and the state's busiest and most prestigious heart practice, the 14-doctor Little Rock Cardiology Clinic, headed by superstar cardiologist Bruce Murphy. MedCath runs similar facilities in Tucson and McAllen, Texas, and is building others in Arizona, California, New Mexico, Ohio, and Texas.

Despite MedCath's growing pains, focused factory is the new mantra of theorists, consultants, entrepreneurs, financial analysts, and even some general hospital executives, who see the future in companies like MedCath, HealthSouth, Intensiva, Pediatrix, Salick, and others. Concentrating on a single product line, they aim to offer convenient one-stop shopping.

Harvard University business professor Regina Herzlinger (1997), who coined the term "focused factory" in her book, *Market-Driven Health Care*, asks why McDonald's can turn out millions of perfect french fries every day, while some hospitals still amputate the wrong legs. People with cancer and other ailments want a total system focused on their needs, she argues, not a broad integrated system that requires traveling from place to place for each service. "The guy who has a narrower range of mission is bound to be better than you are," she says.

Other hospital leaders decry the pure-play trend, though they admit their facilities should provide more efficient care and better customer service. Reginald Ballantyne, III, president of PMH Health Resources in Phoenix and immediate past chairman of the American Hospital Association, calls it "ludicrous and wasteful" for specialty firms to build new hospital beds. Most communities are already overbedded by half and badly need resources to improve primary and preventive services and care for the uninsured. "Many single-specialty hospital facilities appear to be economically motivated or perhaps established to serve the egos of certain specialists," says Ballantyne, whose health system faces a challenge from a MedCath facility scheduled to open this month. "My community needs another hospital about as much as it needs a multimillion-dollar macarena dance hall."

Other observers fear that a proliferation of facilities focusing on well-insured patients with particular conditions could destroy the financial and medical underpinnings of full-service hospitals. Arnold Relman, editor-in-chief emeritus of the *New England Journal of Medicine,* calls the trend "medical gentrification." He worries that freestanding specialty facilities are risky for very sick patients with multiple conditions, for which doctors need a full-treatment arsenal. "It's a selfish skimming off of profitable services without regard to the impact of the total delivery of care."

Commenting on his care at a MedCath Center, Waylon Glover, a 51-year-old construction worker says, "If it gets any better than this, I'd like to see it." He came to the heart hospital on the recommendation of his cardiologist, an investor in the facility, even though it's not in his health plan's network and he had to pay more himself.

"It's the best place to work, and I hope it stays that way," says surgical director C.D. Williams, who's not an investor. "The attitude and qualifications of the people here are superior. We can do everything but transplants. And we can deal with most of the common comorbidities, because we have a full range of specialists."

Some cardiologists who don't practice at the heart hospital question that. "When a heart patient's lungs or kidneys go bad, the pulmonary and renal guys tell me they're at a loss over there," says Steve Greer, Baptist's chief of cardiology. "They can't deal with the problem as rapidly and efficiently as a full-service hospital."

Given the above arguments, what do you see as the pros and cons of integrated delivery systems versus focused factories? How do you see these developments evolving in the future?

Adapted from **Meyer, H. "Focused Factories" Hospitals & Health Networks, *Vol. 72, No 7, by permission, April 5, 1998, Copyright, 1998, American Hospital Publishing, Inc.***

insurance of any kind during 1995—again unchanged from the previous year (U.S. Bureau of the Census, 1997). While most people were covered by private insurance (70.3% in 1995), the fact that most private insurance is employment-based means that any increase in the unemployment rate would increase the percentage of the population without health insurance presenting significant stress on provider reimbursement.

Health care expenditures now exceed $1 trillion, accounting for 13.8% of the gross domestic product, and these expenditures are expected to increase to nearly $1.5 trillion by the year 2002, representing 15% of the gross domestic product. When adjusted for inflation, this increase accounts for a 3.5% annual growth, just 1% to 2.5% lower than the rate of growth during the late 1980s and early 1990s, again placing significant strain on provider organizations (Thorpe, 1997).

Several initiatives are underway that will have important implications for the financing and reimbursement of health services. The increasing visibility that the United States is the only industrialized country (with the exception of South Africa) that does not guarantee financial access to health care for all of its citizens has resulted in a growing interest, at both national and state levels, in expanding financial access to assure a basic set of benefits for all Americans, or at least segments of the population (e.g., mothers and children). Major considerations in developing such a program are what benefits should be considered ba-

sic, what the benefits will cost, how they should be financed, and what incentives should be developed for the delivery system to provide cost-effective care in meeting the increased demand.

Moreover, in the unrelenting effort to contain costs, Medicare will allow a wider range of private health care plans to enroll beneficiaries, and states who manage the Medicaid program will move in similar directions. These approaches will offer wide choice of health care plans to beneficiaries, but, at the same time, provide an opportunity for these programs to operate with a stake in controlling costs. One consequence of this may be cost-shifting and care-shifting responsibilities to other institutions—mainly the families (Estes, Swan, & associates, 1993). For example, shorter hospital stays and limited nursing home care benefits require that care be shifted to the responsibility of family units. Families who already share a significant burden in terms of child-rearing responsibilities, as well as both husband and wife working, present a significant challenge. Thus, while the cost may be contained within health services, the cost to other institutions within our society may be significant.

As the percentage of gross national product devoted to health spending grows, and as health premiums increase, continued pressure will be placed on accountability and cost-cutting and cost-shifting initiatives. Employers and other large purchasers will resist demands for rate increases by HMOs and other health care providers. Given the movement to redefine health care as a commodity, larger purchasers "want the healthcare industry (under whatever configuration) to cut costs—*the way the rest of corporate American has done*" [italics added] (Winslow, 1998). This expectation will force clinicians and health services managers to work together more closely to figure out at what point in the continuum of patient care the greatest value is added. Increasingly, this will be in outpatient settings, in the workplace, and in homes. As noted later, it will involve fundamental transitions in managerial roles.

Social Experimentation, Evaluation, and Learning

Evaluation, experimentation, and learning will extend beyond technology assessment to encompass a wide variety of new approaches, programs, and organizations for delivering more cost-effective health care. The demands for greater accountability under an environment of constrained resources will push the health care system further in the direction of Campbell's classic "experimenting society," in which new demonstration programs are rigorously evaluated. Emphasis will be placed not only on results but also on the process by which the results are obtained and the ability to link this knowledge to improved decision making.

A contemporary application of this becomes operational with the focus on "micro-units" of caregivers and support staff who work together daily to treat illness and injuries and promote the health and well-being of a defined population (Nelson, Batalden, Mohr, & Plume, 1998). The approach is very similar to an approach known as Clinical Firm Trials Research, which was initiated in the 1980s at the Cleveland Metro Health Center and, more recently, ongoing in several hospitals throughout the country. Firm research provides an opportunity to evaluate various changes in programmatic initiatives in the delivery of health care with the rigors of a randomized clinical trial.

An important effect of this research is that health services managers will be increasingly part of a continual organizational learning effort—that is, the capacity or processes within the organization to maintain or improve performance based on experience (Barnsley, Lemieux-Charles, & McKinney, 1998). This

activity involves knowledge acquisition, "development of creation of skills, insights, relationships, knowledge sharing, dissemination to others of what has been acquired by some, and knowledge utilization, integration of the learning so that it is assimilated, broadly available, and can be generalized to new institutions" (DiBella, Novis, & Gould, 1996).

As clinicians move toward evidenced-based medicine, managers will equally be involved with evidence-based management. Under this approach, managers will play an important role in the initiation and facilitation of the evaluation and learning process as well as the mediation of the relationship between the evaluators and organizational personnel and the implementation and use of evaluation results for improved decision making (Veney & Kaluzny, 1998).

In the initiation stage, managers will be responsible for determining the purposes of the evaluation. Is the organization willing to commit the resources required for valid evaluation? What are the likely payoffs? Are ulterior or covert purposes involved? These are some of the questions that managers will have to articulate and assess. In addition, managers will be faced with the issue of selecting an inside or outside group to conduct the evaluation. At the same time, the manager must determine whether and when the organization is ready for the evaluation. Premature evaluation serves no one's ends. The manager will also play an important role in facilitating the implementation of the evaluation. This is particularly true in regard to formulating program objectives, which should be clearly understood by all involved.

The manager can also play an important role in mediating relationships between program staff members and evaluators. These relationships are frequently characterized by conflict. Program staff understandably view their activities as beneficial and as contributing to the organization's goals. Evaluators, on the other hand, are charged with maintaining the integrity of the evaluation design and taking an independent view as to whether or not and to what degree the program's objectives have been achieved. Further, the evaluation may consume resources that program staff members feel may be better spent on direct services. Managers can help minimize these conflicts by ensuring that sufficient time is allocated for discussion

Table 15.1. Environmental Trends

	Past (1960s–1980s)	Present (2000)	Future (2000 and beyond)
Social norms and expectations	Provider dominated	Changing consumer expectations	Deprofessionalization and shared accountability
Demographics and epidemiology	Aging of population not an issue; infectious diseases	Aging as an emergent issue; chronic diseases	Aging a major focus of activity; diseases of lifestyle and aging; growing ethnic diversity
Technical development, assessment, and outcomes	Rapid development and implementation	Emerging efforts at assessment	Use of randomized trials and metanalysis
Financing and reimbursement	Not an issue; retrospective reimbursement	Emergent concern and shift to prospective reimbursement	Increased financial risk
Organizational arrangement	Cottage industry; large number of individual providers	Systems and emerging organizational forms	Reconfiguration of networks and systems
Social experimentation, evaluation, and learning	Emerging efforts	Pressure on accountability	Collaborative efforts among policy makers, researchers, and managers; evidence-based management

and development of mutual understanding and by engaging in direct problem-solving and conflict-resolution strategies as needed.

Finally, managers play a key role in making use of the evaluation results. Managers who work closely with evaluators can help to ensure that the key questions are being answered in a manner that makes sense to the eventual users. This includes suggesting to the evaluators that the report be written in a language and format understandable to the intended audience.

Past, Present, and Future

Table 15.1 presents each of the major trends involving the organization and the environment. As can be seen, both the organization and the environment are faced with increasing risk and uncertainty. Organizations are increasingly being challenged, requiring greater adaptability and creativity. The future obviously will involve activities that have not been done before and will require efforts that have not yet been tried.

INDIVIDUALS AND GROUPS WITHIN THE ORGANIZATION

As an organization functions within a larger environment, individuals and groups function within a larger organizational setting. This interaction is critical to the overall performance of health care institutions in the future role of managers within these organizations. Several developments likely to affect the interaction of individuals and groups within organizations having profound implications on the managerial role are discussed below.

Changing Role of the Physician

Changing demographics and epidemiology, new technologies and their emphasis on assessment and outcomes, and fundamental changes in the configuration of health services resulting in increased scrutiny of health care costs are redefining the role of the physician and are likely to affect the basic role that physicians will play in the emerging health care system. The implications are expected to be reflected in greater attention to prevention, the incorporation of consumer preferences into medical decision making, and greater involvement in managerial activities, either as a knowledgeable clinician or a physician executive.

The shifting patterns of morbidity and mortality as well as changes in the demographic composition of the population are increasingly forcing medical practice to focus on the treatment of diseases associated with specific lifestyles or behaviors and chronic degenerative diseases of aging. Cardiovascular and pulmonary diseases, trauma, substance abuse, AIDS and other sexually transmitted diseases, cancer, chronic cognitive impairment, and diabetes are among the major health problems facing the population. Today and into the future, prevention will be the primary focus, and the physician will increasingly be at the vanguard of this movement.

Changes in the organization and delivery of health services and the results of health services research efforts are reflected in outcomes research and evidence-based medicine as the basis of clinical decisions. Outcomes research will produce more knowledge about the consequences of alternative treatments for specific conditions and provide recognition of the importance of consumer participation in the choice of treatment options available. The empirical documentation that all treatment is not equal and the explicit recognition that there are trade-offs will give increasing focus to shared decisions.

Finally, the emerging trends within the larger environment will force physicians to become increasingly knowledgeable about and involved with the organizational and managerial environment within which they function. Physicians will become active participants in the decision-making process and will join the growing ranks of physician executives forced to confront and reconcile market-oriented economic self-interest with the values of medical professionalism, emphasizing service to patients. This confrontation will impact medical education, challenging the traditional autonomy of professional education, and require new partnerships with emerging delivery systems and the development of a "new professionalism" sustained by a larger institutional framework

(Frankford & Konrad, 1998) and a new "moral fabric" (Shortell, Waters, Clarke, & Budetti, 1998). The latter is based on practicing population-based medicine, new models of managing and governing physician groups, aligning physician incentives, new care-management practices, and outcomes reporting systems. The challenge for the health services executive is to develop a working partnership with the physician community—one that fully recognizes the role of physicians in the managerial process.

Changing Role of the Nurse

Nursing is the largest single profession in health care and is undergoing profound change given the larger transformation in the financing and delivery of health services. As a profession, nursing has joined the coalition of managers and physicians who can make a difference in the major challenges involved in providing efficient and high-quality health care. This is particularly true in enhancing the clinical integration of care across the continuum.

The changing role of the nurse will be particularly painful since the commercialization and "deprofessionalization" of health services will result in both a redefinition of many traditional functions performed by nurses as well as an overall reduction in the total demand for nurses. However, two factors of the nurses' role will assure their continued contribution and influence to the overall transformation. First, as a professional group and clearly recognizing its heterogeneity, nurses are pervasive throughout the care continuum. While the decreased use of hospitals and competition from alternative providers will reduce the overall demand for nurses within acute care facilities, their role in a variety of ambulatory and long-term care facilities and the expanding role of advance nurse practitioners provide an opportunity to maintain a major presence in the provision of care (Salsberg, Wing, & Brewer, 1998). Moreover, the increased demand for and use of unlicensed assistant personnel will require supervision by registered nursing personnel placing nurses in a critical role in the overall management structures of the delivery organization.

Secondly, the nurse is the primary resource coordinator and, given the greater emphasis on information management, the linking of financial and clinical information will become a critical component in the managerial decision process. Historically involved with case management and active participants in the development of critical paths, the future role is likely to expand into a larger role of "care managers"—that is, the planning, assessment, and coordination of health service for a defined population (Greene & Kelsey, 1998). The role is consistent with the larger trend for clinical integration across the continuum of care. As described by Greene and Kelsey: Care management extends the function and philosophies of case management (managing individual cases) to an entire population . . . and requires a team approach. Typically . . . including nurses, physicians, physician extenders, medical assistants, ancillary providers, nutritionists, psychotherapist and other alternative care providers . . . defining their target population either by disease or by need. Both features clearly place nursing at the center of both conceptual and methodological issues critical to assuring organizational productivity.

Many of the trends affecting physicians will affect the changing role of nurses in the future. The emphasis on cost-effective care, changes in the demographics and epidemiology of the population, and the various organizational arrangements within the larger system will continually challenge the role of nursing within the health care system. To meet the challenge, nursing will demand a larger voice in management and governance. The challenge for management is to join in partnership with nursing and implement appropriate roles for nurses, clearly recognizing their professional heritage as well as their importance to emerging health care issues.

Expanding Role of Allied Health Professionals

Comprising more than 60% of the entire health care workforce and including over 200 distinct disciplinary groups, allied health is the largest, most complex, and fastest growing occupational group in the United States (Pew Health Profession Commission, 1995). Defined broadly, allied health includes all of the health-related disciplines, with the exception of nursing and the so-called MODVOPP disciplines: medicine, osteopathy, dentistry, veterinary medicine, optometry, phar-

macy, and podiatry. This group includes approximately 6 million health professionals providing services in a range of settings including hospitals, clinics, physicians' offices, hospices, extended care facilities, HMOs, community programs, and schools—and over the past decade have experienced severe workforce shortages, particularly in physical and occupational therapy (Jones, Johnson, Beasley, & Johnson, 1996).

As with nursing and medicine, the realities of financing, reimbursement, demography, epidemiology, technology, and organizational arrangements will have profound implications on this group of health care providers with subsequent implications for health services management. Perhaps its distinguishing feature is its heterogeneity, size, and overspecialization, and thus the emerging forces within the larger system will greatly affect the role of this particular group of providers. As described by the Pew Health Professions Commission (1995) in their recommendations for allied health:

> The changing health care workplace will require allied practitioners to work on interdisciplinary teams, rely heavily on health and information technologies, and understand the management, legal and financial perspectives of care delivery. Allied health providers will be expected to attain new knowledge and skill, *to take on multiple function across disciplines and to function with fewer regulatory barriers* [italics added].

Dynamic Nature of Individual and Group Configurations

Effective management recognizes the dynamic nature of disciplinary and interdisciplinary work groups and individuals interacting within the organization. Clearly, the emerging and dynamic roles of nurses, physicians, and the range of other health professionals within the context of the larger trends affecting health services delivery involving "micro-units" concerned with the provision of primary care (Nelson et al., 1998) and long-term care (Christianson, Taylor, & Knutson, 1998) will place a premium on the ability to understand and manage these individual and group configurations.

The implications are substantial. First, the recognition that health services organizations are composed not only of work groups, but also a range of interest groups and coalitions that are constantly shifting in order to compete for resources, provides an opportunity for managers to develop leverage between and among these interest groups and coalitions to enhance the overall operations of the organization. The recognition of these dynamics provides an opportunity to structure situations so that individuals and groups can more effectively monitor and control their own activities.

Secondly, the increasing role of interdisciplinary groups and work units in the provision of health services raises the issue of work group effectiveness and the education of health care providers to function in truly interdisciplinary teams (Baker et al., 1998). While the business of providing health services is usually done within the context of some group setting, the ability of these groups to function effectively is limited by the individual's own disciplinary perspective and lack of appreciation for the dynamics involved as well as other disciplinary perspectives. The overall effectiveness of the group is constantly threatened by the tendency of one disciplinary perspective to dominate and by a fundamental lack of group dynamics.

Finally, given the importance of interdisciplinary activity and the increasing emphasis given to total quality management, which attempts to focus on the horizontal flow of activities within the organizations, individuals will increasingly occupy boundary spanning roles involving various work groups, interest groups, or coalitions. Boundary spanning involves considerable conflict, and increased attention will be given to the development of skills required for communication, negotiation, and conflict management.

Health Services Policy and Management Research

Health services research has come of age and clearly has made major contributions to the policy issues facing the health services system. Moreover, it is likely that the synthesis and dissemination of health services research will play a continuing role in the process of formulating policy, albeit within an environment characterized by political controversy. Future considerations, however, need to be given to the interdisciplinary nature of health services research and the utilization of research by managers.

While clearly the substantive issues facing health services at this point focus on cost containment, increasing attention needs to be paid to the configuration and organizational aspects affecting managerial decision making. The interdisciplinary nature of health services delivery and the critical issues of understanding the process of health services delivery will increasingly place a premium on analytical questions that go beyond simply those of cost and reimbursement. The management of groups, the motivation of personnel, and the integration and coordination of services at various delivery levels and across various organizational forms require the attention of a wide variety of social science disciplines within the health services research community.

A second challenge is the utilization of health services research in the decision-making process. More than anything else, the health services manager of the future must be an innovator, at times a visionary, and always a teacher and mentor applying new learning to improved decision making. A partnership is needed between managers and researchers, whereby the health services research community will be acutely aware, responsive, and have ready access to the substantive issues facing managers, and managers will facilitate such access, and in turn be a beneficiary of greater insight and strategies derived from the learning process. In a sense, this partnership represents an alliance in which both managers and researchers work collaboratively to provide an opportunity to assess performance of ongoing activities, develop predictors of performance, and specify the conditions under which various approaches to health services delivery are most effective. Perhaps most importantly, the development of the partnership provides an opportunity to truly develop meaningful and relevant guidelines for evidence-based management.

Information Management

While emerging trends at the larger environmental level such as outcomes management and the development of guidelines are occurring, it has been recognized that existing data systems within organizations are embarrassingly inadequate to meet the information needs and strategies inherent in many of these important developments. Information systems within health services organizations often have a programmatic or categorical character and thus are greatly hindered in their attempt to integrate clinical outcomes, process of care, and financial information. Existing systems either

- do not collect and store the right information
- are not automated or computerized
- are not integrated, or
- lack sufficiently sophisticated computer hardware, software, and data-entry support to permit retrieval and analysis of information.

To address these problems, health care organizations are investing unprecedented sums of money to develop and implement information systems. In part, this is a function of the growing recognition that improved outcomes and decision making requires such systems but also that various external agencies such as JCAHO and NCQA (McGlynn, 1997) require such activities if the organization is to remain competitive, let alone significantly address the issues of costs. It is estimated that health care expenditures could be cut by $270 billion a year—25% of total expenditures—if medical and health care organizations made an annual investment of $50 billion in information systems ("Bugs and viruses," 1998).

At the national level, equally exciting developments are occurring with the development of the National Information Infrastructure (NII) Initiatives, which is enhancing the telecommunications and computer technology in all sectors of the economy. This network will process, store, and display information in many forms, thus providing information retrieval and processing services on demand. Health will be an integral part of this technology, and will provide communities and organizations to carry out nonclinical and population-based functions of public health, including automatic warning of epidemics. This information would be linked from individual physician offices and emergency rooms, creating an online statistical display for policy makers and international database for diagnosis in treating drug-resistant pneumonia (Lasker, Humphreys, & Braithwaite, 1995).

Past, Present, and Future

Table 15.2 summarizes the trends dealing with individuals and groups within the organizations. As with the environment and larger organizations, individuals and groups within organizations are confronting increasing complexity and uncertainty. The future will require the active participation of physicians, nurses, and allied health professionals, with the major challenge being to motivate and preserve human resources available to the organization. These resources will be increasingly involved in interdisciplinary groups and will be informed by a developing research base that will permit new designs and managerial strategies.

THE MANAGERIAL ROLE

Developments at the environment-organizational level, and the individual-group level of the organization provide a clue to future demands on managers. These demands involve three assumptions and three fundamental implications. The first assumption is that health care will continue to have features of both an economic and social good. Since it is financially impossible to provide unlimited care, there must be a mechanism for allocating resources, and it is likely that this will continue to include some marketplace features. At the same time, health care is an intensely personal, human service, which most Americans believe ought to be available to people in need, who are without the ability to pay for the service. A major responsibility and challenge of health services executives and managers in the years ahead will be to manage the inherent tension between health care as both an economic and a social good.

The second assumption is that the world will not become simpler but, if anything, more complex, ambiguous, and uncertain. If past is prologue, managers of health services organizations will encounter continued, if not increasing, stress; this stress will be reflected in the turnover rates among chief executive officers (CEOs). In 1983 hospital CEO turnover rate, for example, was 12.8%; it rose steadily at an annual rate

Table 15.2. Individual and Group Trends

	Past (1960s–1980s)	Present (2000)	Future (2000 and beyond)
Physicians	Solo practice	Group practice	Corporate practice and active involvement in managerial activity
Nurses	Clinical practice	Emerging as a political force	Active participation in managerial structure and policy
Allied health	Not an issue	Emerging issue	Key participants in teams that manage care across episodes of illness and pathways of wellness
Management research and assessment	Not an issue	Increased recognition	Integral part of managerial and organizational effectiveness
Dynamic nature of groups	Individual and disciplinary groups dominate	Emergence of interdisciplinary groups	Dominance of interdisciplinary groups
Information management	Not an issue	Emerging efforts	Clinical and financial networking; National Information Infrastructure

of 7.5% to peak at 18.4% in 1988. Since then the rate has declined so that in 1998 it was again at 12.1% (Weil, 1998). It is expected that this rate will probably increase in the future as the CEO ranks are filled with individuals of diverse background and training.

The third assumption is that health services executives and managers working together and with other health care providers can create the future for themselves and their organization. It is precisely because health care delivery will become even more complex, ambiguous, and uncertain that it is possible for managers to shape their destiny. The external environment not only influences managerial and organizational decision making, but the decisions made by managers on behalf of their organizations will also help to shape and influence the environment.

From the three assumptions come three fundamental implications, each involving a major transition in the managerial role.

- The first involves a transition from managing an organization to managing a market or network of services and joint ventures. Health services executives of the future will increasingly be called upon to manage across boundaries. This will require increased skills in coalition building, negotiation, and the ability to put together strategic alliances and partnerships to serve defined populations. It will require executives who see any given organization as part of a broader whole.

- For middle managers, it involves a transition from managing a department to managing a continuum of care. In brief, the job of the pharmacy department head, laboratory department head, radiology department head, or any other hospital department head is no longer that of a department head but rather a manager of pharmaceutical, laboratory, or radiology services across the continuum of care—most of which will be provided outside hospital settings. This will require these individuals to discard the hospital mindset and develop a broader community-based approach to delivering services. It will place a premium on interpersonal skills and the ability to develop collaborative relationships.

- The third transition involves moving from a mentality of coordinating services to a new mindset of actively managing quality across the continuum of care. This involves adopting a broader view of one's responsibilities. For example, the main focus is no longer on whether intensive care services are coordinated with those of step-down units but rather on coordinating care along the entire episode of illness or pathway of wellness leading from the patient's home, to the physician's office, to the relatively short stay in the intensive care unit, and back out again to the after-care units and into the home. It does little good to coordinate only part of this continuum of care if it has no resulting lasting value or impact on the overall episode of illness or ultimately the patient's health status. Actively managing quality will require health services managers at all levels to move beyond suboptimization and consider the overall interdependent processes involved in patient care—again, most of which will occur outside the hospital.

Role Performance and Emerging Challenges

The managerial role within health services is perhaps one of the most complex administrative assignments. Role performance will become even more challenging as managers attempt to deal with emerging public-private partnerships, aligning incentives, resource constraints, and increasing emphasis on health and preventive services that are customer focused, information driven, and outcome based. To meet these emerging trends, the managerial role requires

- new knowledge and skill competencies based in practice
- a recognition that the rapidly changing environment and the scope and depth of competencies needed by health services managers cannot be provided only at career entry level and requires a lifelong commitment
- a recognition that managerial competencies must be shared with clinical colleagues to form a partnership to meet the changing demands of the future (Pew Health Professions Commission, 1995).

Adequate role performance requires a new managerial image of the organization—not one of a "hierarchy of roles," but a "portfolio of dynamic processes" (Ghoshal & Bartlett, 1995). Cutting across departmental and organizational boundaries, the managers of these processes require new skills and competencies in leadership, coalition building, quality improvement and assurance, sensitivity to cost-quality relationships, research utilization, innovation, and problem solving. Specifically, managers must reaffirm their commitment to leadership as a set of processes that creates organizations in the first place or adopts them to significantly changing circumstances. As described by Kotter (1996), leadership defines what the future should look like, aligns people with that vision, and inspires them to make it happen despite obstacles.

Equally critical will be new skills and competencies in coalition building and a perspective that facilitates networking and partnerships among both public and private organizations. Given the emergence of various alliance-type arrangements involving various specialty and primary care providers along with expanding outsourcing arrangements, managers of the future will need skill and vision to integrate the clinical professions and institutions into organizations that provide predictable, cost-effective care. The managerial role here will require group leadership skills, coalition building, negotiation, and conflict management, as well as an overarching systems perspective.

A third competency is in the area of policy and political acuity. While currently managers know how to make improvements, they often lack access to the levers to change the system. Often they are not rewarded for doing the right thing and are punished for thinking globally. Managers of the future will require political skills including interagency analysis, coalition building, and understanding the realities of partisan politics.

Similarly, the entire area of quality improvement and assurance will be fundamental to role performance in the future. Purchasers—whether individual consumers, third-party payers, or governmental units—increasingly demand accountability of health services providers for an appropriate return on investment and increasingly expressed in terms of improved health status and outcome. To function within this set of expectations, managers will require skills in the area of quantitative, statistical, and epidemiological reasoning; outcome interpretation; and application.

Future role performance also requires that managers have a sensitivity to the cost-quality relationship. Individual consumers, third-party payers, and governmental units increasingly demand the provision of health services within the constraints of budgetary limits in all their diversity. Increasingly managers will be called upon to demonstrate their abilities in budget-based resource management, resources creation and allocation, and management within limits and constraints.

New dimensions of role performance are also required in **organizational learning** and innovation. Future role performance will require practitioners to have skills in the area of health services research, management assessment, and application. Many health services managers fail to recognize problems that are, in fact, researchable and fail to apply knowledge from existing research to enhance organizational performance. There is a serious and growing need for managers to become informed consumers of health services management research to improve organizational performance and services outcomes. Finally, future role performance requires that managers apply knowledge to assure benefit. In an area where the demand for greater productivity and improved outcomes with finite resource limitations predominate, the health services administrator must create workable solutions to operational and system problems.

Another challenge facing the future of role performance of the administrator is the recognition that, given the rapidly changing environment, the scope and depth of competencies needed by health service administrators cannot be provided only at career entry level. The acquisition of new competencies will be needed throughout their entire careers. Health services managers will increasingly come from a variety of educational backgrounds, and thus enhanced lifelong learning is required to equip the manager to address the issues in a rapidly changing environment.

Finally, role performance in the future will increasingly require the support and participation of clinical professions. Clinicians have increasing impact on the management of the health service system. Thus, if the managerial role is to meet its expectations, it must join in a partnership with the clinicians exposing them to the basic core of the organization and policy knowledge to support role performance in the future. At a minimum, clinical colleagues require a basic understanding of the health services system and the impact of clinical practice and decision making an organization, delivery, and cost (Nolan, 1998).

Preparing Future Managers

Health services managers are playing an increasing role in all segments of the health services delivery system. Initially developed to improve the management of large acute care hospitals, the demand for professional administrators has expanded greatly to include all the private and public organizations that are involved in financing, regulating, assessing, supplying, assisting, and generating policies for health services. While limited training is provided at the undergraduate and doctoral levels, major effort in health services education is at the master's degree. Although commonly referred to as the MHA, the degrees conferred include health management specialization within the MBA, MPH, MPA, MS, MA, MSHA, and others. The degrees reflect a variety of settings in which the programs are based, including schools of medicine, public health, management, public affairs, and graduate schools. Moreover, the commercialization of health services has been accompanied by the increase in the number of individuals with generic business training as measured by the number of new associates joining the American College of Healthcare Executives (ACHE). For example, in 1970, only 6.57% of the new associates had generic business degrees (no formal training in health services management) compared with 14.73% in 1997, with the largest percentage (26.26%) occurring in 1993 (Weil, 1998). In the public sector alone, it is estimated that only 20% of the public health administrators have formal professional training (Boedigheimer & Gebbie, 1998).

To meet the changing challenges and opportunities, several strategies need to be considered (Pew Health Professions Commission, 1995):

- *Core Curriculum Reform:* Develop an integrated core curriculum that embraces the new competencies, including leadership, coalition building, a community perspective, quality improvement, and the principles of organizational learning. These must be presented in an integrated manner—not as freestanding courses, but as modules that can be "mixed and matched" to meet the learning needs of the student. Moreover, these content areas must be linked to personal assessment such that the role of the manager becomes part of a larger socialization process that begins with the very initiation of the educational experience.

  The development of educational materials and methods must emphasize adaptability and the development of skills to manage the characteristics of the health care system of the future. Given the demographic changes in the community and the workforce composition of health service organizations, it is imperative that students and academic faculty reflect this diversity.

- *Quality Partnerships between University and Practice Personnel:* Expand the university-practice interface to assure the relevance of health services administration curricula to broader health care fields and return the research and educational products that yield improved administrator and organizational performance. The practitioner-academic interface requires a major expansion of the range or provider organizations involved and a redefinition of the mutual benefits accruing to each party. Special emphasis needs to be given to identifying and establishing a broad range of relationships with operating health services organizations, particularly those exhibiting the characteristics of the system of the future, and using these as teaching and research models and focal points for training administrators. Idealized relationships with the future include:

  - experiential learning opportunities such as mentoring, internships, residencies, postgraduate fellowships, and administrator training programs

  - middle-management congresses by academic programs for provider organizations participating in experiential learning programs

  - executive-in-residence or visiting-health-care-executive programs bringing operational managers to the classroom

  - leadership forums for multidisciplinary management teams from health care organizations, providing them with training in areas of self-identified skill and competency deficiencies

  - collaborative research efforts between faculty and health care systems that focus on operational problems

- *Stage Career Competency and Professional Development:* Management education for health services management must be tied to critical career transitions and linked to specific competencies. Given the dynamics of the health care system, managers will be in constant need to update and expand their ability to function within the system. Relevant content areas include epidemiology, biostatistics, negotiation skills, health behavior, the organization and management sciences, preparation in community development, and training in ethics and principles of social justice (Halverson, Kaluzny, Mays, & House, 1997; Boedigheimer & Gebbie, 1998).

  The temptation is to "add" new courses in an attempt to meet the knowledge needs of practicing executives. Perhaps a more efficient approach is to introduce such content into existing learning situations familiar to the student (Batalden, 1998). For example, rather than requiring a separate course on ethics, ethical content would be built into many existing courses throughout the curriculum.

- *Management for Clinical Professions:* Health services management programs need to serve as key managerial-policy education resources by supporting and teaching health care organization and management to the clinical professions. This obviously is a collaborative endeavor, taking a variety of forms including joint appointments, collaborative teaching, research, and service activities, but also serving as a resource to prepare clinical faculty to teach their students health services management and policy issues. As our industrial colleagues

Table 15.3. Managerial Trends

	Past (1960s–1970s)	Present (2000)	Future (2000 and beyond)
Role performance and changing values	Coordinating role subordinate to professional providers	Ascendance of managerial ability; financial and strategic expertise	Continued prominence of managers and recognition of role in managing human resources and relationships vs. simply financial resources
Preparing future managers	Relatively isolated from mainstream management and organizational theory	Emerging integration yet differentiated from industrial management	Fully integrated into management training/ lifelong learning/ distance learning

have learned so long ago, the world is too complex to go it alone.

- *Distance Learning Opportunities:* Whether the student is a clinician interested in management or a manager who is interested in further preparation, all are extremely busy, and many are inaccessible to conventional teaching modalities and traditional residential educational programs. Through teleconferencing, ·the information highway complemented with two-way television, it is possible to provide state-of-the-art education to thousands of students throughout the country and the world (Ibrahim, House, & Levine, 1995).

Past, Present, and Future

Table 15.3 presents the summary of trends dealing with the managerial role. As can be seen, the role has made a number of major transitions, and more will be required to meet the challenges of the new millennium and beyond. The field is rich with challenges and opportunities, and as never before, the manager is truly a significant player in determining the future provision of health services.

Returning to Mrs. Peterson and whether hers was an isolated event or chronic system problem, health care managers are likely to face elements of all four future scenarios as they deal with the organization and the environment, individuals and groups within

the organization, and their own roles. The challenge will be to identify tractable elements within each option and their inevitable combinations and to direct limited resources and energy to those elements that make a difference in the provision of health services. Issues of quality and efficiency will remain paramount, confounded by fundamental moral and ethical choices heretofore considered only in the abstract. Our ability and contribution to determining the future provision of health services will depend on a critical mix of abilities, insight, and courage. Failure to meet the challenge will sideline managers to simply observing rather than influencing the future and ensure that others will repeat the events experienced by Mrs. Peterson in the years ahead.

Discussion Questions

1. Recalling the four alternative futures presented at the beginning of the chapter, speculate on the implications of each scenario as it affects efforts at cost containment, changing the organization's culture, and the role of management.
2. Design an idealized educational program for incumbent managers to enhance their overall effectiveness. Be specific about the types of problems you anticipate and how the training program will resolve or mitigate these problems.

3. Compare and contrast how an organized delivery system would be most likely to respond to the challenges outlined in this chapter. Compare the most likely responses of the organized delivery system with those of an individual hospital/health department or group practice. Specifically address issues related to cost containment, changing social norms and demographic composition, technology development and social experimentation, changing roles of physicians and nurses, organizational culture, and the incorporation of women and minorities into management positions.

4. Return to the opening case regarding Mrs. Peterson, what mechanism and/or strategies might one use to prevent or minimize the problem encountered? What are the advantages and disadvantages of each, and how feasible are these under the various scenarios?

References

American Cancer Society. (1998). *Facts & figures.* Atlanta: American Cancer Society, 1999.

Amick, B., Levine, S., Tarlov, A., & Walsh, D. (1995). *Society and health.* Oxford: Oxford University Press.

Baker, R., Gelmon, S., Headrick, L., Knapp, M., Norman, L., Quinn, D., & Neuhauser, D. (1998, Winter). Collaborating for improvement in health professional education. *Quality Management in Health Care, 6*(2), 1–11.

Barnsley, J., Lemieux-Charles, L., & McKinney, M. M. (1998). Integrating learning into integrated delivery systems. *Health Care Management Review, 23*(1), 18–28.

Batalden, P. B. (1998). If improvement of the quality and value of health and health care is the goal, why focus on health professional development? *Quality Management in Health Care, 6*(2), 52–61.

Bezold, C. (1996, January 15). Four futures: Alternative scenarios for health care in the 21st century. *Medicine & Health PERSPECTIVES,* 1–4.

Boedigheimer, S. F., & Gebbie, K. M. (1998, April 27). *Preparing currently employed public health administrators for changes in the health systems.* (Final draft). New York: Columbia University Center for Health Policy and Health Services Research.

Bugs and viruses. (1998, February 28). *The Economist,* pp. 66–67.

Campbell, D. T. (1969). Reforms as experiments. *American Psychologist, 24,* 409–429.

Campbell, P. (1997, May). Population projections: States, 1995–2025. *Current population reports,* Census Bureau, Issues, 25–1131.

Cassileth, B. (1998). *The alternative medicine handbook.* New York: W. W. Norton.

Cassileth, B., & Chapman, C. (1996, March 15). "Alternative and Complementary Cancer Therapies", *Cancer,* Vol. 77, 6, pp. 1026–1034.

Christianson, J., Taylor, R., & Knutson, D. (1998). *Restructuring chronic illness management.* San Francisco: Jossey-Bass.

Diagnosis and reporting of HIV and AIDS in states with integrated and AIDS surveillance—United States, January 1994–June 1997. (1998, April 24). *Morbidity and Mortality Weekly Report, 47*(15), 309–314.

DiBella, A. J., Novis, E. C., & Gould, J. M. (1996). Understanding organizational learning capability. *Journal of Management Studies, 33*(3), 361–79.

Ellrodt, G., Cook, D., Lee, J., Cho, M., Hunt, D., & Weingarton, S. (1997, November 26). Evidence-based disease management. *Journal of the American Medical Association, 208*(20), 1687–1692.

Epstein, A. M., Seage, G., III, Weissman, J. S., Cleary, P. D., Fowler, F. J., Gatsonis, C., Massagli, M. P., Stone, V. E., Coltin, K., Craven, D. E., Goldberg, J., & MaKadon, H. (1995, Summer). Costs of medical care and out-of-pocket expenditures for persons with AIDS in the Boston Health Study. *Inquiry, 32*(2), 211.

Ernst, R. L., & Hay, J. W. (1984, August). The U.S. economic and social costs of Alzheimer's disease revisited. *American Journal of Public Health, 84*(8), 1261–1264.

Estes, C., Swan, J., & associates. (1993). *The long-term care crisis: Elders trapped in the no-care zone.* Newbury Park, CA: Sage, Newberry.

Fletcher, S. (1997). Whither scientific deliberation in health policy recommendations? Alice in breast cancer screening wonderland. *New England Journal of Medicine, 336*(16), 1180.

Frankford, D. M., & Konrad, T. R. (1998, February). Responsive medical professionalism: Integrating education, practice, and community in a market-driven era. *Academic Medicine, 73*(2).

Ghoshal, S., & Bartlett, C. A. (1995, January-February). Changing the role of top management: Beyond structure to processes. *Harvard Business Review, 73*(1).

Glasser, R. J. (1998, March). The doctor is not in. *Harpers Magazine,* 35–41.

Goldsmith, J.C. (1992, May/June). The reshaping of healthcare. *Healthcare Forum Journal,* 14–27.

Greene, B., & Kelsey, D. (1998). From case management to medical care management. In E. O'Neil, & J. Coffman (Eds.), *Strategies for the future of nursing.* San Francisco: Jossey-Bass.

Halverson, P. K., Mays, G., Kaluzny, A. D., & House, R. M. (1997, Spring). Developing leaders in public health: The role of executive training programs. *The Journal of Health Administration Education, 15*(2).

Halverson, P. K., Mays, G.P., Kaluzny, A. D., & Richards, T. B. (1997). Not-so-strange bedfellows: Models of interaction between managed care plans and public health agencies. *The Milbank Quarterly, 75*(1).

Health Care Advisory Board. (1997). *The great product enterprise: Future state for the American health system.* Washington DC: Author.

Herzlinger, R. (1997). *Market driven health care, who wins, who loses in the transformation of America's largest service industry.* Reading, MA: Addison-Wesley Publishing.

Hurley, R. (1998). Approaching the slippery slope: Managed care as industrialization of medical practice. In P. Boyle (Ed.), *Rationing sanity: The ethos of mental health.* Washington, DC: Georgetown University.

Ibrahim, M. A., House, R. M., & Levine, R. H. (1995). Educating the public health work force for the 21st century. *Family Community Health, 18*(3), Aspen Publishers, Inc., pp. 17–25.

Jones, W., Johnson, J., Beasley, L., & Johnson, J. (1996, Summer). Allied health workforce shortages: The systemic barriers to response. *Journal of Allied Health, 25*(3), 219–232.

Kaluzny, A., Warnecke, R., & associates. (1996). *Managing a health care alliance: Improving community*

cancer care. San Francisco, CA: Josee-Bass Publishers.

Kaluzny, A. D., Zuckerman, H., & Rabiner, D. (1998, June). Interorganizational factors affecting the delivery of primary care to older Americans. *Health Services Research, 33*(2), Part II, 381–401.

Kotter, J. P. (1996). *Leading change.* Boston: Harvard Business School Press, pp. 25–30.

Lamb, S., Greenlick, M., & McCarty, D. (Eds.). (1998). *Bridging the gap between practice and research: Forging partnerships with community-Based drug and alcohol treatment programs.* Washington, DC: National Academy Press.

Lasker, R., Humphreys, B., & Braithwaite, W. (1995, July 6). *Making a powerful connection: The health of the public and the national information infrastructure.* Report of the U.S. Public Health Service, Public Health Data Policy Coordinating Committee. Retrieved August 14, 1995, from the World Wide Web: http://www.nnlm.nlm.nih.gov/fed/phs/powerful.html.

McGlynn, E. A. (1997). Six challenges in measuring the quality of health care. *Health Affairs, 16*(3), 7–21.

McLaughlin, C. P., & Kaluzny, A. D. (1997). Total quality management issues in managed care. *Journal of Health Care Finance, 24*(1), Aspen Publishers, Inc., pp. 10–16.

Meyer, H. (1998). Focused factories. *Hospitals and Health Networks, 72*(7).

National Center for Health Statistics. (1997). *Health, United States, 1996–97 and injury chartbook.* Hyattsville, MD: Author.

Nelson, E., Batalden, P., Mohr, J., & Plume, S. (1998). Building a quality future. *Frontiers of Health Services Management, 15*(1), 3–32.

Nolan, T. (1998, February 15). Understanding medical systems. *Annals of Internal Medicine, 128*(4), 293–298.

Pew Health Professions Commission. (1995, November). *Critical challenges: Revitalizing the health profession for the twenty first century.* The Third Report of the Pew Health Professions Commission. San Francisco, CA.

Resident population, by age and sex: 1990 to 1996. (1997). *Statistical abstract of the United States, 1997*

(117th ed.). (No. 14, p.21). Washington, DC: Government Printing Office.

Salsberg, E., Wing, P., & Brewer, C. (1998). Projecting the future supply and demand for registered nurses. In E. O'Neil, & J. Coffman (Eds.), *Strategies for the future of nursing.* San Francisco: Jossey-Bass.

Satinsky, M. (1997). *The foundation of integrated care: Facing the challenges of change.* Chicago: American Hospital Publishing.

Shortell, S. M., Gillies, R. R., Anderson, D. A., Morgan-Erickson, K., & Mitchell, J.B. (1996). *Remaking health care in America: Building organized delivery systems.* San Francisco: Jossey-Bass.

Shortell, S.M., Waters, T. M., Clarke, K. B . W., & Budetti, P. P. (1998). Physicians as double agents: Maintaining trust in an era of multiple accountabilities. *Journal of the American Medical Association, 280*(12), 1102–1108.

Thorpe, D. (1997, April). *Emerging health trends: Changes in the growth in health care spending: Implications for consumers.* Prepared for The National Coalition on Health Care, Institute for Health Services Research, Tulane University. New Orleans, LA.

U.S. Bureau of the Census. (1997, March). *How we're changing: Demographic state of the nation: 1997* (Series P23-193). Washington, DC: U.S. Department of Commerce, Current Population Reports, Special Studies.

U.S. Government Accounting Office. (1998, January). *Alzheimer's disease: Estimates of prevalence in the United States* (GAO/HEHS-98-16). Washington, DC: U.S. Government Accounting Office.

Veney, J., & Kaluzny, A. (1998). *Evaluation and decision-making for health service programs* (3rd ed.). Chicago: Health Administration Press.

Weil, P. (1998). American College of Health Care Executives. Personnal communication.

Weiner, B., & Alexander, J. (1998). The challenges of governing public-private community health partnerships. *Health Care Management Review, 23*(2), 39–55.

Weinstein, M. M. (1998, May 31). Whiplash: In health care, be careful what you wish for. *The New York Times,* Late Edition, p. 4.1.

Winslow, R. (1998, May 19). Health-care inflation revives in Minneapolis despite cost-cutting. *The Wall Street Journal,* section 1A.

Zuckerman, H.S., Hilberman, D. W., Andersen, R. M., Burns, L. R., Alexander, J. A., & Torrens, P. (1998). Physicians and organizations: Strange bedfellows or a marriage made in heaven? *Frontiers of Health Services Management, 14,* 3.

Zuckerman, H. S., & Kaluzny, A. (1991). Strategic alliances in health care: The challenges of cooperation. *Frontiers of Healthcare Management, 7,* 3–23.

GLOSSARY

Absolute power   A source of competitive advantage grounded in the overall size and/or resources of an organization.

Accommodation   Giving the other party in a conflict what they want without resistance; capitulation.

Accountability   The responsibility for actions or decisions.

Acquisition   The purchase of one company by another; the assets and liabilities of the seller are combined with those of the purchaser.

Adaptation   An organization's adjustment to changes in its environment.

Adaptation Function   Within the open system view, this is one of the key management functions. The adaptation function helps the organization to anticipate and adjust to needed changes.

Administrative Conflict   Awareness by the involved parties that there are controversies about how task accomplishment will proceed.

Alliance Problems vs. Symptoms   This distinction highlights that there is often disagreement as to why alliances fail, and that this disagreement is often rooted in mistaking a root cause for a mere symptom.

Alliance Process   This refers to the flow of activities in the life cycle of a strategic alliance.

Alliance Risk   The risk that the alliance will fail. Must be balanced against the expected rewards.

Alliances   Informal, voluntary agreements among individuals or groups of similar or complimentary interests for purposes of achieving objectives.

Analyzing Work   Breaking work into distinct tasks in the horizontal and vertical division of labor.

Approaches to Work Design   The two primary approaches to work design are psychological and technical.

Arbitrator   Manager who intervenes in a dispute as a third party by taking high control over the outcome but not the process of the dispute.

Aspiration Level   A challenging but attainable outcome a negotiator would ideally like to achieve in the negotiation; target; goal.

Assessment for Design   Important stage in preparing to redesign an organization to identify strengths and weaknesses in relation to the mission. It includes consideration of the mission, external environment, internal organization, culture, human resources, and political processes.

Attribution Theory   A theory that holds that a manager's selection of a leadership style depends upon the way in which follower behavior is perceived and interpreted. Managers notice some things and are unaware of others; what is perceived is always filtered through a manager's distinctive cognitive frame and reshaped by it.

Authority   A source of power in organizations which is formally sanctioned, often expressed by the role or position of an individual within the organizational hierarchy.

Avoidance   A response to conflict that consists of ignoring it and taking no action to resolve it.

Awareness   the initial stage of the organizational change process in which individuals recognize that there is a discrepancy or gap between what the organization or work unit is currently doing and what it should or could be doing.

Bargaining Zone   In a negotiation, the set of agreements both parties prefer over impasse, found by determining the range of outcomes across which negotiators' reservation prices overlap; if there is no overlap, the bargaining zone is negative.

Behavior and Performance Norms   Behavior norms are rules that standardize how people act at work on a day-to-day basis, while performance norms are rules that standardize employee output by governing the amount and quality of work.

Behavioral Masking   Behavioral masking, known as "free riding" or "social loafing," occurs when individuals in large teams are able to maintain a sense of anonymity and gain from the work of the group without making a suitable contribution. When behavioral masking occurs, a member of the team obtains the benefits of group membership but does not accept a proportional share of the costs of membership.

Behavioral Perspective   A theoretical "school" of leadership focused on describing the behaviors of leaders (style) and their differential effectiveness.

Benchmarking   is the process of establishing operating targets based on the leading performance standards for the industry.

Best Alternative to a Negotiated Agreement (BATNA) What a negotiator will do if a negotiation ends in an impasse.

Biological Organisms   One of the metaphors of health care organizations. This metaphor identifies health care organizations as biological organizations that must adapt to their environments in the process of birth, growth, decline, and eventual death.

Boundary Spanning   The management role that facilitates adaptation and change of the organization in response to changes in the external environment.

Boundary Spanning Function   Another key function of the health care organization as a system. (See *Adaptation Function* previous page.) The boundary spanning function focuses on the interface between the organization and its external environment.

Brains   The metaphor of organizations as brains places emphasis on the importance of learning, intelligence, and information processing.

Building and Maintenance Roles   Building and maintenance roles are social-emotional behaviors aimed at helping the interpersonal functioning of the team. These behaviors are necessary to keep group members feeling good about the team and interacting effectively with one another.

Bureaucratic Organization   An organization structured on bureaucratic principles with clear roles, lines of

authority and accountability, procedures, rules, and policies for how work is performed and several levels in the hierarchy.

Bureaucratic Theory   Classical bureaucratic theory is consistent with the closed system approach to organizations. Building on five key characteristics, the bureaucratic organizational form can achieve technical superiority under certain stable conditions.

Buyer Threats   Threats from buyers, which depend on the market structure, environmental changes, and the relative competitive advantages of buyers and rivals.

Centralization and Decentralization   Centralization occurs when decision making is concentrated at the top of the organization. Decentralization occurs when decision making is delegated or decentralized to lower levels in the organization.

Change   Health care organizations must have the capacity for change and innovation. For most health services organizations, the abilities to create and manage change and to innovate as needed represent the key differences between short-run existence and long-run viability.

Charismatic Leadership   A social relationship between a leader and followers in which the leader presents a revolutionary idea or transcendent image. The follower accepts this course of action not because of its rational likelihood of success, but because of an emotional attachment to the extraordinary qualities of the leader.

Clinical Guidelines or Protocols   Whereas critical pathways standardize the treatment approach for a given clinical condition, clinical guidelines standardize the decision process for adopting a treatment approach. Clinical guidelines address the appropriateness of care by specifying the indications for either tests or treatments. Various government agencies and professional associations are involved in the development of guidelines.

Clinical Mentality   The cognitive frame of clinicians (e.g., physician or nurse) developed through professional education and experience. Clinicians are thought to have a "mentality" that differs from managers.

Closed System   The closed system view assumes that at least parts of an organization can be sealed off from the external environment. The need for predictability, order, and efficiency is consistent with a closed system view of an organization. Contrast with *open systems view.*

Coalitions   See **Alliances.**

Collectivist-Democratic Organization   Authority lies with the collective. There is no identifiable manager or hierarchy, and decision making is by consensus.

Communication   The creation or exchange of understanding between sender(s) and receiver(s). Effective communication plays a vital role in both programming and feedback coordination mechanisms.

Communication Channels   The channels or methods of communication are the means by which messages are transmitted. Channels include face-to-face or telephone conversations involving individual and/or groups of senders and receivers, e-mail, facsimile messages, letters, memos, policy statements, operating room schedules, reports, electronic message boards, web pages, video teleconferences, newspapers, television and radio commercial spots, and newsletters for internal or external distribution.

Communication Networks   Patterns of downward, upward, horizontal, and diagonal communication flows within organizations combined into patterns called *communication networks,* which are communicators interconnected by communication channels (Scott et al., 1981, p. 165). The five common networks are chain, Y, wheel, circle, and all-channel.

Communication Structure   The communication structure is the network that develops in teams that allows members to exchange information. The speed and accuracy of the team communication are determined by this structure.

Community Care Networks   An integrated system of medical care, public health, and human service organizations that is formed to: (1) serve a common population defined at the community level; (2) provide consistent and coordinated access to services across care settings and along the continuum of care; (3) implement mechanisms for ensuring accountability to patients and to the general public; (4) manage the delivery of services within the context of fixed financial resources, such as through risk-adjusted capitation payments or global budgets; and (5) pursue the objective of improving community health status as well as the health status of enrolled populations.

Compatible Issues   Issues for which negotiating parties have the same preferences.

Competition   Parallel striving by multiple parties toward a goal that all parties cannot reach simultaneously.

Competitive Advantage   The characteristics of a firm that enable it to outperform its rivals; could be called "key success factors" as well.

Concentration   An expression that characterizes the degree to which a small number of competitors control a market (by capturing market shares).

Conflict   Occurs when a concern of one party is frustrated, or is perceived to be frustrated, by another party.

Confrontation Meeting   Brings together a large segment of the organization for problem identification and action planning in the event of an immediate threat or a need for rapid action in order to provide direction in a short time period.

Consolidation   The pattern of competitors combining, usually through merger and acquisition, into larger and larger organizational arrangements.

Contingency Perspective   A theoretical "school" that holds that the most effective leadership style is dependent upon a series of contingencies, the most important being: characteristics of the leader (e.g., his or her preferences and competencies), characteristics of followers (e.g., their level of maturity and motivation), and the nature of the situation in which leader and follower interact (e.g., time).

Contingency Theory   Posits that the selection of the most appropriate form of organization is dependent upon the particular circumstances of the environment in which the organization operates. Contingency theorists do not advocate an either/or approach but rather view the process as a continuum from more or less bureaucratic (i.e., mechanistic) to more or less organic forms.

Contingency View of Coordination   Recognizes that organizations typically use some combination of various coordination mechanisms, but that a particular mechanism or combination of mechanisms will achieve different levels of success depending upon characteristics of specific situations. A contingency approach to intraorganizational coordination requires that managers match the most appropriate coordinating mechanism or mechanisms to a given situation.

Continuing Education   Provides health services personnel with the knowledge required to keep themselves and their organizations aware of new technology and service delivery programs.

Continuous Improvement   Commitment to quality is a hallmark of successful organization. Recognizing the centrality of quality not only internally but also in terms of the perceptions and expectations of key external constituencies and stakeholders is leading health care organizations toward the principles of continuous quality improvement (CQI) and total quality management (TQM).

Continuous Quality Improvement (CQI) A participative, systematic approach to planning and implementing a continuous organizational improvement process.

Cooptation Attempts to gain the support of a political faction by appointing influential members of such factions to legitimate roles (e.g. special committees, task forces, board of trustees) in a context supportive of the organization.

Coordinating Mechanisms Mechanisms for managing the interconnectedness of work.

Coordination A means of dealing with interdependencies by effectively linking together the various parts of an organization or by linking together two or more organizations pursuing a common goal. This conscious activity is aimed at achieving unity and harmony of effort in pursuit of shared objectives within an organization or among organizations participating in a multiorganizational arrangement of some kind.

Cope with Uncertainties A source of power for individuals and groups by virtue of their ability to handle nonroutine and unpredictable factors that influence the day-to-day operations and strategies of an organization (see **Uncertainty**).

Cost Effectiveness Is a composite measure that takes into account the degree of goal attainment and the costs to achieve them. To compare the overall cost-effectiveness of a set of alternative strategies, a common unit of measurement, such as cost per life saved, is used to summarize the likelihood and benefits and costs of achieving all possible outcomes under each strategy.

Cost Reduction vs. Revenue Enhancement This distinction highlights that the strategic intent behind alliances may differ on fundamental dimensions, such as cost versus value, and that such differences imply different bases for evaluating the success of an alliance.

Countervailing Power A strategy whereby buyers (or sellers) seek to increase their competitive advantage relative to sellers (or buyers), usually by use of power strategies to counteract the power of the other.

Critical Pathways Also known as *clinical pathways, care maps,* and *critical paths,* critical pathways are plans for managing patient care "that display goals for patients and provide the corresponding ideal sequence and timing of staff actions to achieve those goals with optimal efficiency" (Pearson et al., 1995). Thus for a given diagnosis or condition, a critical pathway specifies the work activities in advance.

Cultural Assessment The assessment of an organization's culture through questions such as, "What is it like to work here?" Indications of culture can be derived from employees favorite stories about heroes, traditions, and language used. Organizations may be multicultural and have strong or weak cultures.

Decision Making Decision making is a process by which teams attempt to apply all available information to the problem at hand so as to make correct decisions. Some of the problems that prevent good decision making are free riders, polarization, and groupthink.

Declining Market A market in which there is an absolute decline in growth over a sustained period of time.

Delphi Technique The Delphi technique is a structured group decision-making method that elicits group members' opinions prior to judgments about those opinions. Through this technique, alternative ideas get to the table and are objectively debated by the team members, thereby decreasing the chance of groupthink.

Design Outcome Design outcome is the organization chart produced at the end of the design process that represents who has authority to make which decisions. It is usually transitory because of changes in the external and internal environments.

Design Preparation The activities preceding organizational design including assessment for design.

Design Process The process of rethinking how authority, responsibility, and accountability should be distributed in an organization.

Designing Individual Jobs Individual jobs can be designed with an eye to motivation, skill requirements, or information flow.

Designing Work Groups to Address Coordination Needs Coordination is simplified when interconnected tasks are assigned to members of a single work group.

Direct Supervision A way of coordinating work that occurs when someone takes responsibility for the work of others, including issuing them instructions and monitoring their actions. Direct supervision entails some form of hierarchy within the organization.

Direct Work Effort that directly contributes to the accomplishment of an organization's goals.

Distributive Dimension of Negotiation The dimension along which any gain to one party necessarily corresponds to an equivalent loss for another party; the negotiated outcome stated in terms of the relative distribution among the individual parties of the resources being negotiated.

Diversity Training Provides individuals with new experiences and data to disconfirm old belief structures and replace them with fairer judgments regarding gender, ethnicity, race or sexual orientation.

Divisional Design The organization is divided into several operating units, and decision making is decentralized to these units.

Effectiveness In organizations is the degree to which organizational goals and objectives are successfully met.

Efficiency Is defined as the cost per unit of output.

Emerging Market A newly formed or reformed market in which there remains a high degree of uncertainty as to the essential characteristics of the market or the strategic behaviors of the competitors.

Emotional Conflict Awareness of interpersonal incompatibilities among those working together on a task; characterized by negative emotions and dislike of the other person.

Empowerment Empowerment is a strategy in which employees are given information, knowledge, and power to make decisions when the traditional hierarchical management structure and command and control-management techniques are no longer viable. Teams, when used as an extension of the general employee empowerment strategy, occur along four dimensions: potency, meaningfulness, autonomy, and consequences.

Entrant Threats Threats that new competitors will enter the market, where entry is dependent on the height of entry barriers.

Entry Barrier A market/industry characteristic that moderates the rate at which new rivals enter the market/industry.

Environmental Assessment Assessment of the main factors in the external environment that influence how the organization can operate.

Environmental Barriers to Communication Characteristics of an organization and its environmental context that block, filter, or distort communications. Such barriers can be nothing more than the fact that people have too little time to communicate carefully. Other environmental barriers include the organization's managerial philosophy, multiplicity of its hierarchical levels, and power/status relationships between senders and receivers.

Environmental Context The environmental context of a team refers to the external factors that may affect team performance. Examples of these factors are other teams along with the intergroup relationships and conflict that exist, organizational resources, top management support, and the reward and incentive systems.

Equality Fairness Norm A guiding rule stating that every negotiating party should get the same absolute amount of resources in a negotiation.

Equity Fairness Norm A guiding rule stating that negotiating parties should be allocated an amount of resources proportional to their inputs along some relevant dimension.

Ethnic Composition The relative size and distribution of defined ethnic groups within a given population or community. A broad range of constructs may be used in defining ethnic groups, including origin, culture, and race—but most definitions are constructed from self-reported indicators of group membership.

Evidence-Based Management The continual identification and application of available scientific knowledge to improve administrative decision making in health care or other industries. Scientific knowledge may include information about optimal clinical staffing levels, compensation and incentive structures, organization and team design, health care financing arrangements, health care demand and supply projections, consumer preferences, cost-effectiveness information regarding health technologies and services, and information regarding the adoption and diffusion of clinical practices and technologies.

Evidence-Based Medicine The systematic identification and application of available scientific information for clinical decision making by health care professionals. Scientific information includes findings related to process and outcome-based measures of quality, as well as findings related to cost and cost-effectiveness. This process is supported by various mechanisms including clinical practice guidelines, clinical information systems, computer-based medical records, practice profiling and provider feedback mechanisms, health care report cards, and performance measurement systems.

External Environment One key to an organization's success is having a good understanding of its external environment. Depending on these attributes (of the external environment), organizations might choose different strategies, structures, and processes to compete successfully.

Feedback   Feedback approaches to coordination entail the exchange of information among staff usually while work is being carried out. Feedback approaches permit staff to change or modify work activities in response to unexpected requirements. Feedback also refers to the part of the communication process through which sender and receiver engage in a two-way process of communication. It reverses the sender and receiver roles so that information can be shared, recycled, and fine-tuned to achieve an unambiguous and mutual understanding in the communication process.

Feedback Approaches to Coordination   Managing interconnections among tasks through interaction and communication among those who perform those tasks.

Formal and Informal Leadership   Leadership refers to the ability of individuals to influence other members toward the achievement of the team's goals. Teams may have multiple leaders. Formal leaders have legitimate authority over the team, and since their power has been granted by the organization, these leaders have the ability to use formal rewards and sanctions to support their authority. Informal leaders, on the other hand, are not recognized by the organization and therefore have no legitimate authority; however, they are able to influence the group members and should be considered a powerful force.

Formal Authority System   Rights and obligations which create a field of influence within which an individual or department can legitimately operate with the formal support of those with whom they work.

Formal Groups   Formal groups are formally organized work teams that operate within an organizational context and interact with a larger organization or organizational subunit. These groups are intact social systems with boundaries, interdependence among members, and differentiated member roles.

Four-Firm Ratio   The sum of shares of the top four firms in a market, defined by their relative market shares; this is an indicator of market concentration.

Fragmented Market   A market in which no firm has sufficient market share to have a strong influence on the strategic behaviors of competitors.

Functional Design   The organization is divided into departments according to the function to be performed (e.g., finance, nursing, pharmacy, purchasing and so on).

Future Scenarios   A set of descriptive profiles that forecasts the performance of a given product,

organization, market, or industry over an established period of time. Profiles are based on (1) the extrapolation of current and past performance trends, (2) expectations of future market developments, and (3) assumptions about key managerial decisions that are made during the period. Alternative performance profiles are generated by varying key assumptions, expectations, and managerial decisions across all plausible values. Scenarios are used to facilitate organizational strategic planning under uncertainty by identifying the range of possible outcomes associated with each potential action.

Gender Gap   The way in which one gender perceives themselves along a set of dimensions (e.g., aspects of the managerial role, leadership style) versus how they are perceived by the other gender.

Goal Accomplishment   The primary objective of leadership; exercising leadership in order to accomplish goals that are so large and/or complex that they cannot be achieved by individuals working alone.

Governance Function   When viewed from the systems approach, this is one of six key functions. This area is being given increasing attention because of the important public trust and social accountability responsibilities of health services organizations.

Groupthink   Groupthink is a phenomenon that occurs in groups when the desire for harmony and consensus overrides members' efforts to appraise group judgments and decisions realistically. In other words, groupthink occurs when maintaining the pleasant atmosphere of the team becomes more important to members than coming up with good decisions. Self-censorship, collective rationalization, stereotyping others, and pressures to conform are some of the signs that groupthink may be present.

Growth/share Matrix   A graphical representation of and tool for analyzing the businesses/divisions within a multibusiness company; businesses/divisions are arrayed by market share and market growth rate; the matrix was first developed by the Boston Consulting Group.

Herfindahl-Hirschman Index   The sum of the squared shares of competitors within a market (often multiplied by 10,000); this is an indicator of market concentration.

Holograms   Another metaphor for health care organizations. This is an object in which each of the parts contains the entire essence of the overall object or image. Designing health services organizations as holograms emphasizes the need for flexibility, creativity, change, and innovation.

Horizontal Division of Labor Dividing work into tasks to be completed by different people at the same level of the organization.

Horizontal Expansion A power strategy whereby firms that are in the same industry/market are linked operationally to gain market share and operational synergies; horizontal expansion can occur by: (1) acquisition and merger, (2) building new capacity/facilities, and/or (3) strategically aligning with competitors.

Horizontal Integration The process of combining organizations within the same industry under a common ownership or management structure. This strategy is typically used to consolidate production processes and thereby achieve economies of scale, and/or to aggregate the market shares of individual organizations and thereby achieve enhanced market power.

Human Relations School The focus of the human relations school is on the individual. This is one of the classical perspectives on organizations and has been applied in the health care sector to emphasize the usefulness of participatory decision making.

Human Resources Assessment An assessment of the availability of individuals with appropriate knowledge and skills to carry out the mission of the organization.

Human Resources Change Strategies Concerned with changing the attitudes, values, skills, and behaviors of personnel within the organization.

Hybrid Organization An organization that combines two or more firms to achieve coordination or control, but without the use of ownership arrangements (the mingling of assets and liabilities).

Identification The second stage of the change process that involves an attempt to address the discrepancies or performance gap identified in the awareness stage.

Implementation Stage of the organizational change process that involves the very presence or operations of the change within the organization or the relevant work unit within the organization.

Industrial Organization A field of economics that involves the study of how market structures and processes affect the behaviors and strategies of competitors as they seek to meet consumer demands.

Influence Actions that, either directly or indirectly, cause a change in the behavior and/or attitudes of another individual or group. The primary effect of leadership.

Influence Systems Political activity and informal systems of power that often arise in attempts to influence decisions and activities outside the formal system of authority.

Informal Communication Coexisting with formal communication flows and networks within organizations are informal communication flows, which have their own networks. Like informal organization structures, informal communication flows and networks result from the interpersonal relationships in organizations.

Informal Groups Informal groups are not recognized by the organization but are found in all organizations. They may have a positive effect on the organization, but they can also be powerful enough to undermine the formal authority structure of the organization.

Innovation A change that is new to the organization adopting it (use of a new product, service, method, or strategy in business practice).

Inquisitor Manager who intervenes in a dispute as a third party by taking high control over both the process and outcome of the dispute.

Institutional Theory Institutional theorists emphasize that organizations face environments characterized by external norms, rules, and requirements that the organization must conform to in order to receive legitimacy and support.

Institutionalization Stage of the change process in which change is integrated into the ongoing activities of the organization.

Integration Structures and processes that tie the various units of an organization together so as to increase coordination and collaboration.

Integrative Dimension of Negotiation The dimension along which one party can gain without another party necessarily incurring an equivalent loss; allows mutually beneficial outcomes to be discovered.

Integrators Individuals who, because of specialized knowledge and because they represent a central source of information, are able to facilitate coordination. Examples of effective integrators are found among all health professionals. In most health care organizations, individual nurses, regardless of formal position, often function as integrators linking physicians to the organization's formal administrative structure.

Interconnectedness of Work Interdependencies among tasks, where the completion of one task depends upon the completion of another.

Interdependence   The condition of mutual dependence between or among people and organizational units (including entire organizations) that exists whenever work activities are interconnected in some manner—physically or intellectually.

Interdependency   Whenever one actor does not entirely control all the conditions necessary for the achievement of an action or for obtaining the outcomes desired from the action.

Interests   Aims and objectives of individuals or groups that can differ from and compete with larger organizational goals and objectives or from the aims and objectives of other individuals or groups.

Intergroup Conflict   Intergroup conflict occurs when different teams interact, and disagreements occur between the groups. Most intergroup conflict is due to factors related to interdependence among work groups. For example, when two groups are dependent upon each other to do their work, conflicts can easily result when information-transfer procedures are ineffective or lacking.

Internal Environment   The conditions within an organization including culture, stakeholder relationships, structures, and processes.

Interorganization Relations   An organization's formal and informal relationships with other firms and regulatory agencies.

Interorganizational Relationships   As the health services environment grows in complexity and accelerates its rate of change, a key component of many organizations' strategies is to form relationships with other organizations.

Interpersonal Conflict   Conflict between two or more individuals.

Intragroup Conflict   Conflict among members of the same group.

Intrapersonal Conflict   Conflict within one person who is attempting to choose among multiple options in making a decision.

Job Skill and Knowledge Requirements   The skills and knowledge required for the successful completion of a particular job.

Just-in-time management (JIT)   A managerial strategy designed to achieve operational efficiencies by reducing the need for excess or "slack" human, capital, and intellectual resources. Reductions in slack are achieved by implementing processes to secure resources rapidly on an "as-needed" basis rather than maintaining large resource inventories for future use. Similarly, operational processes within the organization are engineered to produce both internally consumed products and externally consumed products at the time of demand.

LEAD Model   A model suggesting that leadership style can be described along two dimensions: the amount of attention accorded to developing/sustaining relationships, and the amount of attention accorded to accomplishing tasks. The most appropriate style is a function of individual/group maturity.

Leadership   Providing direction in group activities and influencing others to achieve common goals.

Leadership Match Model   The first comprehensive model of leadership style. The underlying theory holds that leaders are unable to alter their style to any appreciable degree. Hence, leadership effectiveness depends not on fitting one's style to the situation (as most contingency theories hold), but rather selecting situations that are conducive to one's style.

Leadership Role   One of the roles of a manager: intentionally influencing individuals and groups in order to accomplish a goal.

Leadership Styles (S1, S2, S3, and S4)   S1 is a leadership style characterized by a large amount of attention accorded to task accomplishment, and little accorded to building/sustaining relationships with followers. S2 is a leadership style characterized by a large amount of attention accorded to both relationships and task. S3 is a leadership style characterized by a large amount of attention accorded to building/sustaining relationships and little accorded to accomplishing tasks. S4 is a leadership style that accords little attention to either relationships or task. (See *LEAD Model*.)

Learning Organization   An organization skilled at creating, acquiring, and transferring knowledge, and at modifying its behavior to reflect new knowledge and insights.

Levels of Organization Design   Organization design may be considered at different levels including for a position, work group, cluster or work groups, total organization, network of organization, and a system.

Linking Pins   People who serve formally as links between various units in the organization—similar to integrators (Likert, 1967, p. 156). Horizontally, in such situations, there are certain organizational participants who are members of two separate groups and serve as coordinating agents between them. On the vertical axis, individuals serve as linking pins between their level and those above and below.

Machines Another metaphor for health services organizations that emphasizes bureaucratic traits.

Macro Approach When selecting the "unit of analysis" in research and observations on organizations, the macro approach leads us to emphasize the organization as a social system in the context of other organizations.

Maintenance Function The maintenance function is concerned with both the physical and human infrastructure of the organization. As the rate of change accelerates and as the external environment becomes more threatening, greater demands are placed on the maintenance functions of health services organizations.

Management Function Management is a distinct function that cuts across all the other functions and subsystems. In a sense, it is the "head" that organizes, directs, and oversees all of the other functions.

Management Teams Management teams coordinate and provide direction to the subunits under their jurisdiction. They may exist at the board, senior management, or departmental level.

Management Work Decision making about the organizational context within which work is performed.

Managerial Office A hierarchically superordinate office, occupied by a manager, in an organization or organizational component.

Managerial Roles A collection of expectations attached to an office. Role expectations are defined by the office's charter (job description) in addition to the expectations of superiors, peers, and subordinates. The aspects of managerial roles can be conceptualized in a variety of ways.

Managing Across Boundaries In the changing health care system where continuity of care is becoming more and more essential, the ability to manage across boundaries between and among organizations is becoming increasingly crucial.

Market Share The proportion of a market that is controlled by a given competitor.

Market Structure The characteristics of markets that determine the overall strength and patterns of competition.

Matrix Design A matrix design is characterized by a dual-authority system. Each worker is accountable to two bosses, each able to exercise authority over the worker.

Mature Market A market in which there is sustained moderate, flat, or even slightly declining growth.

Mediator A third party to a dispute who intervenes by taking high control over the process but not the outcome of the dispute.

Merger The combination of companies whereby the assets and liabilities of each are intermingled.

Micro Approach In the micro approach, the emphasis is on organizational behavior to understand organizations. The unit of analysis is the individual, the group, or the department units.

Mission and Values The encompassing ideas of the organization that define its purpose and its principles.

Mission/Goals The organization's mission and associated goals largely dictate the major tasks to be carried out and the kinds of technologies and human resources to be employed.

Monopolistic Market A market in which one firm has a significant (perhaps total) share of the market; many monopoly markets, however, are also "contestable" in that entry barriers are sufficiently low to cause a monopolistic to act as if the market were competitive.

Motivating Potential of Jobs A job's motivating potential score (MPS) is affected by the skill variety, task identity, task significance, and autonomy and feedback experienced by performing a particular job, which depends in turn on the design of that job.

Multiskilled Employees Employees whose jobs are designed to encompass multiple tasks in the horizontal division of labor, with the goal of either making the work more meaningful, simplifying coordination, or both.

Mutual Adjustment A way of coordinating work that occurs through informal communications among individuals who are not in a hierarchical relationship to one another; for example, two physicians sharing information about a patient's clinical condition.

Need Fairness Norm A guiding rule stating that negotiating parties should receive an amount of resources proportional to their need for them.

Negotiation The process whereby two or more parties decide what each will give and take in an exchange between them.

Niche Strategy A strategy of differentiating oneself in order to target a particular sector of a market.

Nominal Group Technique Nominal group technique is a group decision-making and problem-solving technique that elicits group members' opinions prior to judgments about those opinions. The technique is particularly effective for setting goals and priorities, and gaining a better understanding of complex issues.

Office   An office is point in organizational space to which a role is attached (collection of expectations).

Oligopolistic Market   A market in which there are a small number of firms, and the competitors believe that their rivals have sufficient market power to influence their long-term survival; they therefore consciously adapt their strategies in response to their assessments of rival competitive advantages and expected strategic maneuvers.

Open System   This view emphasizes that organizations are parts of the external environment and, as such, must continually change and adapt to meet the challenges posed by the environment. The need for openness, adaptability, and innovation is consistent with an open system view.

Organization Behavior   See **Micro Approach**.

Organization Design   In contrast with work design, organization design focuses on the overall allocation of power and authority, information processing, and decision-making rules within the organization and how individual work groups, departments, or divisions are themselves linked together.

Organization Learning   A method by which organizations continuously improve performance by ensuring that each member continuously develops knowledge, skills, and motivations that are linked with the organization's central mission and objectives.

Organization Structure   The apportionment of responsibility and authority among members of an organization; the architecture of an organization.

Organization Theory   Organization theory involves the systematic examination of the ways that organizations function. Over time a number of major "perspectives" of how organizations work have evolved including: classical bureaucratic theory, the scientific management school, etc. These perspectives can be used to gain insight into the structure and functioning of health services organizations.

Organizational Effectiveness   The extent to which an organization accomplishes its basic objectives and maintains its viability.

Organized Delivery System   An integrated network of health care providers, supported by a health care financing and administrative entity, that competes to assume clinical and financial responsibility for the health of defined populations of health care consumers. A continuum of health care services is available through the network of affiliated providers.

Outcome Measures of Quality   In health care delivery assess changes that occur in the health outcomes of the person receiving the service that can be attributed to the quality of the services performed.

Outcomes Assessments   A way of systematically collecting, monitoring, and reporting performance results. Through such assessments, managers from different organizations or units can detect and attend to undesirable variation in outputs (by changing or modifying work activities as needed over time or relative to competitors).

Ownership vs. Control   This distinction refers to the fact that greater ownership stakes do not necessarily result in greater control of an alliance. Control indicates influence, and an influence can come from many sources, of which ownership is only one.

Pace strategy   A strategy whereby a competitor seeks competitive advantage through the use of timing, aggressiveness, and risk-taking behaviors.

Parallel Design   The parallel design retains a functional design that has responsibility for routine activities but also has a parallel side responsible for solving complex problems.

Partner Orientation   A summary characterization of the degree to which an alliance partner is interested in working cooperatively with his/her partner.

Path-Goal Model   A theory of leadership based on the expectancy theory of motivation. Followers' motivation (which the leader attempts to influence) is seen to be a function of expectancies, instrumentalities, and valences.

Patient-centered Care   A multidisciplinary approach to patient care that centers the design of work around patients' needs.

Performance   Achievement of a desired result.

Performance Gap   Deficiencies in the performance of an organization. This begins the initial stage in the change process within organizations.

Performance Strategy   A strategy whereby a competitor seeks competitive advantage through superior operational and/or strategic performance.

Personal Barriers to Communication   Barriers that arise from the nature of people, especially in their interaction with others that apply equally to communication within organizations and between them and their external stakeholders. Examples include people distorting the encoding or decoding of their messages according to their frames of reference or their beliefs and values. People may also consciously or unconsciously engage in selective perception, or permit their emotions—such as fear or jealousy—to influence their communications.

Personal Roles   Personal roles refer to those roles that individuals assume in groups that mainly satisfy individual needs and are thus unrelated to the group's goals. It is important for team leaders to understand personal roles because they may detract from team performance.

Playing Fields   Another analogy for health care (and other) organizations. Health services organizations require the inputs of a variety of highly trained professions who each bring his or her own "culture" to the organization. The challenge is to create a larger overall sense of organizational identity and culture that can embrace the individual cultures of the different health professionals.

Political Games   The exercise of power in the form of political influence expressed as a set of "games," each with its own structure and rules that are played outside the legitimate system of authority.

Political Model of Organizations   Model of organizational behavior that emphasizes the existence of power and influence other than that vested in the formal authority system.

Political Process Assessment   Assessing the nature of the informal organization including who are the key leaders and how communication flows.

Political Systems   Organizations can also be viewed as political systems in which various groups and actors vie for control of important resources. See *Playing Fields* above.

Politics   Domain of activity in which participants attempt to influence organizational decisions and activities in ways that are not sanctioned by either the formal authority system of the organization, its accepted ideology, or certified expertise.

Pooled Interdependence   Occurs when individuals and units are related but do not bear a close connection; they simply contribute separately in some way to the larger whole.

Pooling vs. Trading Alliances   Pooling alliances reflect two or more organizations contributing similar resources for mutual gain, whereas trading alliances are based on the notion of combining dissimilar—but complementary—resources.

Population Ecology Theory   Population ecologists argue that the environment "selects out" certain organizations for survival. Organizational success is more dependent upon environmental selection than managerial decision making and implementation.

Population-Based Management   In the managed care environment, health care organizations are increasingly being called upon to work to improve the health status of whole populations or some subset of the public.

Porter Model   A framework developed by Michael Porter of Harvard University to analyze the five main forces that affect competition in a market.

Portfolio strategy   A power strategy whereby firms (either under the same ownership or within a strategic alliance) are managed financially by a parent company in order to achieve synergies and greater competitive advantage.

Position strategy   A strategy whereby a competitor seeks competitive advantage by projecting value to consumers; they do this by pursuing a: (1) low-cost position, (2) differentiated position, and/or (3) market niche.

Power   Ability (or potential) to exert actions that either directly or indirectly cause a change in the behavior and/or attitudes of another individual or group. The potential to exercise influence. As power increases, so does the probability of getting others to think or act in a certain way.

Power strategy   A strategy whereby a competitor seeks competitive advantage by building/acquiring greater size and/or resources.

Pressing   Using relatively contentious tactics in a conflict situation to achieve one's goals without regard for the other party's outcome.

Process Consultation   Involves an outside consultant helping a client to perceive, understand, and act upon process events that are occurring within the organization. Focus is put on communications, role and function of group members, group problem solving and decision making group norms, and the use of leadership and authority.

Process Measures of Quality   Focus on evidence relating to the quality of the performer's activities in carrying out the work.

Production Function   The production function provides the product or the service and is at the center of most organizational activity.

Productivity   Is defined as the ratio of outputs to inputs.

Product-Line or Program Design Product-line management is defined as the placement of a person in charge of all aspects of a given product or group of products (for example, all health care for a segment of the population such as women, children, or the elderly).

Programming Programming approaches to coordination seek to clarify work responsibilities and activities in advance of the performance of work, as well as specify the outputs of the work process and the skills required to perform the work. Programming approaches essentially standardize work activities for all expected requirements.

Programming Approaches to Coordination Managing interconnections among tasks by prespecifying the nature and sequence of tasks, and who is to perform them.

Project-Management Design A structural means for coordinating a large amount of talent and resources for a given period on a specific project (Cleland & King, 1997). For example, a health care organization may wish to organize services into a comprehensive home health care program for the chronically ill by forming a team organized around the focus of the program—home services for the chronically ill. Team members would be drawn from nursing, social services, respiratory therapy, occupational therapy, pharmacy, and physicians specializing in chronic disease. To market the program and to handle finance and reimbursement issues, expertise would be provided by team members drawn from the organization's administration. A project manager would be responsible for coordinating the activities of team members.

Psychic Prison Organizations can also be viewed as places where people are trapped by their own perceptions, ideas, and beliefs whether consciously or unconsciously. Often this is reflected in the tendency to avoid conflict, to avoid anxiety-provoking situations, or to strive to maintain one's sense of identity and self-esteem.

Psychological Approach to Work Design Designing work with a focus on worker motivation.

Quality Assurance Refers to the formal and systematic exercise of identifying, monitoring and overcoming problems in health care delivery.

Quality Improvement Is a management philosophy to improve the level of performance of key processes in the organization by focusing on the most important processes to improve, setting high standards for performance outcomes, and using statistical methods and tools to measure current performance, interpret it, and take corrective action when necessary.

Rational Model of Organizations Model of organizational behavior that emphasizes that managers orchestrate the activities of a team whose members all subscribe to a common set of goals and objectives.

Reactivity To performance criteria refers to the tendency for evaluated persons to react in ways to maximize achieving positive evaluations of their performance rather than to achieve the best performance.

Reciprocal Interdependence Occurs when individuals and units bear a close relationship, such that they mutually depend on each other to achieve given tastes.

Relative Power A source of competitive advantage that is grounded in a competitor's local market power (based on market share) relative to that of its local rivals.

Reservation Price The point at which a negotiator is indifferent between an impasse and an agreement, stated in terms of whatever units are being negotiated (e.g., dollars).

Resource Acquisition Refers to the ability of an organization to successfully obtain capital and other types of resources needed.

Resource Dependence Theory The resource dependence theory emphasizes the importance of the organization's abilities to secure needed resources from its environment in order to survive.

Responsibility Charting Technique that identifies decision-making patterns among a set of actors—individuals, units, departments, or divisions within the organization. It provides an opportunity to compare responses of a specific participant about that person's role in a decision with the response of one or more participants about the same participant role, to compare responses across all actors on a specific decision, to examine responses of each actor across a set of decisions, and to compare actual decision patterns with desired activity.

Risk Taking Characterizes proactive and far-reaching actions of health care organizations to step out of the traditional modes of action and develop new programs and services or modify their ways of carrying out their mission and the delivery of care.

Rival Threats Threats from competitors in the market, which depend on the market structure, environmental changes, and the relative competitive advantages of rivals.

Role Differentiation Role differentiation refers to the specialization of work activities in an organization.

Scientific Management A technical approach to work design that attempts to divide jobs narrowly, and to separate management work from direct work.

Scientific Management School   Closely related to the classical bureaucratic approach with an emphasis on span of control, unity of command, appropriate delegation of authority, departmentalization, and the use of work methods to improve efficiency.

Seller Threats   Threats from sellers, which depend on the market structure, environmental changes, and the relative competitive advantages of sellers and rivals.

Sequential Interdependence   Occurs when one person or unit depends on another for resources or information to accomplish a task.

Shared Vision   A common picture of the future an organization seeks to create that draws people together around a common identity and sense of destiny.

Social Experimentation   A collection of methods used for evaluating the performance of programs, services, or other interventions at the population level.

Social Norms and Expectations   A common set of knowledge, values , and beliefs that is shared by a group of individuals and that shapes the decision making and behavior of group members.

Sources of Power   Notion that power can be derived from personal attributes such as sensitivity, articulateness, self-confidence, and aggressiveness, or from structural sources such as where individuals stand in the division of labor and the communications system of the organization.

Stages of Change or Innovation   This process involves awareness, identification, implementation, and institutionalization.

Stages of Team Development   Stages of team development refer to predictable developmental milestones through which teams proceed. The pace at which teams progress through these stages is dependent upon a number of internal and external factors, and the teams may become stymied within a stage or regress to earlier stages of development. Each stage is characterized by different member behaviors and attitudes and requires specific management emphases.

Stakeholder Mapping   Provides a systematic assessment of the variance among personnel as stakeholders using stakeholder identification, stakeholder ranking based on attitudes toward change, and assortment of each stakeholder's power within the organization to shape and affect its ultimate utilization.

Standardization of Outputs   A way of coordinating work that specifies the product or expected performance, with the process of how to perform the work left to the worker.

Standardization of Work Processes   A way of coordinating work that programs or specifies the content of work. Health care organizations standardize work processes when possible, such as standard admission and discharge procedures or standard methods of performing laboratory tests.

Standardization of Worker Skills   A way of coordinating work that occurs when neither work processes nor output can be standardized by standardizing the training of workers.

Status Differences   Status is the measure of worth conferred on an individual by a group. Status differences refer to variations in the worth of individuals and groups in organizations, and are seen throughout organizations.

Strategic Alliance   Any formal agreement between two or more organizations for purposes of ongoing cooperation and mutual gain.

Strategic Management   Those aspects of management within a firm that link strategy analysis and planning to operational management.

Strategic Management Perspective   The strategic management perspective emphasizes the importance of positioning the organization relative to its environment and competitors in order to achieve its objectives and assure its survival.

Strategy   An integrating set of ideas and concepts that guide an organization in its attempts to achieve competitive advantage over rivals.

Stretching   Refers to a style of management and organizational culture in which very high performance standards are set with the deliberate intent to "stretch" people to their fullest capability.

Structural Change Strategies   Concerned with the fundamental design and structure of health services organizations. This involves approaches that change organizational structure, reporting relationships, use of integrating mechanisms within the institution, management and clinical information systems, and financial systems.

Structural Measures of Quality   Assess those organizational features or participants' characteristics that are presumed to have a positive impact on organizational performance.

Substitution Threats   Threats from firms that produce products and services that differ from, but perform the same function as, those of extant competitors in the market; the threats depend on the market structure, environmental changes, and the relative competitive advantages of rivals and of those firms that produce substitute products and services.

Support Work   Work that does not directly result in achievement of an organization goal, but which is needed for effective accomplishment of other work.

Survey Feedback   Provides a mechanism for systematically gathering data on the ongoing social-psychological conditions of the organization and confronting work groups with the findings.

Symbiotic vs. Competitive Interdependence   This distinction highlights that alliances often have mixed motives, whereby parties can create joint value, but often will compete in the claiming of that value.

Synergies   The result of two or more competitors (either under the same ownership or within a strategic alliance) combining activities in order to achieve greater competitive advantage than is possible were they to operate separately.

Task Analysis   Method used for facilitating technical change and improving performance that focuses on the redesign of tasks within the organization.

Task Content Conflict   Disagreements about the content of a task being performed by organizational members.

Task Design   Task design refers to the content and organization of a task or group of tasks for an individual or group. It may also refer to the work processes and technologies necessary to accomplish tasks.

Task Interdependence   Task interdependence refers to the interconnections between tasks, or more specifically, the degree to which team members must rely on one another to perform work effectively.

Task Inventory Approach to Work Design   A technical approach to work design that inventories the tasks and skills needed for particular jobs.

Task-Oriented Roles   Task-oriented roles are roles and functions assumed by team members that help to accomplish team goals and reinforce team norms.

Team Cohesiveness   Team cohesiveness is the extent to which team members are committed to the group task, attracted to each other, or motivated to stay in the group.

Team Composition   Team composition refers to the membership of a team, particularly in relation to variations in gender, age, professional status, and other factors that may affect team performance.

Team Development   Strategies that attempt to remove barriers to group effectiveness, develop self-sufficiency in managing group process, and facilitate the change process.

Team Productivity   Team productivity is the quantifiable measurement of a team's effectiveness in terms of output and efficiency.

Technical Approach to Work Design   Designing work with a focus on skill requirements and information flow.

Technology Assessment   A class of evaluative methods used to examine the technical, economic, health, and social consequences of technological applications. In the health setting, these methods are used to evaluate health technologies in terms of safety, efficacy, effectiveness, cost, cost-effectiveness, legality, and ethics—both in absolute terms and in comparison with competing technologies.

Total Quality Management (TQM)   A participative, systematic approach to planning and implementing continuous improvement in quality.

Trait Perspective   A theoretical "school" of leadership holding that personal traits (attributes/characteristics) have a significant effect on leadership effectiveness and success.

Transactional Leadership   Clarification of the roles followers must execute in order to reach their personal goals while fulfilling the goals of the organization. The objective of this type of leadership is to get followers to comply by the rules of the game as presently played.

Transformational Leadership   Leadership behavior directed toward upsetting the status quo, seeking to alter both the goal and nature of manager-follower interactions. The objective of this type of leadership is to work with followers to alter the rules of the game.

Turbulent Environment   This refers to the situation whereby an organization is facing rapidly changing external circumstances and greater interconnectedness and interdependence between itself and other organizations.

Tyrants   Organizations can behave as tyrants or as instruments of domination that exploit their employees and others either unconsciously or by intent.

Uncertainty   Inability of organizations or managers to accurately predict the consequences of an action or the future state of an organization and its environment.

Uncertainty Inherent in Work   The degree of uncertainty inherent in work affects task and coordination requirements.

Uncertainty Reduction   An important benefit of strategic alliances, when compared to alternative approaches to

growth, given the exit options typically found in alliance agreements.

Vertical Division of Labor Dividing work into tasks—management, direct, and support work—to be completed by people at different levels of the organization.

Vertical Integration The process of combining organizations that contribute to the production process of a given good or service under a common ownership or management structure. The combined organizations may include the primary producer, suppliers to the production process (including suppliers of both human and capital resources), distributors and retailers of the finished product, and/or consumers. This strategy is typically used to achieve production efficiencies by reducing transaction costs, and to achieve market power by internalizing markets for supplies and/or finished products.

Work Group/Work Design Health care organizations vary in the way that work is organized. How people are grouped together to accomplish the organization's mission is usually a function of the organization's technology and environment.

Work Requirements Personal attributes and skills required for the successful completion of an identifiable element of work.

AUTHOR INDEX

SUBJECT INDEX